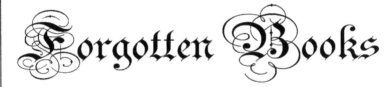

ISBN 978-1-5282-4150-2
PIBN 10919918

English
Français
Deutsche
Italiano
Español
Português

www.forgottenbooks.com

Mythology Photography **Fiction**
Fishing Christianity **Art** Cooking
Essays Buddhism Freemasonry
Medicine **Biology** Music **Ancient**
Egypt Evolution Carpentry Physics
Dance Geology **Mathematics** Fitness
Shakespeare **Folklore** Yoga Marketing
Confidence Immortality Biographies
Poetry **Psychology** Witchcraft
Electronics Chemistry History **Law**
Accounting **Philosophy** Anthropology
Alchemy Drama Quantum Mechanics
Atheism Sexual Health **Ancient History**
Entrepreneurship Languages Sport
Paleontology Needlework Islam
Metaphysics Investment Archaeology
Parenting Statistics Criminology
Motivational

THE JOURNAL
OF THE
MEDICAL ASSOCIATION OF GEORGIA

DEVOTED TO THE WELFARE OF THE MEDICAL ASSOCIATION OF GEORGIA
PUBLISHED MONTHLY under direction of the Council

| Volume XXV | Atlanta, Ga., January, 1936 | Number 1 |

THE TREATMENT BY THE GENERAL PRACTITIONER OF THE MORE COMMON DISEASES OF THE NERVOUS SYSTEM*

LEWELLYS F. BARKER, M.D.
Baltimore, Maryland

When I was invited by Dr. Paullin, the Chairman of the Lectureship Committee, to deliver the Abner W. Calhoun Lecture for this year it occurred to me that a topic bearing upon diseases of the nervous system might be appropriate, since the eye, in which Dr. Calhoun was so interested during his lifetime, is in reality a part of the nervous system. I understand that the audience is composed largely of general practitioners, men who work in the country as well as men who work in cities and towns, so I have decided to deal with the commoner diseases of the nervous system rather than with those that are only very rarely met with.

Examination of the Nervous Functions As A Part of the General Study of All Patients

In recent years, since specialization in medicine has become rampant, there has been too great a tendency among men engaged in general practice to neglect the routine examination of certain organs and organ-systems when studying patients in their every day work. They are prone to think of the main symptoms of which a patient complains, to confine their examinations largely to the parts of the body to which these symptoms appear to point, and to fail to make a sufficiently comprehensive examination of other parts. This is, of course, a lamentable error, since a careful general examination may re-

veal the presence of disturbances of even greater importance to the patient than the disturbances of the parts to which the examination is restricted. Thus, for example, if a patient complains of pains in and swellings of the joints, the clinical study dare not be limited to an investigation of the locomotor system alone but must be extended so as to embrace examinations of the sites in which focal infections are common (tonsils, teeth, paranasal sinuses, etc.) as well as of certain metabolic functions (especially uric acid metabolism). Or, again, if a patient complain of shortness of breath, the clinical examination must extend beyond studies of the respiratory and circulatory organs to other parts as well in order to determine all the factors that may be concerned in the origin of the dyspnea. I choose these two simple examples merely as illustrative, though a hundred might easily be cited.

The general practitioner of today should feel it his duty to make, in every patient for whom he cares, an examination that is sufficiently comprehensive to determine the presence or absence of important symptoms or physical signs in all the organs and organ-systems of the body if he expects to be successful in his work. For it must be very humiliating to a physician to overlook anything that is important and easily ascertainable and to have it pointed out to him later by someone who takes the trouble to follow the general rule just mentioned. I do not mean that the general practitioner can be expected to make use of all the methods of the medical specialists; he can, however, through a careful taking of the history of the patient, through his general physical examination, and by means of a few routine laboratory tests, get the clues to the general situation of his patient and, as a result, he

*Abner W. Calhoun Lecture before the Medical Association of Georgia, Atlanta, May 8, 1935.

will know whether the aid of a specialist in one or another domain may be desirable.

Many practitioners feel that neurology and psychiatry are such specialized domains that they are incompetent to pass judgment upon the presence or absence of pathological neuropsychiatric elements in a given patient. But this, too, is a grave mistake. Every doctor, today, should be able in the course of a few minutes to determine, at least in the great majority of patients, whether any marked nervous or mental symptom or sign is present or absent. Rough tests for the presence or absence of anesthesia to touch, pain or temperature stimuli, of disturbances of vision, hearing, taste or smell, of motor weakness, motor irritation, muscular incoordination, or muscular atrophy, and of disturbances of the reflexes (pupillary reflexes, tendon reflexes, and cutaneous reflexes) take only a very little time. On the mental side, the general conversation with the patient will quickly reveal the multitudinous complaints of the neurasthenic, the vacillation and indecision of the psychasthenic, or the vagaries of the hysterical. And clues to the presence or absence of symptoms suggestive of a hypochondriasis, of a manic-depressive disturbance (elation or depression), of a schizophrenic disturbance (dementia praecox), or of a paranoid disturbance will often be obtained by listening to the answers to three simple questions: (1) Are you sick? (2) Have you been sad, blue or gloomy? and (3) Have other people treated you well? If, in reply to the first question, the patient says there is nothing wrong except the one or two symptoms he has mentioned you will know he is probably not hypochondrical, whereas, if he says that his "duodenum is plugged up" or that he has to watch every stool that he passes to look at its form, color, and quantity, or if he details other bizarre symptoms, you will at once suspect that you may be dealing with a hypochondriacal psychopath. Or, if in answer to the second question, the patient says that he has been blue, gloomy and depressed and has had weeping spells, a melancholic tendency will be manifest, whereas if he laughs, is jolly and says he does not know what it is to be blue, melancholia can be ruled out, though

if he talks rapidly and at great length, turning quickly from one topic to another, an elevative trend will be evident. Again, if in answer to the third question, "Have others treated you well?" he hesitates and says, "Well, I don't know about that," you will find it worth-while to make further enquiries with the purpose of eliciting any paranoid ideas that exist.

Organic and Functional Disorders of the Nervous System

If nervous or mental symptoms are found to be present in a patient, it is the physician's duty to try to determine in how far they depend upon organic changes in the nervous system and in how far upon merely functional disturbances. He must try to find out the origin and nature of all the abnormal signs and symptoms that are present in any given case. If true non-hysterical anesthesias are demonstrable, if paralyses or muscular weaknesses present are accompanied by muscular atrophy or by fibrillation, or if there be definite changes in the superficial or deep reflexes such as a positive Babinski reaction, an Argyll-Robertson pupil or persistent absence of the knee jerks one can feel very sure that he is dealing with an organic disease of the nervous system, in which event he will, after gathering all the data, try to determine, first, just what parts of the peripheral or central nervous system are diseased (localizing diagnosis) and will only later try to decide as to the cause of the lesions (etiological diagnosis). I have seen many mistakes in diagnosis made because of failure to follow this important rule; one should not, for example, jump to the conclusion that he is dealing with a multiple neuritis before he has ruled out the possibility of locomotor ataxia due to syphilis, nor should he assume that a troublesome headache is due merely to migraine before the eyegrounds have been examined for choked discs that point to increased intracranial pressure due possibly to a developing brain tumor.

Only after a careful examination has ruled out the presence of objective signs that make one suspicious of organic disease should one entertain the idea that the nervous disorder is functional in nature, and even then one will keep in mind the fact that signs of an organic disorder may later develop and will make tests at intervals later on to make sure. Certain organic diseases at their inception may be very deceptive, and if the general practitioner be in doubt as to the presence or absence of organic disease, and especially if the symptoms that he thinks are functional do not respond to the usual forms of therapy, he will do well to ask for the privilege of a consultation with a neurological specialist.

Patients should, when ill, always consult their family physicians first, however, for the tendency of some persons to go directly to some specialist is detrimental to the patient's own interests. The family physician knows better than a consultant the home life of the patient, the circumstances in which he lives, and the details of his personal relationships. And the wise family practitioner will know when he needs the help of a specialist in consultation far better than the patient himself can know. Moreover, if a specialist is needed, the family doctor will know the right person to call, a matter in which families of patients are rarely able properly to decide. If more than one specialistic examination be indicated, the family physician will arrange for it, but he will avoid sending the patient to a whole round of specialists when there is no indication of need of the help of more than one or two. Though every diagnostic survey should be sufficiently comprehensive to avoid the overlooking of anything of real importance, the conscientious practitioner will also consider the pocket-book of the patient and will see to it that it is not unjustifiably drawn upon.

Many patients are prone to be over-anxious and to form all sorts of misconceptions regarding the nature of their symptoms. The wise family doctor will try to estimate the part played by such anxiety and misconceptions in any given case, and will quiet unjustified fears by his tactful reassurance, while at the same time he sees that everything that is really necessary is done.

Disorders of the Nervous System Following Traumata

Brain injuries may follow traumata to the head, fractures of the skull, gun-shot wounds and other injuries. The history of the case, the signs referable to the nose, ears and eyes, palpation, and roentgenograms of the skull will be of help in making the diagnosis. The physician will, of course, be on the lookout especially for any focal symptoms that may point to injuries of specific brain areas.

Even when there is no evidence of fracture of the skull after a trauma to the head, symptoms like headache and vertigo following upon the accident may be due to concussion. The patient should be kept quiet in bed for a few days with the head raised upon pillows and cold compresses or an ice bag applied. If the symptoms persist and are pronounced they may be due to edema of the brain, in which case intravenous injections of hypertonic salt solution may be helpful by diminishing the edema. If, despite these measures, the condition is not ameliorated, the possibility of subarachnoid or subdural hemorrhage may be suspected and the aid of a neurologist or of a neurological surgeon may be required.

Injuries to the spinal cord may follow fracture of the spine (especially in the lumbar region) or dislocation of the spine (especially in the cervical region), and may result in complete or incomplete transverse lesions of the cord with accompanying motor and sensory disturbances. A stab wound or a gun-shot wound may cause a unilateral lesion with Brown-Sequard paralysis. Occasionally, as the result of trauma, hemorrhage into the central canal of the cord (haematomyelia) may occur and give rise to characteristic symptoms, resembling those of syringomyelia. In all such cases the aid of a neurologist or neurosurgeon should be promptly enlisted through whom the general practitioner may receive definite instructions as to the best methods of after care.

Injuries to peripheral nerves may also result from trauma and may often require electrical treatment for some time to prevent atrophy of the muscles supplied pending the regeneration of the injured nerve fibres.

Commoner Diseases of the Nervous System Due to Inflammatory Processes

Though there are a great many varieties of such inflammations I shall refer only to those that are of greatest interest to the general practitioner.

Acute Meningitis.—If a patient, especially a child or younger person, be taken suddenly ill with fever, vomiting, and severe headache, the possibility of meningitis should be thought of. Rigidity and retraction of the neck are prone to appear early and the Kernig sign or Brudzynski's sign may be found to be positive. In such a case lumbar puncture should be done at once and a cell count, and a bacteriological culture made. If cerebrospinal meningitis be epidemic at the time. Flexner's antiserum (20 to 30 cc.) should be injected at once through the puncture needle without awaiting the results of the examination; one may give also 40 cc. intramuscularly. But if there be no epidemic. one may postpone intrathecal treatment until after one determines the type of microorganism (meningococcus, pneumococcus, streptococcus, influenza bacillus or tubercle bacillus responsible for the infection. In all cases of acute meningitis (including tuberculous meningitis) drainage of the subarachnoid space at intervals by repeated lumbar puncture is advocated. In meningococcic meningitis one repeats the intraspinous and intramuscular injections of antimeningococcus serum daily until the infection is overcome. In pneumococcal meningitis Felton's serum may be given by intraspinous injection, or one may inject 20 cc. of a one-half of 1 per cent. solution of optochin hydrochloride into the subarachnoid space, though the family should be informed beforehand of possible danger to the eye-sight.

Epidemic Encephalitis.—In the several epidemics of this disease in the United States since 1918, including the recent epidemic in St. Louis, many methods of treatment have been tried but none has proven to be very efficacious. The lethargic form that we saw in 1918 and later, apparently is quite different from the milder form of the St. Louis epidemic; the etiology of these two forms appears to be different. In the acute stage of epidemic encephalitis, one may try intravenous injections of a 10 per cent aqueous solution of sodium iodide, giving 20 cc. on the first day and, if well borne, 50 cc. on the second day, and thereafter 50 cc. thrice weekly until a liter in all has been given. Intramuscular injection of from 20 to 50 cc.

of serum of patients convalescent from the disease may also be given daily for three or four days. Repeated lumbar puncture with drainage of the subarachnoid space may also be helpful.

In postencephalitic Parkinsonism, a tablet of 1/100 grain of hyoscine hydrobromide given thrice daily by mouth is often very helpful in lessening the rigidity; some patients bear larger doses very well, 1/75, 1/50 or even 1/25 grain tablets. Other patients do better on dried extract of stramonium in pills of 1½ to 4 grains thrice daily. If the hyoscine or stramonium cause much blurring of vision or dryness of the mouth, we give also 1/15 grain of nitrate of pilocarpine with each dose.

Acute Anterior Poliomyelitis.—As soon as the diagnosis is made (preferably in the pre-paralytic stage), 20 to 40 cc. of serum from a convalescent patient may be injected into the subarachnoid space and the same amount subcutaneously. The patient should be isolated for three weeks (though as a rule the disease is transmitted by healthy carriers) and should be kept at absolute rest in bed on a bland diet. Great care should be taken to prevent bed-sores. Attempts are being made to discover some effective method of preventive immunization to be used when the disease is prevalent, but as yet without marked success. For the residual paraylses, warm baths, massage, passive movements and electrical treatments are of some value. If contracture develop surgical intervention or orthopedic appliances may become necessary.

Neuritis.—Inflammations of the peripheral nerves (cerebral and spinal) are as every practitioner knows very common, causing pains, anesthesias. and paralysis of the muscles followed by atrophy and reaction of degeneration. They may follow infections (especially diphtheria, typhoid or influenza); more often they are due to exogenous intoxications (alcohol, lead, arsenic, abortifacients), or to auto-intoxications (as in diabetes or gout); sometimes they are due to food-deficiencies (as in beri-beri and pellagra). The first step in treatment is the elimination of the causative factor if it can be discovered; unfortunately, this is not always possible. the etiology remaining obscure. The localization of the symptoms may give clues as to the causation; thus in neuritis due to lead poisoning, there may be a pure motor disturbance (paralyses of extensors of the forearms without disturbances of sensation) and a bluish tint along the margins of the gums may be visible; in neuritis due to alcoholic or arsenical intoxication, there are often paralyses of the distal muscles of the extremities associated with pains and anesthesias of the hands and feet; in neuritis complicating diphtheritic infection, the soft palate is paralyzed, there is failure of the accommodation of the eyes, and sometimes weakness of the legs; whereas, in the neuritis that sometimes occurs in diabetes mellitus, there are pains in the lower extremities with loss of the knee kicks and ankle jerks (so-called diabetic pseudotabes). In some forms of polyneuritis (especially those due to alcoholism or to acute infections) severe mental disturbances may develop with disorientation, loss of memory for recent events, falsifications of memory and even hallucinations (the so-called Korsakoff psychosis).

In postdiphtheritic paralyses, very large doses of diphtheria antitoxin should be administered; in diabetic neuritis, a diet of low carbohydrate content and the administration of insulin should be continued until the blood sugar reaches normal levels; in the polyneuritis of beri-beri vitamin B_1 should be given in large quantities (yeast, wheat germ, green vegetables, etc.), and to prevent neuritis in pellagrous regions the food should contain plenty of vitamin B_2 (or G) in yeast, egg yolk, cereals, leafy green vegetables and liver.

In all severe cases of neuritis the patient should be kept at rest in bed and should be made to perspire copiously. The pains can usually be sufficiently relieved by the administration of aspirin, though in some cases in which they are particularly severe codein in stiff doses may be required; morphine, if used at all, should be employed only temporarily, for one wants to avoid any possibility of the patient acquiring a drug habit. During convalescence, massage, passive movements and gradually increasing resistive exercises are helpful in improving the nutrition of the muscles and in the prevention of contractures. Electrotherapy also has a place though less stress is laid upon it now than formerly. Iron, quinine and strychnine may be helpful as a part of the general tonic measures to be applied.

Neurosyphilis.—Thanks to the great improvement in recent decades in the treatment and general management of patients who have contracted syphilis we see far less syphilis of the nervous system than we formerly did. If neurosyphilis does occur in the secondary or tertiary stage of the infection, the diagnosis can be confirmed early by means of the Wassermann reaction applied to the blood and to the cerebrospinal fluid. The treatment may be begun with a series of intramuscular injections of bismuth salicylate or of iodo-bismitol (2 cc. ampules), after which a course of intravenous injections of neosalvarsan may be ordered, giving 0.15 Gm. at a dose and gradually increasing to 0.45 Gm. per dose. Such alternate courses of bismuth and neosalvarsan treatments should be kept up for about two years. In addition 15 to 30 drops of saturated solution of iodide of potassium in half a glass of water thrice daily after meals may be administered.

In the treatment of *locomotor ataxia* (*tabes dorsalis*) the same methods should be employed, though it is often advantageous to start with a series of mercurial inunctions, rubbing in 3 or 4 Gm. of blue ointment daily, making the applications to the right arm, the left arm, the right thigh, the left thigh, the chest and the back in cycles. If optic atrophy have already begun, great caution in the use of the neosalvarsan injections should be observed (smaller doses). For the lightning pains of tabes aspirin is serviceable. When there are very severe tabetic crises, subcutaneous injections of 10 or 15 minims of Schlesinger's solution (containing dionine and scopolamine) may be required. If, in spite of thorough antiluetic treatment, the tabetic crises continue to be very severe, section of several posterior roots (Foerster's operation) should be resorted to by a consulting neurosurgeon. When the ataxia is marked, the re-education in movement by the methods of G. Frenkel should be undertaken.

In the treatment of *general paresis (de-*

mentia paralytica) great advances have been made recently by inducing a high grade of fever (hyperpyrexia). The patient is admitted to a hospital, is infected with malaria, and is allowed to have a series of 15 or 18 chills, after which the malarial parasites are killed with quinine. Or high fever may be produced by diathermy or better still by means of the new apparatus devised by the General Electric Company for the production of hyperpyrexia. Subsequent to the fever treatments, injections of bismuth and of tryparsamide may be given over a long period. Many general paretics can now be given a new lease on life and of work by means of such fever treatment.

Multiple Sclerosis.—Though I speak of multiple or disseminated sclerosis under the heading of the inflammatory diseases of the nervous system, we are not certain that the changes are actually inflammatory in nature. It is so common among young people between the ages of 15 and 30 that every general practitioner should be on the lookout for it. Often it is not recognized until the later symptoms like scanning speech, intention tremor, nystagmus, and spastic paralysis have developed, though if a systematic neurological examination had been made earlier the characteristic premonitory signs—loss of abdominal reflexes, weakness of the abdominal muscles and temporal pallor of the optic discs—would have been discovered. Too often, the disease in its earlier stages has been supposed to be hysteria and treated accordingly.

The cause of multiple sclerosis is not known. The effects of treatment are difficult to judge since spontaneous remissions are common. The important thing for the general practitioner is to recognize the existence of this organic disease when it is present, to protect the patient from the mistaken assumption of family or friends that the disorder is merely a functional neurosis, and to do everything possible to protect the patient's general health by attention to the personal hygiene. Drugs are of doubtful value though sodium cacodylate and silver arsphenamine have seemed in some cases to be helpful. Very recently, treatment by induction of artificial fever (malarial inocula-

tion; diathermy. etc.) has been tried, but it is too early. as yet to evaluate the results. The improvements observed may be merely natural remissions in the course of the disease to be followed later by relapses and exacerbations.

Commoner Diseases of the Nervous System Due to Circulatory Disturbances

Cerebral Hemorrhage, Embolism and Thrombosis.—Every general practitioner has to treat cases of apoplexy due to *cerebral hemorrhage*, often accompanied by hemiplegia or aphasia, especially common in older persons who have high blood pressure. In younger people. the "stroke" may be due to *cerebral embolism* (especially when there is disease of the mitral valve of the heart) or to a sudden occlusion of a cerebral artery by a thrombus (*cerebral thrombosis*).

If the 'stroke" is due to cerebral hemorrhage, the patient should be kept at absolute rest in bed with the upper part of the body somewhat elevated and with an ice bag upon the head. One should withdraw from 300 to 500 cc. of blood from a vein at the bend of the elbow and should empty the bowel by means of an enema. No food should be given for 24 hours and even after the patient regains consciousness great caution should be observed in the administration of food and liquids because of the danger of aspiration pneumonia. Should the coma continue longer than 24 hours, food should be administered through a nasal tube or by means of nutrient enemata. No electrical treatments should be begun until several weeks have elapsed. In a few cases—not in many—surgical intervention may be indicated for cerebral hemorrhage. In the after-treatment, attention should be paid to reduction of the height of the blood pressure in hypertensives and to the reduction of weight in the obese, in the hope of lessening the probability of further attacks.

Generalized Cerebral Arteriosclerosis.—In this malady, so common in later life and accompanied by mental hebetude, memory defects, slight speech disturbances, fatiguability, dizziness, depression and irritability. there is but little we can do beyond reduction of the patient's activities, restriction of the intake of meat and of common salt, and reorganization of his habits of living. If senile epilepsy occur, we give phenobarbital in ½ grain doses thrice daily. In some cases of cerebral arteriosclerosis, the steady administration of sodium iodide in doses of five grains in half a glass of water after meals has seemed to be of benefit. All too often, however, the malady progresses in spite of treatment and ultimately a pseudobulbar paralysis or an actual arteriosclerotic dementia may develop. It is easier to prevent arteriosclerosis by hygienic living in earlier life than it is to treat it effectively after it has developed in later life.

Raynaud's Disease.—In this condition there are attacks of vasospasm with pallor and cyanosis (sometimes of spontaneous gangrene) of the fingers and toes. Great advances in treatment have recently been made through the use by Adson and his colleagues of the Mayo Clinic of the operation of sympathetic gangliectomy and ramisection. In milder cases operation may not be necessary, the patients doing well enough when treated medically by protection from exposure to cold, by massage, by general upbuilding and for any disturbances of the general health revealed by a careful general diagnostic survey. But in the severer recalcitrant cases operation upon the sympathetic is strongly to be recommended. Raynaud's disease should of course be sharply differentiated from Buerger's disease (thrombo-angiitis obliterans), in which there is a true inflammation of the arterial walls with obliteration of the lumina of the distal arteries of the feet with disappearance of the arterial pulsations and the occurrence of gangrene.

Atrophic and Degenerative Diseases of the Nervous System

Though there are many of these, I shall refer only to a few that are of especial interest to men engaged in general practice.

Progressive Muscular Atrophy.—This disease is due to a progressive degeneration of the anterior horn cells and of the cells in the motor nuclei in the brain stem. In the *spinal form* (Aran-Duchenne type), the disease begins slowly in middle life with fibrillary twitchings and atrophy in the small muscles of the hands (thenar and hypothenar eminences) and extends to the muscles of the arms and back. In the *bulbar form* (progressive bulbar paralysis) the disease begins with difficulties in pronounciation of words, and difficulty in chewing and in swallowing but it must not be confused with so-called asthenic bulbar paralysis (myasthenia gravis) in which there is no fibrillary twitching; in this latter disease, considerable improvement may follow the administration of glycin (15 Gm.) followed by ephedrine sulphate (¾ grain) given twice daily.

In the *spastic form* of progressive central muscular atrophy (sometimes called amyotrophic lateral sclerosis) there is degeneration of the pyramidal tracts as well as of the anterior horn cells.

Unfortunately we have no effective methods as yet for preventing the progress of these muscular atrophies. We caution against over-fatigue of the weakened muscles, pay attention to the general health, and give strychnine in tonic doses.

Ataxic Paraplegia.—In this disease there is combined sclerosis of the posterior and lateral columns of the spinal cord so that the symptoms are like those of locomotor ataxia, on the one hand, and of spastic spinal paralysis, on the other. The spastic-ataxic gait is the most prominent symptom. The disease is often associated with pernicious anemia. Formerly we were powerless in combatting it; today, like pernicious anemia, it often undergoes marked improvement under stomach-treated-liver therapy.

Pressure Paraplegia.—If the cord be compressed because of tuberculous disease of the spine (Pott's disease) surgical interference has been successful in a small percentage of the cases. It is very important when possible to recognize a tuberculous spondylitis before compression of the cord occurs, for in many such cases by general upbuilding treatment and by the aid of orthopedic appliances one may prevent the development of cord compression.

When the cord is compressed by cancer or other tumor growth the outlook is very unfavorable; one usually is limited to the use of pain-stilling measures.

Tumors of the Central Nervous System

Tumors of the Brain.—Unfortunately, tumors of the brain are not at all uncommon. If recognized early, many of them, now-a-days, can be successfully removed, thanks to the great advances that have been made by neurological surgeons. The general practitioner is the first to see such patients and because of the importance of early diagnosis, he should always keep the possibility of brain tumor in mind in patients who have severe headaches, slow pulse, or visual disturbances. If the general practitioner would always carry an ophthalmoscope in his bag and look at the eye grounds when he has any suspicion of the existence of a brain tumor, he might detect the presence of choked discs (easy to recognize) if they should be present, refer the patient promptly to a neurologist and thus perhaps be instrumental in saving the life of the patient. X-ray plates after air-injection, by the method of Dandy, will often show the precise location of a tumor if it be present.

Tumors of the Spinal Cord or of its Coverings.—When patients have pains that are distributed in areas that correspond to one or more nerve-roots, and especially if the Wassermann reaction be negative and there is no evidence of tuberculosis of the spine, a *meningeal tumor* should be thought of as a possibility and the aid of a neurologist sought, since many meningeal tumors can be successfully removed by surgical operation.

Tumors arising within the spinal cord, especially *glioma*, often give rise to *syringomyelia* in which certain areas of the skin show loss of pain sense and temperature sense, though tactile sense may remain intact. In such cases, surgical interference is of no value except in a few cases in which drainage of the syringomyelic cavity may do good by relieving pressure and thus yielding temporary symptomatic relief. Deep x-ray therapy should be tried since it sometimes stops the pains.

The Epilepsies

Attacks of epilepsy in which patients lose consciousness and exhibit convulsive seizures (tonic and clonic) are met with in the practice of every physician. In a large proportion of the cases, heredity plays an important part and other epileptics will be known among the relatives. Still, epilepsy is sometimes encountered in families in which there is no other history of the disease; in such a case, one would seek a cause other than heredity, such as brain trauma, brain tumor, or sequel of an infection (e.g., scarlet fever, syphilis, or earlier meningitis). In some cases, a reflex origin for epilepsy can be discovered (e.g., intestinal parasites, a foreign body in the ear, or a scar of a peripheral nerve). When the first attack of epilepsy occurs after the age of puberty, the possibility of an organic disease as the cause should not be forgotten.

Besides major epileptic attacks, minor forms (petit mal) occur; these may be seen in patients who never suffer from major attacks. The patients exhibit a brief period (often only a few seconds) of unconsciousness (with or without a preceding aura). Or the patients may stop in the middle of speech for a few seconds, and may complain only of dizziness without becoming unconscious.

Every patient who exhibits epileptiform symptoms (either major or minor) should be subjected to a complete diagnostic survey. If an organic cause be discovered, relief is often possible through neurosurgery. If, however, no organic cause can be detected, if hysteria can also be ruled out, and after any possible reflex causes have been removed, the attacks can often be largely or wholly prevented by the systematic use of certain drugs. Formerly we had to rely chiefly upon bromide therapy, but, now, we use phenobarbital and get much better results. This should be given regularly after each meal and at bed time in doses of from $\frac{3}{4}$ to $1\frac{1}{2}$ grains. Unlike bromide, its prolonged use does not seem to do harm. If the patient remain free of attacks, the dosage may be gradually (never suddenly) reduced, though if the attacks reappear increased doses should be given again. In status epilepticus in which life may be endangered, one gives 15 or 20 grains of chloral hydrate by enema, or better still, perhaps, 6 drachms of paraldehyde by rectum.

The diet of epileptics should consist largely of milk, eggs, green vegetables and fruits with restriction of meat and of common salt. Some children with epilepsy seem to do well upon a so-called ketogenic diet (poor in carbohydrates and proteins and rich in fats like butter, cream and olive oil). Epileptics should be warned against horse-back riding, driving a motor, or swimming alone, or flying an aeroplane, since an attack in such situations might be dangerous. If epileptics marry, it might be wise not to have children.

Migraine

Patients suffering from "migraine" or "sick headache" have periodic attacks of headache, usually unilateral, and often associated with nausea, vomiting and vertigo, each attack lasting from a few hours to one or more days. The frequency of such attacks varies; some have them weekly, some monthly, others at longer intervals. In one group of cases, the attack is announced by a peculiar visual disturbance; a point of light appears before the patient and often spreads or assumes a zig-zag figure (known as "fortification scotoma").

In the treatment, the general personal hygiene of the patient should receive careful attention. For the attack itself one may give 5 grains of aspirin with 5 grains of amidopyrin and $\frac{1}{2}$ grain of codeine, repeating in four or six hours if necessary. Care should be taken not to give amidopyrin over a long period of time because of the danger of agranulocytosis. Recently, the effects of ergotamine tartrate ("gynergen") have been much lauded.

To lessen the frequency of attacks, one may give 1 grain of phenobarbital on rising and at bedtime over long periods. Tablets of calcium gluconate (15 grains) chewed and swallowed after each meal may lessen nervous irritability.

Great care should be taken to overcome any refraction error if it exist by the regular use of suitable lenses.

Sydenham's Chorea

This disturbance of motility is most common as a complication of acute rheumatic fever in young children. The little patient should be kept out of school and, if the attack be severe, rest in bed in a darkened room is desirable. Fowler's solution of arsenic in gradually increasing doses is still a favorite remedy, but care must be taken to avoid giving too much lest arsenical neuritis develop. In obstinate cases, the barbital derivative known as phenylethylhydantoin (nirvanol) may be cautiously tried in 5 to 10 grain doses.

The Common Psychoses

In addition to general paresis (dementia paralytica) to which I have already referred, I wish to mention three forms of psychosis that are not infrequently met with by general practitioners, namely, manic-depressive psychoses, dementia praecox and paranoia.

Manic-Depressive Psychoses.—In these disorders, it is the emotions rather than the intellectual processes that are mainly disturbed; hence they are often spoken of as "affective disorders." Members of certain families are subject to alternate periods of mania and melancholia (circular insanity) and such persons are said to be of cyclothymic temperament.

In *manic states* the mood is elated (euphoria), thinking and motor activities are speeded up (psychomotor acceleration), and there is a tendency to motor excitation.

In *melancholic states* we see just the opposite: the patients are sad, blue, gloomy, depressed and exhibit slowing of thought and of movements (psychomotor retardation); sometimes the depression is so deep that suicide is attempted. Some patients show a mixture of manic and melancholic symptoms.

In mild cases, in which the mood is only a little "high" or a little "low," the patients should be carefully watched by the family physician and given counsel with regard to sleep, to activities and to mode of life. Severe cases of mania or melancholia may require treatment in closed institutions; and commitment in such cases may be necessary. Cases of intermediate severity not requiring commitment will often do well under rest treatment away from their own homes, in a nursing home or hospital, temporarily isolated from family and friends; systematic medical supervision, special nursing, massage, occupation therapy and phenobarbital or barbital in divided doses usually lead to recovery, though the period of illness is often a matter of many months.

In melancholias of the involuntary period intramuscular injection daily of 1 cc. of theelin is said to hasten recovery.

Dementia Praecox.—Three forms of this mental disorder are distinguished:

(1) *Hebephrenia* in which unexplained laziness, dulness, and apathy develop about the time of puberty, along with rather strange behavior and the expression of bizarre ideas;

(2) *Catatonia* in which young people become negativistic, sometimes declining to eat or to cooperate, show carelessness in their personal habits, exhibit peculiar mannerisms and attitudes; and

(3) *Dementia paranoides* in which delusions of persecution develop accompanied by evidences of rapid mental deterioration.

All three forms are included under the general heading of *schizophrenic states*. The general practitioner who suspects the development of such a state in a patient will do well to insist upon immediate consultation with a psychiatrist of experience. The treatment of dementia praecox is notoriously unsatisfactory; most of the patients ultimately become permanent residents in psychiatric institutions.

True Paranoia.—The patient gradually becomes suspicious, thinks that others treat him badly, and "have it in for him"; these ideas develop into fixed delusions of persecution. Many of the patients hear ,voices or see visions. They are prone to be dangerous and should be cared for by commitment to closed institutions.

Idiocies and Imbecilities

All degrees of feeblemindedness exist from slight imbecility to outspoken idiocy. The severer cases should be placed permanently in institutions. The general practitioner's greatest difficulty is in making decisions regarding the care of the so-called "backward child" or the child "difficult to train." In such instances he should arrange for a Binet-Simon intelligence test and should rule out hypothyroidism (cretinism) by testing the basal metabolic rate.

For mild backwardness, there are special schools available. The plans for children of limited intelligence should not be too ambitious.

The Psychoneuroses

The functional nervous disorders known as the psychoneuroses we have always with us, and the general practitioner should early learn the best ways of being helpful to his neurotic patients.

In *neurasthenia*, the patient is irritable and weak, complains of fatiguability, restlessness, insomnia, headache, pressure in the head, difficulty of concentration, fear of incapacitation, palpitation of the heart, lack of appetite and various digestive disturbances. If not promptly treated severe states of anxiety (anxiety neuroses) are prone to develop.

In *hysteria* the patient is prone to behave theatrically, seems to be conscious of an audience that she wishes to impress and craves sympathy. She complains that she "cannot" do things, whereas her friends say she "will not." Often pains, anesthesias, paralyses, loss of voice, inability to stand or walk (astasia-abasia) or even convulsive seizures are reported though careful examinations reveal no evidence of organic disease of the nervous system. The "lump in the throat that cannot be swallowed" (globus hystericus) is a common complaint. The patients are extremely suggestible and outspokenly egotistic. Personality studies by psychoanalysts have thrown much light upon the origin of the hysterical reaction in some patients.

In *psychasthenia* the patients are beset by doubts, fears, and especially by difficulty in making decisions. They may have obsessions that interfere seriously with the conduct of their lives. One psychasthenic man had wanted to marry the woman he loved for over ten years but had never been able to make up his mind to do so; finding that they were really both in love with one another and that there was no reason (except his indecision) for not marrying, I put them both in a taxi-cab, went with them to secure a marriage license and then took them to a clergyman who married them with myself as a witness: *he had to be told what to do!*

In the *traumatic neuroses* and so-called *compensation neuroses* the functional nervous symptoms develop after some injury, usually in persons who carry accident insurance, or in soldiers (as all physicians in the Veterans' Bureau well know).

The *treatment of the psychoneurotic states* can be very rewarding if it be skilfully applied. Whoever undertakes it should know that the sufferings of the neurotic patient are very real; they are not "imaginary" and they are temporarily outside the will power and the morality of the person affected. The physician must see to it that the patient has plenty of time to tell his "whole story" and this may make great demands upon the patience of the listening doctor. But while understanding the sufferings of the neurotic patient and genuinely sympathizing with him, the physician who treats him must try to see to it that his orders are faithfully carried out. If the physician make a thorough general examination before starting the treatment, it will give the patient confidence that nothing important can have been overlooked. Many anxiety neuroses can be prevented by such thorough diagnostic studies followed by an emphatic pronouncement by the physician that the symptoms are not those of any serious organic disease that the patient may have feared. He should not, however, say to him, "There is nothing wrong with you; go home and forget about it," for the patient knows very well that there is something the matter with him and he is right; a functional nervous disturbance is a definitely pathological state that needs to be righted.

Though the milder cases may respond very well to treatment at home or at physicians' offices, the severer cases require separation from home and family for a period in a hospital or nursing home, with rest in bed, suitable diet and nursing, massage, mild sedatives, and regular psychotherapeutic conversations and reeducative methods. The results as a rule are very satisfactory indeed, without the use of hypnosis or of any long drawn out and expensive psychoanalysis. There are many little books that patients suffering from functional neuroses may read with advantage; among them, I may mention J. R. Oliver's "Fear," Josephine Jackson's "Outwitting Our Nerves," A. P. Call's "The Freedom of Life," Strickler and Appel's "Discovering Ourselves," A. F. Riggs' "Just Nerves,' and F. Adler's "Understanding Human Nature." The physician may choose those he thinks most suitable for the individual patient. The doctor himself will enjoy C. P. Emerson's "The Nervous Patient," written especially for the general practitioner.

In cases of compensation neurosis, it is essential to arrive at a permanent settlement of any litigation pending as speedily as possible, since as long as the legal situation remains in doubt, it is exceedingly difficult to influence the neurosis favorably.

When a functional neurosis is superimposed upon an organic disease, the physician should make clear to the patient his exact situation and should assure him that both the organic and the functional features will be given the consideration in the treatment.

And after recovery has gone far enough to permit the patient gradually to resume normal activities, the physician will do well to maintain supervision for a time, having the patient report at regular intervals until self-confidence is fully reestablished. In the making of various readjustments in connection with the patient's family and friends, or with his occupational relationships, the wise general practitioner can often be most serviceable in the prevention of recurrences of nervous breakdowns.

VINYL ETHER OBSTETRIC ANESTHESIA FOR GENERAL PRACTICE

Wesley Bourne, Montreal (*Journal A. M. A.*, Dec. 21. 1935), points out that since the more extended employment of vinyl ether in his clinic there has been no question of untoward effects; its entire suitability for use in obstetrics has become very convincing, and although those patients who have had it by the "open" method have done well enough, there can be no doubt that it is better to administer vinyl ether with oxygen, if for no other reason than that every anesthetist knows something of the benefits of adding oxygen to anesthetic vapors. The extreme volatility of vinyl ether is such that it is very wasteful to give it by the "open" method. It is therefore preferable to employ a closed-system apparatus, fitted for supplying oxygen and for absorbing carbon dioxide, so that a very small quantity of anesthetic will suffice for the longest case; in other words, the longer the anesthesia the smaller will be the quantity used per unit of time, such an apparatus should be cheap and should in a short time more than pay for itself by precluding waste of material. The author concludes that when vinyl ether is used to produce anesthesia sufficient for obstetric procedures, it apparently does not cause liver damage nor does it interfere with muscular activity in the intestine and in the uterus. Vinyl ether seems to be particularly suitable for obstetric anesthesia in general practice on account of its safety for mother and child, its ease of administration, the rapidity of its action, the satisfactory maintenance of any desired degree of narcosis, and the early uneventful recovery.

CHEST CONDITIONS IN INFANTS AND CHILDREN*

WM. WILLIS ANDERSON, M.D.
Atlanta

In the negro infants and young children admitted to the Grady Hospital we are seeing more lobar pneumonia than bronchopneumonia. Lobar pneumonia is diagnosed on finding signs of consolidation, such as dulness, tubular breathing, and shadows of consolidation seen with the fluoroscope or on x-ray films. Not always do the signs of consolidation correspond to the anatomic outlines of the various lobes. At times only a part of a single lobe is involved; at others only portions of two or more lobes. Many times ordinary physical examination disagrees entirely with fluoroscopic and x-ray examinations.

Except in the most recent text-books[1] and in an occasional original publication, the subject of lobar pneumonia in infants and all children has received little consideration.

Last year Cathcart and I[2] reported the study of 100 charts of consecutive admissions of infants and children from birth to twelve years of age whom we had observed on the wards at Grady Hospital and in whom we were able to make a diagnosis of pneumonia of any type. Although we had known that the percentage of lobar pneumonia would be high, we were surprised to find that 85 of the 100 children had lobar pneumonia.

I doubt if this figure represents the relative occurrence of lobar pneumonia outside of the hospital. Perhaps only those children who were acutely ill applied for admission. Perhaps children with bronchopneumonia and bronchitis were treated in the out-patient department or at home. Such a high percentage of lobar pneumonia has not been noted in my private practice. However, hospital patients are studied more carefully, and it is possible that if our private patients were submitted to as careful a scrutiny the percentage would be changed.

Seasonal incidents must also be taken into consideration. A hundred patients at another

*Read before the Medical Association of Georgia, Atlanta, May 8, 1935.

time may show differences. That lobar pneumonia does occur frequently in infants and small children in other localities was noted also by Grulee and Mulherin[3] in their experience from 1922 to 1931 inclusive.

I have noted many times the changes in physical signs from day to day. On one visit one hears rales in one area of the chest, and the following day no rales can be elicited. Even a change in percussion, a rather stable sign in examining an infant's chest, may be noted rather frequently.

A sharp drop in the patient's temperature within 24 to 48 hours after admission has been noted often. For instance, a child admitted with a temperature of 105 will appear extremely ill, perhaps sleeping almost continuously. The next morning he is found sitting up in bed or, more frequently, standing up, with a temperature of 99. After this the fever fluctuates. I am unable to account for this other than by the possible exposure prior to admission and the nursing care he gets in the hospital. I am wondering, however, if this phenomenon may not account for some of the enthusiastic published reports of various treatments of pneumonia, particularly intravenous and subcutaneous injections. I am sure that, had we instituted such measures, we could show sharp declines in temperatures within 24 to 48 hours.

Eight of these hundred children died. This high mortality probably confirms the fear that negro children tolerate pneumonia poorly. Or, again, in dealing with the poorer classes resistance and immunity may be lowered from lack of proper diet and hygiene.

I have not been impressed by the tendency of lobar pneumonia to recur.

Leukocytosis occurred so regularly that I think a child with the signs of coryza and a leukocyte count of 20,000 should be suspected of pneumonia.

We tried to determine by careful questioning the exact onset of the pneumonia (and admit possibilities of error in some of the answers of the negro mothers) and add the period of our observation. In the great majority of cases the child was ill only seven or eight days. This does not include the usual week or ten-day interval allowed for convalescence: the recovery is based on the day that the temperature reached normal and stayed there and when the physical signs began to abate and the child's general condition began to improve. Compared to bronchopneumonia and bronchitis the duration is much shorter. I have seen children with bronchitis moderately ill and coughing all winter. A prolonged illness frequently reflects greatly on the child's general development. A child with an acute illness of only a few days with rapid recovery often suffers no permanent injury. I wonder therefore if it is not generally better for an infant to have frank lobar pneumonia of short duration with rapid recovery than to have some other type of pulmonary infection.

Like many others I have been watching with interest the treatment of pleural empyema in infants and small children by aspirating pus with a large hypodermic syringe and replacing air. From March, 1934, to March, 1935, seven negro children with empyema were observed at the Grady Hospital. One of these suffering also from pneumococcic meningitis died the first day. Of the remaining six, two with unilateral empyema and one with bilateral involvement were cured by aspiration and air replacement alone. The three others were finally referred for thoracotomy. One refused operation and left the hospital against advice: two were cured. I adhere to no hard and fast rule in determining how long a patient with empyema should be treated by aspiration alone, but depend on the progress noted in his condition and the advice of the medical and surgical staff.

A resume of the three cures by aspiration and air replacement follows:

Case 1.—A 19 months old boy was admitted Dec. 29, 1934, with lobar pneumonia of the right lower lobe after an illness of one week. Thirteen days after admission empyema developed. In the aspirated pus diplococci, staphylococci and short-chain streptococci were found. On Jan. 12, 1935, 20 cc. of thick greenish pus was aspirated: 5 cc. on the 15th; 250 cc. on the 18th; 180 cc. on the 22nd; 125 cc. on the 26th. On January 30 and February 22 taps were made but no fluid obtained. After the first two aspirations air equalling approximately the amount of pus withdrawn was re-injected into the pleural cavity. Convalescence was complicated by the development of a bronchial fistula and the lung re-expanded only after eight or nine weeks. During this time the heart and

mediastinal organs were pushed to the opposite side. For this reason he was kept in the hospital until March 18, although he was afebrile and comfortable during the last nine or ten weeks.

Case 2.—A girl, aged 14 months, was admitted Oct. 25, 1934, with left lower lobar pneumonia and empyema. She was acutely ill with a temperature of 104. Her chest was tapped November 1, and 3 cc. of thin greenish purulent fluid showing pneumococci in pure culture obtained. Her chest was again tapped on the 4th, 5 cc. of similar pus being obtained. About three days later the temperature became normal and she made an uneventful recovery. She stayed four weeks in the hospital.

Case 3.—A 7 year old boy was admitted July 17, 1934, with lobar pneumonia of the right base and possible empyema. There were signs of resolving lobar pneumonia in the left lower lobe. He had been ill at home since July 1, during which time his mother stated that he had had fever, difficult breathing and a rattle in his chest. The right pleural cavity was aspirated on July 19, forty-eight hours after admission to the hospital at which time 330 cc. of greenish pus showing pneumococci was removed and a like amount of air introduced. On July 25, signs of empyema developed on the other side and 70 cc. of similar pus was withdrawn from the left pleural cavity. After he developed bilateral empyema no more air was introduced. His chest was aspirated 19 times, 9 times on the right with a removal of 1058 cc. and 10 times on the left with a removal of 450 cc. On August 2, he developed respiratory distress with cyanosis lasting about three days. His temperature was normal from August 14 to September 1. It then varied between 99 and 101 until October 3, when it returned to normal. A skin test on October 10 was positive to 0.1 mg. of tuberculin. Treatment other than aspiration, consisted of general diet, sunshine, ferric ammonium citrate, cod liver oil, two transfusions and one period of digitalization. Altogether his progress though tedious was satisfactory. He was in the hospital a little more than four months.

The three cases in which aspiration alone did not cure empyema were as follows:

Case 4.—A 7 months' old girl weighing 14 pounds was admitted Jan. 31, 1935, with right upper lobar pneumonia, having been ill at home for four days. Her temperature was septic and she was acutely ill until February 10. On the 8th she showed signs of pleural effusion. Her chest was first aspirated on the 12th, 50 cc. of thick greenish pneumococcic pus being withdrawn. Her chest was tapped for 50 cc. of pus three times more and for 120 cc. once. On each aspiration one-half the amount of pus withdrawn was replaced by air. Her condition did not materially improve and operation was recommended. Her mother refused this and took her home against advice on March 4.

Case 5.—A 2 year old boy was admitted on Dec. 12, 1934, with lobar pneumonia of the right lower and middle lobes and possibly of the upper. On the 26th he developed empyema and 70 cc. of pneumococcic pus was removed. During the next six weeks his chest was aspirated ten times, an average of 106 cc. of pus being removed each time. Several times his temperature remained normal four or five days. A rib was resected Feb. 6, 1935, after which he made an uneventful recovery from his empyema. The blood Wassermann was strongly positive and he was treated with bismuth and sulpharsphenamine during his stay in the hospital.

Case 6.—A 2 year old boy admitted to the contagious ward Jan. 20, 1935, with tonsillar diphtheria and lobar pneumonia of the right upper, showed extension of the pneumonic process to the right lower on the 27th, which may have been an early empyema. The pleural cavity was aspirated January 30: 70 cc. of pus yielding streptococci in pure culture was removed. His chest was aspirated nine times during the following five weeks, an average of 85 cc. of pus being removed each time. Pneumococci in pure culture was reported in the pus on February 2. His condition not apparently improving, a rib was resected on March 5. Recovery was uneventful.

Summary

Lobar pneumonia is much more common than bronchopneumonia in infants and children at the Grady Hospital. X-ray is an invaluable adjunct in the diagnosis of lobar pneumonia.

When a baby suffering from a cold shows more than 15,000 leukocytes, pneumonia should be suspected.

It is often possible to cure empyema by repeated aspiration of pus.

REFERENCES

1. Holt's Diseases of Infancy and Childhood, D. Appleton and Co., 1933.
2. Anderson, Wm. Willis, and Cathcart, Don F., Chest Condition in Infants and Children, J. Med. Asso. of Ga., Dec., 1934, 11: 456.
3. Mulherin, Philip, and Grulee, C. G., Lobar Pneumonia in Infants and Young Children, J. Pediatrics, 1932, 1: 593.

Discussion on Paper by Dr. Wm. Willis Anderson

DR. H. P. HARRELL (Augusta): In my opinion a good number of the so-called bronchus pneumonias occurring in young children have really been lobar pneumonias. It is important to try to differentiate lobar pneumonia from bronchopneumonia. The mortality rate in a large series of cases at Edinburgh shows a mortality rate of 54 per cent in bronchopneumonia against a rate of 7 per cent in lobar type.

It should be remembered that in lobar pneumonia in young children you may have the entire lobe of the lung involved, but more often you have a number of small areas involved in one or more lobes. Probably with more careful study with the x-ray we can make more accurate diagnoses. According to most investigators on the category of lobar pneumonia in children, type IV pneumococcus is the cause of most cases; however, this is not accepted by some. Lung punctures reveal that type IV pneumococcus did not predominate in as high a percentage of cases as when the type was made from sputum obtained from the larynx. As we have no specific serum against type IV pneumococcus infection, the serum available is useless for treatment. In lobar pneumonia in children where types I or II pneumococcus is found to be the cause and serum given the mortality rate has not been lower than in cases treated symptomatically.

Aspiration pneumonia: The inhalation of amniotic fluid can cause antenatal and postnatal pneumonia. Ahfeld in 1880 pointed out that the fetus in utero was able to make respiratory movements. Other substances that might be aspirated and cause pneumonia are cod liver oil, dusting powder, mineral oil, various nose drops and food. Hess and others stress the danger of aspirating milk during nasal feedings in premature infants. Good technic in doing nasal feedings is most desirable. Pinkerton reported six cases of aspiration pneumonia in which fatty substances were found at autopsy in the bronchi and lungs. All of the above substances act as an irritant to the bronchi and lungs and this is followed by a superimposed infection causing pneumonia.

Treatment of empyema: It should be emphasized that there is no routine treatment for empyema, every case presents its special problem. In my opinion, aspiration should be tried first in each case. Brennerman and others using aspiration alone report complete cure in 2-3 of their cases. Where there is a rapid re-filling of the chest after aspiration and there is a tendency of the condition becoming chronic I believe it is best in children over two years of age to resort to some kind of closed continuous drainage. One objection to the treatment with repeated aspiration alone is the fact that the patient's stay in the hospital is prolonged. In deciding which kind of treatment is best suited for the patient we have to consider the cost of hospitalization. It is necessary to make numerous x-ray pictures of the chest when treating by aspiration alone. This extra cost has to be considered also.

DR. W. WILLIS ANDERSON (Atlanta): Mr. Chairman: From the viewpoint of a pediatrician studying chest conditions in infants and children, I am impressed with the improved methods of treating empyema. In years gone by we were accustomed to see children with empyema stay in hospital wards for months and months, wasting away and dying—or recurring after we thought them well. One man will report a series of cures, employing one method; another will cure a large majority of patients with simple aspiration of pus. Perhaps they are just being treated with a safer, saner and more wholesome attitude. I should like to pay that tribute to the medical profession in treating empyema.

TREATMENT OF ACUTE LOBAR PNEUMONIA*

Review of Five-Year Records of Pneumonia in Atlanta Hospitals

C. C. AVEN, M.D.
A. WORTH HOBBY, M.D.
Atlanta

Twenty years ago, Osler stated that pneumonia had become the "Captain of the men of death," a phrase applied to tuberculosis and attributed to John Bunyan.

Today the mortality rate remains about the same. Therefore, we ask, has any progress been made in treatment of pneumonia? Is there something wrong with our treatment? Are we omitting something that should be done? Are we over-treating our patients Are we contacting our patients too late? Is our diagnostic skill to be questioned? Are we too prone to follow some treatment hobby? These are the questions we leave with you. Many drugs, biologicals and other remedial agents have their quota of advocates.

To treat any disease intelligently, its etiology and the anatomic cause of death must be known. The cause is well established in pneumonia, but the immediate cause of death arouses our interest. Harlow Brooks attempts to answer this by a review of 200 consecutive fatal cases with careful clinical and anatomic studies. Ante and postmortem typing was done. All cases had as their apparent etiologic factor some form of pneumococcus. Fifty-seven per cent showed definite chronic cardiac disease pre-existing before onset of pneumonia; 38 per cent died from cardiac failure; 36.5 per cent showed acute cardiac lesions; in 14 per cent the heart was recorded as normal or else ignored.

Death may occur from circulatory failure without apparent cardiac impairment. This is due to days, hours, or moments of dilatation of superficial or deep capillary beds and veins. The extent of lung involvement plays only a minor part as a fatal factor, for 25 per cent of the 200 had only one lobe involved.

*Read before the Medical Association of Georgia, Atlanta, May 9, 1935.

Cecil has repeatedly emphasized the early use of serum and has condemned its use without typing. Early usage of serum and typing are frequently incompatible with existing conditions. The ideal opportunity for use of specific serum is in the early stage of a typed case.

Rufus Cole, of the Rockefeller Institute, calls attention to the fact that pneumonia is a group of diseases, each based on specific immunologic characteristics. This gives hope for optimism. He states that types I and II are isolated in Rockefeller Hospital. He offers hope in chemotherapy and serum therapy.

The British Medical Research Council spent three years in the study of serotherapy. Treatment was valuable in reducing mortality and the average duration of illness in type I and type II. In fact, specific treatment is only of value in properly typed cases when used early and in adequate dosage.

Our review of pneumonia in Grady and Georgia Baptist hospitals deals only with acute lobar pneumonia in white patients of all ages.

The series in Georgia Baptist Hospital is much smaller, but probably large enough for some comparisons. Five hundred thirty-two case records were reviewed at Grady Hospital: 319 males and 213 females, with 155 deaths, or 29.1 per cent mortality. At Georgia Baptist Hospital 102 cases studied in the same five-year period reveals about the same findings except a death rate of 44 per cent. Patients on admission to Georgia Baptist Hospital were more desperately ill.

The years, 1930-1934 inclusive, were studied. 1933 revealed the lowest death rate of 21 per cent, while 1934 was highest with 36.3 per cent. Such variations in death rates from year to year provide us with the waves of optimism for some "hobby treatment" if the mortality rate is low. We discard our "pet treatment" if the mortality rate is high.

Attempts were made to ascertain the number of days of illness before hospital admission. We concluded from those recorded that moving seriously ill patients might be serious, or that the more seriously ill ones were those that were hospitalized. The average pre-hospital days was less for those admitted to Grady Hospital than to Georgia Baptist Hospital.

Blood pressure records were noted when charted and those patients with systolic pressures of 100 or less and 150 or more had poor prognoses.

White blood counts were recorded on admission in 444 cases. Those with count of 10,000 or less had a mortality rate of 36 per cent plus; those between 10,000 and 20,-000 a death rate of 26 per cent; those over 20,000, 21 per cent.

Some degree of cyanosis was recorded in 12 per cent and was apparently a bad omen. Delirium was noted in only 4 per cent and bore no direct relation to death rate.

Progress notes made by interns improved from 1930 to 1935. Omissions in the notes account for the absence of some data on important symptoms.

A routine procedure was carried out at Grady Hospital for the past three years with no appreciable change in mortality rate. The review at Georgia Baptist Hospital, of 102 cases, shows a death rate of 44 per cent and a shorter hospital stay. This may be accounted for by removal to the private hospital of moribund cases.

Our desperation in private practice may drive us to do things that our better judgment should forbid.

Observation made at Grady Hospital prove that a certain number of patients pass their crisis without any plan of treatment being instituted. They are admitted after several days illness and suddenly go through crisis without previous treatment. A certain group of patients die irrespective of treatment. Another group seemingly respond to careful nursing and symptomatic care.

These observations and a study of the findings of Harlow Brooks, lead us to believe we would be more justified in treating the patients, forgetting the pneumonia only where specific sera or other special measures can be used properly.

Some of the charts reviewed showed as many as 37 various medications, treatments and baths in one 24-hour period. How is it possible for a patient to survive such treatment? These and other observations

lead us to advise an individual plan of treatment.

Pneumonia is a disease usually of a short, stormy course, therefore, a plan of intensive attention to all the details of general care.

Treatment

Absolute mental and *physical rest* is our aim because death is so uniformly connected with circulatory failure; no company and no unnecessary measures at all. *Fresh air* is essential. A properly ventilated room can usually be had. An ice cap for temperature 102 plus; warm sponge bath; no alcohol rubs. *Oral Hygiene* is important; mild acid solutions are probably best. The *bowels* should be evacuated daily with non-irritating enema; castor oil when necessary.

Sodium citrate is administered unless pulmonary edema develops.

Aromatic spirits of ammonia or *ammonium carbonate* are given every 4 to 5 hours.

Digitalis is given only if auricular fibrillation or flutter be present, or on some other special indication.

Dilaudid grs. 1/64 to grs. 1/32 hypodermatically for control of pain and restlessness; *pantopon* is next choice.

Antipyretics are used in small doses for hyperpyrexia.

Coramine or *caffeine* are stimulants of our choice.

Atropine is used for excessive secretion.

Glucose, 50 cc. of 50 per cent solution, is given intravenously daily followed by 10 units of insulin.

Mustard poultices may be used for the comfort of the patient.

Oxygen produces great relief to certain patients and is preferably used with the use of oxygen tent or chamber.

There is no need for a heavy diet as the disease is of short duration. A high carbohydrate diet with low total intake is preferable. Water, strained soups, broths, with rice or barley, with half milk or cream added; buttermilk, fruit juices, coffee or tea with cream and sugar. Small frequent feedings are preferable.

Diathermy has some strong advocates.

Artificial pneumothorax is being employed with apparent good results in properly selected cases.

Experience is a requisite and the case should be x-rayed to be sure of unilateral disease. It is preferably used in the first 48 hours.

Four hundred cubic centimeters of air is injected, to be repeated every 8 to 12 hours for 2 to 3 doses.

Results are: freedom from pain, tranquil sleep without sedatives; crises in 12 to 36 hours. Duration of illness is thereby shortened and heart muscle is conserved.

Conclusions

1. That very little, if any, progress is being made in the treatment of pneumonia by our polypharmacy methods.

2. That no typing is done in these hospitals.

3. That most patients treated in private

hospitals are moved there as a last resort, and that this is a doubtful procedure.

4. That a routine plan is of doubtful value and is possibly harmful.

5. That pneumothorax is in an experimental stage and a careful study of technique and further observations should be made.

6. That our hope is in chemotherapy and serotherapy.

REFERENCES

1. Cecils Medicine.
2. Osler's Medicine.
3. Brooks, Harlow: The Cause of Death in Pneumonia, J. A. M. A., 103: 1192 (October 20) 1934.
4. Harbin, R. M.: Diathermy in the Abortive Treatment of Pneumonia, J. Med. Assn. of Georgia, 23: 45 (February) 1934.
5. Bethea, Oscar W.: Treatment of Pneumonia, J. Kansas Med. Soc. 35: 445 (December) 1934.
6. Moorman, Lewis J.: Artificial Pneumothorax in the Treatment of Pneumonia, Sou. Med. J., 27: 233 (March) 1934.
7. Sutliff, W. D., and Finland, Maxwell: Type I Pneumococcic Infections with Especial Reference to Specific Serum Treatment, The New Eng. J. of M., 210: 237 (February) 1934.
8. Kyle, John A.: The Prognosis and Treatment of Lobar Pneumonia, The Lancet, 1: 345 (February 18) 1933.
9. Moersch, H. J.: The Treatment of Pneumonia, Proceedings of the Staff Meetings of the Mayo Clinic, 9: 187 (March 28) 1934.
10. Behrend, Albert and Cowper, Roscoe, B. G.: Artificial Pneumothorax in the Treatment of Lobar Pneumonia, J. A. M. A., 102: 1907 (June 9) 1934.
11. Stewart, Harry Eaton, Recent Advances in the Diathermic Treatment of Pneumonia, Radium, 13: 668 (November) 1932.
12. Therapeutic Trials Committee Report: The Serum Treatment of Lobar Pneumonia, The British Medical Journal, 3814 241 (February 10) 1934.
13. A Report of the Therapeutic Trials Committee of the Medical Research Council: The Serum Treatment of Lobar Pneumonia, The Lance, 226: 290 (February 10) 1934.
14. Cole, Rufus: Canad. M. A. J: March) 1934.

Discussion on Paper by Dr. C. C. Aven and Dr. A. Worth Hobby .

DR. H. M. TOLLESON (Eastman): In discussing a paper, particularly an excellent one, as you have just heard, it seems to me that the greatest good that comes from the discussion is to the individual who has the privilege of discussing the paper. After studying the essay, a copy of which was kindly sent to me by Dr. Aven. I was impressed. as you have been, by the clear-cut way in which the subject has been presented. Among the deluge of information which comes to us through numerous investigators, commercial advertising and various textbooks, a paper of this kind seems to be as a beacon or buoy to guide us through this maze of data to which the profession has constant access.

Dr. Aven stated that a survey of cases of pneumonia treated at Bellevue (Harlow Brooks) showed that 38 per cent died from cardiac failure. Louis M. Warfield, in the Journal-Lancet, Volume 54, 1934, raised a question which I think particularly appropriate in this connection. Does the heart fail in acute infections? Does it not seem strange that an organ of the body which can beat seventy-two times a minute from infancy to old age, an organ that, given oxygen, glucose and insulin, can beat almost indefinitely outside the body, could fail as a result of infection within a few days? Does the heart fail, or does the peripheral circulation fail? Does the heart fail because of infection,

if it does fail, or because of lack of nourishment to the heart muscle? When the pulse is accelerated and the apex beat becomes diffuse it does not always indicate cardiac failure. When fluids are taken from the blood stream as in the splanchnic area, pleural cavities, pericardial and peritoneal cavities, the blood volume is lessened. The ventricular contraction is in direct proportion to the amount of ventricular stretch. In other words the venous return rather than the heart is impaired, the blood volume is lessened, the heart does not fill properly and in order to supply the tissues with the proper amount of glucose and oxygen the heart beats faster and with less force. Bacterial infections, of course, play an important part in that the bacterial toxins form histamine or histamine-like substances which is the cause of the damage to the capillary and venule systems which allows the transudation of fluid into the above named areas.

With this in mind I would like to emphasize very emphatically the part of Dr. Aven's treatment where he suggests glucose intravenously. Personally, except in extreme emergencies, I prefer giving glucose by the drop method in considerable more dilution as this places no additional strain on the heart muscle and supplies much needed fluid. I believe that many so-called cases of cardiac failure are due to cardiac starvation as a result of the process outlined above. Digitalis, caffein, or any other commonly used stimulant cannot possibly supply nourishment to the heart muscle. Where stimulants are necessary I believe that coramine is one of the best.

The collapse treatment undoubtedly offers some hope of being a valuable addition to our present treatment, but, of course, is not practical at present for use in general practice. In emergencies oxygen can sometimes be administered to advantage by means of the usual anesthetic machines in general use. In this way, with the mask placed tightly over the patient's nose and mouth, we are able to give him a quick, concentrated supply of oxygen which may at times be life-saving, particularly where the patient has not previously been getting oxygen with an oxygen tent, or where such is not available.

DR. H. L. BARKER (Carrollton): I just want to speak a few words on this important subject from the standpoint of the country town physician who is called out at night to go many miles through the mud to a place where he hasn't modern equipment or even the assistance of a practical nurse.

I think one of our greatest handicaps in the treatment of pneumonia is the fact that we do not see our patients early enough. It has been my observation that where we have an acute pleuritis, with pain, as an early symptom, and we then institute a method to relieve that, not with drugs, that we get much better results and an early crisis.

We know in the treatment of any inflammatory process rest to the part involved is essential. For quite a while we tried strapping the side where this pleurisy was involved. We did not get the results for the simple reason that the opposite side could move outward. Consequently, many of us in our section now are employing a circular bandage high up on the chest, from the costal margin up to the nipple under the breast in females. Get two good men to put it on, and don't think that you will hurt the patient. He will complain for a few minutes, but lace, tie or pin this bandage around him securely. He has plenty of room in the upper chest to breathe. You come right back to the essence of treatment of an inflammatory process by putting to rest the part involved. If the pressure is sufficient, you by pressure force this exudate out,.the patient spits it off. In many cases the patients have 24 to 36 hours of complete crisis in this method, and it is practical; you can use it in any home, and I felt that many of us here, like myself, get out in the country at night and we seek relief, and this is one method of relief that is practical anywhere.

DR. AVARY DIMMOCK (Atlanta): There is an old saying that pneumonia is the old man's friend, but I am quite sure that it is not the young man's friend, because there are a great many deaths among the young people, and it is perfectly evident that the ideal treatment for pneumonia has not been found. I think that all of us who are interested in medicine should continue our efforts to find some method of treatment which will materially reduce the mortality rate.

Dr. Brooks, to whom the essayist referred, stated if he could find how the pneumonia patients died possibly he could find why they died, and some other generation might find some way to prevent them from dying.

For the last three years, in our service at Grady Hospital, we have been using the vaccine treatment in these cases, and while the mortality rate has not been materially reduced, we do feel some encouragement in the use of this particular method of treatment. It seems to me that with the reduction in mortality in some of the larger institutions with a specific treatment for pneumonia, such as using the serum, and with the work of Dr. Alexander Lambert in New York in vaccine treatment, that the expectant treatment alone should at this time give way to some of these other treatments, at least for a longer period of trial.

Dr. Lambert ran a series of cases over the last eight years, using the vaccine treatment in 474 patients and a like number of cases as controls. The vaccinated patients showed a mortality of 24 per cent; the controls showed a mortality of 44 per cent, or a reduction of 20 per cent for the vaccinated cases. He seems to think that this figure is too large and too definite to be charged purely to chance. He did a good deal of work on determining the antibodies in the blood.

DR. C. C. AVEN (Atlanta): In reference to Dr. Barker's treatment of pleurisy pain, I admit that that is the most damaging thing in pneumonia, probably more so than the infection itself. I wish to give Dr. Hobby, my associate, credit for doing the detail work. He could not be here. If you do not believe he worked

in reviewing all the temperatures and blood counts and notes in these cases, just try it.

IN MEMORIAM*

A. J. MOONEY, M.D.
Statesboro

In keeping with a resolution passed by the Association a few years ago, your Committee on Necrology, at this time of the session, when attendance is at its height, when old acquaintances are being renewed, when we look for familiar faces and hand clasps of friends and fail to see those who were with us here a short year ago, I wish to read to you the names of those who have passed to their eternal reward since our last session.

Listen to the roll call of the honored dead:

Austin, William Hubert, Griffin, March 15, 1935, aged 60.

Barfield, Frederick Green, Jacksonville, Florida, December 25, 1934, aged 61.

Bennett, Jesse C., Jefferson, April 19, 1934, aged 65.

Bowers, William L., Camilla, February 8, 1935, aged 69.

Burnett, George W., Whitesburg, June 19, 1934, aged 81.

Campbell, Moses Gatlin, Atlanta, February 15, 1935, aged 74.

Clements, James Wilson, Subligna, June 6, 1934, aged 96.

Collum, Oscar Frederick, McRae, November 14, 1934, aged 52.

Crowe, William A., Smyrna, April 4, 1935, aged 78.

Curtis, Charles McPherson, College Park, May 6, 1934, aged 68.

Day, Julius B. H., Social Circle, September 7, 1934, aged 66.

Dorminy, William David, Fitzgerald, June 4, 1934, aged 63.

Eberhart, Alvin Barney, McDonough, January 4, 1935, aged 44.

Fulcher, Marion O., Waynesboro, January 16, 1935, aged 65.

Griffies, John Calhoun, Burwell (Carrollton), July 26, 1934, aged 74.

Hice, Edward Houston, Rock Springs, August 31, 1934, aged 66.

Holliday, Paul Lovejoy, Athens, April 22, 1934, aged 41.

Houseworth, Delvous, April 18, 1934, aged 64.

Hubbard, Francis Marion, Commerce, November 9, 1934, aged 78.

Murdock, Joseph L., Emerson, January 29, 1935, aged 73.

---

*Memorial address before the Medical Association of Georgia, Atlanta, May 9, 1935.

Nunez, Jackson M., Swainsboro, October 10, 1934, aged 75.

Pirkle, William W., Cumming, June 8, 1934, aged 64.

Rogers, John Mitchell, Barnesville, February 28, 1935, aged 40.

Smith, Ernest Lacy, Eastman, January 28, 1935, aged 70.

Stovall, Albert S. J., Elberton, June 21, 1934, aged 72.

Sutton, William Harry, Midville, October 21, 1934, aged 51.

Waits, William J., Gray, April 25, 1935, aged 67.

Walker, Sidney, Dublin, January 21, 1935, aged 55.

Wallis, George W., Fayetteville, June 17, 1934, aged 73.

Williams, Charles Winn, Cedartown, March 8, 1935, aged 45.

As the great Ecclesiasticus wrote, "Or ever the silver cord be loosed or the golden bowl be broken; or the pitcher broken at the fountain; or the wheel broken at the cistern; then shall the dust return unto earth as it was and the spirit shall return unto God who gave it," so it is with our professional brethren who have passed on. Some were of ripe old age, others at the height of their career and usefulness, while others had just begun their life work of service. How fitting it would be to chronicle for each of them the preparations for service; the outstanding qualifications of each; their various fields of activity; the medical sagas they have written and left behind to mark the blazing trail through the scientific medical and surgical fields which they passed, glorious heritages to their living confreres; of the sick they had healed; of the lame they had caused to walk; of the pain they had alleviated; of the heart aches they had soothed; of the disconsolate who found solace in their sympathy and philosophy; of the homes where they banished sadness and sorrow and brought gladness and joy; of the weak who had been made strong by their wisdom such as only a doctor can minister after a long philosophic study and understanding of the weaknesses and frailties of mankind; of the community leadership they had acquired through capability and respect of their fellow citizens; of the wonderful comfort to the spiritually convicted and penitent; how, through their life work and deeds of mercy they followed in the footsteps of the Great

Redeemer when He said, "Come unto me all you who labor and are heavy laden and I will give you rest." How fitting it would be if such a chronicle could be for each of them and their particular outstanding virtues, but such length would be superfluous.

Their virtues exemplified while among us will furnish to us ideals for our guidance while we still live. As Paul, the Apostle, spoke of the glory of the sun, moon, and stars, and said that each star was different in its glory, so it is with the different virtues exemplified by our departed medical brethren.

Being philosophers, they must have had the fancies and temptations so necessary to the well-rounded life-resistance to develop strength; sorrows to make the joys sweeter; shadows to make the sunshine more welcome, and disappointments to develop stamina. We are thankful for the ideals of the professional life they left us. A philosopher has said, "Ideals are like stars; you will not succeed in touching them with your hands, but like the seafaring man on the trackless waste of waters you will choose them as your guides, and following them, you will reach your destiny." Man, for thousands of years, has endeavored to make a lasting memorial by his handiwork. He has erected monuments with their spires pointing to the heavens; with the labor of slaves he has endeavored to build a structure of stone and granite that would stand as a perpetual record of the might of man and as a marker for ages to come; but the remorseless tooth of time has brought them to an earthly level, and the sands of the desert and the storms of the heavenly elements have defaced them and all but covered them in obscurity. But the story of a well lived life has survived and will continue long after the handiwork of man has gone.

Profiting by the beautiful virtues and ideals left us, let us choose them as our own and, practice them, live such lives of service that we also, familiar as we are with death, will not be afraid and will receive him as a kind messenger sent to summon us after a life of usefulness on earth to a better life in accordance with the greater plan of the Almighty. May they rest in peace.

PERFORATED PEPTIC ULCER*

A Study of 32 Cases

J. C. PATTERSON, M.D.
Cuthbert

This paper deals only with cases in our personal experience. There were 32 cases of acute perforated peptic ulcer that required immediate operations. Their ages varied from 22 to 62 years. There were 26 white and 6 colored; 28 men and 4 women. As near as could be classified there were 27 duodenal and 5 gastric ulcers but two were so near the pyloric ring that it was doubtful on which side they were. This is a ratio of about 1 gastric to 5 duodenal and is slightly higher than most authorities give.

There were 3 deaths. One was a young negro man who was moribund when admitted to the hospital 48 hours after perforation and was operated on by my associate, Dr. W. G. Elliott. Another death was in a white man 36 hours after perforation, who was cyanotic and almost pulseless. Under procaine anesthesia I opened the abdomen, quickly located and put a purse string suture around the perforation but he died in a few hours. Another death was in a negro woman in whom the ulcer had perforated 48 hours previously. On admission the temperature was 100, pulse 140, respiration 40. I operated immediately, closed the perforation and drained the abdomen. She developed a subphrenic abscess which was drained after the manner of Ochsner. She left the hospital with a bacterial endocarditis and died four months later. This, however, gave us a mortality rate of 9.3 per cent, which is considerably lower than most published mortality rates.

About 50 per cent of these patients gave a history of indigestion. Not a single one had been under proper ulcer treatment; not one had had a gastric analysis or a gastro-intestinal x-ray examination. Many of them had taken soda and some had been given medicine by doctors for ulcer. One had just left his doctor's office enroute home when his ulcer perforated. Only one of these pa-

*Read before the Medical Association of Georgia, Atlanta, May 9, 1935.

tients was in my own practice and he had never complained of any indigestion. Two were ploughing in the field and thought pulling at the plough caused the severe pain and another one was lifting a bale of cotton when he felt the pain. This sudden increase in intra-abdominal pressure probably perforated the ulcer.

Etiology

The etiology of ulcers has not been determined. The principal theories as to its origin, namely, the vascular, mechanical, constitutional, infectious and neurogenic have been discussed by many writers. I can add nothing except to say that almost, if not every one of my patients had severe mouth infections, severe pyorrhea or infected teeth. Most of these patients were farmers of the poorer class, most were tobacco users and as the filthy mouth was universal, it is my belief that either as a direct infection from swallowing infected saliva or as a focus of infection, it played its part.

Diagnosis

All of these patients had their onset abruptly and the first characteristic symptoms were severe agonizing pains and extreme board-like rigidity of the abdomen. One can usually make a diagnosis from examination of the abdomen. Pain in the shoulder was present in 30 per cent and in one was so severe that spinal anesthesia did not relieve it but ether was required. In very few cases was I able to demonstrate air under the diaphragm with the x-ray, but I did not feel justified in trying long, as most of the patients were suffering intensely even after they had had one, two and three hypodermics of morphine.

The two most important symptoms are excruciating pain and extreme board-like rigidity of the abdomen. Most patients were nauseated and at first the pulse was not elevated. As time went on and peritonitis set up, the temperature and pulse rose rapidly. In the beginning the only other thing which will cause as much pain is acute pancreatitis. Later the picture can very easily be confused with appendicitis as the root of the mesentery turns the escaping fluid into the right iliac fossa.

Treatment

All of my patients were operated on immediately after admission to the hospital. I did as little as possible to the patient at the time of operation. Most of them were given a spinal anesthesia and the opening in the stomach or duodenum was cauterized with an electric cautery and the wound closed with purse string suture, reinforced with peritoneal sutures and omentum tacked over the suture line. Some were not cauterized. The escaped fluid was aspirated from the pelvic and abdominal cavities with a suction pump. In all of our cases the abdomen was drained, but care was used that the drain did not touch the suture line.

Recently Trout argued against drainage in cases of perforated ulcer. He sent a questionnaire to 100 doctors and their report was: 20 per cent drain all cases, 20 per cent never drain, and 60 per cent drain in late cases where there is pus. He pointed out that the hydrochloric acid in the stomach content acted as an antiseptic and that there were few bacteria in the stomach and upper intestinal tract. He admitted that he was prejudiced against drainage by seeing in consultation four cases which developed gastric or duodenal fistulae from improper drainage. He states that in contemplating whether or not to drain it might be wise to consider the condition of the teeth, tonsils and the like and if the mouth was found to be foul, such a finding might justify drainage of the peritoneal cavity. As all of my cases had foul mouths I felt that it was best to drain them. However, I do believe that it is best to drain the subhepatic space through a stab wound.

As to the question of whether to simply close the ulcer, do a gastro-enterostomy or a partial resection, I think the study of the different mortality rates will show that the simple closure is the safest procedure. Older writers advocated gastro-enterostomy, but time has shown that even if it were not a grave emergency that a gastro-enterostomy, unless there is considerable duodenal obstruction, is not the best operation and it is being largely abandoned. The use of the nasal duodenal tube has largely done away with the necessity of immediate gastro-enterostomy. Many of the continental writers advocate partial gastric resection even in acute perforated ulcers, but they are very skillful in doing resections and I think not so careful of mortality as we are.

Trout stated that in a study of the literature less than 10 per cent of the patients with simple closure have had to have subsequent operations. It being true that a simple operation such as cautery and closure will cure the ulcer, why do a more complicated operation which has a much greater mortality and has more recurrences later?

In my series I had to do a gastro-enterostomy one week after a simple closure in one case. In the others not a single one has had to have any surgery and the vast majority have had no symptoms. My mortality is 9.3 per cent, which is below most of the published mortality rates in this condition. This is due not to my skill but to the fact that my cases are referred from an area of about 30 miles radius where the doctors have recognized an abdominal emergency in the early stages and sent them to the hospital immediately. The higher mortality in some clinics is due to some of the patients coming from long distances and possibly from attempting too much surgery.

I think the greatest factors in the prognosis is the size of the perforation, the soiling therefrom, and the length of time of operation after the perforation. The smaller the perforation and the earlier the time of operation, the better the prognosis.

Prevention of Perforation

It is my impression that where peptic ulcer is recognized and adequately treated perforation is exceedingly rare. In my practice I have never had a perforation in a patient whom I had treated for ulcer. I believe if patients coming to us complaining of indigestion were all thoroughly examined, including gastrointestinal x-ray and gastric analysis, that ulcer would be recognized and the abdominal catastrophe of perforation prevented.

Conclusion

1. I have reported 32 cases of acute perforated peptic ulcer with a mortality of 9.3 per cent.

2. I believe that as little surgery as will adequately close the opening should be done.

3. In the majority of cases drainage of the subhepatic space through a stab wound is advocated.

4. All cases of indigestion should be thoroughly studied in the belief that treatment prevent many acute perforations.

REFERENCES

1. Trout, H. H.: The Treatment of Perforated "Peptic" ulcers, J. A. M. A. 104: 6-9 (Jan. 5) 1935.
2. Lahey, F. H.: The Management of Peptic Ulcer, New England J. M., 205: 321-329 (Aug. 13) 1931.
3. Maxone, A. C.: Perforated Gastric Ulcer, Brit. M. J. 2: 1162 (Dec. 20) 1934.
4. Riess, P.: Zur Perforationsneigung des Ulcus Pepticum, Zentralbl. f. Chir. 52: 2818-2819 (Dec.) 1925.
5. Soderlund, Gustaf: The Surgical Treatment of Perforating Gastric and Duodenal Ulcer, The Practitioner 118: 171-181 (March) 1927.
6. Brenner, E. C.: Perforated Ulcers of the Duodenum, Ann. Surg. 86: 393-400 (Sep.) 1927.
7. Editorial: Control of Peptic Ulcer, J. A. M. A. 104: 1522 (April 27) 1935.
8. Beltran, B. R.: Acute Perforation of a Gastric Ulcer, S. Clin. N. A., 6: 270-372 (Feb.) 1926.
9. Lewisohn, Richard: Late Results in Perforated Gastro-Duodenal Ulcers, Ann. Surg. 87: 855-860 (June) 1928.
10. Gibson, C. L.: Acute Perforations of Stomach and Duodenum, J. A. M. A. 91: 1006-1008 (Oct. 6) 1928.
11. Moynihan, Sir Berkeley G.: Address in Surgical Subjects, Philadelphia, W. B. Saunders, 1928.
12. Patterson, J. C.: Acute Perforation of Gastric and Duodenal Ulcers. J. M. A. Georgia 18: 502-504 (Nov.) 1929.

Discussion on Paper by Dr. J. C. Patterson

DR. WILLIAM H. MYERS (Savannah): Mr. President and Gentlemen: Dr. Patterson's results are so good and his conclusions are so well drawn that there is no fault to be found with anything that he said. I want to emphasize a few of the things that he brought out, which he did not cover completely.

This subject has been discussed for many years. The first time that perforating peptic ulcer was mentioned was in 1793, by Joseph Penada of Padua. In 1880, Mikulicz advocated simple closure; but it was many years before that was attempted, and Heussner closed one in 1892. The treatment is a matter of much debate, as is its cause. If we knew the cause, perhaps we would have a treatment that would be more satisfactory.

Dr. Patterson brought out the fact that the size of the perforation has much to do with the prospect of recovery. Not only is that true, but the location of it, as well. The most satisfactory results are obtained in duodenal perforation, next the pyloric area, and finally, the most fatal area is in the jejunum. So far as the treatment is concerned, the best results are obtained by the men who have the smallest number of cases. I judge that it is due to the fact that the men who have the smaller number of cases are more conservative. In other words, the man who chooses to do a radical operation when a simple one is satisfactory, runs the risk of increasing his mortality.

In reviewing the literature, I took a rather large number of periodicals, and was able to tabulate almost 5,600 cases. In this number, the mortality rate is 23.3 per cent. The best results are by Gilmour and Saint, at Newcastle-upon-Tyne, who had a series of sixty-four cases in which the mortality rate was 4.7 per cent. I could find no results better than that or under 18 per cent, which has been reported by C. L. Gibson of New York. His mortality was 18.4 per cent in 123 cases.

So far as drainage is concerned, the essayist brought out that point. Dr. Trout had circularized these one hundred surgeons, to ascertain their views. I think the question of drainage is a pertinent subject; as a matter of fact, I drain. It seems to me in case of doubt, this is the only thing to do. Trout has

brought out the fact, too, that if you have the laboratory facilities, so that rapid study can be made, you can gain some information from examining the contents of the stomach .

If the acid content is high, you will find the bacterial content low. If the stomach is empty, the bacterial count will usually be low, but the determining factor is the acid content of the stomach.

So far as the mortality is concerned, the highest mortality, of course, comes from peritonitis. The next is from pulmonary complications. These complications come about by the extension of inflammation, as well as by being carried by the lymphatics, producing pneumonia, pulmonary collapse and lung abscess. The next cause of death is subdiaphragmatic abscess. It has been suggested that that abscess is more often produced where drainage is used in the upper abdomen. On the other hand, some have advocated the use of drainage, in order to prevent subdiaphragmatic abscess.

Trout, in studying white American soldiers in the Sandwich Islands, was able to arrive at the conclusion that peptic ulcer was only about half as frequent in the Sandwich Islands among young American soldiers as it is in the United States, but that perforation was four times as frequent there as here. He believed it was due to nostalgia and the kind of alcohol that they drink in that community.

My series of cases is not very large, but I do not believe that we have nearly so many cases of perforating peptic ulcer in and around Savannah as they have around Cuthbert. I am wondering if it is the form of alcohol that they consume in that section, as alcohol seems to have a marked bearing in these cases.

DR. W. W. BATTEY (Augusta): This splendid paper has so completely covered the subject that there is very little left for me to say. However, I thought I might make a few remarks that might be of some interest.

I have not had an opportunity to operate upon as many cases as Dr. Patterson has. I have operated on six cases of perforating peptic ulcer, with the loss of one patient, and that case was seen extremely late.

The diagnosis is, comparatively speaking, easy. The intense agonizing pain, which almost floors the individual, radiating frequently to the right shoulder, with marked abdominal rigidity, the anxious expression, the slow pulse, and subnormal temperature—these symptoms are almost pathognomonic of perforating peptic ulcer.

In regard to treatment, I quite agree with Dr. Patterson that we should not do too much surgery on these patients. I believe that we should operate as quickly as possible, simply closing the ulcer. It may be necessary to do a gastro-enterostomy or some form of pyloroplasty later on. The condition of the patient at that time will justify further surgical work when it does not immediately after a perforation.

Unfortunately, some of these patients do not present a history of a previous ulcer. I remember Dr. Philip Mulherin, upon whom I operated seven or eight years ago, had absolutely no history of a duodenal ulcer, and had an acute perforation.

DR. J. C. PATTERSON (Cuthbert): I have nothing further to say except to thank the gentlemen for discussing the paper. I agree with what they have said about perforation, except I do not think that our brand of alcohol has had very much to do with the perforations. I do not think most of them have been drinkers, but they have been in the poorer class of people, and almost universally they have had infected mouths, and I cannot help believing that has a large part to play in the cause of these ulcers.

The perforation came on suddenly, and the intense agonizing pain caused them to come to the hospital quickly. That is the reason I think I have had so low a mortality.

COMPLICATIONS OF THE TREATMENT OF SYPHILIS IN PREGNANCY*

*Report of Three Cases of Arsenical Encephalitis Complicating Such Treatment† ***

E. BRYANT WOODS, M.D.
Augusta

Syphilis is a very important complication of pregnancy because of the apparent ease with which the causative spirochetes may penetrate the placental barrier and thus infect the fetus. Before the introduction of modern serological tests and the general acceptance of antiluetic treatment by women attending prenatal clinics, syphilis constituted the largest single etiologic factor in stillbirths and accounted for three-fourths of the macerated fetuses, while a still larger number of children were born alive with a stigma of congenital syphilis. The wide-spread dissemination of syphilis among all classes of the population leaves it still a major obstetric problem, and one of vital importance in child health work.

Jeans and Cooke report from a collection of 5,358 pregnant women in four cities an incidence of 9.7 per cent of syphilitic individ-

*Read before the Medical Association of Georgia, Atlanta, May 10, 1935.
†From the Department of Obstetrics of the University of Georgia School of Medicine, Augusta.
**From the Department of Obstetrics and Gynecology, State University of Iowa College of Medicine, Iowa City.

uals. The data from the University of Georgia Clinic in Augusta reveal an incidence of 9.8 per cent in women admitted to the prenatal clinic. Plass has observed that the percentage of syphilis in parous women is somewhat greater than in primigravidas and explains this by assuming that the longer the period since marriage, the greater chance for the infected husband to give the disease to his wife.

Since syphilis is generally a milder disease in women than in men, with the primary lesion often passing unnoticed, and since there may be no primary and secondary manifestations if the disease is contracted at the time of, or shortly after conception, reliance must be placed upon the Wassermann or Kahn serologic reaction, which should be made a part of the antepartum routine. The influence of syphilis upon the fetus depends upon the time of infection in relation to conception and is usually differentiated into three classes as follows: (1) Primary infection which has occurred sometime before conception—the probability of infecting the fetus is great and in proportion to the newness of the infection. (2) The infection which has occurred shortly before conception, or within the first few months of pregnancy—the fetus will almost certainly be involved if not treated. (3) The infection which occurs after the sixth month of pregnancy—the fetus will probably escape, but will be subject to the danger of postnatal infection of the mother.

Treatment of syphilis in the pregnant woman is dictated by consideration for both mother and child, since pregnant women have been found to be unusually susceptible to antisyphilitic therapy; the pregnancy itself exerting a beneficial influence upon the course of a syphilitic infection; and since the prevention of congenital syphilis by intensive treatment of the mother is infinitely more effective than any attempt to eradicate the disease after birth. The routine treatment, as carried out in the syphilis clinic at the University of Georgia, consists of alternating courses of treatment of arsenical preparations and bismuth preparations, the emphasis being given to the former. The initial dose of neoarsphenamine is usually 0.3 Gm. given intravenously and repeated in from five to seven days.

Each course of treatment consists of from six to eight injections. McCord[1] believes that five treatments, with an intravenous arsenical preparation constitutes the low limit of efficacy. Treatment should be begun as early as possible in pregnancy and should be continued in some form throughout the entire gestation period unless complications arise. Attention should be paid to the careful examination of the urine, as albuminuria may be the first sign of a toxemia. Under such circumstances all syphilitic treatment must be stopped and remain in abeyance until the urine is again clear. It is well recognized that, even under ideal conditions, and with every precaution satisfied, reactions will follow the intravenous use of antiluetic arsenicals and accessory drugs.*

Cole and his collaborators[2] are of the opinion that young adults generally are more susceptible to the toxic effects of arsenical injections, and that women are more susceptible than men; an opinion which is also shared by Klaften[3], Pritzi[4], and Ireland[5]. Klaften[3] quotes Meirowsky as having collected data on 23 salvarsan fatalities among women, 14 of whom were pregnant.** The danger seems to be greater early in the course of treatment (Ireland[5], Cole et al[2], Phelps and Washburn[6]) with symptoms more commonly appearing after one to four injections. Cole's[2] statistics indicate that those with latent syphilis are more likely to develop reactions than are those with early lesions, and the common finding in pregnant women is a latent infection, which is discovered only by routine serologic tests. Klaften[3], Pritzi[4], McKelvey and Turner[7], and Clason[8] apparently believe that pregnancy increases the danger of serious reactions. *** Gammeltoft[9] quotes Kristjansen as saying that among all patients treated with salvarsan at Rudolph Bergh's Venerological Hospital during a ten year period, four or five died from salvarsan poisoning, and that three were pregnant women.

Pritzi[4] believes that the danger of toxic reactions increases as term is approached. On the other hand, McCord[1] says: "With an experience of many thousands of doses of all kinds of arsenical preparations given to pregnant women, I have never seen a reaction that approached a fatality; I rarely see a reaction of any kind." The fortunate experience of this observerd may be attributed to the fact that his patients are largely colored women, who, according to certain investigators, Cole et al[2], are more immune to the common toxic effects than are the white women.

In considering the complications which have been encountered in the treatment of syphilis in our clinic, we make note of the following: (1) Bismuth Stomatitis, (2) Bismuth Enteritis, (3) Bismuth Dermatitis, (4) Nitritoid Reaction (5) Arsenical Stomatitis, (6) Arsenical Dermatitis, (7) Arsenical (Hemorrhagic) Encephalitis. The following table (Table I.) presents sixty-five cases having complications in 54,791 antiluetic treatments for the four year period from April 1, 1931, to April 1, 1935, in the University of Georgia Syphilis Clinic. In the 31,174 treatments given to women patients, there were 53 reactions or 0.17 per cent, and in only six instances were these reactions in pregnant women.

*Excluding early febrile sequelae, such as "endotoxic reactions," due to the liberation of the "syphilitic toxin" from the spirochetes by the destructive action of the drug, and the "water fever" due to pyrogenic factors in the water used for solution of the drug.
**This author likewise states that he has observed women who showed salvarsan reactions while pregnant, but who after delivery were given the same drug without observable bad effects.
***Klaften attributes a pernicious influence to menstruation and recommends a reduced dosage during these two physiological states.

TABLE I. A.
REACTIONS (COMPLICATIONS) OF ANTILUETIC TREATMENT
In 54,791 Treatments from April 1, 1931, to April 1, 1935
University of Georgia Syphilis Clinic

	Male	Female	Total
No. of Treatments, Neo.	12,267	15,196	27,463
No. of Treatments, Bi.	11,350	15,978	27,320
Patients with Reaction	12	48	60
No. of Reactions	12	53	65
Percent of Reactions	.0509%	.170%	.118%

There were twelve fatal cases: "six from hemorrhagic encephalitis, five from crustaceous dermatitis exfoliative and one from acute severe arsenical hepatitis; all cases were treated less than six months." Eight of the twelve fatal cases had received no more than four injections. The reported data from other investigators are found in Table II.

TABLE I. B.
REACTIONS OF ANTILUETIC TREATMENT
IN WOMEN
(31,174 Treatments)

Reactions	Number	Number Fatal	Pregnant Women
Bi. Stomatitis	23	1	5
Bi. Diarrhea	4	0	0
Bi. Dermatitis	2	0	0
Bi. Nephritis	1	0	0
Nitritoid Reaction	3	0	1
Arsen. Dermatitis	12	0	0
Arsen. Stomatitis	1	0	0
Arsen. Encephalitis	4	1	0

was adherent to the vessel walls, formed in some places a loose reticulum and in others a solid hyalinized plug. Polymorphonuclear leukocytes were seen invading the vessel walls and infiltrating the surrounding tissues. Small recent punctate hemorrhages were present in several areas. Edema was marked, especially in the white matter of the internal capsule and the corpus callosum.

Case 2. I. B., aged 22 years, was admitted in the eighth lunar month of her first pregnancy, showing a strongly positive Wassermann reaction (with spinal fluid Wasserman 4 plus). She was given three small injections of neoarsphenamine at three day intervals and on the day following the third injection (seven days following the initial injection) the patient was severely nauseated and complained of abdominal pains, headache, backache and dizziness. Following a hypo-

TABLE II.
REACTIONS OF ANTILUETIC TREATMENT AS REPORTED IN THE LITERATURE

Author	Injections	Patients	% Pts. Reacting	Fatalities
Parnell & Fildes (16)	6,588	1,250	6.2	
Cole et al (3)	78,350	1,212	15.3	12
Ireland (5)	20,000	2,100	15-fem. 8-male	0
Klaften (2)				1
Phelps & Washburn (6)	272,354			11

Cole et al[3] in 78,350 injections of the various arsenicals found that 15.3 per cent of the 1,212 patients studied showed one or more arsenical complications of treatment (19.0 per cent of the latent and 14.3 per cent of the early cases).

In the past five years at the State University of Iowa Hospital there have been eight deaths from Hemorrhagic (Arsenical) Encephalitis; all of whom were female and three of whom were pregnant[10]. Abstracts of the histories of these cases are given briefly as follows:

Case 1. K. R., aged 19 years, was found to have a strongly positive Wassermann reaction in the eighth lunar month of pregnancy, having been infected probably a month before conception took place. She was given four two minus doses of gray oil intramuscularly, alternating with each two doses of neoarsphenamine, the latter being three days apart. Two days after the sixth dose of neoarsphenamine she developed a slight headache, continuing on the third post-treatment day with the more severe symptoms of vomiting, spastic paralysis, flaccid paralysis and coma, which finally ended in death about twenty-two hours after the onset of the severe symptoms. Blood pressure was 120/80, and other laboratory examinations were essentially negative. Pathological examination showed a marked involvement of the brain capillaries, which were practically plugged with fibrinous thrombi containing many leukocytes. The fibrin, which

dermic injection of 1-4 grain of morphine sulphate she developed a generalized convulsion during which she scratched her face and bit her lips. Urine obtained by catheter contained no albumin or abnormal cellular elements. There was no edema. Following the convulsion the patient was disorientated and stuporous. The deep reflexes which had been slightly hyperactive became markedly diminished. There was no rigidity of the neck and no skin eruption. The temperature rose rapidly to 102°F. On the next day, early in the morning, the patient developed a severe second convulsion and continued a rapid succession of convulsions, being confined sometimes to only one side of the body and other times being generalized. The blood pressure was 105/50. The ocular fundi were essentially normal. The patient had one generalized convulsion before she died, 29 hours after the initial convulsion. Treatment consisted of intravenous injections of sodium thiosulphate and glucose solution. Autopsy was not permitted, but it was felt that the clinical picture was so similar, except for the convulsions, to that observed in the first case, where the diagnosis had been confirmed by postmortem findings, and where the onset had so closely followed the antiluetic treatment, that there was conclusive evidence of the nature of the disease. The absence of edema and of hypertension together with the nature of the convulsions (unilateral seizures) was entirely unlike eclampsia.

Case 3. A. J. T., aged 22 years, probably infected more than a year previously, a secundigravida, was admitted in the tenth lunar month of a normal pregnancy and found to have a strongly positive Wassermann and Kahn reaction (spinal fluid Wassermann was 4 plus). She was given three injections of neo-arsphenamine at three day intervals and on the day following the last injection was delivered spontaneously of a live child weighing 3193 grams. While the Wassermann reaction on the cord blood was strongly positive, roentgenray films of the long bones revealed no evidence of congenital syphilis. Within a few hours of delivery the patient's temperature rose to 100.6°F., and on the second postpartum day the patient complained of a feeling of general malaise. The pulse was 128, temperature 100.0°F., with a blood pressure of 145/105. The urine showed a moderate trace of albumin with numerous finely granular casts and many pus cells. At 4 P.M. on the second postpartum day the patient became unconscious and at 4:50 P. M., there was a generalized convulsion followed by a marked cyanosis with definite respiratory difficulty. Three more generalized convulsions followed in rapid succession before the patient was brought under the influence of morphine sulphate. Lumbar puncture showed the spinal fluid under normal pressure, but the Pandy reaction was two plus and there were 20 lymphocytes per cubic millimeter. The blood pressure was 160/110. Blood chemistry revealed: uric acid, 5.6; urea nitrogen, 11.9; and creatinine 1.6 mg. per 100 cc. of blood while the CO₂ combining power was 49.1 vol. per cent, and the Van den Bergh was 0.1 mg. per cent. The biceps, triceps; knee-jerks, and tendon achilles reflexes were hyperactive, but the abdominal reflex was absent. Plantar stimulation provoked flexion with slight extension of the great toes. Bilateral ankle clonus was present. Because of the respiratory difficulty, oxygen was administered by nasal tube. At 8:55 P.M. atropine sulphate 1-50 grain was administered to combat excessive mucus secretion in the upper respiratory tract. It was noted that the neck was moderately stiff. Urine obtained by catheter at 9:15 P.M. showed a moderate trace of albumin, many finely and coarsely granular casts, and occasional red and white blood cells. The blood pressure was 120/75, respirations were 24 and the pulse 100 per minute. Chloral hydrate, 20 grains and sodium bromide 40 grains, were given by rectum. On the third postpartum day at 12:30 A.M., the temperature was 105.0°F. (axillary), the pulse 140-160 per minute, and the blood pressure 120/40. Death occurred at 1:35 A.M., the heart stopped one minute after respirations had ceased. The axillary temperature shortly before death was 107°F. The clinical diagnosis included a vascular type of neurosyphilis and hemorrhagic encephalitis. The picture so closely resembled that of the previous proven case of hemorrhagic (arsenical) encephalitis (case 1), the time of onset in relation to the last injection of neoarsphenamine (case 2), the clinical determination of marked central nervous system disturbances and the rapidly fatal outcome, that this seemed the most probable diagnosis. There had been, however, none of the usual prodromata, such as nausea vomiting, headache or dizziness. The late appearance of the first convulsion

(39 hours after delivery) and the absence of earlier evidence of a toxemia of late pregnancy argued against the diagnosis of eclampsia. The typical history for an arsenical reaction and the finding of minute hemorrhages in association with a definite arteritis, together with a questionable presence of edema, seem to justify the diagnosis of arsenical encephalitis.

These three fatalities in a relatively small series of luetic pregnant women under treatment with presumably the safest of the modern arsenicals naturally raises speculation as to the cause of increased susceptibility to the toxic effects of arsenic during gestation.* Nowhere can we find this subject discussed with any thoroughness, and it has seemed advisable to review briefly the available literature.

Pritzi[2] believes that the increased susceptibility is due to changes in the body colloids and lipoids, which are well known to develop during gestation. Eastman[14] has, however, pointed out that the placenta acts as a storage center for injected arsenic, which is then gradually set free in the blood for long periods after the injection and it is possible that this factor is significant, since it involves a more or less continuous introduction of arsenic into the system. This phenomenon may explain the relatively greater therapeutic efficiency of small doses of the arsenicals when used in pregnant women, and may in part explain their apparently greater susceptibility to its pernicious effects. Ireland[8] feels that the altered capillary system found during pregnancy favors the production of lesions by arsenicals which are "doubtless produced by capillary vascular injury or thrombosis." Brittingham and Phinizy[12] and Scott and Moore[4] have suggested that the destructive and dilating action of arsphenamine on the blood vessels is not counteracted by epinephrine because of the arsenical destruction of the suprarenals.

The symptomatology of arsenical hemorrhagic encephalitis varies considerably, but there is usually early evidence of involvement

_____
*In each instance the initial dose was within the 'limit usually recommended, and succeeding doses were not large, being smaller than the maximum dose (0.45 gm) recommended by the Council of German Public Health Service, but somewhat larger than the maximum recommended by Klaften for use in pregnant women. Moreover, injections were made twice weekly instead of once each as is commonly advised. It should also be noted that in two instances the spinal fluid Wassermann reaction was positive despite absence of clinical evidence of cerebrospinal lues. There is no good reason to believe that such patients are especially liable to the appearance of encephalitis.

of the central nervous system, with tonic and clonic convulsions and coma predominating. The convulsive seizures may be generalized or unilateral and are commonly followed by coma which terminates in death. More rarely there may be delirium with fever, vomiting and shock. Prodromata, in the form of nausea and vomiting, headache, restlessness and fever are frequently observed, but their serious significance is not appreciated until other symptoms supervene. In a recent case of exfoliative dermatitis developing shortly after delivery, the prodromata aroused a strong suspicion of early encephalitis, but on the following morning the development of a typical skin rash was associated with rapid disappearance of the mild nervous phenomena. Other symptoms and signs, as enumerated by Phelps and Washburn' include: prostration, tachycardia, nervousness, congestion of the throat and eyes, backache, severe abdominal pain, diarrhea, swelling of the posterior cervical glands, delirium, cyanosis and slight muscular twitchings. In some instances, there may also be a paralysis of certain muscle groups of a flaccid or spastic character.

In pregnant and recently delivered women, the appearance of convulsions and coma naturally arouses a suspicion of eclampsia. However, the usually atypical character of the convulsions, the absence of hypertension and albuminuria, and the history of intravenous arsenical injections within a few days should suggest hemorrhagic encephalitis. Moreover, signs of serious central nervous system involvement quickly appear; the deep reflexes are at first hyperactive, but soon become greatly diminished or absent. Babinski's sign may be positive, squint may appear, disturbances of sensation may be detected, disorientation may be observed and ankle clonus may be elicited. Final diagnosis in doubtful cases may rest upon the postmortem demonstration of edema and small hemorrhages in the brain and spinal cord, as well as in the skin, pericardium and various viscera. Hemorrhages into the central nervous system alone are pathognomonic; they usually appear as small punctate extravasations of blood around the capillaries, but occasionally the coalescence of several such small hemorrhages produces a larger hemorrhagic area. Hyaline

thrombosis of the capillaries is also frequently observed.

Death usually occurs within 96 hours, but Dickens", Phelps and Washburn', and Klaften' have reported patients with symptoms suggesting hemorrhagic encephalitis who recovered completely. Treatment commonly consists in the exhibitions of hypnotics to control the convulsions, venesection, spinal puncture and the intravenous injection of hypertonic solutions of glucose or sodium thiosulphate, but it is doubtful whether anything has much effect upon the course of the disease.

Summary

An attempt has been made to call your attention to the possible complications found in the treatment of syphilis in pregnancy. Emphasis has been placed upon the possible confusion of eclampsia and arsenical encephalitis. Careful watching and daily contact with these patients is necessary in order that prodromal symptoms and minor complications which indicate sensitivity may be recognized, for the early recognition of these with cessation of antileutic treatment is our only effective therapy in such complications. Even though there is some danger of reaction from the medicaments used, the overwhelming benefit derived in the majority of pregnant women, together with the responsibility to the unborn child, leaves only one course open to the conscientious medical practitioner.

BIBLIOGRAPHY
1. McCord, J. R.: Syphilis and Pregnancy. Some results obtained from treatment. An analysis of two hundred and fifty cases. A. J. Syph., 12, 181-186, 1928 (April).
2. Cole, H. N., DeWolf, H., McKuskey, J. M., Miskjian, H. G., Williamson, G. S., Rauschkolb, J. R., Ruch, R. O., and Clark, T.: Toxic Effects Following Use of arsphenamines. J. A. M. A., 97, 897-904, 1931 (Sept. 26).
3. Klaften, E.: Die Prinzipien der antisyphilitischen Behandlung des Schwangeren. Arch f. Gynak, 135, 620-650, 1929.
4. Fritzi, O.: Ein Fall von Salvarsanencephalitis in der Schwangerschaft. Zentralbl. f. Gynak., 52, 2930-2936, 1928 (Nov. 17).
5. Ireland, F. A.: Reactions Following the Administration of the Arsphenamines and Methods of Prevention. A. J. Syph., 16, 22-38, 1932 (Jan.).
6. Phelps, J. R., and Washburn, W. A.: Toxic Effects of Arsenical Compounds Employed in the Treatment of Syphilis in the U. S. Navy. A statistical study of the results of 272,354 injected doses of neoarsphenamine and other compounds of arsenic. U. S. Naval Med. Bull., 28, 659-695, 1930 (July).
7. McKelvey, J. L., and Turner, T. B.: Syphilis and Pregnancy. An analysis of the outcome of pregnancy in relation to the treatment in 943 cases. J. A. M. A., 102, 503-510, 1934, (Feb. 17).
8. Clason, S.: Eklampsie oder Salvarsanergiftung, Drei Todesfälle mit diskutabler Genese. Acta Obst. et Gynec., Scandin. 12, 50-58, 1932.
9. Gemmeltoft, S. A.: Ueber einen Fall von Encephalitis hamorrhagica nach Salvarsanbehandlung wahrend der Schwangerschaft. Acta Obst. et Gynec., Scandin., 9, 167-179, 19XX.
10. Plass, E. D., and Woods, E. B.: Hemorrhagic Encephalitis (Neoarsphenamine) in Obstetrical Patients. Am. Journ. Obst. & Gyn., 29, 509-517, 1935 (April).
(Continued on Page 34)

THE JOURNAL

OF THE

MEDICAL ASSOCIATION OF GEORGIA

Devoted to the Welfare of the Medical Association of Georgia

478 Peachtree Street, N.E., Atlanta, Ga.

JANUARY, 1936

FORCED SPINAL DRAINAGE

A new therapeutic procedure that promises benefit in hitherto refractory conditions often leads to unwarranted optimism and injudicious use. This is especially true if it possesses something of the dramatic, for it is much more likely then to stir the imagination of newspaper reporters both lacking in critical faculties and inadequately advised. Such has been the fate of forced spinal drainage, "brain wash."

The method itself is based on sound physicochemical knowledge and after being subjected to experimental appraisal is now being employed in the treatment of an increasing variety of inflammatory diseases of the central nervous system.

It has been established that a principal factor in the exchange of fluid between the blood and the cerebrospinal fluid is osmosis. The intracranial fluid can be reduced, for example, by elevating the osmotic pressure of the blood with the injection of concentrated (50 per cent) glucose—very helpful at times in reducing intracranial pressure or cerebral edema.

On the other hand an increased passage of fluid from the blood into the fluid spaces of the brain can be effected by giving solutions of low concentration intravenously (0.45 per cent). Since normally the flow in the perivascular spaces is towards the subarachnoid space, and if this space is tapped and permitted to drain, theoretically there should result a flushing out of the perivascular spaces. Experimental work by Kubie demonstrated this to be the case.

Animals with artificially induced infections of the nervous system and treated with forced spinal drainage had a much higher recovery rate than animals thus infected but not treated. In those so treated there was found a marked reduction of the perivascular exudate as compared with the controls.

This procedure has since been rather extensively employed in humans, and although it apparently has been of great benefit in some infectious conditions the data are as yet not sufficient to warrant its widespread use. Nor is it without its dangers. Anything that produces a positive water-balance tends to increase the susceptibility to convulsions and its employment in epileptic subjects has resulted in fatalities. If free drainage is not maintained cerebral edema will result. Such an alteration of blood volume and tissue fluid would be hazardous with severe heart or kidney damage. With the exception of these conditions it seems to result in no harm to the patient.

The best results have been obtained in the acute encephalitic and encephalomyelitic processes. Fair results have been obtained in the subacute and even chronic stages; e.g., Parkinsonian syndrome of chronic epidemic encephalitis. It has also been used in other conditions, but judgment as to its value must be withheld until more convincing evidence is available.

Aside from its therapeutic value it may well be a useful instrument in solving some of the problems of fluid-balance and permeability in relation to the nervous system—problems, the importance of which, only in recent years, is coming to be appreciated. Acute neurological disturbances are frequently seen, the course of which virtually excludes any gross lesion. Edema is the principal factor in many of these. More knowledge of the factors influencing the exchange of fluid and the alteration of the barrier will aid in the prevention of such disturbances and in combating them once developed. By altering the barrier it may become possible to prevent the entrance of harmful substances into the nervous system; or, on the contrary, to permit beneficial substances, e.g., certain antibodies ordinarily held back, to pass through. Certain antibodies are present in the blood and not in the spinal fluid, but when the barrier is altered by producing an aseptic meningitis by injecting horse serum into the subarachnoid spaces, the antibodies appear in the spinal fluid. There is some evidence that the forced drainage itself may increase the capillary permeability. A few observations indicate that the protein content of the spinal fluid is higher at the end of the procedure than at the beginning. Thus it would seem that some of the blood colloids, ordinarily held back, have been washed through; since normally the protein content of the blood is much higher than that of the spinal fluid.

Available, then, is a method offering much therapeutically, and promising aid in solving many mysteries of neurological disturbances. It is unfortunate, however, that a procedure should be so publicised as to convince many laymen that a cure for all disorders of the nervous system has been discovered.

RICHARD B. WILSON, M.D.

QUESTIONNAIRE FOR PHYSICIANS

Within the pages of this JOURNAL will be found a printed page, a replica of the questionnaire mailed to all physicians in Georgia. Several hundred replies have been received at the office of the Secretary. If you have not completed yours, please do so at once, using the original pink sheet or the page in the JOURNAL.

The officers of the Association hope to use this information when obtained to promote the interest and welfare of our members and the people without means to pay for adequate medical care. This survey may be of inestimable value to promote legislation which our profession may sponsor, or to defeat legislation which might be to our detriment.

BOOK REVIEWS

Arthritis and Rheumatoid Conditions: Their Nature and Treatment. By Ralph Pemberton. M.S., M.D., F.A.C.P., Professor of Medicine in the University of Pennsylvania. Cloth. Price $5.50. pp. 445 with 69 engravings' and one colored plate. Second edition, 1935. Lea and Febiger, Philadelphia.

A comprehensive, practical study of arthritis which is easy to read and interesting from cover to cover. This book is conducive to thought and study rather than presenting dogmatic statements and treatment along one line. The attitude expressed throughout the book is well summarized by the following quotation from the author's preface:

"The writer is of the firm opinion that no single or fixed viewpoint can encompass the rheumatoid problem which, despite the fine achievements of the doctrine of focal infection, is not a disease of the specialist in any branch of surgery. Every effort has

been made to avoid undue emphasis upon any one phase of treatment, since it is believed that only wide-angled vision can attain to anything more than sporadic results in any large group of cases."

MASON I. LOWANCE, M.D.

Body Mechanics. By Joel E. Goldwait, M.D., LL.D., Lloyd T. Brown. M.D., Lowing T. Swaim, M.D., John G. Kuhns, M.D. 281 pp. 99 illustrations. Published by J. B. Lippincott Co. This book is written for the benefit of the chronic patient and a method of treatment suggested. The subject of Body Mechanics is covered, giving the normal and various body types and the faulty mechanics. The resultant changes in the viscera and skeleton are discussed at some length. Exercises and braces are recommended for the correction of faulty body mechanics. There are case reports of several of the more disabling diseases which were helped by correcting faulty mechanics. An extensive list of references to current literature is appended.

H. WALKER JERNIGAN, M.D.

Heart Disease in the Tropics: H. O. Gunewardene, M.B., B.S. (Lond.) D.M. R.E. (Cantab.) Butterworth & Co. (India) Ltd. Cloth. 94 pages. $3.00.

This monograph presents in an interesting form, cardiovascular phenomena observed in some tropical diseases. Unfortunately the classification of heart disease is not in accordance with standard nomenclature of the American Heart Association, but American readers can follow the discussion.

However, several interesting points are brought out, such as the unexpectedly high incidence of hypertension in the tropics, the cardiac complications of infestations with Ankylostoma, etc. Rheumatic fever, too, is thought to occur more often than usually supposed.

In his discussion of Ankylostoma heart disease, it seems to me he might explain many of the cardiac symptoms on the basis of the anemia caused by the parasite rather than any specific effect of the parasite upon the heart itself.

The book closes with a discussion of therapeutic procedures and their adaptations to tropical conditions.

JOSEPH C. MASSEE, M.D.

Diabetes Mellitus and Obesity. By Garfield G. Duncan. Price $2.75. pp. 227. Lea & Febiger, Philadelphia. 1935. Recognition of the predisposing influence of obesity to the development of diabetes in adult life has caused the author to include the two subjects, diabetes and obesity in one monograph.

The treatment of the subject, diabetes, presents a bird's eye view of the practical aspects of this condition which should be a helpful introduction to the study of more exhaustive tests.

The subject, obesity, is presented with emphasis upon the importance of its correction, thus avoiding serious and life shortening complications and sequelae. The methods of dietary treatment are explained in sufficient detail.

HAROLD BOWCOCK, M.D.

WOMAN'S AUXILIARY

OFFICERS

President—Mrs. Ernest R. Harris, Winder.
President-Elect—Mrs. Wm. R. Dancy, Savannah.
First Vice-President—Mrs. Hulett H. Askew, Atlanta.
Second Vice-President—Mrs. Warren A. Coleman, Eastman.
Third Vice-President—Mrs. T. J. Ferrell, Waycross.
Recording Secretary—Mrs. W. R. Garner, Gainesville.
Corresponding Secretary—Mrs. S. T. Ross. Winder
Treasurer—Mrs. W. M. Cason, Sandersville.

Historian—Mrs. Marvin F. Haygood, Atlanta.
Parliamentarian—Mrs. Ralph H. Chaney, Augusta.
Committee Chairmen
Health Films—Mrs. A. J. Mooney, Statesboro.
Student Loan Fund—Mrs. Benjamin Bashinski, Macon.
Public Relations—Mrs. J. A. Redfearn, Albany.
Press and Publicity—Mrs. J. Harry Rogers, Atlanta.
Jane Todd Crawford Memorial—Mrs. Eustace A. Allen. Atlanta.
Research in Romance of Medicine—Mrs. D. N. Thompson, Elberton.

SOUTHERN AUXILIARY MEETING

The Woman's Auxiliary to the Southern Medical Association met in St. Louis, Missouri, November 20, 21, 1935.

The important decisions of the preconvention Executive Board meeting were to increase the budget to permit necessary committee work and to revise the Constitution and By-Laws.

The luncheon and opening meeting were held at noon November 20th. So many attended that tables were placed in halls. Mrs. Bonar White, Atlanta, the President, presided. Invocation was given by Mrs. D. McBride, Oklahoma City. Welcomes by the President of the St. Louis Auxiliary, Mrs. J. M. Trigg, and by the President of Missouri Auxiliary, Mrs. M. P. Neal. Mrs. John A. Beals, of Mississippi, responded.

Dr. H. Marshall Taylor, President of the Southern Medical Association, spoke on membership and complimented the Auxiliary on its service to the medical profession. Dr. A. W. Harold, Louisiana, one of the Advisors, talked on the way the Auxiliary members could serve as a reserve force in legislation when requested by the medical profession.

Mrs. Rogers N. Herbert, Tennessee, President of the National Auxiliary, gave an address on "Concentration, Cooperation, Consecration."

Mrs. White made three group introductions—the Hostess Committees, the Officers and Chairmen of the Auxiliary, the State Presidents.

After announcements of business and committee appointments, distinguished guests and members were introduced by Mrs. R. C. Kory, Arkansas. These included the founder of the National and Southern Auxiliaries, nine National officers and chairmen, past National and Southern Presidents, and the wife of the President of the Southern Medical Association, Mrs. H. M. Taylor.

A Round Table Conference with Mrs. F. N. Haggard, Texas, First Vice-President of the Auxiliary, presiding, followed. Plans and suggestions on organization were given by Mrs. Bonar White, Georgia; on Health Education by Mrs. V. E. Holcombe, W. Virginia; on Hygeia by Mrs. Rogers Herbert, Tennessee; on History and Archive by Mrs. William Hibbitts, Arkansas.

Soon after adjournment, all visitors attended a tea and fashion show given by the Woman's Club of St. Louis University School of Medicine, and at 9:00 P.M. the reception and ball of the Southern Medical Association. The night previous, they attended the general session of the Southern Medical Association.

The twelfth annual session was called to order by the President on Thursday, November 21st, at 9:30 A.M., and an invocation offered by Dr. Arnold Lowe, of St. Louis.

The most important items of this meeting were the Memorial Services; the address of Dr. Seale Harris, Chairman of the Advisors; an outline of a suggested set-up for membership and financing from Mr. Loranz, as submitted by the Southern Council; (the latter were, by motion, referred to the Auxiliary's Executive Board and Advisors). The reports of officers and chairmen and the address of the National Chairman of Public Relations, Mrs. David S. Long, and State reports. The records show 190 auxiliaries and 5,299 members.

Mrs. Long explained public relations work in the Auxiliary, methods of carrying it out, suggested programs and activities which various states had developed; a stimulating and informing address.

Mrs. S. A. Collom, Sr., read an excellent paper on *Romance of Medicine* and explained the work which her committee had done in research and the material available for members to use in program work.

Many telegrams and letters were received;

nine of the twelve Southern Auxiliary presidents were in attendance.

Many expressions of appreciation of the work of the President and administration were made.

A telegram was sent to the incoming President, Mrs. Oliver W. Hill, of Knoxville, Tennessee, who was absent due to illness in her family.

The following officers were elected and installed:

President—Mrs. Oliver W. Hill, Knoxville, Tennessee.

President-Elect—Mrs. Frank N. Haggard, San Antonio, Texas.

First Vice-President—Mrs. S. M. Prunty, Parkersburg, W. Virginia.

Second Vice-President—Mrs. J. M. Trigg, St. Louis, Missouri.

Recording Secretary—Mrs. C. B. Erickson, Shreveport, Louisiana.

Corresponding Secretary—Mrs. W. A. Shelton, Knoxville, Tennessee.

Treasurer—Mrs. E. W. Veal, Jacksonville, Florida.

Historian—Mrs. Harvey F. Garrison, Jackson, Mississippi.

Parliamentarian—Mrs. P. J. Caldwell, Huntsville, Ala.

In the absence of the President, Mrs. White presented the gavel and good wishes to the First Vice-President, Mrs. S. M. Prunty, who made several announcements, appointed time for the meeting of the Post-Convention Board and adjourned.

The St. Louis Medical Auxiliary entertained the Auxiliary at luncheon at the St. Louis Medical Society Building and a ride about the city.

Sixth District

The Woman's Auxiliary to the Sixth District Medical Society met December 4th at the Dempsey Hotel in Macon. Mrs. J. Lon King, of Macon, was elected President for the ensuing year.

Other officers named were Mrs. James I. Garrard, of Milledgeville, President-Elect; Mrs. Ralph Newton, of Macon, Secretary-Treasurer; and Mrs. T. E. Vickers, Harrison, Parliamentarian.

Mrs. W. M. Cason, of Sandersville, the retiring President, presided. The Rev. Albert G. Harris, Pastor of the First Presbyterian church of Macon, gave the invocation. Mrs. Ernest Corn, President of the Bibb County Auxiliary, welcomed the members. Mrs. Richard Binion, of Milledgeville, responded.

Mrs. C. H. Jones, of Macon, gave two delightful vocal selections, "Thanksgiving Hymn" and an original composition, "The Little White House Down in Georgia," with Mrs. Raleigh Drake accompanying her on the piano.

Speakers at the morning session were Dr. James E. Paullin, of Atlanta, President of the Medical Association of Georgia; Dr. Edgar D. Shanks, of Atlanta, Secretary-Treasurer of the State organization; and Dr. Benj. Bashinski, of Macon.

Auxiliary reports were given by Mrs. Ernest Corn, Bibb County; Mrs. Sam Anderson, Milledgeville; Mrs. E. B. Claxton, Laurens County; and Mrs. O. D. Lennard, Washington County. Mrs. Lennard also reported as Scrap-Book chairman.

After the business session, luncheon was served at the Dempsey Tavern.

Clarke County

Mrs. Ernest R. Harris, President of the Georgia Auxiliary, attended the recent meeting of the Clarke County Auxiliary, held in Athens. Mrs. Harris made an excellent talk on the work of the Auxiliary and also the possibilities of the Auxiliary in the future. She explained the duty of each officer and gave the members of the Clarke County Auxiliary many helpful suggestions for their future work.

Plans for the March program were discussed at the meeting. During that month the Auxiliary is to have a program honoring the members of the Clarke County Medical Society.

It was voted to double the amount to be given to the Student Loan Fund this year.

Mrs. Carl Holliday, Hygeia Chairman, asked each member to get at least one subscription to Hygeia during the year. Several have responded and Mrs. Holliday expects to send in a new list of subscribers each month.

Mrs. S. S. Smith, Health Chairman, reported that she was getting health literature to all the Parent-Teacher Associations, both white and colored, to be used at their monthly meetings.

Mrs. H. M. Fullilove was appointed Scrap-Book Chairman for the Auxiliary.

Fulton County

The Fulton County Auxiliary met Friday, December 6th, at the Academy of Medicine, with the President, Mrs. Calhoun McDougall, presiding. Mrs. W. W. Anderson, Secretary; Mrs. Leland Baggett, Treasurer. Committee chairmen gave reports.

Mrs. Charles Boynton, Program Chairman, introduced Dr. Dunbar Roy, who entertained the guests with a most charming and informal talk.

GEORGIA DEPARTMENT OF PUBLIC HEALTH

T. F. ABERCROMBIE, M.D., Director

DIAGNOSIS AND TREATMENT OF TUBERCULOSIS

A brief review of the essentials of the diagnosis and treatment of tuberculosis is undertaken. The literature concerning these aspects of tuberculosis is so voluminous that it would seem unnecessary to say anything about either of them, yet, because it is known that there is considerable haziness and confusion in the minds of many, it seems advisable to try to clear up certain points.

Diagnosis

Careful inquiry into the family history should be made in every case and if there has been prolonged familial or household contact with a case of open tuberculosis very strong suspicion that your patient has tuberculosis should be entertained if he has one or more of the following symptoms. These symptoms are due to toxemia and may be caused by other diseases. When they are present the possibility of their being due to tuberculosis should be suspected even when there has been no known exposure to tuberculous infection. They are: Lack of initiative, unusual fatigue or easy exhaustion, loss of strength and nerve instability. Loss of weight in tuberculosis is usually associated with digestive disturbances and is not of much significance unless it is fairly rapid and recent. Mere underweight of long duration without symptoms should not be considered as a symptom of tuberculosis. Elevation of temperature is common and may occur at any time of day or night and may be considered of no importance if not 99° F. or over in men and 99.6° F. or more in women and it should be remembered that a physiological rise in temperature frequently occurs in women a week or two before, or during and through menstruation. Night sweats, although they may be due to other causes, should lead us to at least suspect tuberculosis. Pleurisy, repeated pneumonias and attacks of "influenza," frequent chest colds, chronic cough with or without expectoration and blood spitting may be due to tuberculosis. Depending upon the character and extent of lesions in the lung there may or may not be impairment of breath sounds, percussion note, or rales.

The Tuberculin Test: Inasmuch as a considerable number of persons do not react to tuberculin, this test should be made in all suspected cases. There are two methods in common use: the Von Pirquet and the Mantoux.

In the Von Pirquet, a small drop of undiluted old tuberculin is placed on the properly cleansed skin of the flexor surface of the forearm about two inches below the bend of the elbow and through the drop of tuberculin a small abrasion is made on the skin with a sterile needle or with a special instrument made for this purpose. Bleeding should be avoided. With proper technique this test furnishes about the same results as 0.01 milligram of old tuberculin or the first dose of purified protein derivative tuberculin (P.P.D.) by the Mantoux method.

In the Mantoux or intradermal method, which is the one of choice with most operators, the required amount of properly diluted tuberculin is introduced very carefully into the skin (not under it, but between the layers of it) by means of a sharp, medium beveled 26 gauge hypodermic needle attached to a tuberculin syringe. When employing old tuberculin (O.T.) dilutions of it are made with sterile normal saline solution so that for the first dose each 0.1 cc. of the dilution will contain 0.01 milligram of old tuberculin and for the second dose each 0.1 cc. of the dilution will contain 1.0 milligram of tuberculin. In each instance the amount of solution to be injected into the skin is 0.1 cc. The new P.P.D. tuberculin is a standardized preparation and its use is advised whenever possible. It is furnished by its manufacturers in packages of first test strength and second test strength tablets with sufficient buffered diluent and directions for making the required dilutions. As with the O.T. dilutions the amount injected into the skin is exactly 0.1 cc., but the stronger dilution contains 250 times the tuberculin the first dose does. The second dose of P.P.D. produces about the same results as does the second or 1.0 milligram dose of O.T.

When the tuberculin is properly introduced into the skin a wheal is instantly raised. It is important to make the injection intradermally because a dose easily tolerated in the skin may cause a severe systemic reaction when given subcutaneously. If a raised indurated reddened area 5 millimeters or more in diameter is shown 48 to 72 hours after the intradermal test is made it is called positive and *may be considered as indicating that there has been at some time an infection by tubercle bacilli but it never alone proves*

that tuberculous disease is present. If no reaction is produced by the first or weaker
dose, the 1.0 milligram O.T., or the second
test strength dose of P.P.D. is given and if
after 48 hours or under 72 there is still no
reaction, it is highly improbable that the person tested has tuberculosis. An exception is
terminal tuberculosis.

Sputum examinations should be made
whenever there is cough and expectoration and especially in suspected tuberculosis.
Preferably such examinations should be made
by the concentration method. If negative results are obtained in several examinations—
five or more—guinea pig inoculation should
be made. If tubercle bacilli can be discovered by these examinations a diagnosis of
tuberculosis is, of course, justifiable, but *dis-
missing the possibility of tuberculosis because
of negative sputum examinations is never justified. Sputum examinations are of value
only when they give positive results.*

X-ray has proven itself of such distinct
value in showing pathology in the lung before ·it can be discovered in any other way
and in disclosing the nature and extent of
the lesions to physicians trained in its use
that no chest case may be considered adequately examined unless Roentgenographic
or fluoroscopic study has been made.

Treatment

*Do not postpone treatment of a sick per-
son just because a positive diagnosis of tuberculosis cannot be made.* Rest is an essential
part of treatment of the ill no matter what
infection may be responsible. We often witness the loss of a splendid opportunity to
easily recover from what was later proved
to be tuberculosis merely because we could
not find tubercle bacilli in the sputum and
waited too long before insisting on strict bed
care because we were not certain the patient
had tuberculosis. *In active tuberculosis rest
in bed is the very foundation of treatment.*
It should be maintained 24 hours every day,
if arrest of disease is to result, as long as may
be necessary. Usually this requires many
months and it should be continued for several weeks after the subsidence of all clinical
and x-ray evidence of disease. And following the period of strict bed care these cases
should be most painstakingly managed or
instructed so that the time they are allowed
to sit up or the activities they are permitted
to indulge in will be carefully regulated so
that they may not lose what they have
gained. It should be remembered that a dangerous period is after the symptoms have subsided and the patient looks and feels well and
therefore is lulled, as is often the physician,
too, into a sense of false security. It should

also be remembered that every person who develops tuberculosis and has healed or arrested
it must, if he expects not to have a relapse
alter his whole manner of living for the future and that a part of a well established
regime is a regular daily rest-in-bed period.
The physician failing to carefully instruct
his patients when they have unhealed lesions
of the necessity of rest in bed until they
are healed and, when the lesions are arrested,
of the equal necessity, if they are to remain
healed, of part time rest, part time very limited physical activity and avoidance of all ex-
cesses for a long indefinite period, injures
himself and his patients.

Well ventilated and lighted quarters
should be provided in which windows are
kept open day and night the whole year
through. An abundant well balanced diet
is required, but it is unnecessary, and often
harmful, to stuff patients with milk and raw
eggs. Three to six glasses of milk daily is
sufficient with eggs as the patient prefers
them.

Direct sunlight should not be used in active tuberculosis in either children or adults.
Such treatment can be very dangerous. In
adults who are not ill, and in children especially, an outdoor life, much of it in the
sunshine, is health-giving and health preserving.

Drugs do not cure tuberculosis. They are
employed to control ·conditions such as severe cough, insomnia, digestive disturbances,
pain, etc. Ordinarily they are unnecessary
and the use of them should be discouraged
as much as possible.

Artificial pneumothorax, phrenic nerve in-
terruptions and other lung compression methods have an exceedingly valuable place in the
treatment of tuberculosis, often converting
apparently hopeless into curable cases and by
closing cavities and checking expectoration
limit the·spread of infection. Lung compression should be used whenever possible in the
cases which do not respond well to ordinary
bed care and to make it available to greater
extent more physicians should have adequate
training in their use and indications and in
the management of tuberculosis as well. Because of the wide and sometimes extravagant
publicity recently given to these measures
there is a tendency to accept them as cures
for tuberculosis. *They aid in curing tuberculosis only when used in conjunction with the
previously discussed measures and established
principles.*

Children with pulmonary tuberculosis are
treated as adults accordingly as symptoms
· and x-ray evidence of disease demand. Those
with tuberculous lesions in other parts of the

body should have bed care until the symptoms of toxemia are relieved: When there is no evidence of toxemia, no symptoms of disease, they may be regarded as normal children, even though they may be underweight and have occasional rises of temperature, being kept under observation so that at the first manifestation of tuberculous disease they may be placed under treatment.

H. C. SCHENCK, M.D.. Chief.
Division of Tuberculosis Control.

COMPLICATIONS OF THE TREATMENT OF SYPHILIS IN PREGNANCY

(Continued from Page 27)

11. Letter from Berlin, Dec. 29, 1929. Criteria for the use of arsphenamine preparations. J. A. M. A., 92, 489-490, 1929 (Feb. 9).
12. Eastman, N. J.: The Arsenic Content of the Human Placenta Following Arsphenamine Therapy. A. J. Obst. and Gynec., 21, 60-64, 1931.
13. Brittingham, J. W., and Phiniay, T.: Hemorrhagic Encephalitis After Neoarsphenamine. J. A. M. A., 96, 2021-2023, 1931 (June 13).
14. Scott, E., and Moore, R. A.: Fatalities Following the Use of Arsphenamine. A. J. Spyh., 12, 253-262, 1928 (April).
15. Dickens, P. F.: A Case of Hemorrhagic Encephalitis, Neoarsphenamine Poisoning, with Recovery. U. S. Naval Med. Bull., 26, 192-195, 1928 (Jan.).

Discussion on Paper by Dr. E. Bryant Woods

DR. AMEY CHAPPELL (Atlanta): Any paper which shows the importance of correct treatment for syphilis during pregnancy is valuable. I take pleasure in expressing to Dr. Woods appreciation for this contribution.

It is interesting to note that the incidence of syphilis in women who attended the prenatal clinic at the University of Georgia was 9.8 per cent, whereas in a similar clinic conducted in the colored division of Grady Hospital in Atlanta, the incidence was 15 per cent.

Whenever antiluetic treatment is given, occasional reactions occur. The number of these reactions depends on the condition of the patient, the drug used and its quantity, and perhaps most of all on how that drug is prepared and given. The fact that there were on an average less than two reactions in a thousand treatments given at the University of Georgia is worthy of comment and commendation.

As to the cases of encephalitis which occurred at the University of Iowa Hospital and which are reported in detail. I believe these were due to too frequent administration of neoarsphenamine. In each of these cases the drug had been given at three day intervals.

The paper as a whole emphasizes two important points and because of their importance I shall repeat them here.

First, the necessity for a Wassermann test on every pregnant woman. Second, the need of continuous, adequate antiluetic treatment through the entire pregnancy once the diagnosis of syphilis is made, with careful and intelligent administration of the drugs.

COUNTIES REPORTING FOR 1936

Baldwin County Medical Society

The Baldwin County Medical Society announces the following officers for 1936:
President—S. A. Anderson, Milledgeville.
Vice-President—L. S. Bailey, Milledgeville.
Secretary-Treasurer—C. B. Fulghum, Milledgeville.
Censors—H. D. Allen, R. W. Bradford, and Geo. L. Echols.
Delegate—Richard Binion, Milledgeville.
Alternate Delegate—R. E. Evans, Milledgeville.

Cherokee County Medical Society.

The Cherokee County Medical Society announces the following officers for 1936:
President—R. M. Moore, Waleska.
Vice-President—N. J. Coker, Canton.
Secretary-Treasurer—Geo. C. Brooke, Canton.
Delegate—J. T. Pettit, Canton.
Alternate Delegate—J. P. Turk, Nelson.
Censors—Grady N. Coker, J. T. Pettit and J. P. Turk.

Clayton-Fayette Counties Medical Society

The Clayton-Fayette Counties Medical Society announces the following officers for 1936:
President—E. C. Seawright, Fayetteville.
Vice-President—J. R. Wallace, Lovejoy.
Secretary-Treasurer—T. J. Busey, Fayetteville.
Delegate—J. A. S. Chambers, Inman.
Alternate Delegate—H. D. Kemper, Jonesboro.

Hall County Medical Society

The Hall County Medical Society announces the following officers for 1936:
President—E. W. Grove, Gainesville.
Vice-President—J. M. Hulsey, Gainesville.
Secretary-Treasurer—Hartwell Joiner, Gainesville.
Delegate—J. H. Downey, Gainesville.
Alternate Delegate—R. L. Rogers, Gainesville.
Censors—J. K. Burns. Hartwell Joiner and W. C. Kennedy.

Tri County Society
(Calhoun, Early, Miller)

The Tri County Medical Society announces the following officers for 1936:
President—E. B. Baughn. Colquitt.
Vice-President—C. R. Barksdale, Blakely.
Secretary-Treasurer—J. G. Standifer, Blakely.
Delegate—W. O. Shepard, Bluffton..
Alternate Delegate—W. H. Wall, Blakely.

Whitfield County Medical Society

The Whitfield County Medical Society announces the following officers for 1936:
President—E. O. Shellhorse, Dalton.
Vice-President—F. B. Easley, Dalton.
Secretary-Treasurer—H. J. Ault, Dalton.
Delegate—J. C. Rollins, Dalton.
Alternate Delegate—D. L. Wood, Dalton.

Walker County Medical Society

The Walker County Medical Society announces the following officers for 1936:

President—R. M. Coulter, LaFayette.
Vice-President—C. W. Stephenson, Ringgold.
Secretary-Treasurer—Chas. W. Folsom, LaFayette.
Delegate—S. B. Kitchens, LaFayette.
Alternate Delegate—O. B. Murray, Rossville.

Dougherty County Medical Society

The Dougherty County Medical Society announces the following officers for 1936:

President—Alex R. Freeman, Albany.
Vice-President—Frank E. Thomas, Albany.
Secretary-Treasurer—I. M. Lucas, Albany.
Delegate—H. M. McKemie, Albany.
Alternate Delegate—Frank E. Thomas, Albany
Censors—A. H. Hilsman, J. C. Keaton and J. A. Redfearn.

Randolph County Medical Society

The Randolph County Medical Society announces the following officers for 1936:

President—Loren Gary, Jr., Shellman.
Vice-President—E. C. McCurdy, Shellman.
Secretary-Treasurer—W. G. Elliott, Cuthbert.
Delegate—W. G. Elliott, Cuthbert.
Censor—T. F. Harper, Coleman.

Richmond County Medical Society

The Richmond County Medical Society announces the following officers for 1936:

President—Edgar R. Pund, Augusta.
Vice-President—J. H. Sherman, Augusta.
Secretary-Treasurer—R. C. McGahee, Augusta.
Delegate—G. Lombard Kelly, Augusta.
Delegate—Ralph H. Chaney, Augusta.
Alternate Delegate—W. J. Cranston, Augusta.
Alternate Delegate—A. A. Davidson, Augusta.

Fulton County Medical Society

The Fulton County Medical Society announces the following officers for 1936:

President—Grady E. Clay, Atlanta.
President-Elect—H. C. Sauls, Atlanta.
Vice-President—Geo. F. Eubanks, Atlanta.
Secretary-Treasurer—M. T. Harrison, Atlanta.
Delegate—C. C. Aven, Atlanta.
Delegate—T. C. Davison, Atlanta.
Delegate—Edgar F. Fincher, Jr., Atlanta.
Delegate—Ed H. Greene, Atlanta.
Delegate—Cyrus W. Strickler, Atlanta.
Delegate—Grady E. Clay, Atlanta.
Delegate—H. C. Sauls, Atlanta.
Trustee—Major F. Fowler, Atlanta.
Judicial Council—L. G. Baggett, Atlanta.
Judicial Council—J. R. Childs, Atlanta.
Judicial Council—Glenville Giddings, Atlanta.

Thomas County Medical Society

The Thomas County Medical Society announces the following officers for 1936:

President—Harry Ainsworth, Thomasville.
Vice-President—J. N. Isler, Meigs.
Secretary-Treasurer—Rudolph Bell, Thomasville.

Floyd County Medical Society

The Floyd County Medical Society announces the following officers for 1936:

President—J. L. Garrard, Rome.
Vice-President—R. M. Harbin, Jr., Rome.
Secretary-Treasurer—Ralph N. Johnson, Rome.
Delegate—B. V. Elmore, Rome.
Alternate Delegate—W. P. Harbin, Jr., Rome.

Spalding County Medical Society

The Spalding County Medical Society announces the following officers for 1936:

President—T. I. Hawkins, Griffin.
Vice-President—Geo. L. Walker, Griffin.
Secretary-Treasurer—H. J. Copeland, Griffin.
Delegate—A. H. Frye, Griffin.
Alternate Delegate—H. J. Copeland, Griffin.

Georgia Medical Society
(Chatham County)

The Georgia Medical Society announces the following officers for 1936:

President—C. F. Holton, Savannah.
President-Elect—Geo. H. Faggart, Savannah.
Vice-President—S. E. Bray, Savannah.
Secretary-Treasurer—Otto W. Schwalb, Savannah.
Delegate—A. A. Morrison, Savannah.
Delegate—J. C. Metts, Savannah.
Alternate Delegate—H. J. Morrison, Savannah.
Alternate Delegate—J. K. Quattlebaum, Savannah.

Habersham County Medical Society

The Habersham County Medical Society announces the following officers for 1936:

President—Robert B. Lamb, Demorest.
Vice-President—H. E. Crow, Alto.
Secretary-Treasurer—O. N. Harden, Cornelia.

NEWS ITEMS

The Third District Medical Society held its fall meeting in Cordele. Dr. Chas. A. Greer, Oglethorpe, was elected Secretary-Treasurer for life.

Dr. Lansing Lee, Augusta, spoke before a meeting of the Rotary Club, Augusta, on December 17th on "The Potential Prolongation of the Average Human Life."

Dr. Chas. O. Rainey, Camilla, Mitchell County Commissioner of Health, was elected President of the Georgia Public Health Association on December 14th: Dr. W. W. Brown, Athens, Vice-President; Dr. M. E. Winchester, Brunswick, Secretary-Treasurer.

The Georgia Pediatric Society held its third annual meeting on December 12th. Dr. Wm. Willis Anderson, Atlanta, President of the Society, presided.

Dr. Jas. E. Paullin, Atlanta, President of the Association, spoke before a meeting of the Georgia Public Health Association in Atlanta, December 13th on "The Practicing Physician and the Public Health."

Dr. Lon Grove Atlanta, was elected President of the Staff of Wesley Memorial Hospital, Emory University, December 13th; Dr. Vernon E. Powell, Atlanta, Vice-President; Dr. H. H. Allen, Decatur, re-elected Secretary.

Dr. F. C. Mims, Atlanta, was elected Worshipful Master of the Morningside Masonic Lodge.

Dr. H. W. Birdsong, Athens, has been appointed local surgeon for the Seaboard Air Line Railroad.

The Tri County Medical Society met at Blakely on December 11th. Officers were elected for the ensuing year. The next meeting of the Society will be held at Edison on February 12th.

The Burke-Jenkins-Screven (Counties) Medical Society met at Millen on December 5th. A Dutch dinner was served at the Wayside Hotel. Memorial services for Dr. William Robert Lovett, Sylvania, deceased, were held. The scientific program consisted of titles for papers as follows: *Acute Pelvic Infections*" by Dr. Q. A. Mulkey, Millen; *The Mechanical Management of Fractures of the Arm, Forearm, Leg and Thigh*," Dr. Cleveland Thompson, Millen.

The Southeastern Surgical Congress will hold its seventh annual assembly at the Roosevelt Hotel, New Orleans, Louisiana, March 9, 10, 11, 1936. The following surgeons have accepted places on the program: Dr. Arthur E. Hertzler, Halstead, Kan.; Dr. Chevalier L. Jackson, Philadelphia, Pa.; Dr. Francis E. Lejeune, New Orleans, La.; Dr. Arthur W. Allen, Boston, Mass.; Dr. John F. Erdman, New York City; Dr. Jennings C. Litzenberg, Minneapolis, Minn.; Dr. Joseph E. King, New York City; Dr. Fred Rankin, Lexington, Ky.; Dr. Carl C. Howard, Glasgow, Ky.; Dr. George W. Crile, Cleveland, O.; Dr. Garnett W. Quillian, Atlanta; Dr. Paul G. Flothow, Seattle, Wash.; Dr. Alan C. Woods, Baltimore, Md.; Dr. Virgil S. Counseller, Mayo Clinic, Rochester, Minn.; Dr. Alfred A. Strauss, Chicago, Ill.; Dr. W. D. Haggard, Nashville, Tenn.; Dr. Roger G. Doughty, Columbia, S. C.; Dr. Thos. E. Cormody, Denver, Col.; Dr. Chas. O. Bates, Greenville, S. C.; Dr. Guy A. Caldwell, Shreveport, La.; Dr. Gerry R. Holden, Jacksonville, Fla.; Dr. Emmerich von Haam, New Orleans, La.; Dr. Roger S. Anderson, Seattle, Wash.; Dr. Augustus Street, Vicksburg, Miss.; Dr. James S. McLester, Birmingham, Ala.; and Dr. Edgar Fincher, Jr., Atlanta. Other speakers will be on the program.

The Piedmont Hospital Clinical Society, Atlanta, held its annual meeting on December 9th. Officers

elected for the ensuing year were: Dr. John B. Duncan, President; Dr. Wm. Willis Anderson, Vice-President; Dr. Guy C. Hewell, re-elected Secretary.

The Macon Hospital, through its Executive Committee, has appointed Dr. T. Oscar Vinson and Dr. Robert W. McAllister house physicians and surgeons. Interns selected were: Dr. John Gallemore, Dr. John Bradley, both of Macon; Dr. Frank Houser, Scott, Ga.; and Dr. Wendell P. Harris, San Francisco, Cal.

The Floyd County Medical Society held its annual banquet at the Greystone Hotel, Rome, on December 20th. Dr. Geo. B. Smith, Rome, spoke on *Medical Notes from the Pacific Coast.*

The Clinical Society of the New York Polyclinic Medical School and Hospital, New York City, met on November 4th. The program consisted of titles for papers as follows: *Contributory Causes of Coronary Thrombosis*, by Cadis Phipps, M.D., Tufts College Medical School, Boston; the discussion was led by T. Stuart Hart, M.D., and Louis Gross, M.D. *Endothelial Tumors*, Dean Lewis, M.D., Johns Hopkins University School of Medicine, Baltimore; discussion led by Fred Waldorf Stewart, M.D., Nathan Chandler Foot, M.D., and David M. Bosworth. Contributions to the December 2nd meeting were: *Changing Methods in Radiation Therapy in Malignant Diseases of the Uterus*, by William P. Healy, M.D., of the Memorial Hospital; discussion was led by Maurice Lenz, M.D., William Cameron, M.D., and Malcolm Campbell, M.D. *Surgery of the Pancreas*, by Allen O. Whipple, M.D., of the Presbyterian Hospital; the discussion was led by William Barclay Parsons, M.D., Ralph Colp, M.D., and Edward L. Kellogg, M.D.

The Third District Medical Society held its fifty-seventh semi-annual meeting in Cordele on November 13th. The scientific program was especially practical. Visitors on the scientific program were: Dr. Thos. L. Ross and Dr. O. R. Thompson, both of Macon. Other visitors were: Dr. Carl S. Pittman, Tifton; Dr. W. A. Newman and Dr. Chas. H. Richardson, Macon. Officers elected for the ensuing year: Dr. J. E. Walker, Columbus, President; Dr. R. M. Ware, Fitzgerald, Vice-President; and Dr. Chas. A. Greer, Oglethorpe, Secretary for life. The visitors and members were entertained to a banquet at the Sewanee Hotel. The next meeting of the Society will be held at Cuthbert on June 10th.

The Scientific Exhibit at the Savannah session, to be held April 21, 22, 23, 24, 1936, will be in charge of the following committeemen: Dr. Mark S. Dougherty, Atlanta, General Chairman; Dr. Lee Howard, Savannah, Local Chairman; Dr. Everett L. Bishop, Atlanta; Dr. J. L. Campbell, Atlanta; Dr. John L. Elliott, Savannah; Dr. William P. Harbin, Jr., Rome; Dr. William F. Jenkins, Columbus; Dr. Roy R. Kracke, Emory University; Dr. Fred A. Mettler, Augusta; Dr. E. B. Saye, Macon; Dr. T. F. Sellers, Atlanta; Dr. H. F. Sharpley, Jr., Savannah; and Dr. Ernest F. Wahl, Thomasville.

The Randolph County Medical Society met at the Patterson Hospital, Cuthbert, on January 2nd.

The Georgia Pediatric Society held its third annual scientific meeting in Atlanta on December 12th. The next meeting will be held at Savannah in April.

Dr. Joseph C. Read announces the removal of his office to 412 Medical Arts Building, Atlanta.

The Coffee County Medical Society met at Douglas on December 31st. Dr. T. H. Johnston, Douglas, Secretary-Treasurer, made a report covering the activities of the Society for 1935. Eleven papers were read during the year at the Society's ten meetings. Dr. T. H. Clark and Dr. B. O. Quillian, both of Douglas, were appointed on the Program Committee. Speakers and subjects will be selected for each of the scheduled meetings for 1936. Officers elected for the ensuing year were: Dr. J. G. Crovatt, Douglas, President; Dr. T. H. Johnston, Douglas, Secretary-Treasurer; Dr. Sage Harper, Wray, Delegate; Dr. T. H. Clark, Douglas, Alternate Delegate.

The staff meeting of the Emory University Hospital was held on January 6th. Cases reported were: *Bleeding Peptic Ulcer*, by Dr. E. Van Buren and Dr. Henry Poer, Atlanta; *Insulin Shock* and *Vincent's Infection of Lung*, Dr. Mark S. Dougherty, Atlanta.

Dr. Wm. W. Odom, Lyons, has resumed his practice after being confined to his home for several months following an automobile accident which occurred near Savannah.

The Georgia Medical Society, Savannah, held its regular meeting on December 10th. Officers were elected for the ensuing year.

Dr. Earl Floyd, Atlanta, Professor of Urology at Emory University School of Medicine, was elected President of the American Urological Association at its annual meeting in Nashville, Tenn., on December 6th.

The staff meeting of the Crawford W. Long Memorial Hospital, Atlanta, was held on January 9th. Officers were elected for the year. Dr. L. C. Fischer discussed surgical cases, especially intestinal obstruction.

The Habersham County Medical Society met on December 12th. Officers were elected for the ensuing year.

If interested in a location for a general practitioner, write the Secretary-Treasurer.

MARRIAGE

Dr. Harry Eugene Teasley, Hartwell, to Miss Nancy Dorothy Massey, Orlando, Fla. Married in Orlando on December 25, 1935.

OBITUARY

Dr. James Robert Cranford, Sasser; member; Emory University School of Medicine, Emory University, 1895; aged 65; died at his home on November 29, 1935. He was a successful practicing physician, devoted to his work, patients and family. Dr. Cranford was widely known and did a vast amount of charity work. He was public spirited and always rendered the very best service for his home town and community. Surviving him are his widow, two daughters, Mrs. C. S. Forrester, Donalsonville; and Mrs H. F. Smith, Sasser. Funeral services were conducted from the home by Rev. R. H. Forrester, Leesburg, and Rev. Stanaland, Donalsonville. Burial was in the Shellman cemetery.

Dr. Guy Leslie Austin, Pavo; member; University of the South Medical Department, Sewanee, Tenn., 1906; aged 56; died at his home on December 11, 1935. He was born and reared near Pavo. Dr. Austin served in the medical corps of the United States Army during the World War. He had practiced for twenty-nine years and was known for a number of years as one of the best and most active practicing physicians in South Georgia. Dr. Austin was a member of the Thomas County Medical Society, Second District Medical Society, the American Medical Association, Masonic lodge and the Methodist church. Surviving him are his widow, his mother, Mrs. F. M. Austin, Pavo; five sisters, Mrs. Fred Brown, Eton; Mrs. N. A. Sellers and Mrs. Carroll Ford, both of Jacksonville, Fla.; Mrs. Frank Patrick, Quitman; and Miss Marion Austin, Atlanta; two brothers, Fred Austin, Eton, and Roy Austin, Havana, Cuba. Rev. Robert Kerr conducted the funeral services from the residence. Interment was in Lebonen cemetery near Pavo.

Dr. Marion W. Jinks, Suwanee; Georgia College of Eclectic Medicine and Surgery, Atlanta, 1910; aged 66; died at his home on December 3, 1935. He was a member of one of the pioneer families of Gwinnett county, member of the Masonic lodge and Methodist church. Surviving him are his widow, one son, William Jinks; sister, Miss Alpha Jinks. Rev. N. O. L. Powell conducted the funeral services from the Trinity Methodist church and burial was in the churchyard.

Dr. Marion Cicero McClain, Marble Hill; member; University of Georgia School of Medicine, Augusta, 1887; aged 76; died at his home on December 25, 1935. He was born and reared in Jasper and had practiced medicine in Jasper, Marble Hill and Clarkston for more than a half century. Dr. McClain was a leading physician of his section and took a part in all civic and religious activities. He was a charter member and one of the organizers of the Marble Hill Masonic lodge, a member of the Cherokee County Medical Society and the Jasper Methodist church. Surviving him are two daughters; Mrs. F. C. Owen, Walhalla, S. C., and Mrs. J. A. Chandler, Greenville, S. C.; two sons, F. W. and M. B. McClain, both of Jasper. Funeral services were conducted by Rev. D. S. Patterson from the Jasper Methodist church and interment was in the churchyard.

RADIO ADVERTISING
(Copy of Letter)

Federal Communications Commission,
Washington, D. C.

Gentlemen:

When "Dr. Brinkley" 'was refused permission to broadcast his daily talks on the prostate gland over the radio the medical profession then realized that the U. S. Radio Commission was endeavoring to protect the health of the nation as well as arranging radio broadcast to be instructive and entertaining.

Yet, there is another source of radio broadcasting that influences the public, thereby being just as detrimental to the health of the people of our nation as were the broadcasts of "Dr. Brinkley." This source comes from the well trained announcers having people believe that they cannot get enough vitamins unless they eat Smith Brothers cough drops; another that B. C. is a safe method to relieve headaches, etc. All of these broadcasts, of course, make such patent medicines a household remedy and their constant use is being detrimental to the health of our people and any such broadcast should be discontinued and I feel that it is within your power to do so.

I have been instructed to make the above protest, although local, I feel that it expresses the sentiments of physicians in general.

Yours for saner broadcasts over the radio.

RUDOLPH BELL, M.D., Sec'y.-Treas.
Thomas County Medical Society.

Thomasville, Ga.
December 21, 1935.

WANTED:—Internist for group clinic; two years hospital training or equivalent. Must interpret electrocardiograms. Send complete qualifications with first letter. Write "T", care of The Journal.

WANTED:—Eye, ear, nose and throat man for group clinic. Send complete qualifications with first letter. Write "T", care of The Journal.

MEDICAL SURVEY IN GEORGIA

QUESTIONNAIRE FOR PHYSICIANS*

.te_____193____   County_____

ban practitioner _____Rural practitioner _____

hite_____   Colored_____

)w long have you practiced medicine?_____years. How long at present location?_____

What was your **approximate net income** from the practice of medicine for the past year? $_____

What was the **approximate expense** for the year in earning this amount? $_____

What is the approximate amount of your uncollected accounts for the past year? $_____

How much considered good? $_____ How much worthless? $_____

Are you a member of your county medical society? : Yes_____ No_____

Have you attended regularly within the past three years meetings of your county, district or state medical

societies or other medical meetings? : Yes_____ No_____, If so, which? : County_____

District_____ State_____ National_____

Have you within the past five years had post-graduate medical instruction? Yes_____ No_____.

If so, where and length of time_____

Are laboratory and hospital facilities available in your county? : Yes_____ No_____

Describe _____

Approximately what per cent of your practice within the past year was charity?_____

Do you also furnish drugs free to charity patients? : Yes_____ No_____

If so, what was the estimated monetary value for the past year? $_____

Does your county make any provision for the payment to physicians for the care of charity patients? :

Yes_____ No_____

If so, what?_____

What suggestions have you to offer for the improvement of the health of your community and to increase

the financial returns from medical practice? :**_____

*Do not sign your name_____   **If additional space is required, use reverse side of this sheet.

Mail to DR. EDGAR D. SHANKS, Sec'y.-Treas., Medical Association of Georgia,
Doctors' Bldg., 478 Peachtree Street, N.E., Atlanta

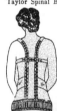
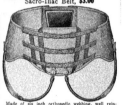

THE JOURNAL
OF THE
MEDICAL ASSOCIATION OF GEORGIA

DEVOTED TO THE WELFARE OF THE MEDICAL ASSOCIATION OF GEORGIA
PUBLISHED MONTHLY under direction of the Council

| Volume XXV | Atlanta, Ga., February, 1936 | Number 2 |

CARCINOMA OF THE COLON*

Case Report

FRANK K. BOLAND, M.D.
Atlanta

It is estimated by Dr. J. L. Campbell, of the Cancer Commission of the Medical Association of Georgia, that of approximately 1800 deaths from cancer in the State in 1934, 5 per cent or 90 deaths were due to carcinoma of the colon. Members of the medical profession appear to be especially likely to have the disease.

Considering the middle of the transverse colon as the dividing line, the two sides of the colon develop from different embryological elements, the right colon arising from the midgut, and the left colon from the hindgut. The two sides differ in anatomy and physiology, and likewise carcinoma of the colon on the two sides presents differences in pathology and symptomatology.

The lumen of the cecum and right colon is somewhat larger than the lumen on the left side. This is one of the reasons why obstruction is commoner on the left side than on the right. The sigmoid is the narrowest part of the large intestine, and is the most frequent site of obstruction by malignant disease.

The lymphatic supply of the right colon is richer than that of the left, to which is attributed later metastasis from this side than from the left side. Formerly it was believed that abundant lymphatic drainage favored rapid metastasis. It is true, however, that metastasis from carcinoma of the descending colon is earlier than from the ascending

colon. It is also true that metastasis does not take place in every case of cancer of the colon, and is less common in the colon than in any other part of the alimentary canal.

The function of the right colon is mainly the absorption of water. The contents of this portion, therefore, are largely liquid, another factor in the rarity of obstruction on the right side. The function of the left colon is mainly storage. Its contents usually are dry and hard, which helps promote obstruction.

Hemorrhage from carcinoma of the left colon occurs more often than from the right, on account of hardened feces in the left side. Ulceration of the tumor in the right side is commoner, a fact which probably is responsible for an equal amount of bleeding from this side. It should be remembered that hemorrhage from cancer of the rectum occurs earlier in the course of the disease than from cancer of the large intestine.

Carcinoma attacks the descending colon more frequently than the ascending colon. The tumor generally is single, but may be multiple, and may be preceded by polypoid formation. On the right side the mass is more apt to be of the large, soft, adenoid type, giving rise to anemia, intoxication and dehydration. Intestinal obstruction is rare, and usually is due to volvulus or intussusception. In most cases carcinoma on the left side is of the scirrhus, fibroid type, the napkin-ring variety, prone to produce obstruction. Another variation has been described, mucoid adeno-carcinoma, but this is met more commonly in the rectum.

There is a time in the life history of every malignant growth when it is only large enough to be visible to the naked eye, or barely palpable to the examining finger. At

*Read before the Medical Association of Georgia, Atlanta, May 8, 1935.

this stage the mass generally is circumscribed, and has not spread to neighboring or distant organs or tissues. It is a matter of daily occurrence to recognize such tumors when they appear on or near the surface of the body, in the breast, or in some cavity accessible to touch or sight. When such a lesion takes root in the stomach or colon, however, it must attain considerable size, or cause conspicuous signs, such as pain, hemorrhage or obstruction before attention is drawn to it.

Through skillful use of the roentgen-ray, the medical profession possesses a means of diagnosis of cancer of the stomach and colon in many cases before clinical evidence has appeared. If the periodic examination of apparently healthy persons over forty years of age could be made to include a thorough gastro-intestinal roentgen-ray series, with barium enema, it is believed that symptomless malignancies of the alimentary tract could be detected early enough in a sufficiently large group of cases to render marked improvement in the mortality statistics of carcinoma. For the present the prohibitive cost of such examination precludes the probability of attempting to make such progress in diagnosis. The large number of negative findings which would be reported no doubt would discourage the continuation of the procedure. The percentage of negative reports, however, would not exceed that which now results from Wassermann tests.

Patients afflicted with carcinoma of the colon may be divided into three groups. First, are those patients who suffer from more or less characteristic symptoms of the disease for months or years, but who do not seek medical advice until the lesion is too far advanced for surgical aid, or only some form of palliative treatment can be offered. Second, are patients who apparently are in fair health and are not aware of the presence of a serious disease until they suddenly present symptoms of intestinal obstruction or peritonitis, or suffer from profuse hemorrhage. These patients usually require colostomy for immediate relief, which may or may not be followed later by successful resection of the malignant growth.

With the dissemination of knowledge among the laity concerning cancer, fortunately the number of patients of the first group is considerably smaller than in former times. At any rate failure to recognize them earlier cannot be laid at the door of the medical profession. Until periodic health examinations become more efficient there always will be patients of the second group, those whose first symptoms come on as a bolt out of a clear sky.

It is the third group to which we owe special study. This is the largest class and includes patients in whom carcinoma of the colon grows under the eye of the attending physician or surgeon. As a rule the disease develops slowly but exhibits signs and symptoms which should excite suspicion and should suggest resort to the confirmatory evidence of the sigmoidoscope or the roentgen-ray.

A patient of the cancer age, and there is no limit, complaining of weakness, some loss of appetite and weight, and showing anemia, should be suspected of having malignant disease, no matter whether localizing signs are present or not. Anemia from cancer of the colon may exist without visible loss of blood. When such a patient complains of borborygmus or vague abdominal pain, or tells of a recent change in bowel habits, colonic cancer should be considered and the patient's history be elicited and heard most carefully. It is so easy to take a hurried history, or none at all, and prescribe a diet and a laxative.

The symptoms may be referred to the stomach, but this is unusual. The abdominal distress, which may be mild or severe, is apt to be diagnosed "intestinal indigestion" or "chronic appendicitis." Cancer in the right colon may simulate acute appendicitis and be subjected to laparotomy, a fortunate circumstance in either event. Intermittent diarrhea with periods of normal bowel movements and without a tendency to constipation may be noted frequently in cancer of the right segment.

Probably the earliest sign of the disease in the descending colon is constipation, which may also indicate cancer of the splenic flexure. Close quizzing on the part of the examiner often is necessary to ascertain whether or not the patient's bowel habits have undergone any recent change. What may be considered constipation by one patient may be regarded as normal by another. If diarrhea exists the influence of 'purgatives should be investigated. The shape and character of the stools are of little significance. Flattened or ribbon-like stools, so frequently described, are seldom seen.

Palpation of a tumor on the left side is rarely possible, but is common on the right. A full-blown, text-book picture case of colonic cancer usually is recognized all too easily. Our aim should be early diagnosis while there is possibility of cure. Other diseases of the colon liable to be confounded with carcinoma are comparatively infrequent, but often are not discovered until laparotomy is performed. The commonest of these are ulcerative colitis, tuberculosis, diverticulitis and abscess of the appendix, or a chronic inflammatory and thickened retrocecal appendix.

The importance of the examining finger and the sigmoidoscope cannot be overrated as diagnostic aids, in the study of diseases of the colon. Whenever possible, suspicious tissue should be removed through the sigmoidoscope for biopsy. The value of roentgenology has been mentioned. In a group of 102 organic lesions of the large bowel examined by the roentgen-ray at the Mayo Clinic, a correct interpretation was made in 99 cases. Such results as these require unusual training, experience, diligence and patience, and do not reward the efforts of the novice.

In neglected cases of cancer of the colon, the surgical management usually narrows down to the treatment of acute intestinal obstruction, which means enterostomy or colostomy. Often this is the only operative procedure ever carried out; occasionally it is possible to go back later for radical resection of the tumor.

Peritonitis is the commonest cause of death from resection of a malignant growth of the colon. Lately prophylactic injection of intraperitoneal vaccine a few days prior to

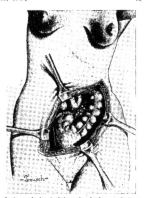

Carcinoma of colon simulating pedunculated tumor of uterus.

operation apparently has reduced the incidence and severity of this complication.

Surgical judgment and experience must decide whether or not a tumor can be removed safely, with reasonable expectation of a satisfactory result. An operation which might be performed safely by one surgeon might not turn out so well in the hands of another surgeon. Indurated mesenteric lymph nodes need not necessarily interdict excision of the growth. Often such glands are inflammatory. Even demonstrable metastatic involvement of other organs should not always preclude removal of the original tumor. Death from metastasis may be less painful and less distressing than death caused by an unremoved primary lesion.

The method of anastomosis to follow after excision, often is a problem, about which able surgeons disagree. The method should be made to fit the conditions present. Lateral anastomosis is the safest, and the easiest to perform. End-to-end anastomosis is the most logical type, although occasionally end-to-side is to be preferred. The Mikulicz method is excellent in certain cases of obstruction.

As emphasized by Jones[1], the maintenance of adequate blood supply and the relief
of the pressure of distention on the line of
sutures is more important than the type of
anastomosis. The blood supply is less apt
to be damaged by lateral anastomosis than
by the end-to-end method, and pressure on
the sutures is diminished by an enterostomy
or colostomy above the site of anastomosis.
The persistence of the fecal fistula thus established is shortened by bringing the tube
through a flap of omentum.

A faultlessly performed operation for carcinoma of the colon may add months or
years to the life of the patient, but the credit
of prolonging life in most instances will belong to the physician who recognizes the
disease in its beginning, when extensive and
brilliant operations may not be necessary.

Case Report

An undiagnosed case of carcinoma of the colon,
with unusual findings, is reported:

The patient was a white woman, 52 years old,
first seen in August, 1934. She had had five children,
and twelve years previously had perineum repaired,
and lacerated cervix uteri amputated. At the same time
radium was introduced into the uterus as treatment
for asthma, from which she had suffered for many
years. Asthma was not relieved, and later her tonsils
were removed, which did not help the asthma. A
few months later the asthma apparently was cured by
taking some kind of 'shots.'" The use of radium
did not stop menstruation, but menstruation ceased
two years later.

The patient lost thirty pounds in weight during
the past few months, and believed it was due to the
fact that during the last year and a half she was having all her teeth removed by degrees, and was not
able to take sufficient food. For the past twelve
months she suffered from attacks of abdominal pain,
starting in the region of the uterus, and extending to
both sides, morphia sometimes being necessary for relief. For several months she had noticed a movable
lump the size of an orange just above the uterus.
Her appetite was fair, she had headaches and some
indigestion, and lately was more constipated than
formerly. Her chest was negative, urine negative, blood
pressure 110-70, erythrocytes 4,370,000, hemoglobin
76 per cent.

Pelvic examination showed the tumor she had noticed, which also could be palpated through the abdomen. The mass appeared to be attached either to
the uterus or left ovary, and was thought to be either
a pedunculated fibroid of the uterus or an ovarian cyst.
The attacks of abdominal pain were ascribed as possibly due to such a movable tumor being twisted on
its pedicle, and the loss of weight suggested malignancy. Digital examination of the rectum revealed

The first evidences of a rectosigmoid carcinoma may be a slight disturbance of gastric digestion associated with pylorospasm, or its earliest symptoms may be mistaken for that scapegoat colitis; an unexplained anemia, together with occult blood in the feces, may signify an early cancer of the hepatic flexure; and the signs of a mild appendicitis may upon exploration disclose an early carcinoma of the cecum.

I believe that if we will keep in mind the possibility of carcinoma of the colon in all patients who have an unexplained bodily deterioration or anemia, or who have persistent, though slight, digestive disturbances, then more patients will be brought to operation earlier, as the latter is the only hope we have to offer them.

DR. J. J. CLARK (Atlanta) : I have been interested for a good many years in the early diagnosis of cancer of the colon and stomach. I am sorry to say that as yet it seems that the early diagnosis of either of these cancers is really out of our hands, because the patients ordinarily do not present themselves early enough in their disease to have symptoms which would necessitate a roentgenological study.

In studying the colon, there are one or two things that should always be kept in mind. Dr. Traylor just mentioned one very important fact. That is, when the pathology suggests colonic disease, begin the study by means of a colon enema and you will not incite an acute obstruction.

When you do decide to examine the colon, you should have everything in your favor. The colon should be empty. The majority of these patients have been vomiting, and of course their stomachs and intestines are fairly empty. Many times they have been given a large number of different kinds of enemas in an effort to open the bowels. Be sure that the colon is not filled with watery enemas, glycerin, turpentine, or whatever you may use, because frequently that makes a barium study of the colon nearly impossible.

The study should be made under a fluoroscope, watching the colon fill from the rectum upwards, so you can examine practically every inch of the entire bowel.

Many times when this is done, the sigmoid will fill up completely and obliterate the descending colon, particularly that part which lies in the pelvis. So after this examination has been done, allow your patient to evacuate the enema and re-examine him. You will be surprised that most of them will only empty the lower rectum and sigmoid, and sometimes pathology which is hidden by the barium filling the sigmoid loops will come into view at this second examination.

Then as a help, after the examination has gone this far, if you reintroduce a rectal tube and inflate the colon slowly with air, giving what is known as a contrast enema, many of these lesions will come into view very quickly.

I should like to use three of Dr. Boland's slides to illustrate the points I have made.

(Slide) This type of patient illustrates exactly what would have happened had a barium meal been given from above. That obstruction is well within the reach of the finger, from the rectal examination. The bowel is very, very narrow; and, as Dr. Boland said, the proximal half of the contents of the colon are liquid and commence to get solid as they pass the transverse colon. You know many patients complain of hard, dry stools following the barium meal, and you can imagine what would have happened to this patient, having a dry hard stool reach this area. You would have had obstruction.

(Slide) Here is another case with a napkin-ring type of carcinoma. Of course the barium meal above would have immediately brought on obstruction. At the same time I wish to warn you, if you give the enema and you encounter a lesion like this or the one before, it is essential that you spend considerable time, maybe an hour or two, siphoning off your barium solution, in order that your enema will not incite obstruction.

(Slide) This last film illustrates what a small lesion an early carcinoma of the colon may be. You will notice this thin linear haustration; just a little sliver running out there, with another haustration above, perfectly normal. This was a small carcinoma originating just above the cecum. It takes careful search to find these lesions, but I believe the majority of them can be found if they are carefully looked for.

DR. LON W. GROVE (Atlanta) : In my exhibit upstairs, I am showing fifteen cases of carcinoma of the colon and rectum, taken from my private files. There are two or three things that I want to emphasize in this discussion. The first is, early diagnosis. Notwithstanding improved x-ray diagnoses, more proctoscopic studies and all that has been said about early diagnosis of cancer, seven of these fifteen cases came in after there was evidence of metastasis. The remaining cases were subjected to radical excision of the growth, all done by the graded or multiple stage technique. There have been two deaths, one following a colostomy in a patient who was completely obstructed when admitted, and one following the combined abdominal-perineal resection, after the method advised by Rankin.

The graded operation is the second thought I want to emphasize. These cases require careful handling. So often they come in with either a complete obstruction or if not complete, a high degree of obstruction, and if they are subjected to much surgery at that time, the mortality is high. As the result of the obstruction, there is always some inflammatory reaction about the growth, and the mere handling of these growths is sufficient to produce a peritonitis in a large per cent of cases. Those with symptoms of obstruction should all have a decompression operation as a preliminary procedure, either a cecostomy or some form of colostomy, to be followed later by the radical operation.

There is another point which Rankin has emphasized, and Lahey has more recently emphasized:

that these patients should not be pushed too rapidly from one step of the graded technique to the other. I am sure that the case we lost with obstruction was due to this. The family complained of the expense in the care of the patient, and the permanent colostomy was done earlier than it should have been.

The cases with growths above the recto-sigmoid junction have all been operated upon by the modified Mikulicz technique, which has decided advantages over the old Mikulicz. With the old technique there was no effort made to remove the gland bearing portion of the mesentery supplying the growth, while in the improved or modified Mikulicz, the colon is thoroughly mobilized and a wide V section of the mesentery is removed, which makes it as radical an operation as can be done. This is an extraperitoneal excision of the growth, and it carries a much lower mortality than we could possibly expect from any of the methods of primary resection. Lahey has recently reported fifty-nine consecutive cases without a death.

DR. JACK G. STANDIFER (Blakely): You have heard this subject discussed mainly from the viewpoint of the surgeon. I believe a few words from a country doctor might be applicable. In the past few months it has been my privilege to see two cases of carcinoma of the colon. The first was a physician who has since died. For some reason, the doctor never mentioned his condition to anyone until it had progressed so far that nothing could be done and it was only in the very last stages that I saw him. An unusual condition was presented in this case, which proved to be a carcinoma of the sigmoid, in that a fistulous tract ruptured into the bladder and for the last few weeks, he passed gas and fecal matter in his urine.

The second case was that of a lady about 52 years old, who complained of some irregularity of the bowels and a slowly increasing constipation. I was fortunate in being able to make an early and at least tentative diagnosis of carcinoma of the colon and sent her to a hospital. A series of operations were performed. Although there was a small fecal fistula for a time, she completely recovered and appears to be a well woman.

I mention this from the standpoint of a general practitioner, for we are the boys out on the firing line. If we do not recognize these conditions early, no matter how good the surgeon may be, it is exactly as Dr. Boland has said: if they come too late, it's just too bad.

DR. FRANK K. BOLAND (Atlanta): The main object of my paper was to urge increased efforts on the part of all of us toward making more early diagnoses in this most serious disease. It seems to be a disease especially liable to attack doctors.

I did not have time to go into many details of treatment and operative procedures. I am glad Dr. Grove brought out some of these, especially in reference to going after these cases rather carefully, method-

ically, and not rushing in to do a radical resection immediately. Of course a great many of these cases come to us completely obstructed, or almost so, and require preliminary colostomy or enterostomy.

I wish to pay special tribute to Dr. J. J. Clark for the valuable assistance he has been to me in the study of these cases. As brought out by him, and in my paper also, the roentgen-ray study does not mean just taking a picture, as we would of ourselves or our family. It means a careful, diligent investigation, sometimes going over a period of two or three days, with a lot of manipulations. There is nothing so important in the diagnosis of carcinoma of the colon as roentgen-ray study.

LARYNGEAL TUBERCULOSIS*

LOUIS C. ROUGLIN, M.D.
Atlanta

Laryngeal tuberculosis is a most important disease, both to the laryngologist and the tuberculosis specialist as it plays an important role in the diagnosis, prognosis and treatment of the patient.

Laryngeal tuberculosis is evidence of a general lowered resistance and is almost always secondary to pulmonary tuberculosis. It may occur at any age of life, but is most common between the ages of 20 and 40. Males are more frequently affected than females and with the exception of occupations that have a direct tendency to produce irritation, it apparently has no relation to vocation or social status of the patient.

The areas of the larynx most commonly involved are the posterior commissure, in the interarytenoid area, the anterior surface of the arytenoid bodies and the vocal processes. Next in order are the vocal cords, the ventricular bands, and lastly the epiglottis. It is important to bear in mind that the disease is most curable when it is just around the margin of the posterior commissure, yet it is this area which is most commonly overlooked.

Etiology

The tubercle bacillus as the sole causative factor in tuberculous laryngitis was conclusively shown by Virchow in 1865 and Heinze in 1879, but the route of invasion has produced some controversy. Two theo-

*Read before the Medical Association of Georgia, Atlanta, May 9, 1935.

ries as to the mode of infection have been considered. Inasmuch as it usually appears first where the sputum is most liable to collect and cling, some consider the infected sputum to be the principal etiological factor. Others believe that the infection is borne to the larynx by means of the blood and lymph vessels, as the disease will often develop in those with pulmonary tuberculosis in which there is no expectoration. In my opinion, both factors play an important role in the production of the disease.

Histologically the lesion is an inflammatory response to a toxic irritant, and the pathologic changes in the larynx assume the same protean forms as in tuberculosis in other organs. A spherical area is formed of whirling layers of modified cells resembling epithelial cells, known as epitheloid cells, these cells have engulfed one or more tubercle bacilli. Near the center, there are one or more multinuclear giant cells of Langhan's in which the bacilli are often found. A zone of small round lymphocytes surround the periphery, coagulation necrosis occurs in its center and when the epithelium becomes involved an ulcer is the result.

The progress of this disease may be divided into the stages of infiltration, ulceration and perichondritis. The most favorable are those which do not reach a state of deep ulceration, the least favorable are those in which the tissues of both within and without the larynx are involved and with little or no evidence of fibrous tissue formation.

The lesion is healed by the deposit of calcium salts in the necrotic areas and the fibrous tissue which develops from fixed connective tissue cells and probably by the epitheloid cells changing into fibroblasts. Such healing processes are encouraged by an increased blood supply.

It must be borne in mind that a tuberculous invasion of the throat may occur without any subjective symptoms. The most suggestive symptom is a slight but persistent huskiness which eventually progresses into a rough whisper, often combined with a rattling incomplete cough. As the disease progresses, symptoms of slight discomfort or pain maybe referred to the throat, and lastly

the most distressing symptoms of pain on swallowing, dysphagia, spasm and choking develop.

Diagnosis:—There is no disease of the larynx that tuberculous laryngitis may not simulate, from the simple catarrhal inflamation of the smokers throat to cancer. In all laryngeal cases of any duration, where syphilis and cancer is ruled out, an x-ray examination, as well as a physical examination of the lungs should be required. The probability of mixed syphilis and tuberculosis should be kept in mind, as well as mixed carcinoma cases. To the trained laryngologist, especially when pulmonary disease is present, there should scarcely be any room for doubt in making a diagnosis.

Differential Diagnosis:—Carcinoma usually occurs in middle life or later. It is more frequently unilateral, while tuberculosis is generally bilateral. Carcinoma is usually more localized, smaller and, most frequently affects the vocal cords. In syphilis the generalized edema of the larynx is more pronounced and the syphilitic lesion generally destroys the identity of the structure.

Prognosis—The average patient with tuberculosis never has a laryngeal examination until the disease is far advanced, and his general condition so grave, that at best, treatment can only be palliative. There exists a prevalent opinion that little or nothing can be done for these patients, and while it is true that the ultimate fate of the patient will depend on his general condition, early diagnosis and treatment of the larynx by relieving pain and other annoying symptoms may be a great factor in prolonging life and even in the production of an ultimate cure.

Treatment—It is obviously hard to determine how much value one can attribute to local treatment in any given case. The resistance of the patient must be primarily considered, as the disease is due to and associated with pulmonary tuberculosis. The general medical treatment then is all important. As for the laryngeal inflammation, the treatment depends on the condition of the patient, as well as on the degree of pathology present. An early diagnosis is most essential. Every tuberculous patient should be considered a potential laryngeal case and thorough routine examinations of that organ should be made. Many cases can be prevented by correction and early attention to other pathological processes that may lead to superficial loss of epithelium and pave the way for sputum infections Hypertrophied turbinates, chronically infected tonsils, adenoids and sinusitis should be corrected. Rest, complete physical and vocal, and with suitable applications of heliotherapy has proven beneficial and curative in many of my cases. When that fails to give satisfactory response, then the galvanocautery is the treatment of choice.

The galvanocautery has superseded all other topical methods of treatment, such as injections, curetting, applications of trichloracetic or lactic acid. Tuberculous laryngitis heals not by the destruction of all the tuberculous tissue but by the development of an inflammatory zone, in which newly formed blood vessels and fibroblasts are produced which hastens cicatrization. The operation in trained hands is a relatively minor procedure. It should preferably be done by the indirect method, the direct method is disagreeable to the patient due to the pressure of the laryngoscope; he invariably complains of sore throat for three or more days. There are no contraindications to the galvanocautery, except marked asthenia, pregnancy, hypertension, or very high degree of temperature. It is of healing and curative value in early cases with moderate ulceration and relieves pain and suffering in advanced cases.

Summary

1. All tuberculous patients are potential tuberculous laryngitis cases.

2. A plea is made for routine, systematic and competent laryngeal examination of all tuberculous patients.

3. An early diagnosis is essential, and when made, may become a dominant factor in the relief and ultimate cure of the disease.

4. Local applications, such as lactic acid or other caustics, are of doubtful value.

5. Hospitalization, complete vocal rest and

heliotherapy, will prove adequate for relief in suitable cases.

6. When the above fail to give results, galvanocautery is the best known method today for giving immediate relief and is a potent factor in the ultimate improvement in the general condition of the patient.

307 Candler Building.

Discussion on Paper by Dr. Louis C. Rouglin

DR. B. H. MINCHEW (Waycross): Dr. Rouglin's paper has a double significance, and has more merit than the usual discussion of laryngeal tuberculosis. The fine things he said with regard to secondary manifestations in the larynx, carry with them a warning for an early diagnosis of a more severe condition.

We are too prone to think of a manifestation of this character coming only after pulmonary tuberculosis has reached a very apparent stage. This is not true. We can have a tuberculous laryngitis with little manifestations in the chest. There is one of the dangers of a conservative estimation of the condition we see in the throat, and there, too, comes the value of a man's research and ability in the matter of diagnosis.

I was particularly glad to hear him say what he did about perfect rest and relaxation of the patient. I am sure that he knows, and we all should know, that the patient is not going to get well by local treatment. We have got to see that the patient is placed in the hands of one who knows how to treat pulmonary tuberculosis, and obtain the full cooperation of the patient toward that end.

I was glad to hear him say something about the removal of other foci of infection. I think this should be done, but great care and caution should be exercised in doing it. I do not believe that we should employ any type of operation under a general anesthetic. If it is the tonsils that are to be removed, the operation should certainly be done under local anesthesia, and the enucleation, dissection or what not should be done with just as little trauma as possible.

I do not believe treatment that he has shown necessary in some of these cases can be carried on by most of us. When I find a case of tuberculous laryngitis and recognize that more radical treatment is necessary, I refer the case to someone with technical skill developed from experience and a fine delicate touch and technic.

DR. DUNBAR ROY (Atlanta): May I be permitted to say a few words on this very important subject?

In the first place, I want to congratulate Dr. Rouglin on his most excellent and concise paper upon this subject. I feel that it is really a subject which ought to be brought before a general medical society more frequently than it is.

After forty-two years of practice, after seeing many hundreds of these cases in private practice and also in the clinic, I have never yet seen a case of primary tuberculosis of the larynx, and this agrees with the best men in the country who have carried out this work in laryngology.

The question of diagnosis in these cases is not when an ulceration has started, but it is a question of when the larynx seemingly is involved. I do not believe that there is ever an involvement of the larynx without there being an involvement of the lungs. You may not discover it, through all of your fine methods of diagnosis, your x-ray and even your sputum examination, because frequently long before there is the presence of the tubercle bacillus, you have an involvement of both of the lungs and also of the larynx. When you have an ulceration of the larynx, it is not very difficult, if there are the other conditions present in the lung, to make your diagnosis, but the great question is in the early stages and what I call the pre-tubercular stage. It is in those stages where the method of diagnosis and the ability to diagnose a laryngeal involvement is one of the most difficult things that I know of, and it is just at this point that the man with experience is a man that is able to make a diagnosis from a certain degree of redness and a certain degree of less redness.

You cannot get it from text-books, and you cannot get it from papers or discussions. It is a question of experience in most all of the cases that come to us in the medical world. And for this reason, the longer I practice, the more I realize that it is a question of experience in diagnosing these cases.

As to the question of diagnosis and the question of treatment. A good many years ago I was at the meeting of the Laryngological Society in New York, and Sir Sinclair Thompson, of London, England, who perhaps has written more upon laryngeal tuberculosis than any other man in the world, and who is certainly one of the most acute observers, in discussing this subject said: "I have a case under observation which has been completely cured, and this case was completely cured by absolute rest for one year. He was not allowed to speak or to use his vocal cords, he did everything by writing upon a pad. That patient, gentlemen, is myself, who stands before you, a case cured by Sinclair Thompson himself."

A relationship between a tuberculous laryngitis and a tuberculous condition in the lungs is one of the most important things that can exist. It is in just such cases as these where there should be the greatest amount of fellowship, you might say, between the internist and the laryngologist, because it is in the lungs where this condition first starts.

They speak of the interarytenoid cartilages and the thickening at this point. There is no man who can make a diagnosis from that condition. I have seen it in normal individuals. Some people have a spongy and enlarged condition in the arytenoids, and if a diagnosis was made that such was a tuberculous condition, in many cases the observer would be wrong. So that in itself is not a positive diagnosis.

In the treatment of these conditions, with the ques-

tion of ulceration, as Dr. Rouglin has said, there isn't anything better than the use of the galvano-cautery, but that requires exceedingly skillful hands for its use, and when there is ulceration, you do get a certain amount of marked benefit in these laryngeal cases. But you must remember that it is from the lungs and the cure of the condition in the lungs that you must expect to get a cure in the laryngeal condition.

One of the worst features about a laryngeal tuberculosis, just as a laryngeal cancer, is that intense and severe pain, which is almost unbearable, and you do not want a patient under the influence of an anodyne, and you try everything that is possible to make the patient comfortable in the present condition in which he exists. The blocking off of the inferior laryngeal does do a good deal of good for a few days, but it returns again, and to my mind one of the greatest problems that I have ever had, is to relieve a patient when he has a marked laryngeal tuberculosis accompanied by this very intense pain.

In relieving the pain I found nothing better than the use of the intralaryngeal syringe, with a solution of 2 grains of quinacol, 2 grains of menthol, and 10 grains of orthoform in olive oil. If injected into the larynx of a patient with severe pain and severe inflammatory conditions, I have found nothing that will relieve the patient as much as such an injection. The beauty about it is that you can get a long medicine dropper, with just a rubber tip on the end, and it takes but a few days for the patient to put that back at the base of the tongue and inhale this fluid and get almost instantaneous relief. Orthoform is a local anesthetic, and very few men seem to use it. You can use a powder, but it is always irritating in the larynx. You can use it, gentlemen, in cases of severe pain, not as a curative, because that must come from the lungs. Whenever the patient begins to be hoarse for four or five months and he loses flesh and has a little cough at night and there is a little rise of temperature in the afternoon, it does not matter what the larynx shows, that man is headed for a tuberculous condition, and that is the time when the internist and laryngologist should work together.

DR. MURDOCK EQUEN (Atlanta, Ga.): This paper by Dr. Rouglin is a most important one and it has been well presented.

Laryngeal tuberculosis must be considered a complication of a pulmonary lesion and not a clinical entity. Dr. Dabinsky of Otisville has probably done more work in laryngeal tuberculosis than anyone else in this country, having charge of the tuberculous patients of that institution for some years, and his findings have been very interesting. He states that twenty years ago 25 per cent of all patients with pulmonary tuberculosis were headed for laryngeal tuberculosis. Since lung collapse therapy has come into use this menace has been reduced to around 14 per cent. He compiled some interesting statistics of over 5,000 individuals who had their lungs collapsed, and only twelve people out of that 5.000 developed laryngeal tuberculosis. This gives an idea of the value of lung collapse in the prevention of laryngeal tuberculosis. He states that whenever you collapse a lung, you are probably preventing a laryngeal tuberculosis.

In laryngeal tuberculosis there is always a previous pulmonary lesion. You must look for the organism in the sputum which will eventually be found. A tuberculous patient may also have other lesions of the larynx. Carcinoma and syphilis may be superimposed on a tuberculous larynx, or may be found in a tuberculous patient whose glottis has not been invaded by the tubercle bacillus. Dr. Beck of Chicago reported several larynges which he removed and which showed carcinoma, tuberculosis and syphilis.

About the cautery, I have found these cases get along better if the new intravenous solution, evipal, is used. The patient is asleep before cauterization is begun and awakens very rapidly afterward. He remains asleep only about fifteen minutes. If you are cauterizing a larynx, the vocal cords snap together thus exposing the normal cord to the cautery. It is impossible to give ether on account of the lung lesion and the danger of an explosion. One may recall how sensitive the larynx is when one accidentally aspirates food while eating and how violent the coughing which followed. Even with the extensive application of cocaine it is impossible to abolish the laryngeal reflex completely.

Dr. Joseph Greene, of Asheville, has shown us that a large part of the larynx may be cauterized with the electric cautery, the patient recovering. I saw a case he demonstrated in Roanoke, Virginia, in which practically no epiglottis remained. There are those who think the epiglottis plays an important part in preventing the entry of food into the larynx and trachea, but these patients learn to swallow without the use of the epiglottis.

In the consideration of the treatment, the consensus of opinion today seems to be that lung collapse, plus the cautery, are the most important procedures, local treatment being only of palliative value. Cauterization should be done extensively, and their lungs collapsed early.

Dr. Roy mentioned Mr. St. Clair Thompson of London. His idea is that the actual cautery is the most important part of any type of treatment. Vocal rest has been recommended in the acute and sub-acute forms, but after there has been scar tissue formation the use of the vocal cords to a moderate degree does not injure the individual.

When there is extensive ulceration and pain of the larynx, the injection of the superior laryngeal nerve after the method of Boulay's is most valuable. Novocain is suitable for a temporary anesthesia of the larynx, but alcohol is necessary for a prolonged one.

DR. LOUIS C. ROUGLIN (Atlanta): I want to thank the gentlemen who have so kindly discussed my paper. We are practically all of one accord, that an early diagnosis is essential. It is not difficult to

years prior ·to the present admission, but otherwise there was .no .history of any other accident or illness.

The present illness began ten days before admission as a slight headache which gradually increased in severity. This pain seemed most intense in the occiput and radiated forward to the eyes, and backward into the neck. Three days prior to admission the patient's neck began to feel stiff and some pain was experienced when the head was bent forward.

Examination revealed a well-developed, well-nourished negro male apparently in considerable pain. The head was normal. There was slight rigidity of the neck. Kernig's, and Brudzinski's signs were positive. The chest and abdomen were negative except for a slight tenderness over the spleen.

Laboratory reports showed a normal urine; red blood cell count of 4,790,000; white blood cell count 9,300; differential white blood cell count, polymorphonuclear neutrophilic leucocytes, 87; basophilic polymorphonuclear leucocytes, 1; lymphocytes, 6; monocytes, 6. Repeated examinations of blood smears were negative for malaria, and the blood Wassermann was repeatedly negative. Lumbar puncture was first done three days after admission and the pressure was 55mm. Hg., rising to 68 mm. Hg. on pressure over both jugular veins; the cell count was 50; globulin was strongly positive both by the Pandy and Ross-Jones tests; Wassermann test negative; colloidal gold curve was 0000110000; "no growth" reported on culture. Repetition of the lumbar puncture two days later showed a pressure of 8 mm. Hg.; Pandy and Ross-Jones tests positive; cell count 360; culture was reported "contaminated with yeast organisms." A third lumbar puncture done four days later showed a pressure of 20 mm. Hg.; Pandy and Ross-Jones tests positive; cell count 280; culture again reported contaminated with yeast organisms.

The ·temperature ranged between 99° and 101° except ·for a sudden elevation to 104° on the sixth day in the hospital, and a second elevation to 103° on the fourteenth day in the hospital. Pulse rate for the first five days ranged between 60 and 90. There was a pronounced acceleration to 116 during the period of the first febrile rise, and a subsequent drop to 90. Following this the pulse rate gradually increased from 90 to 120. Respirations were between 20 and 30 per minute. The patient became progressively worse and died November 1, 1934, 15 days after admission.

At autopsy the body was that of a well-nourished and well-developed negro male, aged 45, 176 cms. long, and weighing about 70 Kg. External examination revealed nothing unusual except for an external strabismus. The essential pathological findings were in the head. The scalp, skull, dura, and blood sinuses showed nothing unusual. The vessels about the base were thickened and sclerotic. The pia-arachnoid was thickened, opaque, hyperemic, and edematous. The spinal fluid was judged to be normal in amount and the lining of the ventricles was clear. Routine sections of the cerebrum, cerebellum, pons, and medulla showed no noteworthy changes in the gross, except that the pia extending down into the sulci and folds of the brain was also thickened and opaque. Microscopically, sections of the brain showed a nonsuppurative, exudative leptomeningitis extending into the brain substance for a short distance along the course of the larger vessels. The meninges covering the entire surface of the brain and the upper cervical cord were involved. The inflammation consisted of a heavy infiltration of endothelial leucocytes (many of which were vacuolated), lymphocytes, and an occasional giant cell of the foreign body type. Many eosinophilic organisms were present, some free and some phagocyted by endothelial .leucocytes. These organisms were around, about the size of a red blood cell, and all were surrounded by a clear halo. These organisms were more readily apparent in sections stained by a silver impregnation method (Dieterle). There were extensions of the process for short distances into the gray matter of the cortex, along some of the larger vessels, but other than this the microscopic sections of the cortex, basal nuclei, cerebellum, pons, medulla, and upper cervical cord showed nothing unusual. No tubercle bacilli or treponema pallida were found in preparations especially stained for these organisms.

Other pathological findings were: The lungs showed an early suppurative lobular pneumonia of a nonspecific type. The heart weighed 360 Gm., the muscular fibers were hypertrophied and the aorta showed advanced atherosclerosis. The liver, spleen, adrenals, and kidneys showed no noteworthy changes. The prostate was slightly enlarged and microscopic examination showed this was due to a glandular hyperplasia with some cystic dilation of the glands. The esophageal mucosa showed numerous, raised, firm, whitish plaques each about 0.4 cm. in diameter and on microscopic section these showed epithelial hyperplasia with lymphocytic infiltration. The stomach contained a large amount of dark red blood and two ulcers were found on the posterior wall, in the middle 1-3 of the lesser curvature. One of these was a round ulcer about 4.5 cm. in diameter, the other was linear, measuring 1x4 cm. These ulcers extended only a short distance into the submucosa and the margins were not thickened or elevated.

The anatomical diagnoses of the case were: Torula leptomeningitis, suppurative lobular pneumonia, multiple acute peptic ulcers with hemorrhage, chronic esophagitis and leucoplakia of the esophagus, cardiac hypertrophy, prostatic hypertrophy, internal strabismus.

Comment

Cases of torula meningitis are of interest from the standpoint of their rarity and the frequency with which the diagnosis is missed. Such cases present clinically, no characteristic syndrome other than that of a sub-acute to chronic leptomeningitis, but recognition is easy upon a careful examination of the spinal fluid which always contains relatively large numbers of the torula organisms. Unfortunately these are frequently passed over as red blood cells to which they bear a superficial resemblance, or they are ascribed to outside contamination as was done in this case. It seems probable that a larger number of correct diagnoses would be made in these cases of torula infection of the central nervous system if more careful studies of the spinal fluid were made.

According to Freeman[1], the pathologic picture is characteristic. The brain grossly shows an engorgement of the superficial vessels and a thickening of the leptomeninges. Frequently small cysts filled with colloid material are found in the meninges and in the superficial portions of the brain substance, along the course of the larger vessels. Microscopically there is an irregular thickening of the leptomeninges by the proliferation of endothelial leucocytes and fibroblasts and infiltration with varying numbers of lymphocytes and an occasional plasma cell. Polymorphonuclear neutrophilic leucocytes and eosinophilic polymorphonuclear leucocytes are rarely seen. Multinucleated giant cells (foreign body type) are found in varying numbers. Scattered more or less freely in the meshes of tissue, both intra- and extra-cellular are round hyaline bodies, the parasites. There is usually extension into the brain substances along the course of the larger vessels. The reaction closely resembles tuberculosis except for the type of organism present, the difference in the type of giant cells, the absence of caseation in torula meningitis, and the vacuolation and liquefaction about the torula organisms.

All cases of torula meningitis thus far reported have terminated fatally and there is no treatment known to be of any value.

BIBLIOGRAPHY

1. Freeman, Walter: Torula Infection of the Central Nervous System, J. f. Psych. u. Neurol. 43:236, 1931.
2. Watts, J. W.: Torulosis, A Review and Report of Two Cases, Am. J. Path. 8:167 (March) 1932.
3. Rogers, J. B. and Jelsma, F.: Torula Meningo-encephalitis, J. A. M. A., 500:1030 (April 1) 1933.
4. Johns, F. M. and Attaway, C. L.: Torula Meningitis, Report of a Case, Am. J. Clin. Path. 3:459 (November) 1933.
5. Fetchett, M. S. and Weidemann, F. D.: Generalized Torulosis Associated with Hodgkin's Disease, Arch. Path. 18:225 (August) 1934.

Discussion on Paper by Dr. Frank H. Van Wagoner and Dr. Edgar R. Pund

DR. R. S. LEADINGHAM (Atlanta): The conditions under which molds and yeasts become adapted to growth in the body are not well understood. They are not infrequently found in the body passages, sometimes associated with other organisms, sometimes, alone producing low grade inflammatory lesions.

The mucous membrane of the mouth and respiratory tract, tonsillar crypts, tooth root canals, and the external auditory canals are common cites of growth. The monilia and aspergillus are perhaps most commonly isolated from these locations. Last year from one patient with chronic recurring bronchitis we recovered a monilia and a hemolytic streptococcus. Both organisms produced a strongly positive intradermal reaction. and treatment with streptococcus vaccine gave speedy relief.

Yeasts are also common inhabitants of the intestinal tract but probably seldom cause any considerable disturbance. Blastomycosis of the skin may be followed by a generalized infection and lesions resembling tuberculosis be found in the various organs of the body.

Dr. Van Wagoner's case report illustrates a rarer type of infection. and it would be interesting to know from what source the organisms reached the brain and spinal fluid.

DR. FRANK H. VAN WAGONER (Augusta): I want to thank Dr. Leadingham for his excellent discussion. We are very interested in this case in trying to determine the source of infection. As far as any published reports go, no one seems to know just where these organisms come from or why in these rare cases they become pathogenic for the human body. It has been suggested a number of times that the portal of entry is through the lungs, and in this case there was a suppurative bronchopneumonia. However, the reaction in the lung was in no way similar to the reaction in the meninges, and on careful study of the sections of the lung we were not able to find any of the torula organisms there. As far as the lesions in the esophagus and stomach were concerned, they appeared to be the ordinary routine leukoplakia and acute gastric erosions. Those were the only three possible sources of entry that we found, and we could not incriminate any of them.

As far as this man's past history was concerned, on careful questioning he stated that he had never been ill a day in his life except for a contusion on the abdomen some two years ago, and so we can safely say his past history was very nearly completely negative.

HONOR ROLL FOR 1936

1. Randolph County, Dr. W. G. Elliott, Cuthbert, October 30, 1935.

2. Dougherty County, Dr. I. M. Lucas, Albany, December 27, 1935.

RELATION OF DRUGS TO THE LEUKOPENIC STATE*

ROY R. KRACKE, M.D.
FRANCIS P. PARKER, M.D.
Emory University

Agranulocytosis, or acute fulminant granulopenia, is a condition that has for its basic pathology a diminution, or disappearance, of the white blood cells, which apparently occurs in a definite sequence of events. The granulocytes and monocytes disappear first, then the lymphocytes become markedly decreased in number. Therefore, agranulocytosis is a disease characterized by diminution in all white cells. If the total white cell count of a patient is only six hundred lymphocytes, it is obvious that not only are the granulocytes involved, but the monocytes and some lymphocytes as well. Also, it is true that a patient may have a white cell count of 2,000 per cubic millimeter of blood and all of the cells be lymphocytes. Such a blood picture can still be construed as being a case of typical agranulocytosis.

Often-times the differential diagnosis between granulopenia and other leukopenic states is difficult. For example, in aplastic anemia is seen a marked leukopenia accompanied, however, by a correspondingly severe anemia with thrombocytopenia. In an acute case of agranulocytosis the red cells are not affected, but in some cases the thrombocytes become markedly decreased, especially in the terminal stages. In the aleukemic forms of leukemia there is also a marked diminution in the number of white cells, even to as low as 1,000 per cu. mm. The diagnosis can be made by observing the immaturity of the few remaining circulating leukocytes. If we continue to adhere to the original definition of agranulocytosis then we must consider it a disease characterized by a profound depression of the leukocytes with the red cells and blood platelets relatively unaffected.

Agranulocytosis was first described thirteen years ago in Germany, and eleven years ago in the United States. We have pointed

*Read before the Medical Association of Georgia, Atlanta, May 9, 1935.

out in previous publications the number of cases that have occurred in the United States. The deaths now number over 2,000, according to the United States Bureau of Vital Statistics. In Germany the disease seems quite prevalent, and probably it is widespread throughout Europe. However, during this same period there have been reported only fifteen cases in Great Britain. Hall, in a recent communication, states that the condition, in all probability, is much more common in England than these figures would suggest. Apparently the disease is worldwide in its distribution at this time, and certainly is seen more frequently in those countries in which modern drugs are in common use.

Our previous studies have shown that it occurs in people of all ages, but mainly in women of middle and old age. It occurs extremely infrequently among negroes, and when such cases are observed, there is usually a definite etiology such as the administration of neoarsphenamine.

It has occurred in people of the better class in the United States. Whether or not this type of person is unusually addicted to the use of modern drugs is open to question. We have shown in previous studies that the disease has a peculiar distribution among physicians, dentists, nurses and relatives of physicians. We believe this distribution can be explained by the fact that those people are more prone to use some of the more complex recently advocated drugs. Since the drug theory of etiology has become widespread and generally recognized by the medical profession, the number of cases at this time apparently are on the decline.

When agranulocytosis was first recognized in the United States and Germany, efforts were made by investigators to determine its etiology. Efforts were made to produce the disease by the injection of various bacteria, and the list of organisms includes practically all of those that have been recovered from the blood streams of patients. In no instance has agranulocytosis been produced in animals by the injection of any of these bacteria, whether dead or living.

Our attention was focused on a causal relationship to drug administration through a study of a patient that was admitted to the Emory University Hospital in 1931. The woman had a white cell count of 500 with a severe methemoglobinemia which was undoubtedly due to the long continued use of phenacetin. After studying the chemical structure of phenacetin we then investigated the drug history in all previous cases that we had observed and found that eight out of nine patients had taken one of the coal-tar drugs in considerable quantity prior to the clinical onset of the disease. We reported our findings in June, 1931[3], and that was the first publication pointing out the relationship between drug administration and agranulocytosis. We attempted also to produce the disease in laboratory animals by the injection and feeding of amidopyrine, phenacetin and allonal, but we were unable to produce it in rabbits, and all subsequent efforts to reproduce agranulocytosis in lower animals by ourselves and other investigators have been uniformly unsuccessful.

Our work was apparently unnoticed in the literature for approximately two years, and in 1933, Madison and Squier[2] reported their important clinical observations in which they showed that all of their fourteen cases of granulopenia had received amidopyrine prior to their clinical onset and further demonstrated that if the drug was removed, the mortality rate was considerably decreased. They had the courage to administer amidopyrine to two recovered cases and in both patients produced a recurrence of the disease. They then attempted to produce the condition in rabbits by the feeding of allonal, but were, in general, unsuccessful.

At the same time[3] we reported eleven cases of agranulocytosis which had been preceded by the administration of amidopyrine and other benzene ring drugs. Since these publications there have been reported 187 cases of agranulocytosis following the use of drugs. The following list states the number of cases and the drug incriminated in each instance: amidopyrine, 169; arsphenamine, 4; dinitrophenol, 7; neostibosan, 1; phenacetin, 2; gold salts, 4.

In all of the reported cases, drugs that contained the benzene ring with the attached NH[2], or amine group, have been incriminated,

while those that contain the ring without the attached NH[2] group, such as aspirin, are apparently harmless. The chief indictment is against amidopyrine. Amidopyrine differs from the other benzene ring drugs mainly by reason of its so-called pyrazolon attachment. In a recent article, Herz is inclined to lay the blame upon the pyrazolon attachment instead of the benzene ring. As we have subsequently pointed out, however, this conception is not tenable. It may be stated here that the six sided benzene ring, C^6H^6, is the only chemical with which we are capable of producing agranulocytosis in lower animals. In our theory concerning this, we advance the hypothesis that the NH[2] attachment is necessary merely because it facilitates ease of oxidation and further that benzene is probably oxidized either at the site of injection or in the gastro-intestinal tract to one of its oxidation products such as quinone.

We have further presented the hypothesis that when a benzamine drug is introduced into the gastro-intestinal tract, that it possibly undergoes oxidation to quinone, or hydroquinone, and that this substance is actually responsible for the depression of the bone marrow. Lately we have been able to oxidize amidopyrine and many of its combinations to quinone and have produced the disease in rabbits by injection of quinone.

Therefore, at this time it seems reasonable that all of those drugs that contain the benzene ring with the amine attachment, are potentially capable of producing the disease in both men and lower animals. These include mainly amidopyrine, dinitrophenol and phenacetin, and the gold salts have been reported as producing the disease in cases of tuberculosis.

The gold salts have as their central structure this benzamine ring with the attached gold molecule. The same is true of neostibosan used in the treatment of kala-azar. Arsphenamine is capable of producing the disease as well as other forms of bone marrow aplasia. Arsphenamine has for its central structure a double benzene ring with the arsenic attached, and it seems probable that its depressant action is due to its benzamine structure.

Unfortunately, amidopyrine has been

combined with different types of barbituric acid preparations, or barbiturates, by various manufacturers and this has resulted in the market being flooded with over one hundred different preparations containing amidopyrine as their essential ingredient.*

*A partial list of proprietary preparations that contain, or did contain amidopyrine:

Allonal, alphebin, amarbital, am-phen-al, ampydin, amytal compound, amido-neonal, amidophen, amidos, amidotal, amifeine, benzedo compound capsules, cibalgine, cinochopyrine, compral, cronal, dysco, gardan, gynalgos, hexin, ipralidon, kalms, lumodrin, midol, mylin, neonal compound, neurodyne, nod, optalidon, peralga, phenamidal, pyramidon, pyraminal.

Confirmation of this work has been reported from several countries, mainly Holland, Germany and Denmark. A group of workers in Copenhagen have reported no less than 40 cases following the use of amidopyrine or some of its combinations.

Many questions have arisen in connection with the drug relationship to agranulocytosis, and one of these has been its mechanism of action. Another question that can not be answered satisfactorily is why an occasional person develops the disease, whereas hundreds of others apparently show no ill effect from the use of the drug. We can only state that an occasional individual probably has a bone marrow sensitivity, or factors in the gastrointestinal tract in the oxidation of drugs that play an important part in the mechanism of its production.

Others seem to believe that the mechanism is an allergic one. There is little experimental, or clinical evidence to support this view. Many patients have been intradermally or patch tested with the various drugs without positive results.

It is believed also that the barbiturates are possibly involved in the process; however, there is little evidence to support that conception. We know of no case that has followed the sole administration of a barbiturate; and there are many instances of prolonged administration of drugs of this class followed by no leukocyte depression. A barbiturate is a straight chain carbon compound and does not contain the benzene ring.

A summation of opinions on this question indicates almost unanimous agreement that benzene ring drugs produce agranulocytosis.

It is probably equally true that some cases do not follow administration of drugs. For example, Heck studied one typical case carefully for a drug history and was unable to elicit any evidence thereof. Fitzhugh reviewed the histories of twenty-six patients and found that seventeen gave a drug history. In the remainder he was unable to state with certainty whether or not they had taken drugs. In two living patients he was unable to definitely rule out the administration of amidopyrine.

Johns[5] recently stated, "Of the ten cases I have seen I do not know of any that have not taken coal-tar compounds of one sort or another." Beck[8] who has had the disease resulting from allonal administration, has uncovered drug administration in all of her cases. Sturgis[6] found that of the nine cases studied at the University of Michigan, seven had followed the use of amidopyrine. He then gave amidopyrine to three who had recovered and this was followed by a profound leukopenia within four hours. Then he gave it to two healthy people without leukocyte depression occurring. He also gave barbital to a recovered patient and no leukocyte depression occurred. He states that from these observations it was apparent that certain individuals have an idiosyncrasy to amidopyrine. Sturgis further emphasized that in a large majority of patients amidopyrine may be taken in large doses without harmful effects and he sums up his attitude in the following statement: "With additional experience I am more and more convinced that amidopyrine is a precipitating factor in agranulocytosis. I am very ready to admit, however, that this syndrome can occur in persons who have never taken this drug."

What should be our attitude toward the use of amidopyrine and its combinations? These are admittedly very valuable drugs. Should they be discarded and their use be entirely discontinued? The Council on Pharmacy and Chemistry of the American Medical Association expresses the most desirable course in which they admit the dangers of amidopyrine, and recommend specifically the use of aspirin and codein, or a straight barbiturate; if it becomes necessary to use amidopyrine preparations it should be done as sparingly as possible, and under well controlled conditions, including a study of the leukocyte count for depression. The Canadian Medical Association Journal states that the coal-tar drugs as a whole should be used with caution. They recommend further the careful taking of histories with reference to drug administration.

The relationship of coal-tar drug administration to agranulocytosis has been generally accepted and demonstrated throughout this country and in some foreign countries. It does not seem logical to adopt an extreme view and discontinue the use of these drugs, but on the other hand they should be used and prescribed by physicians with considerable caution and only in those patients who can be kept under observation. This work indicates the necessity for drastic revision of our laws governing the sale of proprietary remedies. It seems advisable that this class of drugs be placed under the same rules and regulations as governs the dispensing of narcotics and should be available only on non-refillable physician's prescriptions. Some states have already passed such laws. It is hoped that the new Federal bill regulating the sale of proprietary and patent remedies will include measures to prevent the widespread and indiscriminate sale of drugs of this class.

The relationship of drugs to other leukopenic states should be mentioned. There is ample evidence to indicate a close relationship between leukopenic states in agranulocytosis and other blood dyscrasias. We saw a young girl with a white cell count of 600, and hemolytic streptococci in the blood stream, recover from an attack and four weeks later died with acute leukemia and a white cell count of 130,000. The increasing number of cases of myeloid leukemia that eventuate into the aleukemic state illustrates the tremendous range of bone marrow activity that may be seen in the same patient. Cases of aplastic anemia and aleukemic leukemia should be carefully questioned as to ingestion or contact with benzamine ring substances. One may become poisoned from benzene by inhalation, ingestion or by injection, as has been so well pointed out by Alice Hamilton[1].

German workers have reported the injection of mice with aniline over a long period of time and in some of the animals profound leukopenias were produced. In others there developed typical myeloid leukemias. We have been impressed by the possible association of some type of benzene poisoning to aplastic anemia. It behooves all of us, therefore, to take careful histories in our studies of these unusual and atypical blood dyscrasias characterized by the leukopenic state.

Treatment

The cause of agranulocytosis leads directly to the question of its treatment, since it has been shown by Madison and Squier[2] that the mortality rate of their cases was much lower in that group in which benzamine drugs were not used therapeutically. The first therapeutic procedure is to forbid the use of these drugs. If sedatives are required, aspirin, codeine, and the barbiturates should be used.

It seems questionable whether radiation therapy to the long bones is of value. Radiation has been advocated by many writers. When a damaged bone marrow is struggling to deliver a sufficient number of white cells to maintain life, its exposure to any so-called stimulating influence, is fraught with danger. Furthermore, there is wide divergence of opinion as to what radiation does to the immature cells of the marrow. Its influence may be one of destruction instead of stimulation, especially in view of the variation in reactivity of different bone marrows.

Lately there has been constant search for a specific agent that would stimulate the marrow cell production and regulate the output. Among those suggested are the nucleic acid products, of which a considerable number are available. The most recent one of this group now widely used, is pentnucleotide.

We have used this product in a considerable number of cases and it is our impression that it is of no value whatever since our mortality rate has not been lowered with its use. There is no experimental evidence to indicate that it is capable of raising the leukocyte count in either normal or leukopenic animals.

If there exists an agent capable of stimulating and regulating bone marrow production, it probably is to be found in the form of liver extract. We treated a woman whose total white cell count was 800 lymphocytes, with daily injections of Lederle solid liver extract, the daily dose being equivalent to 100 grams of liver, and obtained a leukocytosis of 30,000 on the fifth day, with recovery. We have had similar experiences with other patients with leukopenia. We strongly recommend the treatment of agranulocytosis by daily injections of liver extract.

It must be remembered that when the patient with this disease presents himself to the physician and the diagnosis is made, that the disease probably has existed for some days before the onset of clinical symptoms, and it is not unusual to first see the patient at a time when he is already overwhelmed with localized and generalized infections, and one should be cautious in claiming curative results in a disease characterized by such severe and widespread infections.

Progress has been made in ten years in the study of this disease; certainly, great progress in the study of its causes, but less in methods of its treatment. Perhaps the time will come when there will be no need for treatment if we are cautious in using pain relieving drugs, and prohibit their unrestricted use by the laity. The disease then may disappear from the face of the earth, and figures seem to indicate that this is now happening.

BIBLIOGRAPHY

1. Kracke, R. R.: "The Experimental Production of Agranulocytosis." Am. Jour. Clin. Path.: 2:11-30. 1932.
2. Madison, F. W., and Squier, T. L.: "The Etiology of Primary Granulocytopenia (Agranulocytic Angina)." Jour. Am. Med. Assn: 102:755-739. 1934.
3. Kracke, R. R., and Parker, F. P.: "The Etiology of Granulopenia (Agranulocytosis). With Particular Reference to Drugs Containing the Benzene Ring." Jour. Lab. and Clin. Med.: 19:799-818. 1934.
4. Johns, F. M.: Personal Communication. 1934.
5. Beck, R. C.: Personal Communication. 1934.
6. Sturgis, C.: Personal Communication. 1934.
7. Hamilton, Alice: "Industrial Poisons in the United States." MacMillan. 1925.

Discussion on Paper by Drs. Kracke and Parker

DR. CHARLES C. HINTON (Macon): I enjoy hearing Dr. Kracke talk on this subject, because I think there is no one in this section of the country who is as well qualified to discuss it.

I do not believe that the benzene-ring is by any means the primary factor in the causation of agranu-

locytosis. We used the benzene-ring drugs for many years before 1922, and it does seem that we would have picked up individuals who had sensitiveness or susceptibility to the drug in the bone marrow.

I believe that it has a very important part in a secondary agranulocytosis. Just as in the red blood cell side of the picture we have polycythemia vera, and we have normal red blood counts and primary and secondary anemias, I think the weight of evidence in the future is going to show that white cell changes follow similar lines. We have leukemias, monocytic, lymphatic, splenomyelogenous; we have responses to intoxications, infections and normal leukocyte counts; we have leukopenias due to infections that have been known for a long time, and we have the leukopenias in which the blockage is primarily in the neutrophilic leukocyte system.

R. P. Custer, of Philadelphia, claims that he can distinguish in bone marrow examinations between the agranulocytoses that are due to drugs and those that are primary, and due to a cessation in the production of the granulocytes.

Henry Jackson, of Boston, who has done a great work along this line, reports a number of cases that could be carefully studied as to their use of the drugs. He gave 26 per cent of his cases which he thought had evidence in favor of amidopyrine or some similar drug being responsible. He was willing to grant that they were very probably due to it. There are others in which attacks followed the use of benzene-ring drugs. Recovery was made, and benzene-ring drugs were given in larger doses, without any recurrence of attacks; and there were others in whom leaving off the benzene-ring drugs for quite a long time, secondary attacks did come.

In the six cases that I have seen, one was due to pancreatic carcinoma, and though I did not know of the drug theory at the time, I questioned this man's wife since and she says that he never took anything of the kind. He was a physician, however, and could have taken the drugs without her knowing it.

There were two typical cases with the ulcerations in the mouth, vagina, bladder, and pararectal abscesses. Of one of these I do not know the drug history. He lived outside of the state and I have not seen him since he recovered. The other patient states positively that she never used any of these drugs at all.

The fourth one was probably associated with endocrine disturbances, as she had recurrences of marked granulopenia, with absence of the neutrophils at two menstrual cycles before she died.

The fifth one was a woman who had used pyramidon quite freely for a number of months, several years in fact, before she developed the disease. She had a prolonged attack of it for two or three months before she died.

The last one is a case of anemia, and has a very marked diminution of the red cells and hemoglobin as well as a marked neutropenia.

DR. GEORGE L. ECHOLS (Hardwick): I do not come up here to add anything to your paper, Doctor, but to raise a question. In the state hospital in Milledgeville, one of the problems that we have to deal with at this time is that of drug delirium and confused states. We have much more of that now than in the past. The reason is obvious. You have your patients who develop acute psychoses, and you have to keep them at home or in crowded mental hospitals, and the only recourse is to keep your patient quiet with drugs. You do not see the ill effects much because you have one or two cases a year, while I have many.

I wonder if there is any relationship between confused states and these drug cases, the drug delirium, and so forth, with this agranulocytosis you are talking about. I wonder if there has been any work done along that line, and if any work should be done to investigate further.

We are well prepared to do that work at Milledgeville. We have ample clinical material that you folks are sending us, and it is not your fault that you are sending them to us. It is your misfortune, but mainly the misfortune of the patient.

Due to our very rich clinical material, we have unusually good laboratory facilities, and we have the men who are capable of making the observations, if this would be of any service. I am sure the state hospital is at your disposal, and Dr. Oden and his staff would be very glad, I think, to have any suggestions.

DR. C. K. WALL (Thomasville): This question of agranulocytosis in the past few years has come to the attention of the profession in our part of the state. In the hospital at Thomasville we have had ten or twelve cases since 1925 or 1926. I have been called in on them secondarily, as my work is primarily surgical, as the medical men call us in to give transfusions.

I was very much interested in Dr. Kracke's paper, and the amount of work he has done on this subject. I think he is due a lot of credit. Dr. Hinton states that we have been using benzene drugs for a number of years but haven't been seeing this particular disease. I think we have seen it and did not know what it was. The cases I have seen in consultation, eight or nine, practically all came in with a primary symptom of sore throat. The ages were from a child of six to an old doctor of seventy-six.

Our mortality has been a hundred per cent. The only thing we have found that did any particular good was pentnucleotide. The transfusion seems to help temporarily. It gives you a bridging over for the time being until you can get your pentnucleotide to your patient and raise your blood count. Any disease that is this ravaging in its effect certainly merits the most concentrated attention we can give it.

Evidently the drugs are not causative agents in all cases. One was a child of six years who came in with a sore throat of streptococcus origin. That child had not been taking amidopyrine. We do not know what the old doctor had taken. Another was a case of the town sexton, not the type of person who would have gotten the drug. I think we will have to look further than this drug group for the etiology of it.

In looking back over these cases, you will find the symptoms come in cycles. The symptoms we have seen are secondary to the primary underlying cause. This anemia sets in and they will go to bed and stay in bed three or four days or a week, and nature in its turn comes to the aid of the patient and he gets better, but in our cases, after a painstaking history, we find they have had several attacks before they are finally brought to the hospital.

I hope somebody will devise some treatment more effective than ours.

DR. ROY R. KRACKE (Atlanta): Concerning many cases of agranulocytosis in which it is difficult to obtain a history of drug administration, I should like to stress the difficulty of obtaining a history of drug administration. In attempting to collect data on this point from eleven patients, we found that approximately half of these had taken drugs of this class before their disease developed and it required the most intensive work and detailed investigation to find this out in the other half. We have even had to go to prescription files and to physicians' records, and we have also looked up their accounts in drug stores, and even then we have had to chemically analyze drugs after we have found out that certain patients were taking them, in order to find out what they contained. Only by painstaking work can a drug history be uncovered in some of these patients. To merely question the relatives of a deceased patient as to whether or not they have had drugs, is of no value.

Furthermore, we are confronted with the large number of proprietary and patented compounds containing amidopyrine which patients take from time to time without the knowledge of their physician. Among the hundreds of preparations on the druggists' shelves, we have no way of knowing which may or may not contain it.

It is my opinion that this disease did not exist to any appreciable extent before 1922, in this country. It is so easy of diagnosis, so outstanding in its clinical manifestations, that men of the caliber of Osler and other men of that time would, no doubt, have recognized it.

It may be pointed out that amidopyrine has been on the market for fifty years or more. It was only in 1922 that this drug came to be a central ingredient in so many of the proprietary preparations, and the drug virtually flooded the country at that time.

Relative to the hormone theory, or the relation of menstruation to this disease, many cases have been reported in which the attack seemed to occur at the time of menstruation. On investigation, however, many of these are women that have had severe pain.

at the time of menstruation and have resorted to self-medication at that time.

I do not have any data relative to the relationship of drug therapy in mental states to agranulocytosis, but in an institution like the one at Milledgeville there should be a great opportunity to carry out a very detailed study as to the effect of many of these drugs in those patients that have received them over a long period of time.

The last speaker introduced the question of treatment. Our experience has been similar to his; that is, we have used the nucleotide products and found our mortality rate to be the same, and apparently they have been of little value. In our more recent cases, however, we have used liver extract, and if there is a preparation that has value in this disease I think it is the injectable preparation of liver extract.

SCIENTIFIC MANAGEMENT OF ANAL FISSURE*

CHAS. E. HALL, M.D.
Atlanta

Anal fissure, which consists of a break, tear or ulcer in the anal mucosa, is a condition of common occurrence, and though seemingly a simple, insignificant lesion, it may cause excruciating pain and considerable disability. Fifteen to 25 per cent of the patients seen by the proctologist are suffering with this condition. In a recent series of a thousand rectal cases, both private and clinic cases, 251 cases of anal fissure were encountered.

All fissures do not present the same pathologic characteristics, consequently treatment must be varied according to the condition present. In general, successful management will depend upon three factors: First, determination of the etiological agent; second, understanding of the disease present; and third, an accurate knowledge of the anatomical structure and physiological function of the anal canal.

From an etiologic standpoint, fissures may be separated into two groups, the traumatic and the non-traumatic. Non-traumatic fissures or ulcers result from some specific underlying infection of the peri-anal skin and the anal mucous membrane. The more common infections causing this condition are:

epidermophytosis, chancroid, chancre, secondary lues, gonorrhea, tuberculosis and granuloma. The diagnosis of these various infections depends upon the history, the clinical manifestations and various laboratory procedures, such as smears, cultures and blood tests. Treatment of these infectious fissures must necessarily include the proper therapy for the underlying causative disease.

The great majority of fissures are traumatic in origin, resulting from constipation, straining at stool, passing of foreign bodies in the stools, or rough instrumentation of the anus and rectum.

Most of the traumatic fissures are located in the posterior mid-line, due to the anatomical arrangement of the fibers of the external sphincter muscle. Only a few of the fibers encircle the anus at this point, most of them deviating posteriorly on either side to reach their attachment to the coccyx, thus leaving a potential weak spot in the posterior commissure.

For the purpose of treatment the simple traumatic fissures are classified into two groups, the acute and the chronic. This classification is made according to the disease present, and the fissure considered acute if it is one of short duration, without the presence of purulent infection, connecting sinuses, a sentinel skin tab or induration of the surrounding tissues.

This type of fissure is characterized by severe pain and marked spasm of the sphincter; consequently, treatment must be directed toward the relief of pain and relaxation of the sphincter. It has been proved conclusively that the sensory nerve supply of the anal mucosa is intimately associated with the motor nerve supply of the sphincter ani; so that any painful lesion of the anus causes increased contraction of the sphincter, which, in turn, results in exaggeration of the pain and delay in the healing process. Bearing this physiologic fact in mind, one must direct treatment toward the complete relief of pain, which will result in sufficient relaxation of the muscle spasm to allow the fissure to heal.

The use of prolonged local anesthesia, an agent of comparatively recent development,

*Read before the Medical Association of Georgia, Atlanta, May 10, 1935.

has proved very helpful in treating the acute type of traumatic fissure. Some of the solutions employed to maintain prolonged anesthesia are: quinine urea hydrochloride, nupercain, benacol, St. Mark's Solution, and diothane.

The treatment which I have found most effective for the acute traumatic fissure is as follows: With antiseptic precautions a small quantity, 2 or 3 cc. of 1 per cent novocain is injected beneath the fissure to obtain immediate anesthesia. For prolonged anesthesia the tissues beneath and surrounding the lesion are then infiltrated with 1 per cent diothane. When the anesthesia is complete the fissure is cauterized with 10 to 20 per cent silver nitrate.

The after treatment consists of ample mineral oil to insure easy bowel actions, hot sitz baths two or three times daily, and daily applications of mild antiseptics such as mercurochrome, merthiolate or S.T. 37. Healing will take place in the majority of cases in ten days to two weeks by these simple measures. If complete healing does not occur in a reasonable length of time, then the fissure must be treated as a chronic lesion.

A traumatic fissure is considered chronic if it is of more than a few days duration and presents one or more of the following pathological characteristics: a sentinel pile or skin tab, purulent infection, connecting sinuses, infected anal crypts with hypertrophied papillae, or induration of the surrounding tissues.

Treatment of this type of fissure, in order to be successful, must not only relieve pain and sphincterospasm, but also must establish adequate drainage. A procedure which I have found most satisfactory is as follows: The involved area is anesthetized by local infiltration, using a small quantity of 1 per cent novocain for immediate effect, plus a sufficient quantity of 1:1000 nupercain solution for prolonged effect. I have found that it is not necessary to use large quantities of solution for the local anesthesia, usually 10 to 15 cc. being quite sufficient. It is not necessary to anesthetize the whole sphincter or the entire anal canal, it being sufficient to anesthetize merely the involved area of tissue. This procedure greatly lessens the possibility of toxic reaction which may occur with the use of larger quantities of anesthetic agents. When the anesthesia is complete a bi-valve anal retractor is inserted and adjusted to give clear view of all structures involved. A careful search is made with a hook-shaped probe for sinuses or involved anal crypts, and any that are found are excised with the scissors. More often than not an infected anal crypt will be located beneath a chronic anal fissure, and adequate drainage will not be obtained unless this crypt be excised. Next, an incision is made with a sharp scalpel, beginning above the fissure at the ano-rectal or papillary line, and extending longitudinally downward to the anus, and thence externally for a distance of one and a half to two inches on the perianal skin. The depth of the incision is approximately one-half inch and is sufficient to sever those fibers of the sphincter which decussate posteriorly. These decussating fibers constitute a definite tendinous-like band which can be clearly demonstrated at operation, and which has been designated the Pecten band. By severing this band of fibers sufficient relaxation is obtained without actually dividing the entire sphincter.

After this incision is made all overhanging edges of skin and mucous membrane, together with the sentinel skin tab, are freely ablated with the scissors. The retractor is now withdrawn and the wound packed with a small piece of vaseline gauze in order to keep the edges of the incision separated and to control the slight hemorrhage present. A firm cotton pad is applied to the anus and the patient confined to bed for twelve to twenty-four hours. The bowels are not confined for any great extent of time, a movement being allowed after twenty-four hours.

Careful postoperative attention is essential for good results, and the surgeon personally should dress the incision daily. The wound edges must be kept separated so that healing will take place from the bottom up by healthy granulation. Mild antiseptics are applied locally and any excessive granulations kept down with silver nitrate. The skin portion of the incision is kept open until the mucous membrane of the anal portion is entirely healed, in order to insure adequate drainage for any infection present. Ample mineral oil to render the stools soft, and frequent hot sitz baths are valuable aids in promoting the healing process. Generally, the patient is able to return to his usual occupation after two or three days and healing is complete in about two weeks.

Discussion on Paper By Dr. Chas. E. Hall

DR. HULETT H. ASKEW (Atlanta) : The first cardinal principle in dealing with a fissure is not to attempt any examination until some procedure has been made to prevent pain. These patients are usually nervous, caused either by the fissure itself or by some previous examination. Therefore, I apply a few drops of 4 to 8 per cent cocaine mixed in KY jelly around the anal outlet and massage this for a few moments before attempting to pass a gloved finger into the rectum. The muscles relax and the patient does not lose confidence. A fair examination can be made without danger by this procedure.

After an external examination has been made and it has been deemed necessary to carry out some surgical procedure, all aseptic precautions being taken around the anal outlet, a swab dipped in 50 per cent carbolic acid in oil is applied to the skin, which is rubbed off with alcohol, to prevent pain from the first needle insertion. It is better to do a local infiltration with 2 per cent novocaine followed by 1:1000 nupercaine, as I am confident that the greater number of patients suffering with fissure need a divulsion at the beginning of treatment. By divulsion I mean a careful and general stretching of the sphincters, which are always spastic. Stretching puts them at rest and improves the venous congestion.

After the above procedure, the uncomplicated fissure-in-ano may often be cured. However, after a complete inspection of the entire anus and rectum is made, the disease noted and no complications seen, the fissures are touched their entire length with the actual cautery. If bleeding hemorrhoids are present, they are injected with 5 per cent carbolic acid in Wesson oil.

The complicated fissure-in-ano is another story demanding a certain degree of surgical judgment, for it is following an operation not thoroughly carried out where we find so many chronic fissures, which have healed with the exception of a persistent crack in the anal opening that defies all ordinary treatment. This crack splits at intervals, bleeds and causes moisture, which in turn frequently causes pruritus and excoriation of the anal skin.

As the first step in the handling of an indurated complicated fissure, with the divulsion complete. An incision deeper than the fissure is started at the apex or distal end of the fissure and carried down one side of the fissure well out into the skin. Another incision is begun at the same starting point as the first

incision and carried down the opposite side of the fissure for the same distance as the first. The outer ends should be at least a quarter of an inch from each other, forming an inverted "V." The two incisions should be connected at their base by another incision and the wedge or triangle shaped piece of skin should be dissected out to the anorectal margin or to the high point of the fissure. The skin, sinus, if one exists, hypertrophied papillae and the entire fissure is included in the dissection. Clean tissue is left. The excised area which is properly cared for—namely, by hot sitz-baths, 1 per cent nupercain ointment, passing of a gloved finger and administering mineral oil, heals rapidly and stays healed, unless there be a hemorrhoid on either side which would in itself prevent healing. In such a patient I always inject these hemorrhoids immediately after the operation with 5 per cent phenol in Wesson oil. The incision within the anal canal must be made to heal first, and it will if a high spot of granulation is not permitted to form, or the skin edges allowed to heal together dividing the incision into upper and lower sections and damming the secretion back into the upper end of the incision.

The after effects of all operations performed in the office for fissure-in-ano were formerly very painful and annoying when the effect of local anesthetics began to wear off, but since the advent of reliable, prolonged local anesthesia that lasts from one day to two weeks, this work is satisfactory. My favorite formula for prolonged local anesthesia consists of:

Nupercaine	0.5%
Benzyl Alcohol	10%
Phenol	1%
Olive Oil	93%

The second best formula is St. Mark's formula or A. B. A. Solution. and consists of:

Anesthesin	3%
Benzyl Alcohol	10%
Ether	10%
Olive Oil	82%

The third best is:

Quinine, Urea Hydrochloride	5%
Procaine	2%

One per cent diothane solution, benacol or 20 per cent ethyl alcohol will accomplish the same purpose.

DR. GEO. L. ECHOLS (Milledgeville) : In handling painful ailments, such as the above, I wish to sound the warning that it is very essential that the physician in charge keep in mind the possibility of doing further damage to the patient by the use of sedative drugs. You general practitioners see your side of the case, but you would certainly be surprised if you observed the cases which my colleagues and myself at the State Hospital receive for treatment. We are getting many cases of bromide intoxication in delirious conditions, and we are also finding very bad results from some of the newer drugs, which are advertised as being entirely harmless.

THE CHRONIC COUGH*

ROBERT C. PENDERGRASS, M.D.
Americus

Every patient with a chronic cough has a right to a thorough examination to determine the cause of this cough. It is so easy to simply prescribe a cough medicine; often more difficult to determine what is causing the cough. The large number of cough syrups on the market is an index to the prevalence of chronic coughs and a monument to our failures in curing them.

Any cough persisting beyond the usual period of an acute disease with which it is associated, if any, may be termed a chronic cough.

The causes of chronic cough are numerous but may be divided into groups as follows:

Group One. Nasal, throat, laryngeal and sinus disease.

Group Two. Disease of the trachea and the bronchi-foreign bodies, asthma, bronchiectasis, tracheobronchial tumors, and so-called "chronic catarrhal bronchitis."

Group Three. Diseases of the lung itself; tuberculosis, spirochetosis, influenza, lung abscess, tumors, foreign bodies, cysts, fungus infections, emphysema, lipoid pneumonia, and tularemia.

Group Four. Diseases of the pleura, pleural effusions, empyema, adhesions, metastatic involvement of the pleura, Ewing's tumor of the ribs with pleural extension, subphrenic abscess with pleural involvement, and calcification of the pleura.

Group Five. Mediastinal disease, tuberculosis of the mediastinal glands, Hodgkins disease, mediastinal tumors and Pott's abscess.

Group Six. Thymus, thyroid disease, persistent thymus, thymoma (a peculiar type of thymic neoplasm), goiter (both cervical and substernal).

Group Seven. Diseases of the esophagus

*Read before the Medical Association of Georgia, Atlanta, May 10, 1935.

much lifting, may have a cough due to heart failure.

A careful physical examination may readily reveal the cause of a chronic cough. I would particularly emphasize the importance of a routine transillumination of the sinuses. This can be done with a small lamp attached to a flash light battery or a rheostat. Inspection of the posterior pharyngeal wall for mucous drippings is equally important. Careful examination of the chest and heart is obviously necessary. If practical, the chest should be examined by x-ray in every case of chronic cough. If transillumination of the sinuses yields any suspicious findings they should be confirmed by x-ray examination. Opaque oils (Lipiodol or Iodochlorol) may be injected into the sinuses or into the trachea in order to gain additional information not available on plain films. Skin tests may reveal an allergy to some food or pollen producing hay fever or asthma with cough.

It is wise to consider first the common causes of chronic cough; if these are eliminated then the unusual causes may be considered. Of the common causes I wish to emphasize the following: First, chronic sinus and tonsillar infections; second, heart failure; third, tuberculosis.

The increasing incidence of cancer should make us always think of this as a possible cause. In children foreign bodies, tuberculosis and bronchiectasis are always to be considered. Bronchiectasis following whooping cough is more common than is generally supposed. Haygood has studied a large number of cases of spirochetal infections of the lung at Alto, sent in with a diagnosis of tuberculosis. Careful sputum studies have established the true nature of these cases.

Whatever the cause of the chronic cough, however t e d i o u s, time-consuming, and troublesome the examination to find this cause, give your patient your best efforts at determining it. Don't give him a bottle of cough medicine and a slap on the back and tell him to come back in two or three weeks if he is not better. The only excuse for prescribing in this manner is the discovery of an incurable condition in which symptomatic relief is the only thing you can offer.

INTRAMEDULLARY TUMORS

Report of Case

J. CALVIN WEAVER, M.D.
Atlanta

When one witnesses the trepidation experienced by many surgeons when approaching the enucleation of a false neuroma either of fibrous or myxomatous tissue growing in the center of a nerve, with the nerve fibres spread around it, it is not surprising, as no one could contemplate with complacency the possibility of such a procedure resulting in wrist-drop or foot-drop or a claw-hand from damage to one or another of the major peripheral nerves.

How much greater should be the concern when approaching an intramedullary spinal cord tumor that can not be felt or seen, and if located accurately, may end in permanent paralysis of one or more limbs and a loss of sphincter control.

Twenty years ago this was the melancholic outlook surrounding an attempted removal of spinal cord tumors. Today, the outlook is more favorable as the result of an orderly procedure based on a special technic, with a carefully worked out anatomical foundation developed particularly by Elsburg as "another evidence of the restless forward march of scientific surgery."

While an all-wise providence seems to have arranged anatomy with an eye toward suitable surgical approaches in general, spinal surgery is no exception and special arrangements of the spinal cord fibres have made the removal of intramedullary tumors possible, though the intramedullary growth naturally is calculated to cause more damage than a tumor growing from the meninges.

It is generally conceded that spinal cord tumors for the most part arise from the meninges. That being the case a familiarity with symptoms of the extramedullary growths will help in recognizing the occasional intramedullary growth.

Symptomatology

Neuralgic pains in the area supplied by a certain nerve, sometimes disappearing to recur later are generally the first symptoms. It usually affects one side, then later passes to the other, persisting for a year or several years before fresh symptoms appear as these tumors are generally of slow growth. If it begins on an anterior or motor root, naturally motor excitement in a localized area will appear, such as tremor or spasm, later followed by degenerative paralysis of the corresponding muscles. Of course, if large enough to compress both motor and sensory roots, there will be found the combination of pain and paralysis and later absence of reflexes. Compression of the spinal cord above the lumbar region results in spastic paralysis with exaggeration of the reflexes. Frequently in the early stage, motor weakness is limited to one leg, with hyperaesthesia or an anesthesia of the opposite leg, constituting the Brown-Sequard syndrome. Bladder and rectal symptoms appear early in the nature of functional disturbance. Beginning with increased desire to urinate, "imperative micturition," it gradually changes to incontinence of the bowel and bladder.

Intramedullary Tumors

There is great difficulty in determining whether a new growth arises within the cord or from the meninges and roots. In tumors of the cord substance, the root symptoms such as unilateral pain and absence of reflexes are not prominent early in the disease. In the cord, there is a resemblance to ascending myelitis. On account of fibres to the feet being deeper in the cord than the ones higher up, foot symptoms are seen early, such as pain in the bottom of foot followed by a drawing of the leg.

Technic

After the orthodox laminectomy has been done and the cord is exposed by opening the dura, an incision is made over the lesion in the posterior column near the median column, the higher the level, the nearer the incision should be to the median line. The arachnoid is first incised and grasped with a fine forceps; then the incision made less than 5 cm. in length. The enlarging and deepening is done with a blunt instrument.

The incision into the cord being made, the operative wound is carefully closed layer by layer to be reopened a week later, when the

Pathological Report (Dr. Bishop)

The pathological sections show edematous vascular neural tissue, moderately cellular and with considerable calcification. The bulk of the tissue is composed of masses of fibrilli with scattered lymphocytes and occasional polys. There seems to be a small area of necrosis and no specially cellular areas.

Final Diagnosis.

Glioma of spinal cord.

Summary

1. A case of an unusually large intramedullary tumor of the spinal cord, glioma in type, is reported in a patient still living four and one-half years after a two-step operation.

2. An attempt is made at a differential diagnosis between an intramedullary tumor and an extramedullary tumor, particularly the early foot symptoms in the intramedullary lesion.

3. Attention is called to the curability of nearly all extramedullary tumors by surgical intervention, and the great improvement and sometimes cure of the intramedullary tumors when handled by the "extrusion" technic as devised by Elsburg.

THE TREATMENT OF PARALYTIC MUSCLES BY ACTIVE AND PASSIVE EXERCISE AND THE IMPORTANCE OF DIET

Report of Case

M. F. CARSON, M.D.

Griffin

A majority of cases of cerebral hemorrhage are due to a rupture of the middle cerebral artery. From this hemorrhage a clot is formed. If the hemorrhage is sufficient and the clot large enough, there is total and complete paralysis of all the muscles of the upper and lower extremities of the opposite side and loss of speech.

Report of Case

A white male physician, aged 62, while sitting in his office August 15, 1934, was taken suddenly with hemiplegia of the right side, followed by loss of speech. Twenty-four hours after the hemorrhage, every muscle in his right arm and right leg was totally paralyzed.

The patient was given the usual saline cathartic, an ice cap to his head and a liquid diet. He was kept in bed, or rather was unable to get out of bed for three weeks. He then became unruly; refused to remain in bed or to confine himself to a liquid diet. He insisted on a substantial diet, saying that a liquid diet of soup would neither make or sustain muscles. He argued that nature would remove the clot by absorption, and that it was his job to take care of his muscles or he would be an invalid; that it was his life and he did not propose to let his muscles atrophy, and he ordered ham, cabbage, corn bread, one-half gallon milk a day, beef juice, oat meal, eggs, toast, etc. He had a man carry him to the bath tub twice a day. He began to massage the affected side, had himself assisted to the porch; a few days later, went to Warm Springs for bathing and repeated the routine every other day for weeks, noting improvement every trip. He made a dozen efforts to walk to town; finally got to his office. He drove his car to make calls, taking off his shoe on the right foot in order to feel the pedal. He walked every day, almost to exhaustion; would stop to rest on doorstep of patients' homes. He would never allow anyone, not even his wife, to assist him in dressing himself, always making the paralyzed hand make the effort; though it failed, he tried again and again until it performed. For the passive exercise he went to the osteopath every day for fourteen months. He went swimming every day. He did not allow anything to interfere with his routine exercise. Every afternoon for twelve months he would throw a rubber ball against a barn two hundred times. After sixteen months of effort, his prediction has come true: nature has practically removed the pressure, his muscles are firm and active, and he is practically well. There is still the crossed condition of the mind and a slight incoordination of some of the muscles.

He took 20 grains of potassium iodide three times daily for ninety days, and has taken six ounces of wheat oil (20 m. daily), and feels confident that the vitamin E in the oil is as much a specific for the muscle cells as the vitamin in cod liver oil is for rickets or bone cells. He has made a gradual recovery, about the same percentage each month for sixteen months, and he is practically well; practicing medicine, driving his own car, making calls day and night.

Comment

Much has been said, much money has been spent and some progress made in the treatment of infantile paralysis in the way of exercising the muscles not affected, proper diet, and especially application of proper braces, but the adult paralytic is "the forgotten man"; very little interest is taken in the treatment of hemiplegia.

It is my opinion that the great majority of hemiplegias, granting that they survive the hemorrhage, should get well or practically well, under proper active, vigorous, intelligent treatment, but it must be started early and kept up vigorously.

THE JOURNAL
OF THE
MEDICAL ASSOCIATION OF GEORGIA
Devoted to the Welfare of the Medical Association of Georgia

478 Peachtree Street, N.E., Atlanta, Ga.

FEBRUARY, 1936

ANEMIA

In the last decade, much progress has been made in the field of hematology. It is obvious, therefore, with all this accumulated data, that space will not permit the discussion of all varieties of anemia. Within the limits assigned, consideration is given to pernicious anemia, the iron deficiency anemias and the anemias associated with pregnancy.

Logical diagnosis of anemia ultimately depends on the determination of the fundamental factor producing the disease and the correlation between these factors and the morphologic and functional changes of the blood. Treatment consists in eliminating these factors, or by some measure compensating for them.

Pernicious anemia is a disease now easily controlled, but a crippling or death dealing one with late or inaccurate diagnosis. It is necessary to recognize its presence early and institute proper and adequate therapy.

Since the momentous work of Whipple and, later, that of Minot and Murphy, it has been demonstrated that there are certain factors influencing the development of pernicious anemia, the outstanding one being the relation between an unidentified substance found in whole liver or liver-extract and the maturation of the red blood cells. This substance will cause the blood of a patient with pernicious anemia to return to normal in the absence of complicating conditions. It remained for Castle and his associates to reveal the relation between stomach disorder and production of pernicious anemia. He clearly showed the presence of a substance in the gastric juice of normal individuals which is absent or present in diminished quantities in patients with pernicious anemia (intrinsic factor of Castle). Further, he demonstrated that this intrinsic factor must react with another unidentified substance, the extrinsic factor of the diet, to form a heat

Chronic hemorrhage seems to be the most common cause of iron deficiency anemia. Constant loss of the metal, over long periods of time, depletes the reserves. The logical therapy is control of all bleeding points. The anemia will slowly respond with adequate iron in the diet, but much more rapidly if additional iron is given as a therapeutic measure.

A disease recently brought to the attention of the profession, and seemingly on the increase, is the anemia of middle-aged women, (idiopathic hypochromic anemia), occurring without excessive loss of blood and despite an ample amount of iron in the diet. These patients regularly show achlorhydria or hypochlorhydria. It has been demonstrated that free hydrochloric acid favors the absorption of iron and this apparently plays an important role in this type of anemia.

Although the red blood cell level may not be depressed in iron deficiency anemia, the cells themselves are functionally inadequate. The morphologic structure is changed so that a Price-Jones curve would show a microcytic anemia in contradistinction to the macrocytic type of red blood cell found to predominate in pernicious anemia and related anemias. As liver promotes proper cell maturation in pernicious anemia so does iron effect maturation in the deficiency anemias. It is worth while noting that iron is in no way effective in macrocytic anemia and liver, likewise, is not effective in microcytic anemia.

Having a knowledge of the factors concerned in the production of the above types of anemia simplifies both diagnosis and treatment of the anemias associated with pregnancy. It must be understood that pregnancy can occur in the presence of a deficiency anemia or pernicious anemia and does not change either the diagnosis or the treatment.

A mild type of anemia is almost always associated with pregnancy and is considered, by most clinicians, to be physiologic. The general assumption is that hydremia is responsible.

Appearing during pregnancy is a macrocytic type of anemia which differs from pernicious anemia in that there is found the presence of free hydrochloric acid in the gastric juice, higher white blood count, the absence of glossitis and the absence of cord changes. This type resembles pernicious anemia in its response to liver therapy, icteric tint to the skin, high color index and the absence of response to iron therapy.

The microcytic anemia (idiopathic hyperchromic anemia) occurring during pregnancy resembles that already described and responds promptly to iron therapy.

Transfusion in any of the above types of anemia may hasten recovery. Particularly is this true when the blood constituents are low and when the anemia appears during a pregnancy.

C. W. STRICKLER, JR., M.D.

THE CANCER PROBLEM IN GEORGIA

Cancer as a health and life problem cannot easily be set aside!

In this issue of the *Journal*, page 67, Mr. Butler Toombs, Chief of the State Bureau of Vital Statistics, presents an analysis of Georgia's cancer mortality the past thirteen years. It is intensely interesting and instructive and we hope it will receive the careful study it deserves.

Thirty years ago tuberculosis was the leading cause of death. Early in the present century an intensive campaign of education was launched by the medical profession and the public press, with the result that the morbidity and mortality from tuberculosis has been so reduced that it can no longer be properly called "The Great White Plague."

What education has done for tuberculosis, it should do for cancer!

In order to place the facts about cancer squarely before the profession and the people of Georgia, the Cancer Commission of the Medical Association of Georgia has undertaken to find out the number of people in the State who have cancer, how and where they are being cared for, and what method is best for securing treatment for the masses who are unable to care for themselves.

In the spring of 1935, questionnaires were sent to 1,560 doctors living in 155 counties of Georgia. These questionnaires were returned by only 350 doctors from 93 counties

—an indication of woeful lack of interest. In this survey, 400 cancer cases were reported as having been treated during 1934. Many of the doctors had not seen a cancer in several years.

It was then decided to complete the hospital survey begun two years ago. Accordingly, questionnaires were sent to 78 hospitals, representing 4,322 beds, where general surgical and cancer patients are admitted. Replies have been received from hospitals having a total of 75 per cent of the available beds. In these hospitals, 1,351 cancer patients, less than 250 of whom were negroes, had been treated in 1934. In Emory University unit of Grady Hospital, where only negroes are admitted, there were 185 cancer patients.

The 1,351 patients treated for cancer represents 25 per cent of Georgia's estimated annual cancer population. The average life of a cancer patient in the South is approximately three years; therefore, in order to estimate the number of living patients with cancer, multiply the number of deaths by three.

In this series there were three times as many women as men. The classification according to location of the lesion in 835 patients was as follows: the buccal cavity, 4 per cent; digestive tract and peritoneum, 16 per cent; female genital organs, 42 per cent; breast, 12 per cent; skin, 11 per cent; all other organs and parts of the body were involved in 17 per cent.

The mortality report from the Bureau of Vital Statistics and the report of cases treated in the various hospitals throughout the State coincide except for cancer of the digestive tract and peritoneum and cancer of the female genital organs. In the Bureau report 39 per cent of deaths are due to cancer of the digestive tract and peritoneum; in the hospital report only 16 per cent of admissions were diagnosed as such. Again, in the Bureau report 21 per cent of deaths are listed as resulting from cancer of the female genital organs; the hospital report shows admissions of 42 per cent for this condition. It is not easy to explain these variations except for the fact that the intensive campaign of education being waged by the Cancer Commission and

GEORGIA DEPARTMENT OF PUBLIC HEALTH

T. F. ABERCROMBIE, M.D., *Director*

CANCER MORTALITY IN GEORGIA

Since 1921 the death rate from cancer in Georgia has shown an average annual increase of 1.1 per 100,000 population. This increase has been decidedly higher for the white population than for the colored. In 1921 there were 1321 more deaths from tuberculosis than from cancer, but in 1934 the number of deaths from tuberculosis exceeded those from cancer by only 10. There are approximately 5,000 people in Georgia suffering from cancer at any given time and over 1,700 of these die every year. Indeed, cancer is now one of the major problems in health and life conservation.

The question is often raised as to whether there is an actual increase in cancer or whether the apparent increase is due to better diagnosis and diagnostic methods. Physicians are reporting more cancer deaths than ever before. It is true that with the lengthening span of life there are more people reaching the age when cancer is more common? We must agree that the increase shown in tables 2 and 3 is proof that the number of cancer deaths is increasing over and above any advance in diagnosis.

Table 2 shows the deaths and death rate per 100,000 population by sex, color and location of the lesion. The total death rate

TABLE 2.—DEATHS AND DEATH RATES PER 100,000 POPULATION, FROM CANCER, BY SEX, AND COLOR, IN GEORGIA: 1930 AND 1934

SUBJECT		BOTH SEXES			MALES			FEMALES		
		Total	White	Col.	Total	White	Col.	Total	White	Col.
		NUMBER								
Cancer Total	1930	1552	1105	447	568	442	126	984	663	321
	1934	1762	1272	490	651	507	144	1111	765	346
Buccal Cavity	1930	79	60	19	51	41	10	28	19	9
	1934	82	71	11	46	42	4	36	29	7
Digestive Tract and Peritoneum	1930	553	399	154	259	187	72	294	212	82
	1934	701	528	173	339	258	81	362	270	92
Female Genital Organs	1930	355	207	148	-----	-----	-----	355	207	148
	1934	378	219	159	-----	-----	-----	378	219	159
Breast	1930	134	93	41	2	-----	2	132	93	39
	1934	160	114	46	5	3	2	155	111	44
Skin	1930	72	68	4	51	48	3	21	20	1
	1934	69	67	2	46	45	1	23	22	1
Unspecified Organs	1930	359	278	81	205	166	39	154	112	42
	1934	372	273	99	215	159	56	157	114	43
		RATE PER 100,000 POPULATION								
Cancer Total	1930	53.3	60.0	41.7	39.5	47.9	24.5	66.6	72.2	57.5
	1934	58.6	66.5	44.7	43.9	53.0	27.4	72.9	80.1	60.7
Buccal Cavity	1930	2.7	3.3	1.8	3.5	4.4	1.9	1.9	2.1	1.6
	1934	2.7	3.7	1.0	3.1	4.4	.8	2.4	3.1	1.2
Digestive Tract and Peritoneum	1930	19.0	21.7	14.4	18.0	20.3	14.0	19.9	23.1	14.7
	1934	23.3	27.6	15.8	22.9	27.0	15.4	23.7	28.3	16.1
Female Genital Organs	1930	-----	-----	-----	-----	-----	-----	24.0	22.5	26.5
	1934	-----	-----	-----	-----	-----	-----	24.8	23.0	27.9
Breast	1930	4.6	5.1	3.8	.1	-----	.4	8.9	10.1	7.0
	1934	5.3	6.0	4.2	.3	.3	.4	10.2	11.6	8.0
Skin	1930	2.5	3.7	.4	3.5	5.2	.6	1.4	2.2	.2
	1934	2.3	3.5	.2	3.1	4.7	.2	1.5	2.3	.2
Unspecified Organs	1930	12.3	15.1	7.5	14.3	18.0	7.6	10.4	12.2	7.5
	1934	12.4	14.3	9.0	14.5	16.6	10.7	10.3	12.0	7.5

for cancer of the buccal cavity for male and the rate for white males remained the sam
female was 2.7 per 100,000 in 1930 and . However, the death rate of 3.1 per cent f
1934. In the colored race both sexes showed a white females in 1934 was 48 per cent high
decrease in their rates for 1934 over 1930; than the rate of 2.1 per cent in 1930. Th

TABLE 3.—DEATHS AND DEATH RATES PER 100,000 POPULATION, FROM CANCER, BY SEX, COLOR AND AGE IN GEORGIA: 1930 AND 1934

AGE AND YEAR		BOTH SEXES			MALES			FEMALES		
		Total	White	Col.	Total	White	Col.	Total	White	C
		NUMBER								
All Ages	1930	1552	1105	447	568	442	126	984	663	32
	1934	1762	1272	490	651	507	144	1111	765	34
Under 5 Years	1930	13	8	5	6	5	1	7	5	
	1934	8	5	3	5	3	2	3	2	
5-14 Years	1930	10	7	3	5	2	3	5	5	—
	1934	16	13	3	11	9	2	5	4	
15-24 Years	1930	28	15	13	17	11	6	11	4	
	1934	38	26	12	19	14	5	19	12	
25-34 Years	1930	77	45	32	13	7	6	64	38	2
	1934	74	42	32	13	7	6	61	35	2
35-44 Years	1930	191	93	98	33	19	14	158	74	8
	1934	217	120	97	46	30	16	171	90	8
45-54 Years	1930	315	178	137	93	53	40	222	125	9
	1934	384	240	144	98	66	32	286	174	11
55-64 Years	1930	347	269	78	146	117	29	201	152	4
	1934	405	311	94	163	125	38	242	186	5
65-74 Years	1930	324	278	46	150	133	17	174	145	2
	1934	383	310	73	191	157	34	192	153	3
75 and Over	1930	242	210	32	104	95	9	138	115	2
	1934	231	201	30	104	95	9	127	106	2
Unknown Age	1930	5	2	3	1	—	1	4	2	
	1934	6	4	2	1	1	—	5	3	
		RATE PER 100,000 POPULATION								
All Ages	1930	53.3	60.0	41.7	39.5	47.9	24.5	66.6	72.2	57
	1934	58.6	66.5	44.7	43.9	53.0	27.4	72.9	80.1	60.
Under 5 Years	1930	4.1	4.0	4.3	3.8	4.9	1.7	4.4	3.0	6.
	1934	2.4	2.4	2.5	3.0	2.8	3.4	1.8	2.0	1.
5-14 Years	1930	1.4	1.6	1.1	1.4	.9	2.3	1.4	2.4	—
	1934	2.2	2.9	1.1	3.1	4.0	1.5	1.4	1.8	.
15-24 Years	1930	4.5	4.0	5.3	5.6	5.9	5.3	3.4	2.1	5.
	1934	5.9	6.6	4.8	6.1	7.2	4.3	5.7	6.1	5.
25-34 Years	1930	18.9	17.1	22.2	6.8	5.5	9.4	29.6	28.0	32.
	1934	17.6	15.4	21.8	6.6	5.3	9.3	27.4	24.9	31.
35-44 Years	1930	56.4	42.2	82.7	20.5	17.3	27.3	88.8	66.8	125.
	1934	62.1	52.5	80.2	27.7	26.4	30.5	93.1	78.2	118.
45-54 Years	1930	118.8	104.8	143.8	68.9	61.0	83.0	170.6	150.5	205.
	1934	140.3	136.1	148.0	70.4	73.3	65.1	212.8	201.6	232.
55-64 Years	1930	227.5	262.8	155.6	177.1	218.9	100.1	272.5	310.6	231.
	1934	257.2	292.7	183.7	191.6	225.6	128.5	334.0	365.7	259.
65-74 Years	1930	409.9	504.9	191.8	370.6	481.2	132.5	451.1	528.8	260.
	1934	469.1	542.4	298.1	457.4	547.9	259.5	481.4	536.9	342.
75 and Over	1930	698.5	907.3	282.6	647.1	886.2	168.2	750.2	925.6	385.
	1934	649.2	836.6	260.6	627.6	854.9	164.8	668.0	820.9	344.
Unknown Age	1930	271.0	207.3	340.9	102.5	—	232.6	460.3	477.3	444.
	1934	311.0	390.2	221.2	98.4	173.0	—	547.6	671.1	429.

increase may be due in part to the present prevalent habit of cigarette-smoking among women.

The only exception to an increase in the white people over the colored is in cancer of the female genital organs. In 1934 the death rate of 27.9 per cent for colored women was 21 per cent higher than the rate of 23.0 per cent for white women. Since 75 per cent of colored births are attended by midwives it is reasonable to assume that the higher mortality rate from cancer of these organs in colored women is due to lack of medical attention during confinement and proper observation for the months immediately after delivery.

Table 3 shows the deaths and death rates per 100,000 population from cancer by age, sex and color. Thirty per cent of colored deaths due to cancer occurred before 45 years of age, in the white race only 16 per cent occurred before the age was reached. Females of both races have a higher percentage of deaths under that age than males. This may be partly accounted for by the fact that 31

TABLE I.

*Deaths and Death Rates Per 100,000 Population
From Cancer, By Color, In Georgia:
1921 to 1934.*

YEAR	Total	NUMBER White	Col.	Total	RATES PER 100,000 POP. White	Col.
1921	1210	803	407	41.8	46.9	34.3
1922	1212	782	430	41.8	45.3	36.6
1923	1263	870	393	43.6	50.0	33.9
1924	1393	913	480	48.0	52.1	41.8
1925	1311	891	420	45.2	50.4	37.0
1926	1257	860	397	43.3	48.2	35.4
1927	1470	995	475	50.6	55.4	42.9
1928	1510	1013	497	52.0	55.9	45.4
1929	1456	988	468	50.1	54.1	43.3
1930	1552	1105	447	53.3	60.0	41.7
1931	1580	1106	474	53.8	59.5	43.9
1932	1531	1052	479	51.7	56.1	44.2
1933	1647	1213	434	55.2	64.0	39.8
1934	1762	1272	490	58.6	66.5	44.7

per cent of the deaths under 45 years were from cancer of the female genital organs.

It has been well said that if everyone, including the lay public, knew what they should know of the available information about cancer the mortality from this disease could be reduced at least 50 per cent. Since, however, the lay public is not now sufficiently educated to recognize the danger signals of cancer the responsibility of lowering the morbidity and mortality from cancer rests with the physician. He is the only one in position to make an early diagnosis and to recognize in any part of the body the presence of sus-

picious lesions which, if allowed to continue, might produce cancer. If, therefore, the mortality from cancer is to be reduced every physician must diligently study the early signs and symptoms of the disease and consider the possibility of a potential malignancy in every suspicious lesion.   BUTLER TOOMBS.

COUNTIES REPORTING FOR 1936

Decatur-Seminole Counties Medical Society

The Decatur-Seminole Counties Medical Society announces the following officers for 1936:

President—E. C. Smith, Donalsonville.

Vice-President—Thomas Chason, Donalsonville.

Secretary-Treasurer—M. A. Ehrlich, Bainbridge.

Delegate—M. A. Ehrlich, Bainbridge.

Alternate Delegate—R. F. Wheat, Bainbridge.

Muscogee County Medical Society

The Muscogee County Medical Society announces the following officers for 1936:

President—John E. Walker, Columbus.

Vice-President—J. L. Spikes, Columbus.

Secretary-Treasurer—Wm. C. Cook, Columbus.

Delegate—Frank Schley, Columbus.

Alternate Delegate—W. F. Jenkins, Columbus.

Glynn County Medical Society

The Glynn County Medical Society announces the following officers for 1936:

President—J. W. Simmons, Brunswick.

Vice-President—J. P. Harrell, Brunswick.

Secretary-Treasurer—T. V. Willis, Brunswick.

Delegate—C. B. Greer, Brunswick.

Censors—J. B. Avera, R. S. Burford and G. W. H. Cheney.

Notice to Physicians Attending Obstetrical Mortalities During 1935

The Committee appointed to Study Maternal Mortality in Georgia is anxious to finish the 1935 survey.

A few physicians have failed to answer questionnaires mailed to them by the Committee. These delinquent returns have delayed the completion of the report which will require considerable time because of the large amount of statistical work to be done, before the report is complete.

The Committee desires and asks for your cooperation and immediate reply to the questionnaires, to avoid an unnecessary amount of correspondence and expenditure of our limited funds.

We thank you for your cooperation and the immediate return of the questionnaires sent to you.

E. D. COLVIN, M.D.,
Chairman.

1040 Ponce de Leon Ave., N.E.,
Atlanta, Georgia.

WOMAN'S AUXILIARY

OFFICERS

President—Mrs. Ernest R. Harris, Winder.
President-Elect—Mrs. Wm. R. Dancy, Savannah.
First Vice-President—Mrs. Hulett H. Askew,
    Atlanta.
Second Vice-President—Mrs. Warren A. Coleman,
    Eastman.
Third Vice-President—Mrs. T. J. Ferrell,
    Waycross.
Recording Secretary—Mrs. W. R. Garner,
    Gainesville.
Corresponding Secretary—Mrs. S. T. Ross,
    Winder
Treasurer—Mrs. W. M. Cason, Sandersville.

Historian—Mrs. Marvin F. Haygood, Atlanta.
Parliamentarian—Mrs. Ralph H. Chaney, Augusta.
    Committee Chairmen
Health Films—Mrs. A. J. Mooney, Statesboro.
Student Loan Fund—Mrs. Benjamin Bashinski,
    Macon.
Public Relations—Mrs. J. A. Redfearn, Albany.
Press and Publicity—Mrs. J. Harry Rogers,
    Atlanta.
Jane Todd Crawford Memorial—Mrs. Eustace A.
    Allen, Atlanta.
Research in Romance of Medicine—Mrs. D. N.
    Thompson, Elberton.

Chatham County Meeting

The annual meeting of the Auxiliary to the Georgia Medical Society was held recently. Officers elected were: Mrs. A. A. Morrison, Jr., President; Mrs. Lehman W. Williams, First Vice-President; Mrs. C. R. Riner, Second Vice-President; Mrs. Harry M. Kandel, Recording Secretary; Mrs. John L. Elliott, Corresponding Secretary; Mrs. Shelton Wilson, Treasurer. Mrs. G. Hugo Johnson, the retiring President, had served the time limit under the Constitution and By-Laws.

Mrs. William R. Dancy, President-Elect of the State Auxiliary, made an urgent appeal for more members and better attendance at the meetings and read a paper by Mrs. J. Bonar White, Atlanta, Ex-President, on "Membership in a Medical Auxiliary."

Mrs. C. R. Riner, Chairman of the Membership Committee, introduced the following new members: Mrs. Luther A. DeLoach, Mrs. John L. Elliott, Mrs. Walter E. Brown, Mrs. Wm. O. Bedingfield, and Mrs. John H. Pinholster.

Miss Irma Frost, accompanied by Mrs. Murray, gave an excellent musical program after the business meeting.

Mrs. W. G. Johnson and Mrs. Shelton E. Wilson, hostesses, assisted by Mrs. Lester Neville, Mrs. H. H. McGee, Mrs. L. W. Williams, Mrs. R. E. Graham and Mrs. J. L. Adams, served refreshments.

President's Report

The following excellent report of activities of the Auxiliary to the Georgia Medical Society during the regime of Mrs. G. Hugo Johnson as published in the *Savannah Evening Press* was read by Mrs. Johnson:

"From the reports of your officers and committees it will be noted that the work for the year has been very satisfactory. Our programs have been interesting and instructive, our meetings well attended, and the newspapers have given splendid publicity to our meetings. We have gained five new members. The auxil-

iary was well represented at the mid-winter and also the mid-summer district meetings. During the mid-summer district meeting we entertained with a luncheon at the Hotel De Soto, at which our state President, Mrs. E. R. Harris, gave a splendid talk. Two of our members attended the State convention at Atlanta and also the Southern Medical convention.

"During the year the Auxiliary sent clothes, money for books, and a Christmas box to a boy at Berry School.

"The Auxiliary has always been interested in the work of the Tuberculosis Association and during the past year it has been our pleasure to assist in their 'mile of dimes' campaign. The Auxiliary also contributed the following to the Sunshine Unit: A large number of canned tomatoes, one spread, two pillow cases, two sheets, candy and paper napkins left over from our card party.

"Ten workers were furnished by the Auxiliary for the campaign of the Bethesda Orphan Home for Boys. The Auxiliary was represented at all meetings of the Health Center and also the Friday morning conferences, when requested. Health films were shown in five schools to 1,005 children. We have contributed to the Student Loan Fund and to the Health Film Library.

"It has been my pleasure as your President to preside at all regular, special and executive board meetings and to assist wherever possible with the work of our various committees. I have made the necessary district and state reports. Your president represented the Auxiliary at the President's reception of the Huntington Club.

"On March 30, the Auxiliary observed Doctor's Day with a dinner and dance at the Shrine Club, for the members of the Medical Society and their wives. Mrs. Charles Usher read Mrs. Bonar White's 'Tribute,' and a very clever skit was presented at this time by Mrs. William Myers. We had splendid publicity and an editorial commending our observance of this day was given in our newspapers. A poem, 'His Mission,' by Dr. Ralph Methven Thompson, was published.

"It is with pride that the President calls attention to the number of its members taking very active and prominent parts in the many civic and welfare organizations of our community.

"I want to take this opportunity to thank the officers and members of the Auxiliary who have helped to make the work for the year a success and to extend to all of you my sincerest wishes for a happy, blessed and prosperous new year. To the incoming president I wish as happy and pleasant a year as I have had. I need hardly mention that you will have the full cooperation of every member of the Auxiliary and that you will find everyone willing and glad to assist you in every way possible."

Ware County Auxiliary

The December meeting of the Auxiliary was held at the home of Mrs. T. J. Ferrell, Waycross. Officers elected for the ensuing year were: Mrs. T. J. Ferrell, President; Mrs. R. C. Walker, Vice-President; Mrs. W. C. Hafford, Secretary; Mrs. H. A. Seaman, Treasurer; Mrs. Kenneth McCullough, Chairman of Program Committee; Mrs. J. L. Walker, Historian; Mrs. C. M. Stephens, Parliamentarian, and Mrs. R. L. Johnson, Publicity Chairman.

Minutes of the previous meeting were read and adopted.

The President thanked the members who took part in the recent Forestry Festival.

Mrs. Ferrell gave an interesting account of her recent trip to California, where she attended the convention of the American College of Surgeons.

Mrs. W. L. Pomeroy and Mrs. W. M. Folks, Waycross, entertained the members at the January meeting.

Mrs. T. J. Ferrell, President, appointed committee chairmen for the new year.

Motion carried to contribute to the Student Loan Fund and to observe "Doctors Day," March 30th. Mrs. J. E. Penland will be Toastmaster.

Mrs. Kenneth McCullough reported a visit to a widow of a charter member of the Ware County Medical Society and the donation of Christmas gifts in the name of the Auxiliary.

Mrs. McCullough spoke on, "Any good thing I can do or any kindness that I can show to any human being let me do it now; let me not defer or neglect it for I shall not pass this way again."

The members enjoyed a social hour.

Fulton County

The Auxiliary met at the Academy of Medicine, 38 Prescott Street, N.E., Atlanta, on January 10th. Mrs. Calhoun McDougall, President; Mrs. Wm. W. Anderson, Secretary, and Mrs. Leland Baggett, Treasurer, submitted their official reports.

Mrs. Crawford Barnett, Chairman of the Ways and Means Committee, will be Chairman of a Bridge Party to be given in the Tea Room at Davison-Paxon Company's store on February 19th.

Mrs. Katherine Salmon, Field Secretary of the Georgia Welfare Board, told of the problems faced by the Board.

Mrs. J. Bonar White, Ex-President of the Auxiliary to the Southern Medical Association, gave a report on the annual convention held at St. Louis last November.

Richmond County

The January meeting of the Auxiliary was held on January 23rd.

Dr. John W. Brittingham, Augusta, spoke on the "Hearts, Good and Bad" and illustrated his talk with lantern slides.

A benefit party to raise money for the Student Loan Fund was given on January 31st.

Visitors during the meeting of the Tenth District Medical Society on February 12th were entertained at a luncheon in the Sun Glow Tea Room.

NEWS ITEMS

The Georgia Medical Society, Savannah, met on January 14th. Dr. S. E. Wilson read a paper on *Regurgitation Renal Colic*; discussion was led by Dr. L. W. Shaw and Dr. H. Y. Righton. Dr. J. W. Daniel reported a case of *Changes in Differential Count in Chronic Malaria*.

Dr. and Mrs. Raymond L. Johnson, Waycross, entertained the members of the Ware County Medical Society in their home on January 8th. Dr. Geo. E. Atwood, Ware County Commissioner of Health, read a scientific paper.

The Fulton County Medical Society met at the Academy of Medicine, Atlanta, January 16th. Dr. Richard B. Wilson reported a case of *Carcinomatosis of Meninges*; Dr. Jas. J. Clark made a clinical talk on *Interlobar Lesions and Their Correct Diagnosis—Illustrated*; Dr. Calvin B. Stewart read a paper entitled *Cancer Prevention*, discussed by Dr. J. L. Campbell, Dr. O. D. Hall and Dr. John F. Denton.

The Georgia Eye, Ear, Nose and Throat Club sponsored a lecture on *Practical and Surgical Ophthalmology* at the Academy of Medicine, Atlanta, by Dr. Clyde E. McDannald of the New York Eye and Ear Infirmary, New York City.

The staff meeting of Grady Hospital, Atlanta, was held on January 14th. Dr. C. W. Strickler reported a case of *Acute Arthritis—Neisserian in Origin*.

The Decatur-Seminole Counties Medical Society met at Bainbridge on January 13th. Dr. C. B. Welch, Attapulgus, read a paper entitled *Infections in the Nose and Throat*; Dr. M. A. Ehrlich, Bainbridge,

Intestinal Allergy. Officers were elected for the ensuing year. The next meeting of the Society will be held at Bainbridge on April 9th.

The Jackson-Barrow Counties Medical Society met at Winder on January 6th. Dr. R. P. Adams, Winder, spoke on *The Existing Laws That Are of Vital Importance to the Physicians as Well as the People.* The last meeting of the Society was held at the Harrison Hotel, Jefferson, on February 3rd.

The staff meeting of the Crawford W. Long Memorial Hospital, Atlanta, was held on January 9th. Officers elected for 1936 were: Dr. Harry W. Ridley, President; Dr. W. W. Daniel, Vice-President; Dr. C. E. Lawrence, Secretary.

The Burke-Jenkins-Screven Counties Medical Society met at the Anthony-Wayne Hotel, Waynesboro, on January 9th. Dr. Reuben L. Kahn, Professor of Bacteriology at the University of Michigan, Ann Arbor, discussed, *Tissue Immunity in Relation to Clinical Medicine.* In addition to Dr. Kahn there were many guests present from the adjoining counties, invited especially to hear Dr. Kahn's lecture.

The E. Bates Block Lecture in Medicine was given before the regular meeting of the Fulton County Medical Society at the Academy of Medicine, Atlanta, on January 23rd, by Dr. Tracy Jackson Putnam, Professor of Neurology at Harvard University School of Medicine, Boston. The subject of his address was, *The Cerebral Circulation and Its Disorders.*

The annual banquet of the medical and surgical staff of the Georgia Baptist Hospital, Atlanta, was held in the dining hall of the nurses' home on January 21st. Officers elected were: Dr. C. C. Aven, President; Dr. W. S. Dorough, First Vice-President; Dr. Olin S. Cofer, Second Vice-President; and Dr. Steven T. Brown, Secretary. Mr. W. D. Barker, Superintendent of the Hospital, made a report of the activities of the Hospital for 1935 as follows: 6,216 persons treated; 647 babies born; 600 treated in the Cancer Clinic; and 98 people on the regular payroll and 98 student nurses.

Dr. Ford Ware announces the removal of his office to 814 Georgia Casualty Building, Macon.

Dr. and Mrs. E. H. Lamb, Cornelia, entertained the members of the Habersham County Medical Society and Woman's Auxiliary in their home on January 9th.

The Clinical Society of the New York Polyclinic Medical School and Hospital, New York City, met on January 6th. The scientific program consisted of: *Surgical Treatment of Primary Carcinoma of the Lung,* by Richard H. Overholt, Lahey Clinic, Boston, Mass.; discussion was led by Dr. Howard Lilien-

and Dr. A. A. Morrison were elected to the Board of Trustees.

Dr. Roy R. Kracke, Emory University, discussed *The Use of Pain-Killing Drugs* at the annual meeting of the Macon Chapter of Emory Alumni in Macon on January 25th.

Dr. Charlie N. Wasden, Macon, has been elected to fellowship in the American College of Surgeons.

The staff meeting of St. Joseph's Infirmary, Atlanta, was held on January 28th. Dr. Herbert Alden reported a case, *Tuberculosis and Tuberculides*. Dinner was served and officers elected for the ensuing year.

The Georgia Medical Society, Savannah, held its annual banquet at Oglethorpe Club on January 28th. Dr. C. F. Holton was installed as President for 1936; Dr. S. E. Bray, Vice-President; Dr. O. W. Schwalb, Secretary-Treasurer. Entertainment Committee consisted of Dr. L. B. Dunn, Chairman; Dr. M. J. Epting, and Dr. W. E. Brown.

Dr. C. F. Holton, Savannah, President of the Georgia Medical Society, spoke at a luncheon meeting of the Exchange Club at Hotel Savannah, January 27th. He stated that "One-third of the colored employees of 61 large corporations and businesses of Savannah suffered from social diseases."

The annual meeting of the Trustees of the John D. Archbold Memorial Hospital, Thomasville, was held on January 22nd. Dr. Fletcher H. Brooks, Medical Director, made a report on the activities of the Hospital for last year.

Dr. Chas. W. Folsom, LaFayette, was recently elected Commissioner of Health for Catoosa and Walker counties.

The Coffee County Medical Society met at the Doucoff Hotel, Douglas, on January 28th. Dr. Ed-Berkeley Neal, New York City, spoke on *Recent Advances in Pediatrics*. This meeting was designated as "Ladies Night." Dinner was served to both members of the Society and Woman's Auxiliary. Dr. T. H. Clark and Dr. B. O. Quillian, Douglas, have been appointed to select titles for papers to be read during the year. Titles for papers to appear on the programs to and including the June meeting have been submitted. The President, Dr. J. G. Crovatt, Douglas, assigned the titles for articles to various members of the Society. The next meeting will be held on February 24th. Dr. T. H. Johnston, Douglas, will speak on *Infant Feeding*; Dr. J. W. Wallace, Douglas, *Communicable Diseases of Children*.

At the annual meeting of the staff of the Ware County Hospital, Waycross, officers elected were: Dr. W. F. Reavis, President; Dr. R. L. Johnson, Vice-President; Dr. A. W. DeLoach, Secretary-Treasurer; Executive Committee—Dr. J. E. Penland, Dr. W. C. Hafford, Dr. C. A. Witmer, Dr. W. D. Mixson, and Dr. D. M. Bradley. The physicians and surgeons of South Georgia are invited to attend a clinic which will be held at the Hospital in March.

Dr. Albert Fleming and Dr. Jas. H. Sawyer, Folkston, entertained the members of the Ware County Medical Society to a shad dinner at Bank's Cafe, Folkston, on February 5th.

The Clarke County Medical Society met at the Georgian Hotel, Athens, on February 7th.

Dr. William C. Cook, Columbus, was the recipient of the medal given on January 23rd by the Columbus Junior Chamber of Commerce. He was selected as the young man who had rendered the greatest service of citizenship to the community during 1935. Dr. Cook served last year as Medical Director of the Kiwanis Child Health and Nutrition Clinic and directed a clinic at Hamp Stevens Memorial church. He was in charge of the Tuberculosis Clinic at the Columbus City Hospital.

The annual meeting of the staff of St. Joseph's Infirmary, Atlanta, was held on January 28th. Officers elected for the ensuing year were: Dr. Murdock Equen, President; Dr. John W. Turner, Vice-President; Dr. Don F. Cathcart, Secretary-Treasurer.

If interested in a good location for a practicing physician, write the Secretary-Treasurer. A good doctor has just died at the place.

The Wise Sanitarium at Plains was damaged by fire on January 30th. The patients were all taken care of by removal to homes and other hospitals. Repairs to the damaged building have almost been completed.

Dr. M. F. Haygood, Hamilton, formerly in charge of the Resettlement Community at Pine Mountain, has accepted the position as director of the Works Progress Administration Medical Clinics in Georgia.

Dr. R. L. Miller, Waynesboro, retired from the practice of medicine on February 1st according to announcement in the Waynesboro Citizen.

Dr. V. H. Bassett, Savannah, spoke before a meeting of the Savannah Historical Research Association, January 29th, on *A Southern Medical Student in the Year 1801*.

OBITUARY

Dr. Benjamin L. Clifton, Millen; member; Southern Medical College, Atlanta, 1885; aged 77; died after an illness of several months duration on June 7, 1935. He was a native of Jenkins County and had practiced medicine there for almost a half century until he retired a few years ago on account of his health. Dr. Clifton was active in affairs for the advancement of his community and held in high esteem by his acquaintances. Surviving him are his widow, four daughters, Misses Allie, Bessie and Sallie Clifton, Millen; Miss Maggie Clifton, Milledgeville; seven sons, H. G., W. R., P. L., Douglas; Lemuel, Joseph and Lester Clifton, all of Jenkins County. Funeral services were conducted from Elam Baptist church by Rev. Palmer Edenfield.

Dr. *James W. Anderson*, Gray; member: Bellevue Hospital Medical College, New York City, 1887; aged 70; died of pneumonia at his home on January 3, 1936. He was a native of Gray and had practiced medicine there for more than 45 years. Dr. Anderson was one of the State's most honorable citizens and liked by his associates. He was a member of the Jones County Medical Society, Masonic lodge and Methodist church. Surviving him are his widow and two daughters: Mrs. Tessie Evans, Atlanta; and Mrs. Carola Corley, Gray. Funeral services were conducted from the Baptist church at Hillsboro. Burial was in the churchyard.

Dr. *Edgar F. Fincher*, Atlanta; member: Atlanta College of Physicians and Surgeons, Atlanta, 1901; aged 66; died at his home on January 7, 1936. He was a native of Gwinnett County and had practiced medicine in Atlanta for 34 years. Dr. Fincher was a prominent physician, took an active interest in civic and religious affairs. He served on the Board of Trustees of Grady Memorial Hospital for a number of years and was on the staff of Piedmont Hospital at the time of his death. Dr. Fincher was a member of the Fulton County Medical Society, Minor Lodge No. 608 of F. and A. M., Scottish Rite Masons, Shrine, and Martha Brown Memorial Methodist church. Surviving him are his widow, one daughter, Mrs. W. H. Trimble; one son, Dr. Edgar F. Fincher, Jr., all of Atlanta. Funeral services were conducted by Dr. H. C. Emory and Dr. W. T. Hunnicutt from the Martha Brown Memorial Methodist church. Burial was in West View Cemetery.

Dr. *A. Pierce Kemp*, Macon; member: Southern Medical College, Atlanta, 1889; aged 67; died of pneumonia in a private hospital in Macon on January 13, 1936. He was born in Woodstock, Cherokee county. Dr. Kemp was the youngest member of his graduating class at the Southern Medical College, being only 20 years of age at the time. He began practice at Roswell, moved to Barnesville, thence to Macon more than thirty years ago as Medical Examiner for the Metropolitan Life Insurance Co. and for many years was physician for the Bibb Manufacturing Company. While he practiced for many of the wealthiest people of Bibb County, he was charitable and untiring in his efforts to cure or relieve many of the poorest people. Dr. Kemp was a member of the

reader is confronted with a series of "case histories" which contain little but the bare facts of the girls' sex experiences and "conclusions" which are in themselves foregone, trite and inconclusive. Of what value is it to know that of 1400 cases of rape, there were some girls who had run away from home, others who came from broken homes? Any thinking person would realize that this would be true, but in how far these conditions represented the major cause of trouble, or how large a contributing factor they were, could not be shown by "case histories" so devoid of facts which would give any insight into the kinds of persons these girls were, or the forces that played their part in molding their characters.

The bare recounting of sordid sex experience upon sex experience, illustrates nothing and to pick out as a casual factor any one sociological fact such as a broken home or lack of parental understanding is unscientific.

It may be helpful to shock certain people into the realization that in nearly every community there exist conditions of badhousing, low wages, drunkenness, mental and physical abnormalities, and break-downs. Some individuals prefer to think that experiences of such girls as those cited by these authors is due to some innate evil tendency rather than to conditions of environment for which every citizen bears at least an indirect responsibility. Some few may be shocked by these so-called "studies" into taking their responsibilities in the matter more seriously, and attempting to correct the evil influences which exist in every community.

The most useful contributions in the book, it seems to me, are the last two chapters on "The Community's Factors and Debts to Girls." In these, the authors reiterate the evidence against such evil social influences as cheap dance halls, indecent theatres and movies, and sex magazines. They call for more careful sex instruction for young people, and raise the question as to the most satisfactory way in which sex instruction may be given.

JOSEPH C. MASSEE, M.D.

The Medical Association of Georgia will hold its eighty-seventh annual session at Hotel De Soto, Savannah, April 21, 22, 23, 24, 1936.

 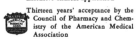
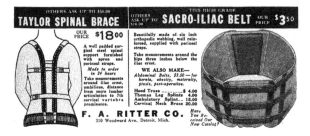

THE JOURNAL
OF THE
MEDICAL ASSOCIATION OF GEORGIA
DEVOTED TO THE WELFARE OF THE MEDICAL ASSOCIATION OF GEORGIA
PUBLISHED MONTHLY under direction of the Council

Volume XXV	Atlanta, Ga., March, 1936	Number 3

THE CONTRIBUTIONS OF CRAWFORD W. LONG AND HIS CONTEMPORARIES TO AMERICAN MEDICINE*

MAX CUTLER, M.D.
Chicago

One hundred years ago there stepped from this very platform a youth of nineteen who was destined to confer upon suffering humanity one of its greatest blessings of all time. Who would have guessed that seven years later this lad was to give to the world the art of anesthesia and by the control of pain at operation, to revolutionize the art and science of surgery—a triumph unsurpassed by any achievement in the history of medicine.

The mystery of pain has been a subject of wonder and speculation by man from the beginning of time. Its cause and its purpose have baffled the mind and failed of satisfactory explanation. Of the birth and death of pain Weir Mitchell has written:

"The Birth of Pain! Let centuries roll away;
Come back with me to nature's primal day.

What will implacable, beyond our ken,
Set this stern fiat for the tribes of men!
This, none shall 'scape, who share our human fates:
One stern democracy of anguish waits
By poor men's cots—within the rich man's gates.

What purpose hath it? Nay, thy quest is vain:
Earth hath no answer: If the baffled brain
Cries, 'tis to warn, to punish—Ah, refrain!
When writhes the child, beneath the surgeon's hand,

What soul shall hope that pain to understand?
Lo! Science falters o'er the hopeless task,
And Love and Faith in vain an answer ask,
When thrilling nerves demand what good is wrought
Where torture clogs the very source of thought

*Crawford W. Long address before the student body, Board of Trustees and faculty of the University of Georgia School of Medicine, Augusta, March 30, 1935.

Whatever triumphs still shall hold the mind,
Whatever gift shall yet enrich mankind,
Ah! here, no hour shall strike through all the years,
No hour as sweet, as when hope, doubt and fears,
'Mid deepening stillness, watched one eager brain,
With God-like will, decree the Death of Pain."

Imagine, if you can, the emotions, the agony and the suffering of patients who had to endure the ordeal of a surgical operation before the days of anesthesia. Untold fortitude on the part of the patient, speed and boldness on the part of the surgeon were essential. Surgeons were pitted one against the other like runners on time and the best surgeon for both patient and onlooker was the one who could break the three minute record for an amputation. It is almost impossible in this generation, to conceive the difference which the introduction of anesthesia has made in operative surgery, and it is difficult to realize that the benefits we now enjoy were not always. Let us attempt to visualize an operation before the days of anesthesia.

"With frightened, imploring eyes she is brought into the amphitheatre and laid upon the table. With the knowledge and merciful regard as to the intensity of the agony which she is to suffer, opiates and stimulants have been freely given her. She is cheered by kindly words and the oft repeated information that it will soon be over. She is enjoined to be calm and still and with assistance at hand to hold her struggling form, the operation is commenced. But of what avail her attempts at fortitude. At the first clean crisp cut of the scalpel she endeavors to leap from the table but force is nigh. Strong men throw themselves upon her and pinion her limbs. Shrieks upon shrieks make their horrible way into the stillness of the room, until the heart of the boldest sinks in his bosom like a lump of lead."

Having attended two bad operations, one on a child in the hospital at Edinburgh, Charles Darwin rushed away before they were completed and was saved from being a doctor by the horror of these spectacles which he says haunted him for many years, Sir James Simpson, shortly after beginning the study of medicine, was so affected by witnessing the agony of a poor highland woman under operation that he resolved to abandon a medical career and seek other occupation. Such were the tortures of the operating room before the days of ether. Little surprise that surgical thought was attempting to find a way out of this dilemma and to perfect some effective method of abolishing pain during surgical operations.

One of the best accounts of the life of Crawford Long comes to us from the pen of his daughter, Frances Long Taylor, who has written the biography of her illustrious father in order that his "grandchildren might know of the Southern gentleman of a vanished day" and with the hope that his example might incite them to noble thoughts and deeds.

Crawford Williamson Long, son of James Long and Elizabeth Ware Long, was born on November 1, 1815, in Danielsville, Georgia, in a two-story house inherited from his grandfather, situated on a high hill overlooking the town. He was allowed to enter Franklin College at the age of fourteen as a special favor to his father who was an intimate friend of the president, Dr. Alonzo Church. Alexander H. Stephens, who was in a more advanced class, was his roommate. In August, 1835, just one hundred years ago, he graduated at the age of nineteen with second honors. The year after graduation was spent in his boyhood home near Danielsville teaching in the town academy. The following year he attended the Medical Department of Transylvania University. Determined to obtain the best medical instruction available in America, he entered the Medical Department of the University of Pennsylvania in 1838, the most renowned of the twenty-eight medical schools then in existence in the United States. After his graduation in 1839 he spent eighteen months

Hypnotism was tried and the extent to which mesmerism was used and accepted by scientific men of the day is truly remarkable. Some of the leading figures in medicine and surgery operated upon patients in the mesmeric sleep and looked upon the mesmeric state as the long waited panacea for the relief of pain in surgery.

At no time did Crawford Long believe in or employ it and said that if the mesmeric state could be produced at all, it was only on those of "strong imagination and weak minds." It has even been recorded that some patients were choked into unconsciousness but this method of anesthesia, being unpopular with both surgeon and patient, was never generally adopted. That there was no lack of ingenuity on the part of the surgical profession in devising methods of anesthesia, is well illustrated by the renowned French surgeon, Dupuytren, who deliberately made such insulting remarks to a lady patient that she fainted and in this condition he operated on her.

According to James Mumford, the story of general anesthesia may be dated back to the year 1799, when, Humphrey Davy, a young practitioner of Clifton, England, discovered the intoxicating properties of nitrous oxide gas. One year later, having proved upon himself the safety of this agent, he suggested that it might be used to advantage during surgical operations. How strange that this most important observation should have remained dormant for forty years for it was not until 1844, two years after Crawford Long's discovery of ether, that nitrous oxide was used as anesthesia for the extraction of a tooth.

The year 1842 found Crawford Long a young doctor, 27 years of age, engaged in the practice of medicine in Jefferson, Georgia. The exhilarating and intoxicating effects of sulphuric ether had been known to the chemists for some years. As was the custom in those days, the "wandering lecturers" in chemistry had traveled to the larger cities in the South and aroused the wonder of the people by exhibiting the effects of these mysterious agents. It was in this manner that the custom of "ether frolics" was introduced and popularized in the South and it is said that there was hardly a gathering of young people which did not end with an "ether frolic" during which the boys and girls would inhale ether for its exhilarating and intoxicating effects. Long had observed upon himself as well as upon others who had inhaled ether, bruises and painful spots (that had been sustained while under its influence) sufficient to produce pain but neither had he experienced such pain nor upon questioning had his friends felt pain from those accidents.

Dr. Long determined to try ether upon the first suitable surgical case and the opportunity came when the now famous Mr. James Venable who lived two miles from Jefferson, consulted Dr. Long seeking removal of two small tumors on the back of his neck. The dread of pain had led the patient to postpone the operation on several previous visits. Knowing the patient to be fond of inhaling ether Dr. Long suggested operating on him while under its influence. The patient consented and the operation was performed the same evening just ninety-three years ago today. The patient experienced no pain and seemed incredulous until the tumor was shown to him. Thus, March 30, 1842, witnessed an event of vast importance to humanity, the first surgical operation ever performed under general anesthesia.

As an inducement to Venable to allow himself to be the subject of such an experiment, Dr. Long's charge for his services was nominal. Two dollars for the operation, and twenty-five cents for the ether.

The next step in the development of anesthesia occurred two years later with a young dentist, Horace Wells, as the central and tragic figure. In December, 1844, the wandering lecturer, Colton, gave a public exhibition of nitrous oxide and invited members of the audience to come down into the amphitheatre and inhale the gas. Dr. Horace Wells, a young dentist, watched the volunteers under the influence of this gas and was impressed with its possibilities. Soon afterwards, he had one of his teeth extracted by a colleague, Dr. Riggs, while under the influence of nitrous oxide administered by the lecturer, Dr. Colton. The experiment was a complete success, but tragedy dogged his footsteps. He attempted to give a public demonstration of this agent and failed. The patient died under the anesthetic and in 1848, Wells took his own life.

It happens, not infrequently, in scientific research that the development of an idea proceeds in parallel fashion independently in the minds of different observers, and so it was with the discovery and the development of ether anesthesia. While Crawford Long was experimenting with ether a young ingenious dentist, William T. G. Morton, pursued the same idea and tried various methods of relieving pain. Deciding that he needed to know more about medicine, he entered the office of Dr. Charles T. Jackson of Boston, a distinguished chemist and a scientist of national reputation. Morton had learned of nitrous oxide from his former partner, Horace Wells, and now Jackson told him of his experience with ether.

In September, 1846, Morton extracted a tooth under ether anesthesia and on October 16, 1846, the first public demonstration of ether was made in the Massachusetts General Hospital, which ended successfully with Dr. Warren's now famous remark, "Gentlemen, this is no humbug." The subsequent events in Morton's life form a tragic chapter in the history of American medicine for unfortunately, his claims of priority and the ensuing ether controversy tend to drown the essential facts of America's greatest contribution to medical science.

Surely in so great a boon to humanity, there is enough honor and glory for all participants. The facts surrounding the discovery of ether are now fully established. That Crawford Long was the first man to use ether for the purpose of producing surgical narcosis is generally agreed upon. Thus Morris Fishbein, in the "Frontiers of Medicine," states: "To Dr. Crawford W. Long goes the credit for first using it in an operation, to Dr. William Morton, the credit for bringing it to public attention and for discovering independently its usefulness." Morton died prematurely of an apoplexy in New York in 1868 in his forty-ninth year.

In connection with Long's memorable contribution to scientific medicine, accomplished singly and without the paraphernalia of the modern research institute, let us consider some other contributions by contemporary pioneers.

In the latter part of the eighteenth century, the life of the frontier doctor was filled with tense and thrilling events. This was before the days of roads and the stage-coach had not yet made its appearance. Calls were made on horse back through trackless regions which often meant absence from home for days and sometimes weeks. It is interesting to consider the peculiarities of the frontier and to reflect upon the influence it had on the development of American medicine. The hardships of the frontier were not without their compensation. Freedom and self-reliance reigned supreme and daring deeds were the order of the day. It was this environment that gave birth to anesthesia, to the first abdominal operation and to the first cesarean section. The surgery of the period was simple and crude and the operations, few in number, were confined to emergency measures. Anesthesia had not been discovered, and operations were usually performed on Sundays in order that both patient and surgeon might derive the benefits of the prayers of the church. There were no trained assistants, and no consultants. Those early years produced men of practical ability who dared to try the untried and put into practice desperate remedies for desperate situations. Let us hear the fascinating story of another of the pioneers in American medicine.

Ephriam McDowell was born in 1771, in Western Virginia under the British flag. He was a Virginian by birth and a Kentuckian by adoption. He lived during an exciting period in American history—the Declaration of Independence and the Revolution. After spending two years in the University of Edinburg he returned without his degree to Danville, Kentucky, counting less than three hundred inhabitants, where he was the only surgeon in the state during most of his active life.

In 1809, McDowell was called to see Mrs. Jane Todd Crawford for a large abdominal tumor. He proposed an operation to her with the understanding that it was in the nature of an experiment. She accepted, and traveled sixty miles on horseback to Danville where under the influence of a large dose of morphine he removed the tumor in twenty-five minutes. The patient recovered so rapidly that on the fifth day he found her making her beds. She lived more than thirty years after the operation. Thus Ephriam McDowell was the first to open the peritoneal cavity and perform ovariotomy. This operation was performed thirty-three years before the first use of ether and sixty years before Lister's introduction of antiseptic surgery. It must be remembered that one hundred and seventy years ago the peritoneal cavity was an unexplored domain and its exposure was taken to mean peritonitis and death. During the subsequent four years he performed two similar operations successfully. Being an extremely modest man, it required much persuasion on the part of his friends to induce him to publish his results. It was not until seven years later that this modest country doctor recorded his deed so simply and briefly and so out of proportion to its importance that it was met with skepticism, distrust and derision. For half a century he was almost completely forgotten, when his countrymen awoke to the realization that in the backwoods of Kentucky there lived and died one of the greatest of American surgeons, the founder of abdominal surgery.

About the time that Crawford Long introduced ether anesthesia, there lived in the beautiful forests of Northern Michigan on an isolated military post a young surgeon of the United States Army, William Beaumont. On June 6, 1822, at the little trading post of Mackinac, a young French Canadian lad was standing in the company's store when a shotgun was accidentally discharged, the whole charge entering St. Martin's body, tearing away a portion of the upper abdominal wall and perforating the stomach. He was attended by young William Beaumont who cared for him at his home for two years. To the astonishment of all, he recovered, but until his death sixty years later, he carried a fistulous opening from the surface of

his abdomen directly into his stomach. Beaumont saw an opportunity to study the workings of the stomach. He could see directly into it and watch its movements. He inserted fragments of food tied to a string and after varying periods removed and analyzed them. He studied the gastric secretions. In 1833 he published the results of his investigations. He showed that gastric juice is secreted into the stomach only when it contains food, and that the gastric juice contains hydrochloric acid. He demonstrated how the stomach mixes the gastric juice with the food, and that the average meal is digested in three to four hours.

William Beaumont, an army doctor on an isolated military post on the outskirts of civilization, thus became the hero of one of the most dramatic and romantic episodes in medical history.

It has been fully established in recent years, but unrecognized by medical history, that the first cesarean section to be executed successfully in this country was performed in 1794 by Dr. Jesse Bennett. Pickrell relates that on January 14, 1794, Jesse Bennett's wife was confined in her first pregnancy. The Bennetts then lived in a frontier settlement in the Shenandoah Valley. Labor was difficult because of a contracted pelvis. The patient chose caeserian section and, stretched on a crude plank table over two barrels, was put under the influence of a large dose of opium. Assisted only by two negro women the courageous frontier surgeon, by one stroke of the knife laid open the abdomen and delivered the child. To the astonishment of all, the mother recovered and the child is said to have reached the age of seventy-five years. When asked why he did not report his case in a medical journal, Bennett replied that "No strange doctors would believe that operation could be done in the Virginia backwoods and the mother live and he'd be damned if he would give them a chance to call him a liar."

Benjamin Waterhouse was born in 1754 in Newport, Rhode Island. At the age of 29, he accepted the chair of Theory and Practice in the newly organized Harvard Medical School. In 1799 he received a copy of Jenner's publication on vaccination, was at once impressed with its importance and promptly published in the Columbian Sentinel of Boston a short account of the new inoculation under the title, "Something Curious in the Medical Line."

For centuries smallpox was the great horror of the human race and of that period, it has been said that no mother counted her children until all had passed through smallpox. No corner of the earth was safe from the plague. MacCauley called it the most terrible of all the ministries of death. It has been reliably estimated that in the eighteenth century alone smallpox killed sixty million men, women and children.

On the 14th day of May, 1796, the young Edward Jenner, a humble village doctor took matter from the hand of a dairy maid who had contracted cowpox while milking and inserted it by two superficial incisions into the arm of James Phipps, a boy of eight, and performed the first vaccination. Six weeks later he introduced into this arm virulent smallpox matter without the slightest effect, for Phipps had been vaccinated. Thus at one stroke, smallpox was destined to become a disease of the past.

After an exhaustive study of the new inoculation, Benjamin Waterhouse, the Jenner of America, proceeded to perform the first vaccinations in the United States upon his own children and a servant boy. Two months later they were sent to a smallpox hospital where they were not only exposed to the disease but inoculated with the virulent matter. The children did not contract the disease and thus the effectiveness of vaccination was first demonstrated in America. Waterhouse requested the Massachusetts Medical Society to organize a vaccination center, but the society took no notice of his communication. Their refusal is not so surprising, for had not the Royal Society of London declined to receive and publish Jenner's brilliant contribution on the ground that he ought not to risk his reputation by presenting to that learned body anything so incredible as vaccination.

In the intense opposition that it encountered, vaccination shared the fate of other great discoveries in medicine. One clergyman for example, declared that vaccination was as old as the bible and the reason Job had so many boils was because the devil had vaccinated him. William Rowley exhibited a boy with a swollen face at one of his lectures with the following explanation. "On this cheek you plainly perceive a protuberance arousing like a sprouting hair. Another corresponding one will shortly spring up on the other side, for this boy is gradually losing human lineaments and his countenance is transmuting into the visage of a cow."

Finally, let us consider another pioneer whose contributions to medicine constitute a milestone in our path of progress. James Marion Sims was born in Lancaster County, South Carolina, in 1813. He was graduated from the University of South Carolina. Years afterward, when he had reached the height of fame, he said of himself, "I never was remarkable for anything while I was in college except good behavior: nobody ever expected anything of myself." He attended Charleston Médical School and was graduated from the Jefferson Medical College of Philadelphia in 1835. After an unsuccessful attempt in practice he settled in Alabama.

It was in Montgomery, Alabama, that Sims was consulted within a short period by three patients suffering from vesico-vaginal fistulae. He realized that they were hopeless, but by accident discovered that by means of a bent pewter spoon he could inspect these wounds. Sims was the first man to properly visualize the lesion and he was immediately convinced that he might cure it. After several unsuccessful attempts his efforts were finally crowned with success when he cured his first patient, even though it required forty operations to rid her of this horrible condition.

Compelled by ill health to seek a cooler climate, he moved to New York City where, after severe trials and humiliations, he established a hospital where he could conduct his work, the Woman's Hospital of the State of New York.

Sims was invited to demonstrate his operation in various European countries where they showered many honors and distinctions upon him. In 1877 he returned to Montgomery to visit his old friends and the scene of his discovery which started him on the road to everlasting fame.

Thus the path of progress in science is marked by landmarks of individual ideas and acts which have erased from the calendar of human afflictions and removed from the catalogue of evils some of the worst enemies of mankind.

Kings and warriors have not suffered from lack of space and attention in the histories of nations. Had any of these pioneers distinguished themselves in battle with prominence at all comparable to their scientific contributions to humanity, the names of all would have been household words and their features properly carved in everlasting statue. How strange the human mind reacts, to shower honor and glory with immense profusion upon the hand that circumstances force to spread death and destruction and the modest man of science, whose gift to humanity stills the suffering and saves the lives of millions, is allowed to sink into obscurity with no acclaim and little public notice.

It is indeed a signal honor to have been invited to deliver the Ether Day address on this momentous occasion and for this unique privilege I am deeply thankful to the trustees and faculty of the University of Georgia, my alma mater.

I should be remiss and ungrateful if I did not at this time acknowledge my debt of gratitude to the University and to the little community of Athens, that one quarter of a century ago gave me a home, opened its schools to me, and sent me on the way to add my humble bit to the combat against human disease. Just seventeen years ago I received, upon this very platform, my bachelors degree. What an honor to be a graduate from the university that can claim the distinction of such illustrious an alumnus as the great benefactor whose memory we are gathered to honor today.

How fitting that the trustees of the University of Georgia have inaugurated this event commemorating the first use of ether as an anesthetic in surgery and honoring the name of Crawford W. Long. Facile pens

and eloquent tongues have tried, but no words have yet succeeded in adequately describing this precious gift to suffering humanity. Of the control of pain by anesthesia Holmes and Bigelow have written:

"In this very hour while I am speaking how many human creatures are cheated of pangs which seem inevitable as the common doom of mortality and lulled by the strange magic of the enchanted goblet, held for a moment to their lips, into a repose which has something of ecstasy in its dreamy slumbers.

"Nature herself is working out the primal curse which doomed the tenderest of her creatures to the sharpest of her trials but the fierce extremity of suffering has been steeped in the waters of forgetfulness and the deepest furrow in the knotted brow of agony has been smoothed forever."

SIGNS AND SYMPTOMS OF EARLY CANCER*

The only hope for the cancer patient is early diagnosis, prompt and efficient treatment. Every week's delay in making the diagnosis and beginning the treatment lessens the chances for recovery by two per cent. A fact that must be kept in mind is, in early cancer of the uterine cervix there is no characteristic sign or symptom; a bloodstained discharge should however arouse suspicion. Too many doctors remember only the statement in the older text-books that: "The three classical signs of cancer of the cervix are pain, hemorrhage and foul smelling discharge." This is true of only the advanced and usually hopeless cases. It is true that an occasional case, not too far advanced, can be salvaged but the percentage is pitifully small. It is a mistake of the older teaching that cancer of the cervix occurs only from middle life on, and while this is true in the majority of cases, it does occur frequently in young women, in those who have borne children, in the nullipara and even in the virgin.

The only sign that early cancer of the

(Continued on Page 84)

*Prepared for the Cancer Commission of the Medical Association of Georgia by John F. Denton, M.D., Atlanta.

THE JOURNAL
OF THE
MEDICAL ASSOCIATION OF GEORGIA
Devoted to the Welfare of the Medical Association of Georgia

478 Peachtree Street, N.E., Atlanta, Ga.

MARCH, 1936

INVITATION

To The Members of The Medical Association, and The Woman's Auxiliary:

On April 21, 1936, The Medical Association of Georgia will again convene in Savannah, the mother city of the State.

As President of The Georgia Medical Society, the mother medical organization of the State, it gives me great pleasure to invite the Georgia doctors and their ladies to come to Savannah.

We are particularly happy that this meeting will be held in April because at that time Savannah will be at its loveliest. The azaleas and wistaria will be in bloom, then too the dogwood trees throughout the city will be in their beautiful foliage. It is worth a special trip to Savannah in the spring to see the beauty of the city at that time.

Dr. Paullin and his program committee have arranged for a wonderful scientific meeting. We in Savannah expect to do our part in making the session successful. We have arranged for the headquarters to be at Hotel DeSoto where the famous Tavern orchestra will play nightly for dances. At the Savannah Hotel the equally famous Rathskellar and Drum Room will offer entertainment to those who wish night life.

For those who like sports Savannah offers five championship golf courses, all of which should be in perfect condition in April. A golf tournament will be held over the links of the Savannah Golf Club, where golf originated in America. This course has been considerably remodeled and is now an exacting test of golf.

A skeet shooting tournament will be held under the direction of Dr. J. F. Chisholm, and trophies will be offered to the winners and runners-up in two classes. Those interested in breaking clay pigeons are especially requested to write Dr. Chisholm at 512 Abercorn Street, Savannah, in advance, so that he may make the necessary arrangements. It is most likely that this tournament will be held at the traps of the General Oglethorpe Hotel on Wilmington Island, a few miles distant from Savannah and itself one of the beauty spots of the county.

For those who are interested in fishing, ample provisions will be made.

The people of Savannah generally, and the doctors and their wives especially, are eagerly awaiting the opportunity to entertain the ladies and gentlemen of the State Association and we trust that every one possible belonging to or affiliated with the Association will attend the Savannah session.

C. F. HOLTON, M.D., *President*
Georgia Medical Society.

Feb. 12, 1936, Savannah, Ga.

CRAWFORD W. LONG DISCOVERER OF ETHER ANESTHESIA

We are fortunate in having the opportunity of reading in the present issue of the JOURNAL an address by Dr. Max Cutler, of Chicago, entitled, "The Contributions of Crawford Long to American Medicine." This address was delivered by Dr. Cutler at the University of Georgia, March 30, 1935, as the principal feature of the exercises commemorating the ninety-third anniversary of the first use of ether as a surgical anesthetic employed by Crawford Long at Jefferson, Georgia, March 30, 1842.

The celebration of this epochal achievement has become an annual event at the University of Georgia and it was appropriate that Dr. Cutler, an alumnus of the university, should be selected to deliver the oration on this occasion. No alumnus of this university of recent years has distinguished himself in medicine more conspicuously than Dr. Cutler. His valuable contributions to the surgery of breast tumors are well known to the profession everywhere. Not only has he become a world authority on this subject, but his ability to express himself both by the written and spoken word is surpassed by few writers and speakers. The JOURNAL takes unusual pleasure in publishing Dr. Cutler's address.

FRANK K. BOLAND, M.D.

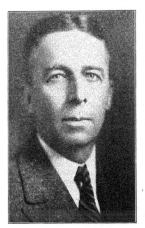

JAMES E. PAULLIN, M.D., Atlanta
President, 1935-36

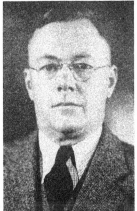

BENJAMIN H. MINCHEW, M.D., Waycross
President-Elect, 1935-36

TRICHOMONAS VAGINALIS INFECTION

During the past few years the importance of the *Trichomonas vaginalis* has been well recognized, particularly in the etiology of leukorrhea and a specific type of vaginitis. This protozoan frequently invades the urethra and bladder with a resulting urethritis and cystitis. Some authorities believe the Trichomonas are capable of reaching the upper genital tract in women and thus cause definite inflammatory changes, but proof of this is lacking at the present time. Also, the organisms have been found inhabiting the colon and rectum and considered the cause of some instances of diarrhea in both sexes. In the male they have been recovered from the urine and prostatic secretion when symptoms suggested, or contact warranted, search for these as a causative agent. In women the infection seems equally as prevalent during pregnancy as at other times, but no significant relation has been found with puerperal infection or abortion.

In the acute stage of vaginitis caused by the Trichomonas vaginalis there is a characteristic diffuse inflammaton of the vaginal mucosa and the pars vaginalis of the cervix with a "strawberry-red" appearance. Also present is a thin, yellowish, purulent, foamy and foul-smelling discharge, often profuse, which is extremely irritating to the surrounding skin. With such a condition as this women complain chiefly of leukorrhea, vaginal burning and irritation, dyspareunia and intense pruritus of the vulva, perineum and anus. Urinary symptoms are frequently associated and at times will be the chief complaint. In the chronic stage the vaginal mucosa shows little or no inflammation, the discharge is not as profuse nor as irritating, and symptoms may be mild or entirely absent. With the chronic type of infection acute exacerbations are prone to occur.

A diagnosis is easily made by microscopic examination of a fresh preparation of the purulent discharge in a few drops of normal saline. Care is necessary to keep the preparation warm and is best examined immediately in order to identify the protozoan by its characteristic jerky movements. The Trichomonas has a pear-shaped body, about twice the size of a polymorphonuclear leukocyte, the active form possessing four flagella. The cystic immobile form is more difficult to recognize. At times the microscopic examination of a fresh specimen of urine will reveal the typical organisms in motion, and such findings may be the first clue to the presence of a Trichomonas infection.

Innumerable methods for treatment of Trichomonas vaginitis have been proposed, the majority of these being equally effective. Probably the most widely used method consists of vigorous vaginal scrubs with tincture of green soap, followed by thorough rinsing with water and the application of one of the various antiseptics or the administration of an antiseptic douche. For local application one of the following can be used: acriflavine 0.5 per cent, gentian violet 1 per cent, ether, or Lugol's solution. The common douches in use are bichloride of mercury 1-5000, lactic acid 2 per cent, sodium perborate, sodium bicarbonate, and boric acid. Recently it has been shown that daily hypertonic (25 per cent) salt douches render the Trichomonas permanently inactive and that this is a simple method which can be effectively carried out by the patient at home. An arsenic tablet preparation "Devegan" (Winthrop), used as a vaginal suppository, two to three tablets daily, has proven equally effective as other methods. Proper treatment for two weeks is usually sufficient. If a cystitis or urethritis is persistent after the vaginitis has cleared, the usual method of treatment with irrigations and instillations is sufficient. Recurrances, however, are not uncommon and these frequently appear following a menstrual period. Therefore, careful observation is necessary, particularly at this time, and if organisms are found treatment should be repeated.

JAMES N. BRAWNER, JR., M.D.

The American Medical Association will hold its eighty-seventh annual session in Kansas City, Missouri, May 11-15, 1936. Official call of the officers of the Association will be published in this Journal in April.

SIGNS AND SYMPTOMS OF EARLY CANCER
(Continued from Page 81)

cervix gives is intermenstrual, painless bleeding or a bloodstained leukorrheal discharge, and this is not characteristic of cancer, for it may be due to other and less harmless causes, such as cervical polyps, fibroids, vaginitis, from an eroded and infected cervix, or from some endocrine disturbance. But any woman, young or old, presenting this symptom should have immediate, thorough and careful examination. There should be no delay in attempts to make a diagnosis because if the bleeding is caused by cancer, it is already well established; for in the very beginning of its growth it gives no sign whatsoever. There is nothing characteristic about the feel or appearance of a cervix with early cancer. There is some bleeding from the eroded or everted area when the surface is sponged which also may occur in inflammatory conditions of the cervix. The only sure way is by removing a section from the suspicious looking area and having a microscopical examination made by a competent and experienced pathologist.

An aid to determine what portion should be removed for microscopical examination is the Schiller test, which is the application to the cervix of Gram's solution. The normal cell, because of its glycogen content, will take on a brown stain, the abnormal cell will not take this stain. Cancer can not be diagnosed by means of this test, but the diseased portions will stand out clearly and from these the biopsy should be taken.

The specimen should be placed in a ten per cent solution of formalin and submitted to a pathologist of wide experience in the examination of tissues, for it is not always an easy matter to detect the transition from inflammatory cells to cancerous ones. With an improper diagnosis some women may be subjected to the radical treatment who do not require it or the treatment for cervicitis may be given when the radical treatment is necessary.

It is Utopian to hope for many cases to be diagnosed and treated in this very early stage, but many more could be found if women could be educated to periodic examinations, particularly those who have borne children or had unnatural discharges.

Better still with such an examination large numbers of cancers could be prevented by having the simpler inflammatory condition cured. It should be the duty of those doctors doing obstetrics to so instruct their patients and not to dismiss them until the cervix is completely healed from trauma of the parturition.

Early diagnosis and prompt and proper treatment means the saving of life that otherwise might be doomed; the cure of cervicitis means the prevention of cancer of the uterine cervix.

PROGRAM
MEDICAL ASSOCIATION OF GEORGIA
1935-1936

EIGHTY-SEVENTH ANNUAL SESSION, SAVANNAH

HOTEL DESOTO, HEADQUARTERS
APRIL 21, 22, 23, 24, 1936

Officers

President	James E. Paullin, Atlanta
President-Elect	B. H. Minchew, Waycross
First Vice-President	James J. Clark, Atlanta
Second Vice-President	Philip R. Stewart, Monroe
Secretary-Treasurer	Edgar D. Shanks, Atlanta
Parliamentarian	John W. Simmons, Brunswick

Delegates to the A. M. A.

William H. Myers (1935-36) ....Savannah
Alternate, Wm. A. Mulherin ....Augusta
Chas. W. Roberts (1935-36) ....Atlanta
Alternate, Marion C. Pruitt ....Atlanta
Olin H. Weaver (1936-37) ....Macon
Alternate, C. K. Sharp ....Arlington

GEORGIA MEDICAL SOCIETY
(Chatham County)
Officers

President	C. F. Holton, Savannah
President-Elect	Geo. H. Faggart, Savannah
Vice-President	S. E. Bray, Savannah
Secretary-Treasurer	O. W. Schwalb, Savannah
Delegate	A. A. Morrison, Savannah
Delegate	J. C. Metts, Savannah
Alternate Delegate	H. J. Morrison, Savannah
Alternate Delegate	J. K. Quattlebaum, Savannah

COMMITTEES
Arrangements

William H. Myers, Savannah, Chairman
Craig Barrow, Savannah
Lee Howard, Savannah
T. P. Waring, Savannah

A. A. Morrison, Savannah
R. V. Martin, Savannah
J. K. Quattlebaum, Savannah

Reception

William R. Dancy, Savannah, Chairman
John L. Elliott, Savannah
H. J. Morrison, Savannah
W. V. Long, Savannah

Transportation

L. A. DeLoach, Savannah, Chairman
D. B. Edwards, Savannah
C. G. Redmond, Savannah

Golf

H. Y. Righton, Savannah, Chairman
M. J. Egan, Savannah
E. J. Whelan, Savannah

Skeet Tournament

J. F. Chisholm, Savannah, Chairman
J. O. Baker, Savannah

Entertainment

J. C. Metts, Savannah, Chairman
E. C. Drmmond, Savannah
Ruskin King, Savannah
C. K. McLaughlin, Savannah
A. J. Waring, Savannah

Finance

G. H. Lang, Savannah, Chairman
Robert Drane, Savannah
H. L. Levington, Savannah
W. A. Cole, Savannah
Charles Usher, Savannah
H. T. Exley, Savannah

Publicity

O. W. Schwalb, Savannah, Chairman
John W. Daniel, Jr., Savannah
J. F. Chisholm, Jr., Savannah

Alumni Dinners
Emory University School of Medicine

E. N. Manor, Savannah, Chairman
L. W. Shaw, Savannah
G. T. Olmstead, Savannah

University of Georgia School of Medicine

J. H. Pinholster, Savannah, Chairman
T. A. Peterson, Savannah
W. O. Bedingfield, Savannah

COUNCIL

J. A. Redfearn, Chairman ....Albany
Grady N. Coker, Clerk ....Canton

Councilors

1.	C. Thompson (1936)	Millen
2.	J. A. Redfearn (1936)	Albany
3.	J. C. Patterson (1936)	Cuthbert
4.	Kenneth S. Hunt (1936)	Griffin
5.	W. A. Selman (1937)	Atlanta
6.	H. G. Weaver (1937)	Macon
7.	M. M. McCord (1937)	Rome
8.	J. E. Penland (1937)	Waycross
9.	Grady N. Coker (1938)	Canton
10.	S. J. Lewis (1938)	Augusta

Vice-Councilors

1. Jas. C. Metts (1936) ....Savannah
2. Chas. H. Watt (1936) ....Thomasville
3. J. Cox Wall (1936)............................Eastman
4. Enoch Callaway (1936)....................LaGrange
5. Marion C. Pruitt (1937) ....Atlanta
6. H. D. Allen (1937) ....Milledgeville
7. H. J. Ault (1937) ....Dalton
8. Wm. W. Turner (1937).....................Nashville
9. J. K. Burns (1938) ....Gainesville
10. W. C. McGeary (1938)......................Madison

Honorary Advisory Board

T. J. McArthur ....President, 1909-1910
Ralston Lattimore ....President, 1913-1914
W. S. Goldsmith.....................President, 1915-1916
J. G. Dean ....President, 1916-1917
E. E. Murphey.......................President, 1917-1918
J. W. Palmer..........................President, 1918-1919
J. M. Smith ....President, 1922-1923
J. W. Daniel ....President, 1923-1924
J. O. Elrod............................President, 1924-1925
F. K. Boland ....President, 1925-1926
V. O. Harvard ....President, 1926-1927
W. A. Mulherin......................President, 1927-1928
C. K. Sharp ....President, 1928-1929
Wm. R. Dancy.......................President, 1929-1930
A. G. Fort.............................President, 1931-1932
M. M. Head ....President, 1932-1933
C. H. Richardson ....President, 1933-1934
Clarence L. Ayers..................President, 1934-1935

COMMITTEES

Scientific Work

S. T. R. Revell, Chairman (1936) ....Louisville
Geo. A. Traylor (1937) ....Augusta
H. C. Sauls (1938) ....Atlanta
Edgar D. Shanks, Secretary-Treasurer............Atlanta

Public Policy and Legislation

Dan Y. Sage, Chairman (1937) ....Atlanta
A. R. Rozar (1936)...................................Macon
C. C. Aven (1938)...................................Atlanta
Edgar D. Shanks, Secretary-Treasurer............Atlanta
T. F. Abercrombie, Director, Department of
   Public Health, State of Georgia....................Atlanta

Medical Defense

Frank K. Boland, Chairman (1938).............Atlanta
J. O. Elrod (1936)..................................Forsyth
Wm. A. Mulherin (1939) ....Augusta
J. A. Redfearn, Chairman of Council.............Albany
Edgar D. Shanks, Secretary-Treasurer............Atlanta

Hospitals

R. H. Oppenheimer, Chairman (1937)...........Atlanta
Arthur D. Little (1936) ....Thomasville
D. Henry Poer (1938)...............................Atlanta
C. D. Whelchel (1939) ....Gainesville
L. P. Holmes (1940) ....Augusta

Abner Wellborn Calhoun Lectureship

Jas. E. Paullin, Chairman (1938) ....Atlanta
H. I. Reynolds (1939) ....Athens

Eugene E. Murphey (1940) ....Augusta
Craig Barrow (1936).............................Savannah
Frank K. Boland (1937)............................Atlanta

Economics

Lewis M. Gaines, Chairman (1940) ....Atlanta
C. W. Roberts (1938) ....Atlanta
C. L. Ridley (1936) ....Macon
Dan Y. Sage (1937) ....Atlanta
J. H. Downey (1939) ....Gainesville

Necrology

A. J. Mooney, Chairman ....Statesboro
Thos. J. McArthur ....Cordele
C. K. Sharp ....Arlington

Medical History of Georgia
Sub-Committee

Frank K. Boland, Chairman........................Atlanta
William R. Dancy................................Savannah
Arthur G. Fort......................................Atlanta
V. H. Bassett.....................................Savannah
Allen H. Bunce......................................Atlanta

Crawford W. Long Memorial Prize

William R. Dancy, Chairman....................Savannah
Stewart R. Roberts.................................Atlanta
V. P. Syndenstricker..............................Augusta
George Bachmann ....Atlanta
Edgar R. Pund ....Augusta

Cancer Commission

Jas. L. Campbell, Chairman.......................Atlanta
William H. Myers ....Savannah
Charles H. Watt................................Thomasville
J. C. Patterson....................................Cuthbert
Kenneth S. Hunt ....Griffin
Charles C. Harrold...................................Macon
W. P. Harbin, Jr.....................................Rome
Kenneth McCullough ....Waycross
Grady N. Coker ....Canton
Ralph H. Chaney....................................Augusta

Advisory—State Board of Health

C. W. Roberts, Chairman..........................Atlanta
Craig Barrow ....Savannah
M. E. Winchester................................Brunswick
M. M. McCord..Rome
Marvin H. Head...................................Zebulon
A. H. Hilsman ....Albany
T. F. Abercrombie..................................Atlanta

Advisory—Woman's Auxiliary

Jas. N. Brawner, Chairman ....Atlanta
J. M. Smith...Valdosta
E. R. Harris...Winder
W. R. Garner....................................Gainesville
Benjamin Bashinski ....Macon

L. G. Hardman Loving Cup

W. A. Selman.......................................Atlanta
Wm. A. Mulherin...................................Augusta
Chas. H. Watt...................................Thomasville
M. M. McCord...Rome

Crawford W. Long Bronze Statue to Cooperate with
Chamber of Commerce, Jefferson, Georgia
Garnett W. Quillian, Chairman..........................Atlanta
Ralph M. Goss ....Athens
D. N. Thompson..Elberton
E. M. McDonald..Winder

Post-Graduate Study
G. Lombard Kelly, Chairman..........................Augusta
Russell H. Oppenheimer..................Emory University
Chas. H. Watt..Thomasville
W. W. Chrisman..Macon

Scientific Exhibit
Mark S. Dougherty, General Chairman..............Atlanta
Lee Howard, Local Chairman..........................Savannah
Everett L. Bishop..Atlanta
J. L. Campbell..Atlanta
John L. Elliott..Savannah
William P. Harbin, Jr..Rome
William F. Jenkins..Columbus
Roy R. Kracke............................Emory University
Fred A. Mettler..Augusta
E. B. Saye..Macon
T. F. Sellers..Atlanta
H. F. Sharpley, Jr..Savannah
Ernest F. Wahl..Thomasville

Prize for Hookworm Control*
W. F. Reavis, Chairman..................................Waycross
E. F. Wahl..Thomasville
H. M. Tolleson..Eastman
*Award by the Ware County Medical Society.

Study of Maternal Mortality and Infant Deaths
E. D. Colvin, Chairman..Atlanta

First District
A. J. Mooney..Statesboro
A. J. Waring..Savannah

Second District
W. L. Wilkinson..Bainbridge
W. W. Jarrell..Thomasville

Third District
Herschel A. Smith..Americus
J. C. Patterson..Cuthbert

Fourth District
H. J. Copeland..Griffin
Emory R. Park..LaGrange

Fifth District
E. D. Colvin..Atlanta
J. R. McCord..Atlanta

Sixth District
Otis R. Thompson..Macon
T. C. Clodfelter,..Eatonton

Seventh District
P. O. Chaudron..Cedartown
W. Mayes Gober..Marietta

Eighth District
M. E. Winchester..Brunswick
E. J. Overstreet..Baxley

Ninth District
Pratt Cheek ....Gainesville
Geo. C. Brooke..Canton

Tenth District
S. S. Smith..Athens
John W. Thurmond, Jr..Augusta
ex officio
T. F. Abercrombie, Director, Department of
Public Health for Georgia..............................Atlanta

Fraternal Delegate to the
Georgia Dental Association
R. Hugh Wood..Atlanta

Fraternal Delegate to the
Georgia Pharmaceutical Association
Glenville Giddings ....Atlanta

Fraternal Delegates to Other State Meetings
To visit Alabama—Wallace H. Clark, LaGrange, and
J. T. McCall, Rome.
To visit Florida—C. F. Holton, Savannah, and Ar-
thur G. Fort, Atlanta.
To visit North Carolina—H. L. Erwin, Dalton, and
C. G. Butler, Gainesville.
To visit South Carolina—Stewart D. Brown, Roys-
ton, and A. O. Meredith, Hartwell.

Fraternal Delegate from the South Carolina
Medical Association
C. O. Bates..Greenville, S. C.

Fraternal Delegate from the Georgia Dental
Association
F. C. Wilson, D.D.S..Savannah

State Board of Health
First District—Cleveland Thompson, Millen, Sept. 1,
1939.
Second District—C. K. Sharp, Arlington, Sept. 1,
1939.
Third District—Mr. R. C. Ellis, Americus, Sept. 1,
1936.
Fourth District—Marvin M. Head, Zebulon, Sept. 1,
1937.
Fifth District—Mr. Robert F. Maddox, Atlanta, Sept.
1, 1936.
Sixth District—A. R. Rozar, Macon, Sept. 1, 1938.
Seventh District—Mather M. McCord, Rome, Sept.
1, 1938.
Eighth District—Henry W. Clements, Adel, Sept. 1'
1938.
Ninth District—L. C. Allen, Hoschton, Sept. 1, 1939.
Tenth District—Wm. A. Mulherin, Augusta, Sept.
1, 1937.

State of Georgia At Large
Pharmaceutical Association
T. C. Marshall, Atlanta, Sept. 1, 1941.
W. T. Edwards, Augusta, Sept. 1, 1941.
Georgia Dental Association
J. G. Williams, D.D.S., Atlanta, 1940.
Paul McGee, D.D.S., Waycross, Sept. 1, 1940.

DISTRICT SOCIETIES
Officers and Meeting Dates
First District
President—Chas. T. Brown, Guyton.

Sec'y-Treas.—Chas. Usher, Savannah.
Third Wednesdays—March and July.
Second District
President—C. K. Wall, Thomasville.
Sec'y-Treas.—J. C. Brim, Pelham.
Second Tuesdays—April and October.
Third District
President—J. E. Walker, Columbus.
Sec'y-Treas.—Chas. A. Greer, Oglethorpe.
Third Wednesday in June—Second Wednesday in November.
Fourth District
President—Enoch Callaway, LaGrange.
Sec'y-Treas.—M. M. Head, Zebulon.
Second Wednesdays—February and August.
Fifth District
President—H.· G. Ansley, Decatur.
Sec'y-Treas.—D. Henry Poer, Atlanta.
No definite date.
Sixth District
President—J. E. New, Dexter.
Sec'y-Treas.—W. W. Chrisman, Macon.
Last Wednesday in June—First Wednesday in December.
Seventh District
President—H. J. Ault, Dalton.
Sec'y-Treas.—William Harbin, Jr., Rome.
First Wednesday in April—Last Wednesday in September.
Eighth District
President—R. L. Johnson, Waycross.
Sec'y-Treas.—Gordon T. Crozier, Valdosta.
Second Tuesdays—April and October.
Ninth District
President—D. H. Garrison, Tate.
Sec'y-Treas.—Pratt Cheek, Gainesville.
Third Wednesdays—March and September.
Tenth District
President—Ralph H. Chaney, Augusta.·
Sec'y-Treas.—Philip R. Stewart, Monroe.
Second Wednesdays—February and August.

DELEGATES TO THE 1936 SESSION

Counties	Names and Addresses
Appling (Altamaha)	
Baldwin	Chas. B. Fulghum, Milledgeville
Bartow	T. Lowry, Cartersville
Ben Hill	Lewis Abrams, Fitzgerald
Bibb	J. B. Kay, Byron
	A. R. Rozar, Macon
Blue Ridge	
Brooks	
Bulloch-Candler-Evans	
Burke	W. C. McCarver, Vidette
Butts	
Carroll	S. F. Scales, Carrolton
Chatham	A. A. Morrison, Savannah
	J. C. Metts, Savannah
Chattooga	R. N. Little, Summerville
Cherokee	J. T. Petti● Canton
Clarke	H. B. Harris, Athens

Clayton-Fayette	J. A. S. Chambers, Inmar
Cobb	W. H. Perkinson, Mariett:
Coffee	Sage, Harper, Wra}
Colquitt	C. C. Brannen, Moultri
Coweta	
Crisp	Chas. Adams, Cordel
Decatur-Seminole	M. A. Ehrlich, Bainbridg
DeKalb	
Dooly	
Dougherty	H. M. McKemie, Alban}
Douglas	C. V. Vansant, Douglasvill
Elbert	D. N. Thompson, Elberto1
Emanuel	C. E. Powell, Swainsbor
Floyd	W. P. Harbin, Jr., Rom
Forsyth	
Franklin	B. T. Smith, Carnesvill
Fulton	C. C. Aven, Atlanta
	Grady E. Clay, Atlanta
	T. C. Davison, Atlanta
	E. F. Fincher, Jr., Atlant
	Ed H. Greene, Atlanta
	H. C. Sauls, Atlanta
	C. W. Strickler, Atlanta
Glynn	C. B. Greer, Brunswicl
Gordon	Z. V. Johnston, Calhou1
Grady	J. V. Rogers, Cair1
Greene	
Gwinnett	
Habersham	M. F. Haygood, Hamilto1
Hall	J. 'H. Downey, Gainesvill
Hancock	C. S. Jernigan, Spart
Harris	
Hart	W. E. McCurry, Hartwel
Henry	J. G. Smith, McDonoug|
Houston-Peach	
Jackson-Barrow	C. B. Almand, Winde
Jasper	
Jefferson	S. T. R. Revell, Louisvill
Jenkins	C. Thompson, Mille1
Jones	
Lamar	
Laurens	
Lowndes (South Georgia Medical Society)	
	G. T. Crozier, Valdost
Macon	Thos. M. Adams, Montezum
McDuffie	J.·R. Wilson, Thomso
Meriwether	
Mitchell	
Monroe	
Montgomery	
Morgan	
Murray	
Muscogee	Frank Schley, Columbu
Newton	
Ocmulgee (Beckley, Dodge, Pulaski)	
	A. R. Bush, Hawkinsvill
Paulding	
Polk	John W. Good, Cedartow
Putnam	
Rabun	J. C. Dover, Clayto
Randolph	W. G. Elliott, Cuthber

Richmond ....G. L. Kelly, Augusta
                                    R. H. Chaney, Augusta
Screven ....
Spalding ....A. H. Frye, Griffin
Stephens ....
Stewart-Webster ....
Sumter.............................J. C. Logan, Plains
Talbot ....
Taliaferro ....
Tattnall .... L. V. Strickland, Cobbtown
Taylor...........................S. H. Bryan, Reynolds
Telfair...........................F. R. Mann, McRae
Terrell ....
Thomas ....
Tift ....C. S. Pittman, Tifton
Toombs ....
Tri-Society (Calhoun, Early, Miller)..................
...............................W. O. Shepard, Bluffton
Tri-Society (Liberty, Long, McIntosh)............
.... I. G. Armistead, Warsaw
Troup ....Enoch Callaway, LaGrange
Turner ....
Upson ....
Walker ....S. B. Kitchens, LaFayette
Walton ....
Ware.......:......................W. F. Reavis, Waycross
Washington ....N. J. Newsom, Sandersville
Wayne ....J. T. Colvin, Jesup
Whitfield ....J. C. Rollins, Dalton
Wilcox ....J. D. Owens, Rochelle
Wilkes ....O. S. Wood, Washington
Warren ....
Worth ....

*This list includes the names of all delegates reported to the Secretary-Treasurer.

ANNOUNCEMENTS

Meetings will be held in the Dining Room, Hotel DeSoto.

Be sure to go to the Registration Desk, present your 1936 membership card and procure a badge immediately on your arrival.

Discussion of papers is open to all members and guests of the Association. It is not limited to those named on the program.

On arising to discuss a paper the speaker will please announce his name and address clearly for the benefit of the Association and stenographer.

Meetings will be called to order at the hour fixed on the program. It is especially desired that the members be prompt in their attendance.

All manuscript should be typewritten, double spaced and on one side of the paper only. Papers must be handed to the Secretary immediately after being read.

IMPORTANT NOTICE!

Delegates must present written credentials to the Committee on Credentials from the House of Delegates to secure Delegates' badges.

Members may not take part in the proceedings until they have registered and procured official badges.

PUBLIC MEETINGS
Eastern Standard Time
Dining Room—Hotel DeSoto

WEDNESDAY, APRIL 22, 9:00 A.M.
Opening meeting
Dining Room—Hotel DeSoto

WEDNESDAY, APRIL 22, 8:00 P.M.
Dining Room—Hotel DeSoto
Presentation of the "Badge of Service" to the President, James Edgar Paullin, Atlanta, by F. Phinizy Calhoun, Atlanta.

The Problem of the Diaphragm
Arthur M. Shipley
Professor of Surgery, University of Maryland School of Medicine and College of Physicians and Surgeons, Baltimore, Maryland.
Introduction by S. T. R. Revell, Louisville.

Management of the Chronic Heart
Jonathan C. Meakins
Professor of Medicine, McGill University Faculty of Medicine, and President of the Canadian Medical Association, Montreal, Quebec, Canada.
Introduction by James Edgar Paullin, Atlanta.

The Influence of the Present-Day Depression Upon the Nutritive State of the American People
James S. McLester
Professor of Medicine, University of Alabama School of Medicine, and President of the American Medical Association, Birmingham, Ala.
Introduction by Lewis M. Gaines, Atlanta.

THURSDAY, APRIL 23, 12:00 Noon
President's Address
The President's Address will be at an open session to which the public and visitors are invited.

Memorial Exercises
A. J. Mooney, Statesboro, Chairman, Committee on Necrology.

ENTERTAINMENTS

TUESDAY, APRIL 21, 9:00 P.M.
Dr. and Mrs. William H. Myers will be at home, 101 East Jones Street, Savannah, in honor of the officers of the Medical Association of Georgia, and of the Woman's Auxiliary.

WEDNESDAY, APRIL 22, 6:00 P.M.
Annual dinner of the alumni of the University of Georgia School of Medicine, Hotel DeSoto.
Annual dinner of the alumni of Emory University School of Medicine, Hotel DeSoto.

THURSDAY, APRIL 23, 12:00 NOON
Annual Luncheon, Georgia Pediatric Society, Hotel

DeSoto. Invited Guest: Warren Quillian, Coral Gables, Florida.

THURSDAY, APRIL 23, 2:00 P.M.

Annual luncheon of the Eye, Ear, Nose & Throat Club of Georgia, Hotel DeSoto. G., H. Lang, Local Chairman.

THURSDAY, APRIL 23, 8:00 P.M.
Banquet—Hotel DeSoto
C. F. Holton, Savannah, Toastmaster
Dance—10:00 to 2:00

SPORTS
Golf

All golf courses will be open to all players. A golf tournament will be held at the Savannah Golf Club.

Fishing

If interested in deep-sea fishing, write to C. F. Holton, DeRenne Apartments, Savannah, President of the Georgia Medical Society.

Trap Shooting

J. F. Chisholm, 512 Abercorn Street, Savannah, will be in charge of a skeet shooting tournament. Trophies will be awarded to winners and runners-up.

MEETING OF THE COUNCIL

The first meeting of the Council will be held in the Gold Room, Hotel DeSoto, Tuesday, April 21, at 6:30 P.M. Each Councilor will render a written report of conditions in each county in his district. Other meetings of the Council will be held on the call of the chairman.

MEETING OF THE HOUSE OF DELEGATES
Gold Room—Hotel DeSoto
TUESDAY, APRIL 21, 2:00 P.M.
Eastern Standard Time

First meeting of the House of Delegates.
1. Call to order by the President.
2. Roll call.
3. Appointment of Reference Committee.
4. Reports of officers:
   President.
   President-Elect.
   Vice-Presidents.
   Parliamentarian.
   Secretary-Treasurer: Financial report.
   Report of Delegates to the A. M. A.
   Preliminary report of the Committee on Medical Economics.
   a. Scientific Work.
   b. Public Policy and Legislation.
   c. Arrangements.
   d. Medical Defense.
   e. Hospitals.
   f. Necrology.
   g. Cancer Commission.
   h. History.
   i. Abner Wellborn Calhoun Lectureship.

   j. Crawford W. Long Memorial Prize.
   k. L. G. Hardman Silver Loving Cup.
   l. Advisory—State Board of Health.
   m. Advisory—Woman's Auxiliary.
   n. Crawford W. Long Bronze Statue.
   o. Special Committees.
5. Reports of Fraternal Delegates.
6. Unfinished business.
7. New business.

TUESDAY, APRIL 21, 8:00 P.M.
Eastern Standard Time

Second meeting of the House of Delegates.
1. Call to order by the President.
2. Reading of minutes.
3. Study of Maternal Mortality—Chairman of Committee.
4. Reports of Committees continued.
5. Unfinished business.
6. New business.

FRIDAY, APRIL 24, 8:00 A.M.
Eastern Standard Time

Third meeting of the House of Delegates.
1. Call to order by the President.
2. Reading of minutes.
3. Reports of committees.
4. Unfinished business.
5. New business.

OFFICIAL REPORTER
Master Reporting Company......................Chicago

PROGRAM

The papers for each meeting must be read as scheduled on the program.

WEDNESDAY, APRIL 22, 9:00 A.M.
Dining Room—Hotel DeSoto
Eastern Standard Time

Call to order by the President, James Edgar Paullin, Atlanta.

Invocation
Rev. C. C. J. Carpenter......................Savannah
Addresses of Welcome
Cornelius F. Holton......................Savannah
President, Georgia Medical Society
Hon. Thomas Gamble......................Savannah
Mayor of Savannah
Response to Addresses of Welcome
William S. Goldsmith......................Atlanta

SCIENTIFIC PAPERS

1. The Dilution and Concentration Tests of Kidney Function.
   W. Edward Storey, Columbus.
   To lead the discussion:
   J. C. Metts, Savannah.
   Geo. L. Walker, Griffin.
2. Fusospirochetal Diseases of the Lung.
   J. P. Tye, Albany.
   To lead the discussion:

H. I. Reynolds, Athens.
J. T. Ross, Macon.

3. *Symposium on Thyroid and Parathyroid Problems.*
(a, b, c, d.)
(a). Chronic Hyperthyroidism with a Persistent
Low Metabolic Rate.
T. C. Davison, Atlanta.
(b). Goiter in Children.
J. Gaston Gay, Atlanta.
(c). Goiter and Iodine.
Ben Hill Clifton, Atlanta.
(d). Hyperparathyroidism—Lantern Slides.
J. Reid Broderick, Savannah.
To lead the discussion:
Robert L. Rhodes, Augusta.
D. Henry Poer, Atlanta.
J. C. Metts, Savannah.
Olin H. Weaver, Macon.

WEDNESDAY, APRIL 22, 12:00 NOON
ABNER WELLBORN CALHOUN LECTURE
*Fundamental Aspects of the Diagnosis and
Treatment of Anemia.*
Wm. Bosworth Castle,
Associate Professor of Medicine, Harvard University
Medical School, Boston, Mass.
Introduction by Eugene E. Murphey, Augusta.

WEDNESDAY, APRIL 22, 2:00 P.M.
Eastern Standard Time
Dining Room—Hotel DeSoto

1. Some Comments Upon the Present-Day Practice of
Rhinolaryngology Based Upon Forty-Two
Years Experience.
Dunbar Roy, Atlanta.
To lead the discussion:
B. H. Minchew, Waycross.
· H. J. Ault, Dalton.

2. Primary Bronchial Carcinoma—Report of Case.
J. D. Gray, Augusta.
To lead the discussion:
Stewart R. Roberts, Atlanta.
Murdock Equen, Atlanta.

3. Appendicitis.
Charles Usher, Savannah.
To lead the discussion:
B. T. Wise, Americus.
Grady N. Coker, Canton.

4. Uretero-Intestinal Anastomosis.
Geo. W. Wright, Augusta.
To lead the discussion:
J. K. Quattlebaum, Savannah.
L. G. Baggett ,Atlanta.

5. Examination of the Prostate.
Rudolph Bell, Thomasville.
To lead the discussion:
Montague L. Boyd, Atlanta.
Wallace L. Bazemore, Macon.

6. A Yardstick for Properly Evaluating the Merits or
Demerits of the Various Methods of Infant
Feeding.
Wm. A. Mulherin, Augusta.
To lead the discussion:
Benjamin Bashinski, Macon.
Mather M. McCord, Rome.

WEDNESDAY, APRIL 22, 8:00 P.M.
Eastern Standard Time
Hotel DeSoto
Presentation of the "Badge of Service" to the Presi-
dent, Dr. James E. Paullin, Atlanta, by ·F. Phinizy
Calhoun, Atlanta.

The Problem of the Diaphragm
Arthur M. Shipley
Professor of Surgery, University of Maryland School
of Medicine and College of Physicians and Surgeons,
Baltimore, Maryland.
Introduction by S. T. R. Revell, Louisville.

Management of the Chronic Heart
Jonathan C. Meakins
Professor of Medicine, McGill University Faculty
of Medicine, and President of the Canadian Medical
Association, Montreal, Quebec, Canada.
Introduction by James Edgar Paullin, Atlanta.

*The Influence of the Present Day Depression Upon
the Nutritive State of the American People*
James S. McLester
Professor of Medicine, University of Alabama School
of Medicine, and President of the American Medical
Association, Birmingham, Ala.
Introduction by Lewis M. Gaines, Atlanta.

THURSDAY, APRIL 23, 9:00 A.M.
Eastern Standard Time
Dining Room—Hotel DeSoto

1. Five Unusual Fractures.
J. H. Mull, Rome.
To lead the discussion:
Kenneth McCullough, Waycross.
Wm. A. Newman, Macon.

2. Chronic Arthritis and Fibrositis.
Hal M. Davison, Atlanta.
Mason I. Lowance, Atlanta.
Crawford F. Barnett, Atlanta.
To lead the discussion:
Ernest F. Wahl, Thomasville.
F. G. Hodgson, Atlanta.

3. Friedman's Modification of the Aschheim-Zondek
Pregnancy Test—Report of 75 Cases.
George F. Klugh, Atlanta.
To lead the discussion:
G. Lombard Kelly, Augusta.
A. J. Ayers, Atlanta.

4. Further Observations on Sleep.
Glenville Giddings, Atlanta.
To lead the discussion:

Jas. N. Brawner, Atlanta.
V. P. Sydenstricker, Augusta.

5. Tumors of the Adult Kidney—Lantern Slides
Showing the Pathologic Changes and the
Pyelographic Deformity.
Earl Floyd, Atlanta.
Jas. L. Pittman, Atlanta.
To lead the discussion:
J. Righton Robertson, Augusta.
W. F. Reavis, Waycross.

6. Public Health Problems in Georgia.
T. F. Abercrombie, Atlanta.
To lead the discussion:
J. D. Applewhite, Macon.
Gordon T. Crozier, Valdosta.

THURSDAY, APRIL 23, 12:00 NOON
Eastern Standard Time
Dining Room—Hotel DeSoto
President's Address
James E. Paullin, Atlanta
President, Medical Association of Georgia

Memorial Exercises
A. J. Mooney, Statesboro
Chairman, Committee on Necrology

THURSDAY, APRIL 23, 2:00 P.M.
Eastern Standard Time
Dining Room—Hotel DeSoto

1. The Use of Atabrine in the Control and Treatment
of Malaria.
M. E. Winchester, Brunswick.
To lead the discussion:
H. M. Tolleson, Eastman.
J. W. Mobley, Jr., Pelham.

2. Psychosis Following the Administration of Atabrine
for Malaria—Report of Nine Cases.
E. W. Allen, Milledgeville.
H. D. Allen, Jr., Milledgeville.
Chas. B. Fulghum, Milledgeville.
To lead the discussion:
Shelton P. Sanford, Savannah.
Geo. L. Echols, Milledgeville.

3. Conservative Obstetrics Will Materially Lower the
Mortality Rate in Eclampsia.
Jas. R. McCord, Atlanta.
To lead the discussion:
D. N. Thompson, Elberton.
O. R. Thompson, Macon.

4. Physiology of Evolution, Menstruation and Preg-
nancy—Lantern Slides.
H. F. Sharpley, Jr., Savannah.
To lead the discussion:
B. T. Beasley, Atlanta.
C. B. Greer, Brunswick.

5. Hemorrhages of the Brain: Their Differentiation
and Treatment.
J. Calvin Weaver, Atlanta.
To lead the discussion:

Richard Binion, Milledgeville.
A. H. Hilsman, Albany.

6. A New Phase of Intestinal Allergy.
M. A. Ehrlich, Bainbridge.
To lead the discussion:
Clarence L. Laws, Atlanta.
H. L. Earl, Sparta.

FRIDAY, APRIL 24, 9:00 A.M.
Eastern Standard Time
Dining Room—Hotel DeSoto

1. Endoscopy as an Aid to the General Practitioner
in the Diagnosis and Treatment of Diseases
of the Respiratory and Upper Alimentary
Tract.
B. McH. Cline, Atlanta.
To lead the discussion:
Ed. S. Wright, Atlanta.
Geo. H. Lang, Savannah.

2. Antitoxin Treatment of Meningococcic Infections
and Meningitis.
Howard J. Morrison, Savannah.
To lead the discussion:
G. W. H. Cheney, Brunswick.
Bradley B. Davis, Gainesville.

3. History of Hysterectomy with a Review of Hyst-
erectomies Performed in the John D. Arch-
bold Memorial Hospital.
Arthur D. Little, Thomasville.
To lead the discussion:
Chas. C. Harrold, Macon.
Guy T. Bernard, Augusta.

4. The Treatment of Myasthenia Gravis.
Wm. A. Smith, Atlanta.
To lead the discussion:
Mercer Blanchard, Columbus.
R. B. Wilson, Atlanta.

5. Congenital Hypertrophic Pyloric Stenosis—A Clini-
cal and Statistical Study of 143 Cases with
Special Reference to Treatment and Results.
R. C. McGahee, Augusta.
To lead the discussion:
A. M. Johnson, Valdosta.

6. The Surgical Correction of Crossed Eyes.
Wm. O. Martin, Jr., Atlanta.
To lead the discussion:
J. F. Chisholm, Savannah.
C. L. Penington, Macon.

ALTERNATE
The Treatment of Osteomyelitis with Bipp and Auto-
genous Vaccine.
Martin T. Meyers, Atlanta.

FRIDAY, APRIL 24, 12:00 NOON
Eastern Standard Time
Election of Officers
President-Elect.
First Vice-President.

Second Vice-President.
Two Delegates to the A. M. A.
Two Alternate Delegates to the A. M. A.
Councilors for the First. Second. Third and Fourth
    Districts.*
Selection of meeting place for 1937.

*Nominated by their respective district societies.

CONSTITUTION AND BY-LAWS

Chapter II. Section 2. No papers or addresses before the Association, except those of the President and invited essayists, shall occupy more than fifteen minutes in their delivery; and no member shall speak longer than five minutes, nor more than once on any subject, provided that each essayist shall have five minutes in which to close the discussion of his paper.

Chapter VIII. Section 1. The deliberations of this Association shall be governed by parliamentary usage as contained in Roberts' Rules of Order, when not in conflict with this Constitution and By-Laws.

Chapter VIII. Section 2. All papers read before the Association shall become its property. Each paper shall be deposited with the Secretary when read, and if this is not done, it shall not be published.

No miscellaneous or business matters will be discussed before the scientific meetings, but will be referred to the House of Delegates.

Resolution Adopted 1921

Resolved. That a member who sends in a title of a paper to be placed on the program and is not present to read the paper shall pay the penalty of not having an opportunity to appear on the program for two years. unless he presents an excuse acceptable to the Committee on Scientific Work.

NOTICE TO MEMBERS PARTICIPATING IN THE SCIENTIFIC EXHIBIT

Three certificates of merit, to be known as first, second and third prizes, will be given by the Committee on Scientific Work to the three outstanding exhibits at this session of the Medical Association of Georgia. These will be judged on the first day of the session.

We are instructed by the President to announce to all essayists that the session of the Scientific Program of the Association will begin on time, and that the above regulations of the By-Laws in reference to the program will be strictly enforced.

Committee on Scientific Work
S. T. R. Revell. Louisville, Chairman.
Geo. A. Traylor, Augusta.
H. C. Sauls. Atlanta.
Edgar D. Shanks, Atlanta. Sec'y-Treas.

IN MEMORIAM*

Anderson, James W., Gray, January 3, 1936, aged 70.
Austin, Guy Leslie, Pavo, December 11, 1935, aged 56.
Bailey, Eugene McKay, Acworth, March 2, 1936, aged 68.
Barron. John M. F., Milner, April 30, 1935, aged 78.
Brice. George P.. Cumming, September 2, 1935, aged 75.
Campbell. John A.. Nahunta, September 20, 1935, aged 51.
Clifton, Benjamin L.. Millen, June 7, 1935, aged 77.
Coleman, Alexander Stuart Matheson, Douglas, November 15, 1935, aged 45.
Cranford, James Robert, Sasser, November 29, 1935, aged 65.
Evans. William Walker, Blakely, May 10, 1935, aged 70.
Fincher, Edgar F., Atlanta, January 7, 1936, aged 66.
Fullilove. Henry Marshall, Athens, November 17, 1935, aged 58.
Griffin, Archie, Valdosta, May 2, 1935, aged 65.
Griffin, William C., Cartersville, July 23, 1935, aged 80.
Harpe, Samuel Melvin, Calhoun, October 27, 1935, aged 72.
Hinton, Charles Crawford, Macon, February 25, 1936, aged 48.
Joiner, Buford O'Neal, Tennille, June 16, 1935, aged 49.
Jones, Abram B., Tyrone, September 6, 1935, aged 59.
Jones, Francis Gilchrist, Atlanta, February 25, 1936, aged 50.
Kelly, John Oliver, Avera, October 31, 1935, aged 54.
Kemp, A. Pierce, Macon, January 13, 1936, aged 67.
King, James M., Metcalf, February 8, 1936, aged 78.
Lester, James A., Fayetteville, June 24, 1935, aged 65.
Lindsay, James Arthur, Cairo, February 8, 1936, aged 63.
Lovett, William Robert, Sylvania, November 11, 1935, aged 73.
McClain, Marion Cicero, December 25, 1935, aged 76.
McDuffie, James Henry, Columbus, November 16, 1935, aged 76.
McMahan, John Walter, Alma, July 30, 1935, aged 60.
Nelson, G. W., Marshallville, February 26, 1936, aged 74.
Osborne, James C., Acworth, March 11, 1936, aged 70.
Peterson, Nichols, Tifton, March 13, 1936, aged 68.
Powell, John H., Atlanta, November 16, 1935, aged 66.
Pumpelly, William Collins, Macon, September 18, 1935, aged 58.
Ridley, Robert Berrien, Atlanta, December 4, 1935, aged 56.
Simmons, Robert Olin. Rome, July 6, 1935, aged 52.
Tracy, John Lunsford, Sylvester, July 19, 1935, aged 61.

Waits, William J., Gray, April 25, 1935, aged 67.
Wall, Homer Augustus, Ochlochnee, January, 27 1936, aged 67.
Westmoreland, Willis F., Atlanta, December 4, 1935, aged 71.
White, John C., Atlanta, September 7, 1935, aged 76.

*This is the list of members who have died since our last annual session as it appears on our records. Please notify the Secretary-Treasurer of any errors or omissions.

THE COMMERCIAL EXHIBIT

A list of commercial exhibitors, names and adresses. is published on page 112. They are all ethical and will put on display only articles and pharmaceuticals which have been accepted by the Council of the A. M. A.

CONSTITUTION AND BY-LAWS OF THE MEDICAL ASSOCIATION OF GEORGIA
BY-LAWS

Constitution

ARTICLE I.—NAME OF THE ASSOCIATION.
The name and title of this organization shall be the Medical Association of Georgia.

ARTICLE II.—PURPOSES OF THE ASSOCIA-TION
The purpose of this Association shall be to federate and bring into one compact organization the entire medical profession of the State of Georgia; to extend medical knowledge and advance medical science; to elevate the standard of medical education and to secure the enactment and enforcement of just medical laws; to promote friendly intercourse among physicians; to guard and foster the material interests of its members and to protect them against imposition; and to enlighten and direct public opinion in regard to the great problems of state and medicine, so that the profession shall become more capable and honorable within itself, and more useful to the public, in the prevention and cure of disease, and in prolonging and adding comfort to life.

ARTICLE III.—COMPONENT SOCIETIES
Component societies shall consist of those county societies which hold charters from this Association.

ARTICLE IV.—COMPOSITION OF THE ASSOCIATION
Section 1. This Association shall consist of members and delegates.

Sec. 2. Members: The members of this Association shall be the members of the component county medical societies to which only white physicians shall be eligible.

Sec. 3. Delegates: Delegates shall be those members who are elected in accordance with this Constitution and By-Laws to represent their respective component societies in the House of Delegates of this Association.

ARTICLE V.—HOUSE OF DELEGATES
The House of Delegates shall be the legislative body of the Association, and shall consist of: (1) delegates elected by the component county societies; (2) the officers of the Association enumerated in Section 1 of Article IX of the Constitution; (3) ex-presidents and delegates to the American Medical Association.

ARTICLE VI.—COUNCIL
The Council shall be the Board of Trustees and Finance Committee of the Association. The Council shall have full authority and power of the House of Delegates between annual sessions, unless the House of Delegates be called into session as provided in the Constitution and By-Laws.

It shall consist of the Councilors, the President, the President-Elect and the Secretary-Treasurer of the Association. Five of its members shall constitute a quorum.

ARTICLE VII.—SESSIONS AND MEETINGS
Sec. 1. The annual sessions shall take place on the second Wednesday in May at such place as shall be designated by the Association, provided that in case of conflict with the meeting of the American Medical Association the Council may change the date by publishing a notice in the Journal of the Medical Asociation of Georgia three months before the session.

Sec. 2. Special meetings of either the Association or the House of Delegates may be called by a two-thirds vote of the Council, or upon the petition of twenty delegates.

ARTICLE VIII.—SECTIONS AND DISTRICT SOCIETIES
Section 1. The House of Delegates may provide for a division of the scientific work of the Association into appropriate sections, and for the organization of such Councilor district societies as will promote the best interests of the profession such societies to be composed exclusively of members of component county societies.

ARTICLE IX.—OFFICERS
Section 1. The officers of this Association shall be a President, President-Elect, two Vice-Presidents, a Secretary-Treasurer, a Parliamentarian, and one Councilor for each congressional district in the state.

Sec. 2. The officers, except the Secretary-Treasurer, Parliamentarian and Councilors, shall be elected annually, provided that after the annual meeting of 1928 a President-Elect and not a President shall be elected annually. The President-Elect shall assume his office as President immediately after the next annual meeting following his election. The terms of the Councilors shall be for three years, as may be arranged, viz: the Councilor for the first, second, third and fourth districts for three years; those for the fifth, sixth, seventh, and eighth districts for one year; those for the ninth and tenth districts for two years. The Secretary-Treasurer shall be elected for a term of five years, and the Parliamentarian for a term of three years. All these officers shall serve until their successors are elected and installed. (1933);

Sec. 3 The officers of this Association shall be elected by ballot at 12 o'clock noon on the third day of the annual session. Nomination for office shall be made orally, but the nominating speech must not exceed two minutes. The Councilors shall be elected at the same time, but on nomination by their respective District Societies at the annual meeting of such Societies preceding the meeting of the Association at which the vacancy occurs. If there is no election on the first ballot, the three names receiving the highest number of ballots shall be voted on, the other names being dropped. If there is no election on the second ballot, the two names receiving the highest number of ballots shall be voted on until an election occurs. Delegates to the American Medical Association shall be elected at the same time and in the same manner.

Sec. 4. The members of the State Board of Health shall be nominated by their respective district societies at the annual meeting of such societies preceding the annual session of this Association, and in failure of nomination by district societies, they may be nominated by the delegates present from each of the district societies, all of which shall be ratified by this Association.

ARTICLE X.—FUNDS AND EXPENSES

Funds shall be raised by an equal per capita assessment on each component society. The amount of the assessment shall not exceed the sum of $10.00 per capita per annum. Funds may be appropriated by the House of Delegates to defray the expenses of the Association, for publications, and for such other purposes as will promote the welfare of the profession. All resolutions appropriating funds must be approved by the Finance Committee before action is taken thereon.

ARTICLE XI.—RATIFICATION

The House of Delegates shall submit all questions before it to the Association for ratification.

ARTICLE XII.—THE SEAL

The Association shall have a common seal, with power to break, change or renew the same at pleasure.

ARTICLE XIII.—AMENDMENTS

Any amendment that may be offered to the Constitution shall lie over until the next annual session; and for its adoption at such session shall require a two-thirds vote of all present and voting.

By-Laws

CHAPTER I.—MEMBERSHIP

Section 1. The name of a physician on the properly certified roster of members of a component society, which has paid its annual assessment, shall be *prima facie* evidence of membership in this Association.

Sec. 2. Any person who is under sentence of suspension or expulsion from a component society or whose name has been dropped from its roll of members, shall not be entitled to any of the rights or benefits of this Association, nor shall he be permitted to take part in any of its proceedings until he has been relieved of such disability.

Sec. 3. Each member in attendance at the annual session, shall enter his name on the registration book, indicating the component society of which he is a member. When his right to membership has been verified by reference to the roster of his society, he shall receive a badge which shall be evidence of his right to all the privileges of membership at that session. No member shall take part in any of the proceedings of an annual session until he has complied with the provisions of this section.

Sec. 4. Any member for old age, length of service, or other good reasons, may, upon recommendation of the Board of Censors, be elected to honorary membership of his county society without dues. Such member shall be enrolled as an honorary member of his county society and the Association, and shall be entitled to all the privileges of the Association.

Sec. 5. In addition to regular and honorary members, upon recommendation of the Board of Censors, associate members and intern members may be elected by any constituent-county society without the payment of dues. The associate members will be such as may be eligible for regular membership, but not in very active practice and usually with a very limited income—also certain salaried physicians and members of the Army, Navy, U. S. Public Health Service, etc. These are privileged to attend and participate in all scientific meetings, but can not hold office and do not receive the Journal or benefits of Medical Defense. Intern members are limited to interns in hospitals and are only privileged to attend and participate in scientific meetings. (1933).

Sec. 6. Any physician applying for membership in a component medical society of this Association, who has previously practiced in a county in which affiliation with a component society is provided, and who moves to another county without having affiliated with the medical society in the jurisdiction of previous residence, before he is admitted to membership, the cause for his lack of affiliation in the society of his previous residence shall be ascertained.

CHAPTER II.—GENERAL MEETINGS

Sec. 1. All registered members may attend and participate in the proceedings and discussions of the general meetings. Visitors duly accredited to represent the Association of other states, or of the District of Columbia, not exceeding two in number for each organization, may attend upon, and participate in the discussion of the general meetings, but shall not have a vote. Such delegates may read papers upon invitation of the Committee on Scientific Work. The general meetings shall be presided over by the President or by one of the Vice-Presidents.

Sec. 2. No papers or addresses before the Association, except those of the President and invited essayists, shall occupy more than fifteen minutes in their delivery; and no member shall speak longer than five minutes, nor more than once on any subject, provided that each essayist shall have five minutes in which to close the discussion of his paper.

Sec. 3. Entertainments. Any social entertainment which may be given by this Association shall be confined to the evening of the second day.

Sec. 4. Guests. Any physician not a resident of this state but a member of his state association, or any distinguished scientist not a physician, may be counted a guest during any annual session on invitation of the President, and shall be accorded the privilege of participating in the scientific work of that session.

CHAPTER III.—HOUSE OF DELEGATES

Section 1. The House of Delegates shall meet on the day preceding the first day of the annual session, the time to be fixed by the Committee on Scientific Work. It may adjourn from time to time as may be necessary to complete its business; provided that its hours shall conflict as little as possible with the general meetings. The order of business shall be arranged as a separate section of the program.

Sec. 2. Each component county society shall be entitled to send to the House of Delegates each year one delegate for every fifty members, and one for each fraction thereof, but each component society which has made its annual report and paid its assessment as provided in this Constitution and By-Laws shall be entitled to one delegate. Should the regular delegate from any county not be present at the meeting, the President shall appoint a substitute from that county to act.

Sec. 3. Twenty delegates present shall constitute a quorum.

Sec. 4. It shall, through its officers, council and otherwise, give diligent attention to and foster the scientific work and spirit of the Association, and shall constantly study and strive to make each annual session a stepping-stone to future ones of higher interest.

Sec. 5. It shall consider and advise as to the material interest of the profession, and of the public in those important matters wherein it is dependent on the profession, and shall use its influence to secure and enforce all proper medical and public health legislation, and to diffuse popular information in relation thereto.

Sec. 6. It shall make careful inquiry into the condition of the profession of each county in the State, and shall have authority to adopt such methods as may be deemed most efficient for building up and increasing the interests in such county societies as already exist, and for organizing the profession in counties where societies do not exist. It shall especially and systematically endeavor to promote friendly intercourse among physicians of the same locality, and shall continue these efforts until, if possible, every physician in every county of the State has been brought under medical society influence.

Sec. 7. It shall encourage post-graduate and research work as well as home study, and shall endeavor to have the results utilized, and intelligently discussed in the county societies.

Sec. 8. It shall divide the State into councilor districts, one for each congressional district, and when the best interests of the Association and profession will be promoted thereby, organize in each a district

medical society, and all members of component county societies and no others shall be members in such district societies.

Sec. 9. It shall have authority to appoint committees for special purposes from among members of the Association who are not members of the House of Delegates. Such committees shall report to the House of Delegates and may be present and participate in the debate thereon.

CHAPTER IV.—DUTIES OF OFFICERS

Section 1. The President shall preside at all meetings of the Association and of the House of Delegates; shall appoint all committees not otherwise provided for, and shall perform such other duties as custom and parliamentary usage may require. He shall be the real head of the profession of the State during his term of office, and as far as practicable, shall visit, by appointment, the various sections of the State and assist the Councilors in building up the county societies, and in making their work more practical and useful.

In order to give him a better opportunity of becoming more fully acquainted with his duties and with the needs of the Association, the President shall be elected one year prior to taking office. During this time he shall be known as President-Elect and shall be ex-officio member of the standing committees, and shall make recommendations at the next annual session.

Sec. 2. The Vice-Presidents shall assist the President in the discharge of his duties. In the event of the President's death, resignation or removal, the Vice-Presidents, in their order, shall succeed him.

Sec. 3. The Secretary-Treasurer shall give bond in. the sum of One Thousand Dollars. He shall demand and receive all funds due the Association, together with the bequests and donations.

Sec. 4. The Secretary-Treasurer shall attend the general meetings of the Association and the meetings of the House of Delegates, and shall keep the minutes of their respective proceedings in separate record books. He shall be ex-officio Secretary of the Council. He shall be custodian of all record-books and papers belonging to the Association. He shall provide for the registration of the members, delegates and accredited visitors at the annual session. He shall, with the co-operation of the secretaries of the component societies, keep a card-index register of all the legal practitioners of the State by counties, noting on each his status in relation to his county society, and on request transmit a copy of this list to the American Medical Association. He shall aid the Councilors in the organization and improvement of the county societies in the extension of the power and usefulness of this Association. He shall conduct the official correspondence, notifying members of meetings, officers of their election, and committees of their appointment as may be ordered by the House of Delegates with the approval of the Association, and shall make an annual report to the Association. He shall supply each component society with the necessary blanks for making their annual reports; shall keep an account with the component societies, charging against each society its assessment and collect the same. Acting with the Committee on Scientific Work, he shall prepare and issue all programs. The amount of his salary shall be fixed by the Association. He shall be editor of the Journal of the Medical Association of Georgia. He shall employ such assistants as may be ordered by the Council or the House of Delegates. He shall annually make a report of his doings to the House of Delegates.

He shall furnish a balance sheet at each annual meeting for the past fiscal year to be published in the Journal. This shall consist of an itemized statement of all financial transactions of the past year, all accounts made, money received and from whom and all moneys disbursed, to whom, and for what purpose, with vouchers attached. A fiscal year includes the period of time between the first day of May and the last day of April.

CHAPTER V.—COUNCIL

Section 1. The Council shall meet on the day preceding the annual session and daily during the session, and at such other times as necessity may require, subject to the approval of the President. It shall meet on the last day of the annual session of the Association to organize and outline work for the ensuing year. It shall elect a chairman and clerk, who, in the absence of the Secretary of the Association, shall keep a record of its proceedings. It shall, through its chairman, make an annual report to the House of Delegates. It shall be the business body of the Association and attend to the business of the Association in the interim between meetings.

Sec. 2. Each Councilor shall be organizer and peacemaker for his district. He shall visit each county in his district at least once a year for the purpose of organizing component societies where none exist, for inquiring into the conditions of the profession, and for improving and increasing the zeal of the county societies and their members. He shall make an annual report of his work and of the condition of the profession of each county in his district at the annual session of the House of Delegates. The necessary traveling expenses incurred by such Councilor in the line of the duties herein imposed may be allowed by the House of Delegates on a properly itemized statement, but this shall not be construed to include his expense in attending the annual session of the Association. Each Councilor may appoint a Vice-Councilor to assist him in the performance of his duties in that district.

Sec. 3. The Council shall be the board of censors of the Association. It shall consider all questions involving the right and standing of members, whether, in relation to other members, to the component societies, or to this Association. All questions of an ethical nature brought before the House of Delegates or the general meeting shall be referred to

the Council without discussion. It shall hear and decide all questions of discipline affecting the conduct of members of a component society, on which an appeal is taken from the decision of an individual Councilor, or to which attention has been called by the Councilor or interested members. It shall hear and decide all questions affecting unethical conduct on the part of any members at any annual session, and its decision in all such matters shall be final when ratified by the Association.

Sec. 4. In sparsely settled sections it shall have authority to organize the physicians of two or more counties into societies, to be suitably designated so as to distinguish them from district societies, and these societies, when organized and chartered, shall be entitled to all rights and privileges provided for component societies until such counties shall be organized separately.

Sec. 5. The Council shall provide for and superintend the publication and distribution of all proceedings, transactions and memoirs of the Association, and shall have authority to appoint such assistants to the editor as it deems necessary. It shall manage and conduct the Journal of the Medical Association of Georgia, which is the organ of the Association, and all money paid into the treasury as dues shall be received as subscriptions to the Journal.

All money received by the Council and its agents, resulting from the discharge of the duties assigned to them, must be paid to the Secretary-Treasurer of the Association. As the Finance Committee it shall annually audit the accounts of the Secretary-Treasurer and other agents of this Association, and present a statement of the same in its annual report to the House of Delegates, which report shall also specify the character and cost of all the publications of the Association during the year, and the amount of all other property belonging to the Association under its control, with such suggestions as it may deem necessary. In the event of a vacancy in the office of the Secretary-Treasurer, the Council shall fill the vacancy until the next annual election.

Sec. 6. All reports on scientific subjects and all scientific discussions and papers heard before the Association, shall be referred to the Journal of the Medical Association of Georgia for publication. The editor, with the consent of the Councilor for the district in which he resides, may curtail or abstract papers or discussions, and the Council may return any paper to its author which it may not consider suitable for publication.

Sec. 7. All commercial exhibits during the annual sessions shall be within the control and direction of the Council.

Sec. 8. In the absence of a Councilor and Vice-Councilor the President is empowered to appoint a representative from the district as acting Councilor, who shall have full rights and power of a Councilor.

Sec. 9. Each Councilor shall render at every session a written report of each county in his district.

Sec. 10. Any member of the Council who fails to

attend two regular successive sessions of the Council, or whose district does not show evidence of the performance of his duties during the year, unless he renders an acceptable excuse to the Council, is subject to have his position declared vacant by the President and a successor appointed by the President.

CHAPTER VI.—COMMITTEES

Section 1.   The standing committees shall be as follows:

A Committee on Scientific Work.

A Committee on Public Policy and Legislation.

A Committee on Arrangements.

A Committee on Medical Defense, and such other committees as may be necessary.

Sec. 2.   The Committee on Scientific Work shall consist of four members of which the Secretary-Treasurer shall be one. The other three members shall be appointed for terms of one, two, and three years, respectively. The vacancy which will occur each year by the expiration of the term of one member shall be filled by the President with an appointment for three years. The member who has the shortest time to serve shall be Chairman. The committee shall determine the character and scope of the scientific proceedings of the Association for each session. Thirty days previous to each annual session it shall prepare and issue a program announcing the order in which papers, discussions and other business shall be presented.

This By-Law shall not prohibit the Committee on Scientific Work from inviting not more than two distinguished members of the national organization to deliver addresses or read papers at any annual meeting.

Sec. 3.   The Committee on Public Policy and Legislation shall consist of three members and the President and Secretary, the Commissioner of Health of the State of Georgia, and a sub-committee of three members from each Councilor District appointed by the chairman when needed. It shall represent the Association in securing and enforcing legislation in the interest of public health and of scientific medicine. It shall keep in touch with professional and public opinion, shall endeavor to shape legislation so as to secure the best results for the whole people, and shall strive to organize professional influence so as to promote the general good of the community in local, state and national affairs and elections.

Sec. 4.   The Committee on Arrangements shall be appointed by the component society in which the annual session is to be held. It shall provide suitable accommodations for the meeting places of the Association and of the House of Delegates and, of their respective committees, and shall have general charge of all arrangements. Its chairman shall report an outline of the arrangements to the Secretary-Treasurer for publication in the program, and shall make additional announcements during the session as occasion may require.

Sec. 5.   The Committee on Medical Defense shall consist of five members, of whom the Chairman of the Council and the Secretary-Treasurer of the Association shall be members. The other members, one of whom shall act as Chairman of the Committee, shall be elected by the Council for a period of five years. Those elected at this meeting (April 19, 1916), shall serve one, three and five years, respectively.

It shall be the duty of the Committee on Medical defense to investigate and defend all damage suits against the Medical Association of Georgia; to investigate all claims of civil malpractice made against its members; to take full charge of such cases, which after investigation, they decide to be proper cases for defense; to defend all such cases in the courts of last resort, to furnish General Counsel and pay court cost usual to such litigation, and reasonable fees for local attorneys as shall be arranged by General Counsel. Provided that any member who has indemnity insurance shall have such insurance bear its portion of the expense. However, they shall not pay, or obligate the Medical Association of Georgia to pay any judgment rendered against any member upon the final determination of any case. They shall be empowered to contract with such agents or attorneys as they may deem necessary for the proper carrying out of this By-Law.

The assistance for defense, as herein provided, shall be available only to members of the Medical Association of Georgia in good standing. Any member who has not paid his annual dues by April 1st shall not be considered in good standing in the application of this By-Law.

Any member or members of the Association threatened with suit for civil malpractice shall immediately communicate with the Secretary of the Association and shall give full and complete information in reference to all the circumstances alleged in the complaint. The Secretary may proceed immediately to investigate the circumstances reported and shall advise with the attorneys or agents employed by the Committee for this purpose. The member sued, or threatened with suit, shall be consulted and shall have the complete confidence of the Committee in all transactions connected with the investigation in question. The Committee shall have the authority to require of a constituent society or the president thereof, the appointment of a committee of investigation in any such case, and it may direct the committee so appointed to report to the Committee on Medical Defense and not to the society from which it was appointed.

The Committee on Medical Defense may also, at its discretion, arrange to prosecute illegal practitioners in the State of Georgia and assist in the enforcement of the Medical Practice Act of this State.

CHAPTER VII.—COUNTY SOCIETIES

Section 1.   All county societies now in affiliation with this Association, or those which may hereafter be organized in the State, which have adopted principles of organization not in conflict with this Con.

stitution and By-Laws, shall on application, receive a charter from and become a component part of this Association.

Sec. 2. As rapidly as can be done after the adoption of this Constitution and By-Laws, a medical society shall be organized in every county in the State in which no component society exists, and charter shall be issued thereto.

Sec. 3. Charters shall be issued only on approval of the Council, and shall be signed by the President and Secretary of this Association. The Association shall have authority to revoke the charter of any component society whose actions are in conflict with the letter or spirit of this Constitution and By-Laws.

Sec. 4. Only one component medical society shall be chartered in any county.

Sec. 5. Each county society shall judge of the qualifications of its own members, but as such societies are the only portals to this Association, every reputable and legally registered white physician who does not practice or claim to practice, nor lend his support to any exclusive system of medicine, shall be eligible to membership. Before a charter is issued to any county society, full and ample notice and opportunity shall be given to every such physician in the county to become a member.

Sec. 6. No matter what the unethical conduct or discipline of the members of the county society may be, both plaintiff and defendant shall have the right to appeal to the Council whose decision shall be final when ratified by the Association.

Sec. 7. In hearing appeals the Council may admit oral or written evidence, as in its judgment will best and most fairly present the facts, but in case of every appeal, both as a board and as individual Councilors in district and county work, efforts at conciliation and compromise shall precede all such hearings.

Sec. 8. When a member in good standing in a component county society moves to another county in this state, he shall be given a written certificate of these facts by the secretary of his society, without cost, for transmission to the secretary of the society in the county to which he moves. Pending his acceptance or rejection by the society in the county to which he moves, such member shall be considered in good standing in the county society from which he was certified and in the Medical Association of Georgia to the end of the period for which his dues have been paid.

Sec. 9. A physician living on or near a county line may hold his membership in that county most convenient for him to attend, on permission of the component society in whose jurisdiction he resides.

Sec. 10. Each component society shall have general direction of the affairs of the profession in its county, and its influence shall be constantly exerted for bettering the scientific, moral and material condition of every physician in the county; and systematic efforts shall be made by each member, and by the society as a whole, to increase the membership until it embraces every qualified physician in the county.

Sec. 11. At some meeting in advance of the annual

session of this Association, each county society shall elect a delegate or delegates to represent it in the House of Delegates of this Association, in the proportion of one delegate to each fifty members, or fraction thereof, and the Secretary of the society shall send a list of such delegates to the Secretary of this Association at least ten days before the annual session.

Sec. 12. The Secretary of each component society shall keep a roster of its members, and of the non-affiliated registered physicians of the county, in which shall be shown the full name, address, college and date of graduation, date of license to practice in this State, and such other information as may be deemed necessary. In keeping such roster the Secretary shall note any changes in the personnel of the profession by death, or by removal to or from the county, and in making his annual report he shall be certain to account for every physician who has lived in the county during the year.

Sec. 13. The Secretary of each component society shall forward its assessment, together with its roster of officers and members, list of delegates, and lists of non-affiliated physicians of the county, to the Secretary of this Association each year, thirty days before the annual session.

Sec. 14. Any county society which fails to pay its assessment, or make the report required, on or before April 1 of each year, shall be held as suspended, and none of its members or delegates shall be permitted to participate in any of the business or proceedings of the Association, or of the House of Delegates, until such requirement has been met.

Sec. 15. The Secretary of each county society shall report to the Journal of the Medical Association of Georgia full minutes of each meeting and forward to it all scientific papers and discussions which the society shall consider worthy of publication.

CHAPTER VIII.—RULES AND ETHICS

Section 1. The deliberations of this Association shall be governed by parliamentary usage as contained in Roberts' Rules of Order, when not in conflict with this Constitution and By-Laws.

Sec. 2. All papers read before the Association shall become its property. Each paper shall be deposited with the Secretary when read, and if this is not done it shall not be published.

Sec. 3. The principles of medical ethics of the American Medical Association shall be those of this Association.

Sec. 4. Any member of this Association, on locating in a new place for practicing his profession may place his professional card, containing name, address, telephone number, and statement as to whether or not his practice will be limited to any particular class of disease, in the local paper for a period of not longer than one month. The placing of such card for this period of time shall not be considered unethical. The use of the word "specialist" by any member in connection with his name in any newspaper, telephone directory, or other public places, shall be considered unethical.

CHAPTER IX.—AMENDMENTS

These By-Laws may be amended at any annual session by a majority vote of the Association after the amendment has lain on the table for one day.

RESOLUTIONS, MEDICAL ASSOCIATION OF GEORGIA

1921

Resolved, That a member who sends in a title of a paper to be placed on the program and is not present to read the paper, shall pay the penalty of not having an opportunity to appear on the program for two years, unless he presents an excuse acceptable to the Committee on Scientific Work.

1922

Be it Resolved, That the House of Delegates recommend that the Committee on Scientific Work make available on the program of the State Association space for two papers from each Councilor district; that a definite time be assigned for reading and discussion of each of these papers, and they be given precedence over all other business. The said papers are to be selected by the Committee on Scientific Work, and, in case a writer does not respond when his name is called, some paper will be substituted and the schedule not deranged. The President ruled that this resolution is only a recommendation and not a law.

1928

Resolved, That the delegates to the A. M. A. elected at this and succeeding meetings of the Medical Association of Georgia be installed January 1st, following their election, and that their term of service run for two years thereafter. And be it further

Resolved, That our delegates be authorized to attend the regular and any called meeting of the House of Delegates of the American Medical Association during the term to which they are elected.

1929

Resolved, That the House of Delegates approve the increase of dues to $7.00 per capita per annum.

Resolved, That the House of Delegates adopt the report of the Council authorizing the Committee on Public Policy and Legislation to spend the necessary amount of money to carry on its work.

Resolved, That in order to expedite the business of the House of Delegates, all reports of special and regular committees of the Association involving matters of public policy, legislation or appropriation of the funds of the Association be submitted in writing to the Secretary of the Association a sufficient time in advance of the regular annual session, about March 15th, to permit of the publication of said recommendations either in the official program prior to the session or in a special circular that shall be mailed to the constituent societies, in order that the delegates may be advised of the proposed changes.

1933

Resolved, That the House of Delegates approve the reduction of dues to $6.00 per capita for the year 1934.

1934

Resolved, That the House of Delegates set the amount of dues at $6.00 per capita for the year 1935.

1935

Resolved, That the House of Delegates set the amount of dues at $6.00 per capita for the year 1936.

PROPOSED AMENDMENTS

Proposed amendment to Article VII, Section 1, of the Constitution and By-Laws by adding after the words American Medical Association in the fifth line the following: "or on petition of the county society of the host city made at least six months before the fixed dates for the annual session." The section when amended will read as follows: "Sec. 1. The annual session shall take place on the second Wednesday in May at such place as shall be designated by the Association, provided that in case of conflict with the meeting of the American Medical Association or on petition of the county society of the host city made at least six months before the fixed dates for the annual session, the Council may change the date by publishing a notice in the Journal of the Medical Association of Georgia three months before the session."

Proposed amendments to ARTICLE VII, SECTION 1, of the Constitution and By-Laws by substituting the word "shall" for the word "may" in the first line. When amended to read as follows: "The House of Delegates shall provide for a division of the scientific work of the Association into appropriate sections, and for the organization of Councilor District Societies to be composed exclusively of members of the component county societies."

Proposed amendment to ARTICLE IX, SECTION 3, part of lines 5, 6, 7, 8, 9, which reads: "The Councilors shall be elected at the same time on nomination by their respective District Societies at the annual meeting of such Societies preceding the session of the Association at which the vacancy occurs." To be changed and amended to read: "The Councilors shall be elected at the same time on nomination by their respective District Societies at the annual meeting of such societies preceding the meeting of the Association at which the vacancy occurs, but if no nomination from the District Society is brought before the Association, the nomination for Councilor may be presented from the floor." The balance of Section 3 to remain unchanged.

STATUE OF DOCTOR CRAWFORD W. LONG TO BE UNVEILED AT DANIELSVILLE

Mr. Lemartine G. Hardman, Jr., will be in charge of the arrangements for unveiling a statue of Dr. Crawford W. Long at Danielsville on Monday, March 30th, at 11:00 A.M., Eastern Standard Time. Dr. Hugh H. Young of Baltimore, Maryland, will be the principal speaker. All members of the Medical Association of Georgia are invited to be present on this occasion.

WOMAN'S AUXILIARY

OFFICERS

President—Mrs. Ernest R. Harris, Winder.
President-Elect—Mrs. Wm. R. Dancy, Savannah.
First Vice-President—Mrs. Hulett H. Askew,
  Atlanta.
Second Vice-President—Mrs. Warren A. Coleman,
  Eastman.
Third Vice-President—Mrs. T. J. Ferrell,
  Waycross.
Recording Secretary—Mrs. W. R. Garner,
  Gainesville.
Corresponding Secretary—Mrs. S. T. Ross.
  Winder
Treasurer—Mrs. W. M. Cason, Sandersville.

Historian—Mrs. Marvin F. Haygood, Atlanta.
Parliamentarian—Mrs. Ralph H. Chaney, Augusta.
  Committee Chairmen
Health Films—Mrs. A. J. Mooney, Statesboro.
Student Loan Fund—Mrs. Benjamin Bashinski,
  Macon.
Public Relations—Mrs. J. A. Redfearn, Albany.
Press and Publicity—Mrs. J. Harry Rogers,
  Atlanta.
Jane Todd Crawford Memorial—Mrs. Eustace A.
  Allen, Atlanta.
Research in Romance of Medicine—Mrs. D. N.
  Thompson, Elberton.

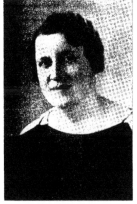

MRS. ERNEST R. HARRIS, Winder
President, 1935-36

this convention and to become a member of
the Auxiliary.

MRS. A. A. MORRISON, JR.,
*President, Woman's Auxiliary to the
Georgia Medical Society.*

CALL TO CONVENTION

The twelfth annual convention of the
Woman's Auxiliary to the Medical Associa-
tion of Georgia, is called to meet at the Hotel
De Soto in Savannah, April 21-24.

Each County Auxiliary is requested to send
its President, two delegates, two alternates
to represent it officially.

State officers, committee chairmen, district
managers and past presidents are asked to attend the Executive Board pre-convention
meeting on Wednesday, April 22nd, 9:00
A.M. at the Hotel De Soto.

All members and every eligible wife are
invited to be present and to enjoy the sessions which will begin each day at 10:00
A.M.

Registration daily, beginning Tuesday at
Hotel De Soto.

MRS. ERNEST R. HARRIS, *President.*

INVITATION

The Woman's Auxiliary to the Georgia
Medical Society cordially invites the Woman's
Auxiliary to the Medical Association of
Georgia to attend the twelfth annual conven-
tion in Savannah, April 21-24.

Arrangements are being made to insure
the success of the meeting and to provide entertainment and amusement.

The wife of every member of the Medical
Association of Georgia is invited to attend

PROGRAM

TWELFTH ANNUAL CONVENTION
WOMAN'S AUXILIARY TO
MEDICAL ASSOCIATION OF GEORGIA
Hotel De Soto, Savannah
April 21, 22, 23, 24, 1936
OFFICERS AND COMMITTEES
Executive Board
President—Mrs. Ernest R. Harris, Winder.
President-Elect—Mrs. W. R. Dancy, Savannah.
First Vice-President—Mrs. H. H. Askew, Atlanta.
Second Vice-President—Mrs. W. A. Coleman, Eastman.
Third Vice-President—Mrs. T. J. Ferrell, Waycross.

Recording Secretary—Mrs. W. R. Garner, Gainesville.
Corresponding Secretary—Mrs. S. T. Ross, Winder.
Treasurer—Mrs. W. M. Cason, Sandersville.
Historian—Mrs. M. F. Haygood, Hamilton.
Parliamentarian—Mrs. R. H. Chaney, Augusta.
Past Presidents of State Auxiliary.

Chairmen of Standing Committees

Organization—Mrs. W. R. Dancy, Savannah.
Health Education—Mrs. H. H. Askew, Atlanta.
Hygeia—Mrs. W. A. Coleman, Eastman.
Scrapbook—Mrs. T. J. Ferrell, Waycross.
Health Films—Mrs. A. J. Mooney, Statesboro.
Student Loan Fund—Mrs. Benjamin Bashinski, Macon.
Legislation—Mrs. Dan Y. Sage, Atlanta.
Press and Publicity—Mrs. J. Harry Rogers, Atlanta.
Jane Todd Crawford Memorial—Mrs. Eustace A. Allen, Atlanta.
Research in Romance of Medicine—Mrs. D. N. Thompson, Elberton.
Public Relations—Mrs. J. A. Redfearn, Albany.

District Managers

First District—Mrs. Cleveland Thompson, Millen.
Second District—Mrs. N. Peterson, Tifton.
Third District—Mrs. E. B. Davis, Byromville.
Fifth District—Mrs. Joseph Yampolsky, Atlanta.
Sixth District—Mrs. J. Lon King, Macon.
Eighth District—Mrs. Conrad Williams, Valdosta.
Ninth District—Mrs. D. H. Garrison, Clarkesville.
Tenth District—Mrs. R. H. Chaney, Augusta.

Conventions and Presidents.

1924—Augusta—(Organization) Mrs. C. W. Roberts, Atlanta, Temporary Chairman.
1925—Atlanta—Mrs. J. N. Brawner, Atlanta.
1926—Albany—Mrs. W. H. Myers, Savannah.
1927—Athens—Mrs. C. W. Roberts, Atlanta.
1928—Savannah—Mrs. Paul Holliday, Athens.
1929—Macon—Mrs. C. C. Hinton, Macon.
1930—Augusta—Mrs. M. T. Benson, Atlanta.
1931—Atlanta—Mrs. C. C. Harrold, Macon.
1932—Savannah—Mrs. Ralston Lattimore, Savannah.
1933—Macon—Mrs. S. T. R. Revell, Louisville.
1934—Augusta—Mrs. J. Bonar White, Atlanta.
1935—Atlanta—Mrs. J. E. Penland, Waycross.

GEORGIA MEDICAL AUXILIARY—
COMMITTEES
Hotel DeSoto, Headquarters
MRS. A. A. MORRISON, JR., Savannah,
President, Georgia Medical Auxiliary

Arrangements

Mrs. Lee Howard, Savannah, General Chairman.
Mrs. A. A. Morrison, Jr., Savannah, Registration and Credentials.
Mrs. W. R. Garner, Gainsville, State Chairman.
Mrs. R. E. Graham, Savannah, Local Chairman.
Mrs. H. M. Kandel, Savannah.
Mrs. S. P. Sanford, Savannah.
Mrs. L. W. Shaw, Savannah.
Mrs. W. E. Brown, Savannah.

Transportation

Mrs. Luther A. DeLoach, Savannah, Chairman.
Mrs. J. T. Burkhalter, Savannah.
Mrs. E. N. Gleaton, Savannah.
Mrs. H. H. McGee, Savannah.

Hospitality

Mrs. L. W. Williams, Savannah, Chairman.
Mrs. Herman W. Hesse, Savannah.
Mrs. H. Y. Righton, Savannah.
Mrs. G. T. Olmstead, Savannah.
Mrs. Chas. Usher, Savannah.
Mrs. Geo. H. Faggart, Savannah.

Publicity·

Mrs. J. Harry Rogers, Atlanta, State Chairman.
Mrs. G. Hugo Johnson, Savannah, Local Chairman.

Health Film

Mrs. A. J. Mooney, Statesboro, State Chairman.
Mrs. R. V. Martin, Savannah, Local Chairman.

Introduction of Officers and Honor Guests

Mrs. Ralston Lattimore, Savannah.

Timekeeper

Mrs. John W. Daniel, Savannah.

PROGRAM
Hotel De Soto, Headquarters
TUESDAY, APRIL 21, 1936
Registration

ENTERTAINMENTS
WEDNESDAY, APRIL 22, 1:30 P.M.
Luncheon at General Oglethorpe Hotel, Wilmington Island.

WEDNESDAY, APRIL 22, 3:30 P.M.
Trip by motor and boat to historic Fort Pulaski.

WEDNESDAY, APRIL 22, EVENING
Informal reception at Hotel De Soto in honor of State officers.

THURSDAY, APRIL 23, 1:30 P.M.
"Get-together luncheon" at Hotel Savannah.

THURSDAY, APRIL 23, 8:30 P.M.
Banquet, Hotel De Soto.

WEDNESDAY, APRIL 22, 9:00 A.M.
Hotel De Soto
Eastern Standard Time
BUSINESS MEETING
Executive Board

PROGRAM
WEDNESDAY, APRIL 22, 10:00 A.M.
Hotel De Soto
Eastern Standard Time
Call to order by the President, Mrs. E. R. Harris, Winder.

Invocation
Rev. Geoffrey Horsefield .... Savannah
Rector. St. Pauls Episcopal Church.
Address of Welcome
Mrs. A. A. Morrison, Jr. .... Savannah
President. Georgia Medical Auxiliary
Response to Address of Welcome
Mrs. J. Wallace Daniel................................ Claxton
Introduction of Distinguished Guests
Mrs. Ralston Lattimore .... Savannah
Medical Organization
James E. Paullin .... Atlanta
President. Medical Association of Georgia.
Address
Program in Auxiliary Work
Mrs. J. Bonar White................................ Atlanta
First Vice-President. American Medical Auxiliary. .
Report of Entertainment Committee
Mrs. L. W. Williams, Chairman ....Savannah
Rules Governing Convention Procedure
Mrs. Ralph H. Chaney. Parliamentarian .... Augusta
Reading of minutes.
Reports of district managers.
Reports of county presidents.
Report of Executive Committee by Chairman.
Report of Credentials Committee by Chairman. Mrs.
R. E. Graham, Savanah.
Appointment of special committees.
Showing of Health Film
Mrs. A. J. Mooney.................................Statesboro

THURSDAY, APRIL 23, 10:00 A.M.
Hotel De Soto
Eastern Standard Time
Call to order by the President. Mrs. E. R. Harris.
Winder.
Invocation
Rev. Samuel McP. Glasgow ....Savannah
Pastor. Independent Presbyterian Church
Address of Welcome
Mrs. G. H. Johnson .... Savannah
Response to Address of Welcome
Mrs. Eugene L. Ward...........................Gainesville
Report of Advisory Committee
Dr. Jas. N. Brawner, Chairman........................ Smyrna
Address
"The Auxiliary as a Unit in Community Activities."
Dr. B. H. Minchew...............................Waycross
President-Elect. Medical Association of Georgia
Reading of minutes.
Report of President.
Reports of other officers.
Report of Auditor.
Report on meeting of the American Medical Auxiliary.
Mrs. J. C. Metts. Savannah.
Report on meeting. Woman's Auxiliary to S. M. A.,
Mrs. L. W. Williams, Savannah.
Reports of chairmen of standing committees.
Report of Resolutions Committee, Chairman.
Report of Courtesy Committee, Chairman.

Report of Credentials Committee, Chairman.
Memorial Services. Mrs. H. W. Birdsong, Athens.
Unfinished business.
New business.
Report of Nominating Committee by Chairman.
Election of officers.
Installation of officers.
Introduction of officers.
Announcement of new President.
Adjournment.

THURSDAY, APRIL 23, 3:00 P.M.
Hotel Savannah
Eastern Standard Time
Post-Convention Board Meeting
Mrs. Wm. R. Dancy, President. Chairman.

RULES TO GOVERN THE CONVENTION
1. To gain recognition, a delegate is requested to
rise. address the chair, give her name and auxiliary.
2. No delegate shall speak more than twice on the
same subject and is limited to two minutes each time.
3. Reports shall not be read from Auxiliaries which
are not represented by delegates but shall be filed with
the Secretary.
4. All original motions or resolutions shall be made
by submitting two copies, one to the Chairman of the
Resolutions Committee and one to the Recording Secretary.
5. Reports of delegates and district managers are
limited to three minutes.
6. No one is entitled to vote before she is registered.
Whispered conversations greatly retard the business of
a meeting.
PLEASE BE PROMPT. Meetings will begin promptly at the time stated in program.

Whereas, death has claimed one of our most valued
members. Lucile Flanders Selden and,
Whereas. her leadership, friendship, cheerfulness and
generous understanding; impartial judgment and willingness to serve we shall ever hold in affectionate re-
membrance, and
Whereas. we, the members of the Bibb County Medical Society, feel a deep sense of our
loss. therefore.
Be it resolved. That we express to the husband our
love and sympathy, and
Be it further resolved, That these Resolutions be
spread upon the Minutes of the Auxiliary, that copies
be sent to the family of our friend and member and
to the Auxiliary page of The Journal of the Medical
Association of Georgia.
                    MRS. CHARLES COTTON HARROLD
                    MRS. JULIUS EMORY CLAY
                    MRS. THOMAS EDWARD ROGERS
                            Committee.
Macon, Ga., Feb. 10, 1936.

GEORGIA DEPARTMENT OF PUBLIC HEALTH

T. F. ABERCROMBIE, M.D., *Director*

BEHAVIOR OF UNDULANT FEVER IN GEORGIA

Undulant fever is not a disease of major importance in Georgia from a public health standpoint. The highest reported annual incidence was 63 cases reported in 1934, while the average for the past three years was 46.

That human infections with Brucella melitensis variety abortus originate from contact with infected animals or from the ingestion of the milk of infected cows, is established beyond controversy. Yet when we consider the high incidence of animal infections and the probability that a large percentage of people are exposed repeatedly through infected milk, meat and animals we are forced to conclude that human susceptibility to this infection is only slight. More remarkable still is the extreme rarity of undulant fever in recognizable form in children who presumably drink more milk than adults. A few years ago, the owner of one of the largest dairies in the State producing raw milk reported an increasing number of abortions among his finest herd of cows. An investigation by the State Department of Agriculture revealed that over 60 per cent of this herd were infected with Brucella abortus. A large part of the output was certified for use by children. Yet upon careful investigation not a single case of human infection was found among the consumers of the milk. This is only one of numerous instances later noted.

Nevertheless, undulant fever is sufficiently common to warrant its consideration in the differential diagnosis of every case of prolonged fever of otherwise undetermined origin. A definite diagnosis based on clinical findings alone is always difficult and often impossible. The symptomatology is usually vague and there is no specific syndrome. Fortunately the serologic or agglutination test in the hands of an experienced technician is highly specific. In fact, all of the cases reported to the State Department of Public Health are confirmed by the serologic test.

For several years reports on all positive tests for undulant fever have been accompanied by a questionnaire to be filled out by the attending physician. While returns are by no means complete, 100 more or less complete case histories have been accumulated since 1931. The writer is now engaged in analyzing these histories. As a preliminary report certain salient items of information thus far obtained are given herewith:

Age—Only 3 per cent were under year of age; 60 per cent occurred in age group of 20 to 45 years; 19 per c were above 50. The youngest was 3 a the oldest 78.

Sex—73 per cent were males and 27 cent females.

Race—89 per cent were white and 11 cent negro.

Occupation—49 per cent were farmers, persons living on farms, or workers wi raw meat products and hides. Infected a mals as well as milk may have been t sources of infection in this group; 51 per ce were made up of persons whose most pro able source of infection was raw cow's mi only.

Consumers of Raw Milk—90 per ce drank some raw cow's milk daily; 2 cent used only pasteurized milk; 5 per ce denied drinking fresh milk of any kind a contact with animals or raw meat produc

Delay in Diagnosis—In the records of cases the interval between date of onset a date of diagnosis was given. The avera interval was 46.2 days. The longest inte val was 294 days and over 100 days in cases.

Symptoms—The following symptoi were reported in over 50 per cent of the ca records:

Fever	100%
Fatigue	95%
Sweating	90%
Loss of weight	86%
Headache	86%
Backache	78%
Chills	73%
Other frequent symptoms were—	
Cough	50%
Constipation	50%
Arthritis	43%
Palpable spleen	35%
Rash	14%

Specific Laboratory Findings—100 cent gave more or less strongly positive se logic tests, that is, complete agglutinati as high as dilution 1:320 of patients' seru 17 per cent showed positive blood cultu for Brucella abortus.

Space does not permit further discussion of this study. The writer plans to publish the completed analysis in detail at a later date.

T. F. SELLERS, M. D.,
Chief, Dept. of Health Lab.

BOOK REVIEWS

Obstetrical Practice by Alfred Beck, Professor of Obstetrics and Gynecology, Long Island College of Medicine; Obstetrician and Gynecologist-In-Chief, Long Island College Hospital, Brooklyn. pp. 702. Illustrations over 1,000. Price $7.00. The Williams and Wilkins Co., Baltimore. 1935.

This book, written primarily for undergraduate students, is a comparatively concise presentation of obstetrical procedures. Its greatest asset is a profusion of illustrations. Most of these are drawings by the author. They are clear and well done and in many cases are so complete that the text seems almost superfluous.

The book is about equally divided between the normal and abnormal. There is included a chapter on the changes of pregnancy from a chronological standpoint. This correlates the embryological development with clinical signs and symptoms and is a valuable addition.

The author's style is simple and clear; amounting almost to an outline in some instances. Theories and controversial points have been largely omitted. While the handling of normal patients is described in detail it is felt that too little consideration is given to the toxemias of pregnancy and to operative obstetrics.

The book will prove valuable for teaching purposes, particularly for junior students. It will also be helpful to the general practitioner who wishes to review and keep his obstetrical work in line with present methods with a minimum of effort.

AMEY CHAPPELL, M.D.

The Medical Treatment of Gall Bladder Disease. By Martin M. Rehfuss, M.D., and Guy M. Nelson, M.D. Pages, 465. Price, $5.50. W. B. Saunders Company, 1935.

The scope of this volume is so wide that it might well be referred to as Biliary Disease.

Admitting that surgery is the most potent weapon in the armamentarium of gallbladder therapy, the medical approach is necessary in those cases where surgery is inadvisable, where the patient will not submit to surgery, and in cases in which surgery has not afforded relief. The chronic nature of the disease is given special consideration, and the authors discuss in a practical way the employment of those methods which have been so successful in the handling of diabetes and tuberculosis.

The fundamental conception as set forth is that gallbladder disease is a medical problem both before and frequently after surgery.

CRAWFORD F. BARNETT, M.D.

Immunology. By Noble Pierce Sherwood, Ph.D., M.D., Professor of Immunology, University of Kansas, Pathologist of the Lawrence Memorial Hospital, Lawrence, Kansas. C. V. Mosby Co., St. Louis, Mo., 1935. Price $6.00; 608 pp., including 84 pages of references.

While the book is written primarily for students, it will form an excellent book for reading for physicians desiring to review immunology in general, without intent to specialize.

It contains a remarkably large number of concise discussions of experimental work done by others. At the end of every chapter there is a summary, or at the end of a series of chapters a summary chapter.

Especially recommended is the chapter on anatomic and physiologic factors in infection and resistance. All the theories of immunity are reviewed. While the book is not in any sense a handbook on technic, the exposition is full enough for this purpose in many chapters, especially those on blood group, the agglutinin reactions and the precipitin tests.

The chapter on toxemia and antitoxins gives an inclusive survey of the use of antitoxins in the various diseases, with a practical application which will be useful for any physician.

There is a thorough analysis of hypersensitiveness in general, an excellent chapter on hypersensitiveness due to infection, with a full discussion of the tuberculin type, and two chapters giving a resume of allergy, including committee recommendations for an allergy clinic.

HAL M. DAVISON, M.D.

The Human Foot. By Dudley J. Morton, M.D. University Press, 2960 Broadway, New York City. Price $3.00.

The human foot, a subject greatly neglected by our profession, so much so, that the irregulars grasped the opportunity to specialize on it, because of the demand by the suffering public. This book is timely and should fill a prominent place in the library of every practitioner. The author treats the subject from an evolutionary-biologic and physiologic point of view, which should be of special valuable interest to the doctor of medicine, who is interested in the scientific treatise of this subject.

The chapters dealing with the anatomy of the foot, as the muscles of the leg, the intrinsic muscles of the foot, are interesting and conform to our knowledge of anatomy, except the chapter concerning the evolution of foot musculature, which is something very new and to my knowledge, original.

Part Two, the physiology of the human foot, is especially noteworthy; the author discusses foot balance, locomotion, the mechanics of the foot in walking and running in an original authoritative way. The drawings, pen and ink sketches, are well done and are accurately diagrammed.

The specialist and the general practitioner will find a great deal of information in Part Three. It describes in an excellent manner the causes of foot troubles, their etiology and constitutional disorders. The treatment of these troubles is covered in three chapters, including the advisory conservative correction and operative removal of obstructions and pathologic conditions.

The contents of the book is educational, comprehensive and of practical application.

THEODORE TOEPEL, M.D.....

COUNTIES REPORTING FOR 1936

Wilkes County Medical Society

The Wilkes County Medical Society announces the following officers for 1936:

President—H. T. Harriss, Washington.
Vice-President—H. M. Sale, Sharon.
Secretary-Treasurer—A. W. Simpson, Washington.
Delegate—O. S. Wood, Washington.
Alternate Delegate—R. J. McNeill, Tignall.
Censors—C. E. Wills and L. R. Casteel.

Cobb County-Medical Society

The .Cobb County Medical Society announces the following officers for 1936:

President—W. G. Crawley, Acworth.
Vice-President—W. C. Mitchell, Smyrna.
Secretary-Treasurer—H. B. Terry, Acworth.
Delegate—W. H. Parkinson, Marietta.
Alternate Delegate—W. M. Gober, Marietta.

Wayne County Medical Society

The Wayne County Medical Society announces the following officers for 1936:

President—T. G. Ritch, Jesup.
Vice-President—J. T. Colvin, Jesup.
Secretary-Treasurer—A. J. Gordon, Jesup.
Delegate—J. T. Colvin, Jesup.
Alternate Delegate—J. A. Leophart, Jesup.

Sumter County Medical Society

The Sumter County Medical Society announces the following officers for 1936:

President—A. C. Primrose, Americus.
Vice-President—R. C. Pendergrass, Americus.
Secretary-Treasurer—Arch Avary, Jr., Ellaville.

Coffee County Medical Society

The Coffee County Medical Society announces the following officers for 1936:

President—J. G. Crovatt, Douglas.
Secretary-Treasurer—T. H. Johnston, Douglas.
Delegate—Sage Harper, Ambrose.
Alternate Delegate—T. H. Clark, Douglas.

Macon County Medical Society

The Macon County Medical Society announces the following officers for 1936:

President—D. B. Frederick, Marshallville.
Vice-President—C. P. Savage, Montezuma.
Secretary-Treasurer—Thos. M. Adams, Montezuma.
Delegate—Thos. M. Adams, Montezuma.
Alternate Delegate—Chas. A. Greer, Oglethorpe.

Chattooga County Medical Society

The Chattooga County Medical Society announces the following officers for 1936:

President—R. B. Talley, Trion.
Vice-President—H. D. Brown, Summerville.
Secretary-Treasurer—Inman Smith, Trion.
Delegate—R. N. Little, Summerville.
Alternate Delegate—N. A. Funderburk, Trion.

Douglas County Medical Society

The Douglas County Medical Society announces the following officers for 1936:

President—C. V. Vansant, Douglasville.
Secretary-Treasurer—R. E. Hamilton, Douglasville.
Delegate—C. V. Vansant, Douglasville.

Monroe County Medical Society

The Monroe County Medical Society announces the following officers for 1936:

President—W. J. Smith, Juliette.
Vice-President—J. O. Elrod, Forsyth.
Secretary-Treasurer—G. H. Alexander, Forsyth.

South Georgia Medical Society
(Lowndes County et al)

The South Georgia Medical Society announces the following officers for 1936:

President—H .W. Clements, Adel.
Secretary-Treasurer—L. R. Hutchinson, Adel.
Delegate—Gordon T. Crozier, Valdosta.

Jenkins County Medical Society

The Jenkins County Medical Society announces the following officers for 1936:

President—H. G. Lee, Millen.
Vice-President—Q. A. Mulkey, Millen.
Secretary-Treasurer—C. Thompson, Millen.
Delegate—C. Thompson, Millen.

Tattnall County Medical Society .

The Tattnall County Medical Society announces the following officers for 1936:

President—J. C. Collins, Collins.
Vice-President—A, C. Branch, Glennville.
Secretary-Treasurer—J. M. Hughes, Glennville.
Delegate—L. V. Strickland, Cobbtown.
Alternate Delegate—J. M. Hughes, Glennville.

Rabun County Medical Society

The Rabun County Medical Society announces the following officers for 1936:

President—J. C. Dover, Clayton.
Secretary-Treasurer—J. A. Green, Clayton.
Delegate—J. C. Dover, Clayton.
Alternate Delegate—J. A. Green, Clayton.

Jefferson County Medical Society

The Jefferson County Medical Society announces the following officers for 1936:

President—J. J. Pilcher, Wrens.
Vice-President—G. L. Carpenter, Wrens.
Secretary-Treasurer—S. T. R. Revell, Louisville.
Delegate—S. T. R. Revell, Louisville.

Polk County Medical Society

The Polk County Medical Society announces the following officers for 1936:

President—S. L. Whitely, Cedartown.
Vice-President—C. V. Wood, Cedartown.
Secretary-Treasurer—Jno. M. McGehee, Cedartown.
Delegate—Jno. W. Good, Cedartown.
Alternate Delegate—C. V. Wood, Cedartown.

Clarke County Medical Society

The Clarke County Medical Society announces the following officers for 1936:

President—W. D. Gholston, Danielsville.
Vice-President—J. Weyman Davis, Athens.
Secretary-Treasurer—Jno. A. Simpson, Athens.
Delegate—H. B. Harris, Athens.
Alternate Delegate—C. H. Bryant, Comer.

Colquitt County Medical Society

The Colquitt County Medical Society announces the following officers for 1936:

President—T. H. Chesnutt, Moultrie.
Vice-President—H. T. Edmondson, Moultrie.
Secretary-Treasurer—R. M. Joiner, Moultrie.
Delegate—C. C. Brannen, Moultrie.
Alternate Delegate—W. R. McGinty, Moultrie.

Washington County Medical Society

The Washington County Medical Society announces the following officers for 1936:

President—N. Overby, Sandersville.
Vice-President—R. L. Taylor, Davisboro.
Secretary-Treasurer—O. D. Lennard, Tennille.
Delegate—N. J. Newsom, Sandersville.
Alternate Delegate—R. L. Taylor, Davisboro.

Hancock County Medical Society

The Hancock County Medical Society announces the following officers for 1936:

President—Horace Darden, Sparta.
Secretary-Treasurer—H. L. Earl, Sparta.
Delegate—C. S. Jernigan, Sparta.
Alternate Delegate—E. H. Hutchings, Sparta.

Hart County Medical Society

The Hart County Medical Society announces the following officers for 1936:

President—J. I. Jenkins, Hartwell.
Vice-President—B. C. Teasley, Hartwell.
Secretary-Treasurer—A. O. Meredith, Hartwell.
Delegate—W. E. McCurry, Hartwell.
Alternate Delegate—B. C. Teasley, Hartwell.
Censors—G. T. Harper, W. E. McCurry, and B. C. Teasley.

Tri County Society
(Liberty, Long, McIntosh)

The Tri County Society announces the following officers for 1936:

President—C. C. Fishburne, Darien.
Vice-President—B. H. Gibson, Allenhurst.
Secretary-Treasurer—T. W. Wellborn, Hinesville.
Delegate—I. G. Armistead, Warsaw.
Alternate Delegate—B. H. Gibson, Allenhurst.

Carroll County Medical Society

The Carroll County Medical Society announces the following officers for 1936:

President—T. M. Spruell, Temple.
Vice-President—H. J. Goodwyn, Carrollton.
Secretary-Treasurer—D. S. Reese, Carrollton.
Delegate—S. F. Scales, Carrollton.

Taylor County Medical Society

The Taylor County Medical Society announces the following officers for 1936:

President—Lewis Beason, Butler.
Vice-President—S. H. Bryan, Reynolds.
Secretary-Treasurer—R. C. Montgomery, Butler.
Delegate—S. H. Bryan, Reynolds.

Tift County Medical Society

The Tift County Medical Society announces the following officers for 1936:

President—M. F. Shaw, Omega.
Vice-President—W. H. Hendricks, Tifton.
Secretary-Treasurer—C. S. Pittman, Tifton.
Delegate—C. S. Pittman, Tifton.

Gordon County Medical Society

The Gordon County Medical Society announces the following officers for 1936:

President—W. R. Barnett, Calhoun.
Secretary-Treasurer—Z. V. Johnston, Calhoun.
Delegate—Z. V. Johnston, Calhoun.
Alternate Delegate—W. R. Barnett, Calhoun.

Lamar County Medical Society

The Lamar County Medical Society announces the following officers for 1936:

President—D. W. Pritchett, Barnesville.
Secretary-Treasurer—S. B. Traylor, Barnesville.

Crisp County Medical Society

The Crisp County Medical Society announces the following officers for 1936:

President—T. J. McArthur, Cordele.
Vice-President—H. J. Williams, Cordele.
Secretary-Treasurer—L. O. Wooten, Cordele.
Delegate—Charles Adams, Cordele.
Alternate Delegate—C. E. McArthur, Cordele.

Wilcox County Medical Society

The Wilcox County Medical Society announces the following officers for 1936:

President—S. R. Mitchell, Pineview.
Vice-President—J. M. C. McAllister, Rochelle.
Secretary-Treasurer—J. D. Owens, Rochelle.
Delegate—J. D. Owens, Rochelle.
Alternate Delegate—J. M. C. McAllister, Rochelle.

Ocmulgee Medical Society
(Bleckley, Dodge, Pulaski)

The Ocmulgee Medical Society announces the following officers for 1936:

President—W. F. Massey, Chester.
Secretary-Treasurer—I. J. Parkerson, Eastman.
Delegate—A. R. Bush, Hawkinsville.
Alternate Delegate—I. J. Parkerson, Eastman.

NEWS ITEMS

The Burke-Jenkins-Screven Counties Medical Society met at Millen on February 12th. Dr. J. M. Byne, Jr., Waynesboro; Dr. J. B. Lewis, Waynesboro; and Dr. A. G. Thurmond, Waynesboro, reported cases of *Septic Sore Throat* with which there were maculopapular rash over the body. Dr. W. W. Hillis, Sardis, reported a case of *Pneumonia* with unusual clinical progress. Dr. H. G. Lee, Millen, reported a case and displayed x-rays of a case of *Intussusception* in a seven months old infant. Dr. J. B. Lewis, Waynesboro, and Dr. Cleveland Thompson, Millen, reported cases of *Osteomyelitis* and emphasized the early symptomatology and necessity for early diagnosis. Dr. C. Thompson discussed the *Autonomic Nervous System* and stressed its relation to clinical medicine and surgery. Dutch dinner was served.

The Coffee County Medical Society met at Douglas on February 25th. Dr. T. H. Johnston, Douglas, spoke on *Infant Feeding*; Dr. J. W. Wallace, Douglas, discussed *Communicable Diseases*. The discussion was led by Dr. I. W. Moorman, Douglas, and Dr. W. F. Sibbett, Douglas.

The office of the Association has been advised that a man about 40 years of age, wore glasses, visited certain doctors, took orders with advance payments, fleeced the physicians out of their money.

The Georgia Medical Society, Savannah, met on February 11th. Dr. Wm. H. Myers read a paper entitled *Do We Want Sickness Insurance?* Dr. L. B. Dunn reported a case *Aneurysm of the Dorsalis Pedis Artery*; Dr. W. O. Bedingfield, *Pelvic Abscess with Unusual Complications*. Refreshments were served.

Dr. N. J. Coker and Dr. Grady N. Coker, Canton, opened their new hospital on Clubhouse Hill at Canton, on February 5th. The hospital is a new brick structure, equipped with modern apparatus for the diagnosis and treatment of diseases. Both of the physicians have an excellent reputation for their success as general practitioners and surgeons.

The Baldwin County Medical Society met at the Milledgeville State Hospital on February 11th. Dr. S. A. Anderson reported three cases of *Upper Respiratory and Sinus Infections* in which vertigo was the chief complaint. Dr. L. P. Longino discussed *Vertigo and Its Relation to Infections of the Mastoid Antrum;* Dr. Chas. B. Fulghum reported cases of *Apparently Mild Coryza Associated with Intense Chest Pain;* Dr. W. G. Miles, *Delirium Following Prolonged Exposure to Cold.*

If interested in a good location for a physician, write the Secretary-Treasurer of the Association.

The Chatham-Savannah Tuberculosis Association

held its annual meeting on February 6th. Dr. John L. Elliott, Medical Director, discussed *Pneumothorax;* Dr. Ruskin King discussed the *New Tuberculin, Purified Protein Derivative.* Dr. A. A. Morrison is First Vice-President; Dr. H. H. McGee, Third Vice-President.

Dr. Arthur G. Fort, Atlanta, spoke on the Voters' Radio Forum, sponsored by the Georgian-American over the Georgian-American Globe Trotter hour on February 1st. A synopsis of address follows: "1. No group is more critical of government and governmental services than the doctor and professional man. No man has the right to criticize unless he backs his criticism with his ballot. 2. Our laws express the opinion of a cross section of the community. It is the duty of the doctor and professional man to add his voice. 3. Physicians, in the pursuit of their duties, meet the needs of every class of people. None is better qualified to know his community need than is the doctor. 4. The doctor and professional man should vote as a protection to himself, and as insurance against the passage of foolish laws which those unfamiliar with the profession frequently introduce. 5. The medical profession in Georgia has attained a high standard over the years, for the protection of society. To maintain these standards, the doctor and professional man must vote."

The staff meeting of the Crawford W. Long Memorial Hospital, Atlanta, was held on February 13th. Dr. Geo. F. Eubanks and Dr. L. B. Robinson reported a case of *Melena Salient Sign.*

Dr. Earl Floyd, Atlanta, was elected President of the Medical Staff of Grady Memorial Hospital on February 11th.

The Fourth District Medical Society met at Griffin on February 12th. The scientific program consisted of titles for papers as follows: *Chemical Burns—Case Report,* Dr. J. G. Smith, McDonough; *Pigmented Moles, Birthmarks and Melanomas,* Dr. Chas. C. Harrold, Macon; *Vaginal Hysterectomy—Illustrated by Moving Pictures,* Dr. Enoch Callaway, LaGrange; *Pneumothorax and Other Measures in the Treatment of Tuberculosis,* Dr. Joseph C. Massee, Atlanta; *Modern Treatment of Pneumonia,* Dr. George L. Walker, Griffin. Officers elected were: Dr. Enoch Callaway, LaGrange, President; Dr. Marvin M. Head, Zebulon, re-elected Secretary-Treasurer. The next meeting of the Society will be held at Warm Springs on August 12th.

The Tattnall County Medical Society met at the Nelson Hotel, Reidsville, February 12th. Cases reported were: *Traumatic Surgery and Laryngeal Diphtheria with Diagnosis and Treatment.*

Dr. Morris Fishbein, Chicago, Editor of the *Journal of the American Medical Association,* spoke on Fads *and Quackery in Healing* in the Glenn Memorial Auditorium under the auspices of the Emory Student Lecture Association on February 24th.

Dr. William E. Mitchell announces the removal of his office to 1111 Medical Arts Building, Atlanta. Practice limited to surgery.

Dr. Newdigate M. Owensby, Atlanta, spoke before a meeting of the Southern Psychiatric Association at New Orleans, on February 23rd. He was quoted in the press as saying: "Mental disorders are increasing because life today is a battle of wits, whereas in the days of our forefathers it was a battle of brawn. Many of us are overtaxing our brain in our battles to outwit the other fellow, and therefore get out of line." Dr. Owensby was further quoted: "That no mental disease is inherited, that only the germs which cause disease are inherited and these germs only infinitesimally attack the brain. A child apes much more than a monkey, because the child's brain is far better. The child often knows more about the parents than the parents about the child."

The officers of the Atlanta Hopkins Society, Dr. Wm. Willis Anderson, Atlanta, President; Dr. Wm. H. Kiser, Jr., Atlanta, Vice-President; and Dr. M. T. Edgerton, Atlanta, Secretary, with the alumni of Johns Hopkins University School of Medicine, Baltimore, entertained Dr. Luther Emmett Holt, Jr., Baltimore, Associate Professor of Pediatrics of the School, at a luncheon given at the Atlanta Athletic Club on February 15th. Dr. Holt spoke on *Research Work in Diseases of Children.*

Dr. Stewart R. Roberts, Dr. Wm. Willis Anderson, Dr. J. L. Campbell and Dr. Everett L. Bishop, all of Atlanta, spoke on *Health Education* before a meeting of the Woman's Auxiliary to the Fulton County Medical Society, at the Academy of Medicine, February 13th.

Dr. Calhoun McDougall, Atlanta, has been elected a member of the Executive Committee of the Medical Interfraternity Conference of the National Association of Medical Fraternity Alumni at a meeting of the organization held in Chicago, February 16th.

Dr. H. G. Huey, Homerville, assumed the responsibility of caring for two ex-slaves, Liverpool Hazzard, age 107; Jane Lewis, age unknown—by paying to each of them $25.00 per month during the remainder of their lives. In addition to the payment of a stipulated sum per month, he has caused to be made numerous repairs on and around the homes of the old negroes according to an announcement published in the *Darien Gazette.*

Dr. T. R. Aycock and Dr. Philip R. Stewart, both of Monroe, have been elected trustees of the Walton County Hospital.

The Georgia Medical Society, Savannah, met on February 25th. Dr. J. C. Patterson, Cuthbert, read a paper entitled *Acid Ulcer with Especial Reference to Acute Perforation;* the discussion was led by Dr. M. J. Egan and Dr. J. K. Quattlebaum, both of Savannah. Dr. C. K. McLaughlin, Savannah, reported a case, *Convergent Strabismus.*

The staff meeting of St. Joseph's Infirmary, Atlanta, was held on February 25th. Dr. Mark S. Dougherty reported a case, *Carcinoma of the Prostate with Early Metastasis;* Dr. Frank K. Boland, *Surgical Complications of Diathesis.*

The Colquitt County Medical Society met at Moultrie on February 18th. Dr. J. R. Paulk, Moultrie, read a paper on *Allergy;* Dr. J. B. Woodall, Moultrie, *Bronchial Asthma.* Officers were elected for 1936.

Dr. Walter R. Holmes, Atlanta, spoke before a meeting of the Spalding County Medical Society on February 18th. Dinner was served at the Strickland and Son Memorial Hospital, Griffin.

Dr. C. C. Aven, Atlanta, was re-elected President of the Atlanta Tuberculosis Association at its annual meeting held on February 20th; Dr. Evert A. Bancker, Jr., Atlanta, Chairman of the Medical Staff.

The staff meeting of Wesley Memorial Hospital, Emory University, was held on March 2nd. Dr. R. B. Wilson and Dr. R. R. Kracke reported a case of *Thrombosis of Spinal Cord;* Dr. R. A. Bartholomew, *Placenta Praevia and Threatened Rupture of the Uterus;* Dr. Dan C. Elkin, *Liver Abscess.*

Dr. H. G. Huey, Homerville, entertained the members of the Ware and Lowndes Counties Medical Societies to dinner at the Woman's Club Room in Homerville on March 4th. An excellent scientific program featured the joint meeting of the Societies.

Dr. Eugene E. Murphey and Dr. V. P. Sydenstricker, both of Augusta, spoke before a meeting of the Science Club at Athens on February 28th.

Dr. J. R. McCord, Atlanta, has been appointed full-time Professor of Obstetrics and Gynecology at Emory University School of Medicine.

Dr. E. A. Bancker, Jr., Atlanta, was appointed Chairman of the Medical Staff of the Atlanta Tuberculosis Association. A silver basket was presented to Dr. George F. Klugh, Atlanta, in recognition of his leadership for two years.

The staff meeting of Grady Hospital, Atlanta, was held on March 10th. Dr. Dan C. Elkin reported a case of *Thyroid Disease;* Dr. C. W. Strickler, Dr. Jack Norris, case of *Acute Pellagra with Pathological Findings.*

The Fulton County Medical Society met at the Academy of Medicine, Atlanta, on March 5th. Dr. Vernon E. Powell reported a case, *Idiosyncrasy to Orange Juice Resembling Cholecystitis;* Dr. Hal M. Davison, Mason Lowance and C. F. Barnett, Jr., clinical talks on the *Use of Calcium and Vitamin Concentrates in Prevention of Colds;* Dr. Edgar G. Ballenger, *Sexual Impotence;* Dr. Hulett H. Askew read a paper, *Rectal Fistula and Its Treatment.* The discussion was led by Dr. Ben H. Clifton, Dr. Chas. E. Hall, Jr., and Dr. W. E. Person.

The Randolph County Medical Society held its regular monthly meeting at the Patterson Hospital, Cuthbert, on March 5th. Dr. W. G. Elliott and Dr. L. R. Massengale reported cases of *Puerperal Sepsis* and *Hypochromic Anemia.*

Dr. Ralph McCord, resident physician in the Ophthalmology, Laryngology and Rhinology Department at Grady Hospital, Atlanta, has been elected to membership in the Floyd County Medical Society of Rome. He will finish his two years of resident service at Grady Hospital on June 30th and will return to Rome where he will be engaged on the staff of the McCall Hospital. Dr. McCord's practice will be limited to diseases of the eye, ear, nose and throat. He was engaged in rotating service at the Piedmont Hospital, Atlanta, before he assumed his duties at Grady Hospital.

Dr. T. F. Sellers, Atlanta, spoke before a meeting of the Smyrna Civic Club, Smyrna, on March 2nd.

The Georgia Medical Society, Savannah, held its regular monthly meeting on March 10th. Dr. Geo. G. Faggart read a paper on *Sinusitis in Children;* the discussion was led by Dr. G. H. Lang and Dr. G. T. Olmstead. Dr. L. J. Rabhan reported a case of *Impotency.*

OBITUARY

Dr. *Samuel Melvin Harpe,* Calhoun; member; University of Georgia School of Medicine, Augusta, 1884; aged 72; died at his home of heart disease on October 27, 1935. He was born in Cherokee county and began the study of medicine under his father, who was a prominent physician during those years. After he graduated in medicine, he practiced in Cherokee county for a number of years and served as physician for the Cherokee Gold Mining Company. Later he moved to Gordon county where he practiced for 27 years. Dr. Harpe was a member of one of the pioneer families of his section. He was recognized by the profession as an able and conscientious practitioner and by the laity as a great doctor and friend. His career covered four eras of transportation, horseback, horse and buggy, automobile and airplane. Dr. Harpe was a member of the Gordon County Medical Society and the Methodist church.

residence by Rev. T. F. Callaway and Rev. J. H. Carswell. Burial was in Horne cemetery near Metcalf.

Dr. G. W. Nelson, Marshallville; member; College of Physicians and Surgeons, Baltimore, Md., 1882; aged 74; died at the home of a friend in Macon on February 26, 1936. He was a prominent physician and did an extensive practice in Macon and Taylor counties for a half century. Dr. Nelson was favorably known for his acts of kindness and a citizen of sterling ability and character. He was a member of the Masonic lodge and Methodist church. Dr. Joseph P. Boone conducted the funeral services from the Burghard O'Connally chapel, Macon. Burial was in Riverside cemetery.

Dr. Francis Gilchrist Jones, Atlanta; member; Atlanta College of Physicians and Surgeons, Atlanta, 1910; aged 50; died at a private hospital in Atlanta on February 25, 1936. He was born in Jacksonville, Florida, and moved to Atlanta with his parents while a youth. Dr. Jones graduated from the Boy's High School of Atlanta in 1903 and received his bachelor of arts degree from Washington and Lee. He served as an intern at Grady Hospital, Atlanta, and then began the practice of medicine as a general practitioner, later limited his practice to dermatology. Dr. Jones made an enviable reputation in the treatment of skin diseases. He was a member of the Fulton County Medical Society, Piedmont Lodge No. 447, F. & A. M., and the First Presbyterian church. Surviving him are his widow, one son, F. G. Jones, Jr.; one daughter, Mrs. Susan J. Medlock; his parents, Mr. and Mrs. Robert H. Jones, Sr., Atlanta; one brother, Robert H. Jones, Jr., Atlanta. Funeral services were conducted from Spring Hill chapel by Dr. J. Sprole Lyons. Interment was in West View cemetery. Members of the Piedmont Lodge No. 447 F. & A. M. and the Fulton County Medical Society formed an honorary escort.

Dr. John W. Taylor, Luthersville; Emory University School of Medicine, Emory University, 1875; aged 82; died at his home on February 25, 1936. He practiced medicine for almost fifty years and retired from active practice a few years ago on account of his advanced age. Dr. Taylor served as postmaster of Luthersville for many years. He was a prominent and useful citizen. Surviving him are three daughters, Mrs. D. L. Holman, Columbus; Mrs. Bryant Hatchett, Greenville; Miss Janie Taylor, Luthersville; four sons, W. A. Taylor, Luthersville; Dr. H. W. Taylor and Lovett Taylor of Savannah; J. E. Taylor, Texas. Rev. G. W. Davis conducted the funeral services from the Methodist church and interment was in the churchyard.

Dr. Eugene McKay Bailey, Acworth; member; Emory University School of Medicine, Emory University, 1890; aged 68; died in a private hospital in Atlanta on March 2, 1936, of heart disease. He practiced at Acworth for more than forty years, was a leader in civic and religious activities. Surviving him are his widow, two nephews and a half brother. Dr. Bailey was a member of the Cobb County Medical Society, American Medical Association and the Methodist church. Rev. R. P. Segar assisted by Rev. J. C. Collum and Rev. J. L. Plexico, conducted the funeral services from the Methodist church.

RESOLUTIONS ON THE DEATH OF DR. E. F. FINCHER, SR.*

On the evening of January 6, 1936, he lay down to rest and in the small hours of the morning awoke unexpectedly to the dawning of a brighter day.

He faced the winds of life, and with an eye towards the everlasting, threw his handful of seed on high.

His inherent quality compounded of integrity and sweetness, has caused a multitude of friends and patients to bemoan the passing of this ideal, beloved physician.

Dr. Fincher first saw the light of day on June 10, 1869, in Gwinnett County, Georgia.

His early life was the life of the average country boy.

He attended the Decatur, Georgia, High School, and obtained his college training in the refined, wholesome atmosphere of Emory College, Oxford, Ga., where he received his diploma in 1895. The refining influence of this college life stayed with him throughout the remainder of his days.

Leaving Emory College he secured a position on the teaching staff of Clinton College, Kentucky, where he remained a year.

He was destined to live in a medical atmosphere, so returned to Atlanta for the study of medicine and entered the Atlanta Medical College. From this school he graduated in 1900 and located in East Atlanta where he carried on his practice until called to his reward.

He was in a sense a pioneer in this locality, rapidly built up a loyal following, his life being a successful one from any angle viewed.

For thirty years he was a member of the Martha Brown Memorial Church (Methodist), for several years was a member of the board of stewards, was one time a trustee of Grady Hospital, was appointed on several important committees by the City of Atlanta and was on the bond commission at the time of his death.

He was president of the East Atlanta Bank. He was a Mason and a Shriner.

On December 28, 1897, he married Miss Grace Maddox, daughter of Dr. G. W. Maddox, of Stone Mountain, Ga., whose abiding faith in him, coupled with an abundance of old time sweetness, spurred him on to bigger and better things.

There were four children resulting from this marriage: one son, Edgar, Jr., followed in his father's footsteps and has won for himself a most creditable position in the medical world.

*Read and adopted by the Fulton County Medical Society, February 20, 1936.

The hardships of a general suburban and rural practice, combined with several attacks of influenza, kept him from reaching his allotted three score and ten, yet he was among those "who saw life steadily and saw it whole."

He was refined as a woman, was clean in mind, never grew old, and "was one in a thousand to carry unto the end the freshness of the morning and the bouyant heart of youth."

No more appropriate summary of his life could be made than this: "This brave and tender man in every storm of life was oak and rock, but in the sunshine he was love and flower.".

Whereas, the Fulton County Medical Society has lost a valued member.

Whereas, those members who knew and loved him are grieved by his going away.

Be it Resolved: that this sketch be spread upon the minutes of the Society, that our deep and sincere sympathy in their loss be extended to his wife and children, that a copy of these resolutions be sent to his family, that they be published in the Society Bulletin and in the JOURNAL OF THE MEDICAL ASSOCIATION OF GEORGIA.

Committee:
EMMETT WARD, M.D.
J. R. CHILDS, M.D.
J. CALVIN WEAVER, M.D., Chairman.

Psychoanalytic Observations in Cardiac Disorders. The Menningers have made an interesting contribution (Am. Heart J. 11: 10, Jan., 1936) to the cardiac neuroses. One may not accept their hypotheses as widely applicable, and they cite a case of a cardiologist in his 40's who was relieved for several years of the symptoms of angina and, after returning to practice, dropped dead of coronary disease. Even though an expert psychoanalyst may not be required, one is reminded of Paul White's famous remark that if he had to turn part of the study of a patient over to an assistant, he would take the history and allow the assistant to make the physical examination of the patient's heart.

Abstract by L. Minor Blackford, M.D.

SAVANNAH SESSION
COMMERCIAL EXHIBIT

1. Lea & Febiger, 600 South Washington Square, Philadelphia, Pa.
2. C. B. Fleet Company, Lynchburg, Va,
4. Philip Morris & Company, 119 Fifth Avenue, New York City.
5-6. Wachtel's Physician Supply Company, 408-41 Bull Street, Savannah, Ga.
6½. Mead Johnson & Company, Evansville, Indiana
7. Butler Island Dairy, T. L. Huston, Owner, Brunswick, Ga.
8. Lederle Laboratories, 30 Rockefeller Plaza, New York City.
9. J. A. Majors Company, 1301 Tulane Avenue, New Orleans, La.
10-11. Vegex, Incorporated and Vitamin Food Co. 122 Hudson Street, New York City.
14. Surgical Selling Company, 139 Forrest Avenue N.E., Atlanta, Ga.
15. M. & R. Dietetic Laboratories, Columbus, Ohio
16. American Surgical Supplies, Inc., 23 Houston Street, N.E., Atlanta, Ga.
17. Holland-Rantos Company, 37-41 East 18th Street, New York City.
18. The Harrower Laboratory, Inc., Glendale, California.
20. General Electric X-Ray Corporation, 205 Spring Street, Atlanta, Ga.
21. Max Wocher & Son Company, 29-31 West Sixth Street, Cincinnati, Ohio.
22. S. & H. X-Ray Company, 429 Peachtree Street N.E., Atlanta, Ga.
22½. H. G. Fischer & Company, 2323-2337 Wabansia Avenue, Chicago, Ill.
23-24. Estes Surgical Supply Company, 56 Auburn Avenue, N.E., Atlanta, Ga.

The medical staff of the Menninger Clinic will conduct its second annual postgraduate course on Neuropsychiatry in General Practice, April 20-25, 1936 at the Menninger Clinic, Topeka, Kansas. An introduction to the fields of neurology and psychiatry will be given by the members of the staff.

THE JOURNAL

OF THE

MEDICAL ASSOCIATION OF GEORGIA

DEVOTED TO THE WELFARE OF THE MEDICAL ASSOCIATION OF GEORGIA
PUBLISHED MONTHLY under direction of the Council

| Volume XXV | Atlanta, Ga., April, 1936 | Number 4 |

ACUTE APPENDICITIS*†

Factors Influencing the Mortality

DANIEL C. ELKIN, M.D.
WADLEY GLENN, M.D.
Atlanta

At the first meeting of the Association of American Physicians, approximately fifty years ago, Reginald H. Fitz, of Boston, read his classic paper on *"Perforating Inflammation of the Vermiform Appendix; with Special Reference to its Early Diagnosis and Treatment."* It was not received with great enthusiasm, and the discussors seemed a bit confused by Fitz' positive remarks, but coming as it did from the Professor of Pathological Anatomy at Harvard, and backed by clear and irrefutable autopsy findings, it eventually attracted worldwide attention and was the beginning of definite knowledge of this disease. Fitz pointed out the cardinal symptoms and signs upon which a diagnosis could be made, urged early operation, deplored the use of cathartics, and illustrated, usually by autopsy findings, the clinical course of appendicitis.

Since that time there have been innumerable and vigorous debates concerning the proper treatment, and some 10,000 papers, for the most part concerned with diagnosis and operative technic, have been written. There is now no doubt as to the value of early operation, but the mortality is rising. The number of deaths per 100,000 population in the United States from appendicitis has increased from 9.7 in 1900 to 13.4 in 1920, and to 15.2 in 1929. In Atlanta the

*Read before the Medical Association of Georgia, Atlanta, May 9, 1935.
†From the Department of Surgery, Emory University School of Medicine.

mortality from appendicitis of all types is 4.4 per cent, or about 21 per 100,000 of population. Attempts have been made to educate the lay public regarding the danger of cathartics and the value of early operation. In spite of this, the mortality has risen 30 per cent since 1905, and 20,000 people, for the most part young and vigorous, die annually of this disease in the United States.

It is our purpose in this paper to report our personal experience in the treatment of appendicitis in a well controlled group of patients. The experience of others, particularly in the comparison of statistics, is usually confusing. This is probably due to the difference in classification. Then, too, there is no uniform opinion in regard to the treatment of all types of appendicitis, only that operation is advisable in the early stages.

The patients on which this report is based were all negroes, and all were treated under our direction at the Emory University division of the Grady Hospital. This type of patient is ideal for the study of acute appendicitis, particularly in its late stage, since it is well known that the negro fears hospitals and will only submit to opertaion after all medication has failed. Ninety per cent had taken cathartics, and the percentage of peritonitis was, therefore, high.

Our interest in this subject was stimulated by the report of Boland on acute appendicitis treated in the same hospital from 1927 to 1931, inclusive. In that period 286 patients were operated upon with 42 deaths, a mortality of 14 per cent. It was then the practice of the hospital to operate on all patients as soon as the diagnosis was made, regardless of the stage of the disease. The rule was 'granted a diagnosis of appendicitis, operate." The mortality seemed astoundingly high, even in this class of patients. In 1932 we decided to change the method of handling these patients in the hospital. The rule, to operate on every patient as soon as the diagnosis was made, was altered so as to individualize each case, and to determine, as far as possible, the stage of the disease, and the pathologic changes within the abdomen.

One member of the resident staff was assigned to see and make careful notes on each patient with appendicitis. Only in this way can statistical data of any value be obtained, for records, once they are old and cold, are frequently misleading.

It was found that the duration of the disease in hours was unreliable as a measure of severity, although the appendix was rarely ruptured under eighteen hours. When the process appeared to be limited to the appendix, or where the symptoms and signs indicated that perforation had only lately occurred and the peritonitis was limited to the appendiceal region, immediate operation was performed. One hundred and forty-eight cases of this type were operated upon with two deaths, a mortality of 1.3 per cent.

Where the disease was of several days duration and a *localized* tender mass was present, either in the right lower abdomen or in the pelvis, the treatment was that advocated by Ochsner in 1902. The patient was placed in Fowler's position, hot stupes were applied to the abdomen, nothing was given by mouth, and 50 grams of glucose and 4,000 cc. of physiologic salt solution were given intravenously daily. Morphine was given routinely every four hours. No cathartics or enemas were given. If there was vomiting or distention, a small tube was introduced into the stomach through the nose, and kept in place.

Most patients of this type responded favorably to treatment in that there was an early and rapid drop in temperature, pulse and leucocytosis. Nausea soon ceased, and distention became less marked. In twelve of the patients treated, the inflammatory process completely subsided, and the patients were dismissed without operation, but advised to return immediately if abdominal pain returned, or in three months, in any event, for appendectomy. Where the inflammatory mass did not subside, but gave evidence of abscess formation, operation was usually done in five

to seven days after the onset of the illness. We have felt that to operate merely because a mass was present was extremely unwise, since a mass may subside without progressing to suppuration, or if suppuration did occur, ample time should be given to allow protective barriers to form. The danger in such treatment lies in the fact that secondary rupture of the abscess may occur, usually with fatal outcome. Thirty-two cases were so treated, with four deaths, a mortality of 12.5 per cent. We believe that if every patient with an inflammatory mass or abscess were treated by immediate operation, the mortality would be much higher. When an abscess was treated by operation, no attempt was made to remove the appendix unless it presented in the wound.

The patients that showed evidence of spreading peritonitis were by far the most difficult to treat, for in them the highest mortality was to be expected. These patients had, as a rule, been sick for over forty-eight hours and had taken cathartics. Vomiting was usually marked, with distention, dehydration, an elevated pulse and temperature. Peristalsis was usually absent or slight. The rigidity and tenderness had extended beyond the right lower quadrant to the lower abdomen or the whole abdomen.

In most instances the deferred operative treatment, as described by Ochsner, was carried out in cases of this type. The patients were placed in Fowler's position, and hot stupes applied to the abdomen. Nothing was given by mouth and glucose and saline were given intravenously. The stomach was usually drained by a small nasal tube. Morphine was given routinely in sufficient amounts to allay pain and apprehension. As a rule improvement was noted in that the temperature and pulse dropped, distention became less marked and the abdomen less rigid. One of three courses may be taken by a patient in this condition. First, the peritonitis may subside entirely; second, one or more localized abscesses may develop; or third, the process may continue and the patient die. It is this third type which is most difficult to treat, and frequently they have been operated upon with the idea, usually erroneous, that an operation may offer hope in an otherwise hopeless condition.

Eighty-two patients with peritonitis of varying degree were treated with 15 deaths, a mortality of 18 per cent. While this is admittedly high, and accounts for most of the deaths, it compares favorably with statistics of other clinics and, when compared with former methods of treatment in our own clinic, shows a drop in mortality rate of 50 per cent.

There are undoubtedly other factors influencing the mortality, not the least among them being the idea that every graduate of a medical school can at least perform this operation, when as a matter of fact it frequently requires fine skill and experienced judgment. Then, too, it is extremely difficult to defer operation in late cases when family, friends, and even well-intentioned colleagues are urging it. The value of such a procedure is best illustrated by the following operative statistics in patients of the same type, in the same hospital: the first treated by immediate operation in all instances, and the second by deferred operation in cases of peritonitis.

Type	1925			1932, 1933, 1934		
	No.	Died	%	No.	Died	%
Simple acute,	26	2	7.8	148	2	1.3
Peritonitis,	· 30	9	30	82	15	18
Total acute,	56	11	20	230	17	7.6
Interval,	28	0	0	49	0	0
1927-1931,	286	42	14			

Ninety-five per cent of the operations were done by members of the resident staff. As a rule the McBurney incision, or some modification of it, was used, on the basis that it offered a more direct approach, was less likely to spread infection through handling of small intestine, and was better suited for drainage. Where an abscess was present, the incision was made through the nearest line of approach, in several instances through the rectum. No unusual methods of treatment were carried out, such as lavage of the peritoneal cavity with saline, or antiseptics. In only one instance was enterostomy performed. In two cases with peritonitis, the appendix was removed and the abdomen closed without drainage. Both patients recovered, and we are inclined to believe that this method, so successful in the hands of Shipley, deserves consideration.

All patients with peritonitis, or even acute appendicitis without peritonitis, were treated postoperatively by the Ochsner method until the temperature was practically normal, the abdomen soft, and until peristalsis had returned to normal. If such treatment is of value before operation, it certainly is of more value after the appendix is removed and dormant infection is awakened.

We have become thoroughly convinced of the advantages of these methods. We likewise feel that, while the advantages of early operation should be taught to doctors and laymen, the treatment of peritonitis is an entirely different problem, which should be treated in an entirely different manner, and that to treat both by the same method has resulted in a definite rise in the death rate of appendicitis.

Discussion on Paper by Drs. Elkin and Glenn

DR. T. C. DAVISON (Atlanta) : This paper should not be allowed to pass unchallenged. Dr. Elkin should have stated that the increase in mortality following operations for appendicitis is due largely to the fact that the patient too often gets to the surgeon too late, and not due to the operative procedure.

Dr. Elkin advocates the prolongation of the waiting period in late cases. It will increase the mortality rate still further if doctors keep patients at home too long. If these patients are to be watched, by all means they should be in a hospital and under the eye of a competent surgeon.

DR. R. M. HARBIN, JR., (Rome) : Dr. Elkin's subject has been and promises to continue to be of perpetual importance. The wide diversity in surgical judgment, technic and post-operative care serves well to illustrate that the ideal has not yet been attained. However, the result of the management he has just set forth as compared with previous records in the same hospital is certainly a step forward in this perplexing situation.

The Ochsner technic would obviously have a wider range of usefulness in negro patients because surgical practice is confronted with later stages of pathology in such patients than is usually observed. But in a more general surgical practice the results might not be so convincing.

Reports, heretofore, of this particular method, show varying degrees of success because the principal difficulty seems to lie in the judgment of waiting and the lack of proper facilities to determine the intensity and spread of the disease. Physical signs are often unreliable. The diagnosis of acute appendicitis is often easy, but differentiation of the stages of pathological developments is often impossible.

We have kept no accurate records on the Ochsner method although it has been practiced in a few instances, partly because of uncertain diagnosis and secondly because our statistics seem to justify prompt operation. In a series of 1,080 cases of acute appendicitis taken from the records of the Harbin Hospital, a total mortality rate of 2.8 per cent is shown with no case dying without operation. Our procedure has been to operate as soon as a diagnosis has been made. Excluding negroes who constituted 3 per cent of the total number of cases the mortality rate was 2.4 per cent. Our death rate for negroes has been 29 per cent which is greatly in excess of that reported by Dr. Elkin.

DR. ROBERT L. RHODES (Augusta): I want to back up what Dr. Elkin has said and also Dr. Davison's explanation. That is that these patients ought to be in the hospital, but in the stage of a spreading or diffuse peritonitis, the treatment as outlined by Dr. Elkin and watchful waiting is the thing that lowers the mortality. We can not drain the peritoneal cavity. We drain a localized area, but not the peritoneal cavity. You get well of infections by immunity, and not otherwise.

On Monday night, two days ago, I operated on a two-year-old infant for acute appendicitis. The turbid peritoneal fluid showed a staphylococcus, but a careful examination of the appendix did not show a perforation. The abdomen was closed without drainage. I have for years closed such patients without drainage. If there is perforation, that is a different story. If you are dealing with a localized walled off abscess, you can drain that abscess, because nature has built an area around it, but with diffuse peritonitis we do not drain.

Development of a New Blood Supply to the Heart by Operation. Claude S. Beck, M.D., Cleveland, Ohio, Annals of Surgery, November, 1935. The heart was given a new blood supply by grafting tissue upon the heart muscle. Experimentally the tissue used was skeletal muscle, parietal pericardium, pericardial fat and omentum. Vascular anastomosis developed between grafts and the heart when the blood supply to the heart was reduced by occluding the coronary arteries. It is possible to occlude both coronary arteries and have the heart survive. The blood supply came through the grafted tissues. This work was based upon experimentation carried out over a period of years. The purpose of the experimental work was to save the human heart in cases of coronary sclerosis. This purpose apparently has been achieved. Beck has operated upon nine patients with coronary sclerosis. Pectoral muscle, pericardium and adjacent fat were grafted upon the heart. The results were encouraging. Angina pectoris has been completely relieved. Exercise tolerance has been increased. Patients have felt better. Perhaps a new field of surgery has been opened up by this work.

Abstract by Dan C. Elkin, M.D., Atlanta.

Program for the eighty-seventh annual session of the Medical Associaiton of Georgia was published in the March issue of the JOURNAL, pages 85-94; Constitution and By-Laws on pages 94-100.

one-half of one per cent. The chief cause of death following acute appendicitis is septic peritonitis. In Boland's review of 4,270 cases of appendicitis in Atlanta in a five-year period (1927-1931), 60 per cent of the total deaths were due to peritonitis. Thus the "drainage" group constitutes the serious cases and it is to this group that our attention should be concentrated if we expect to lower the mortality. J. M. T. Finney, Jr., reports a series of 240 cases of ruptured appendicitis with immediate operation and drainage with a mortality of 22 per cent. Maes reports 299 cases of appendectomy with drainage, 180 of these having a primary caecostomy, with a mortality of 19 per cent. Christopher and Jennings reviewed 183 cases of immediate operation and drainage with a mortality of 16 per cent. Sworn and Fitzgibbon report 231 cases with mortality of 19 per cent. The Charity Hospital in New Orleans from 1910 to 1929 had 1,252 cases of ruptured appendicitis or drainage cases and using the plan of immediate operation, report a mortality of 25 per cent. The average mortality rate of the reported cases of septic peritonitis in which immediate operation and drainage was the treatment instituted is approximately 25 per cent—one patient out of every four dying. In Boland's review of Atlanta cases there were 335 cases of peritonitis of which 110 died, a mortality rate of 33 per cent. This is more forcefully illustrated by the realization that one person out of every three having peritonitis and treated by immediate operation and drainage died. In a series of 48 cases of diffuse peritonitis reported by Dixon at the Mayo Clinic in which drainage alone without appendectomy was performed the mortality was 10 per cent.. He called attention to the additional risk attached to the removal of a perforated appendix in the presence of coexisting peritonitis. While the advocates of the deferred operation and Ochsner treatment are in the minority, their mortality rate is much lower. Deal reported a series of 247 cases of ruptured appendicitis treated by deferred operation with a mortality of 4.45 per cent. Stanton reviewed 113 cases of diffuse peritonitis; 31 having an immediate operation with a mortality of 42 per cent, and the remaining 82 having a deferred operation with a mortality of 8.5 per cent. Coller and Potter reported a mortality of 9.38 per cent following the use of the Ochsner treatment. Guerry, reporting 123 cases of diffuse peritonitis in which operation was deferred, had a mortality of only 1.6 per cent.

operated upon within 24 hours of onset. The absence of cases of ruptured appendicitis in this first 24-hour period is conspicuous.

In the mortality review under postoperative medication, the terms supportive and catharsis need amplification. Supportive treat-

CHART No. I

	Peritoneal contamination	Local peritonitis and abscess	Diffuse peritonitis	Total
Number cases	3	47	53	103
Caecostomy or Enterostomy....	0	2	7 (4 died)	9
Drainage without appendectomy	0	5	6 (1 died)	11
Cases died	0	2	21	23
Mortality rate	0%	4.25%	39.64%	22.35%

Chart No. 1 presents 103 cases that were treated by immediate operation upon entrance to the White Division of Grady Hospital with a mortality rate of 22.35 per cent. Three cases are included in which a gangrenous appendix was ruptured during operation with peritoneal contamination or potential peritonitis. Of the remaining 100 cases, 53 were classified as having diffuse peritonitis and 47 cases as having local peritonitis of abscess formation. The mortality rate in the former group was 39.64 per cent while that of the latter group was only 4.25 per cent.

ment included fluids subcutaneously or intravenously, morphine generously, heat to abdomen, nothing by mouth, and stimulants as indicated. The cases listed under catharsis received calomel in small doses immediately after operation. It is believed by some that this procedure offers prophylaxis against paralytic ileus. The occurrence of ileus in four cases treated thusly makes an interesting observation.

Case No. 1 illustrates the hazard of draining a pelvic abscess through the abdominal wall. Had the patient been drained through

CHART No. II

Age	1-10	11-20	21-30	31-40	41-50	51-60	60+	Total
No. cases	14	39	22	9	6	10	3	103
Died	1	5	5	4	1	4	3	23
Mortality rate	7.1%	12%	22%	36%	16%	40%	100%	22.33%

Chart No. II shows the age of incidence with mortality in decades. The mortality of 7.1 per cent in the first decade is unusually low but this is explained by the fact that only one child seen was under five years of age. The highest mortality belongs to the extremes of life while the highest incidence is in the 2nd and 3rd decades.

the rectum, as was possible in this case, death might not have occurred.

Conclusions: The greatest service the medical profession can render in combating peritonitis is the same service rendered in combating typhoid fever, malaria, diphtheria, and smallpox—by preventing its occurrence. This may be affected; first, by increased diligence

CHART No. III

Days	1 (1-24 hrs.)	2 (25-48 hrs.)	3 49-72 hrs.)	4 (73-96 hrs.)	5	6	7	Total
No. cases	1	30	24	23	10	5	6	99

Average pre-operative duration 3.6 days; 73 per cent gave history of taking purgative. In Chart No. III the pre-operative duration is shown and it is of interest to note that only one case of ruptured appendicitis was

in impressing the public of the danger in the use of purgatives or sedatives for the relief of abdominal pain; and secondly, by reemphasizing necessity of operation for acute appendicitis in the first 24 hours.

When confronted with a case of peritonitis for curative treatment, it would seem that the better procedure would avoid immediate operation. Deal has stated "when the appendix has caused a peritonitis we should center our thoughts on the peritonitis and the con-

Deferred operation requires a more careful study of the patient and a greater need for diagnostic acumen than the practice of routine laparotomy, but the saving of life as evidenced by a lowered mortality rate by this method in the hands of different surgeons in

MORTALITY REVIEW

No.	Age	Pre-operative medication	Pre-operative duration	Post-operative medication	Comment
1.	54	Purgative	4th day	Supportive	Drainage only. Complete localization of pelvic abscess after 5 days. Reopened from above for drainage. Died 12 hrs. later. Sepsis and shock.
2.	66	Purgative	2nd day	Supportive	Died 5th P. O. day. Uremia.
3.	65	None	4th day	Supportive	Died 3rd P. O. day. Uremia.
4.	36	Purgative	?	Supportive	Died 3rd P. O. day. Diabetic Acidosis.
5.	11	Purgative	4th day	Supportive	Died 24 hrs. P. O. Sepsis and shock.
6.	2	Purgative	4th day	Supportive	Died 24 hrs. P. O. Sepsis and shock.
7.	24	Purgative	6th day	Supportive	2 days P. O. (Drainage only.) Sepsis.
8.	20	?	3rd day	Supportive	Died 3 days P. O. Sepsis.
9.	51	Purgative	3rd day	Supportive	Died 24 hrs. P. O. Sepsis and shock.
10.	28	Opiate	4th day	Supportive	Died 7 hrs. P. O. Sepsis and shock.
11.	23	Purgative	2nd day	Supportive	Died 24 hrs. P. O. Caecostomy. Sepsis and shock.
12.	11	Purgative	?	Supportive	Died 2 days P. O. Sepsis.
13.	13	Purgative	2nd day	Supportive	Died 3 days P. O. Sepsis.
14.	58	?	3rd day	?	Caecostomy. Fecal fistula. Chronic sepsis, 5 transfusions. Died 98 days P. O. Sepsis.
15.	55	Purgative	4th day	Catharsis	Died 3 days P. O. Enterostomy. Sepsis.
16.	18	?	7th day	Catharsis	Died 5 days P. O. Sepsis.
17.	35	None	5th day	Catharsis	Died 10th P. O. 2nd Closure. Shock.
18.	21	Purgative	2nd day	Catharsis	Ileus. 2nd enterostomy after 5 days. Died 26th P. O. day. Sepsis.
19.	22	Purgative	2nd day	Catharsis	Ileus. 2nd enterostomy after 4 days. Died immediately. Sepsis and shock.
20.	32	Purgative	2nd day	Catharsis	Ileus. Died 7th P. O. day.
21.	71	Purgative	31st day	Catharsis	Ileus. Died 7th P. O. day.
22.	39	None	?	Catharsis	Died P. O. Sepsis and shock.
23.	42	?	2nd day	Catharsis	Died 24 days P. O. Fecal fistula and sepsis.

dition of the patient and forget the appendix." Operation here can do little to control or limit the septic process but can do much to hasten its extension. Deaver coined the term "forbidding peritonitis" and Richardson described this so well "as cases too early for the late operation and too late for the early operation." Physiological and anatomical rest are essential here for a lowered mortality rate. This may be best achieved by the Ochsner regime which includes nothing by mouth, morphine generously, fluids with glucose subcutaneously, Fowler's position, hot applications to abdomen and the stomach tube and rectal tube if necessary. The action of peristaltic stimulants in the presence of peritonitis is unphysiological and definitely contraindicated.

widely separated localities, is a challenge to those of us who accept the responsibility of treating a patient suffering with this serious malady—septic peritonitis.

REFERENCES

1. Yates, Jno. L.: Local Effects of Peritoneal Drainage. Surg.-Gynec. & Obst. 1: 473, 1905.
2. Fowler, Geo. R.: Diffuse Septic Peritonitis With Special Reference to a New Method of Treatment, namely the Elevated Head and Trunk Posture to Facilitate Drainage with the Pelvis," N. Y. Medical Record, 57: 617, 1900.
3. Deaver, Jno. B.: Appendiceal Pus. J. A. M. A. 33: 197 (July 22) 1899.
4. Ochsner, A. J.: Appendicitis. J. A. M. A. 33: 192 (July 22) 1899.
5. Ochsner, A. J.: A Handbook of Appendicitis. Chicago. G. P. Englehard & Co., 1902.
6. Ochsner, A. J.: Appendicitis (Summary), Jour. Mich. Med. Soc., 3: 371, 1904.
7. Finney, J. M. T.: Five Successful Cases of General Suppurative Peritonitis Treated by a New Method. Bul. Johns Hopkins Hosp. 8: 141-143 (July) 1897.
8. McBurney, Charles: Treatment of General Septic Peritonitis. Ann. Surg. 18: 42 (July) 1893.
9. Finney, J. M. T. Jr.: An Analysis of Complications and Deaths Occurring in Appendicitis. Am. J. Surg. 20: 772-799 (June) 1933.
10. Orr, T. G.: A Rational Treatment of Acute Peritonitis. South. Surgeon 2: 102-109 (June) 1933.

11. Ochsner Alton: The Conservative Treatment of Appendiceal Peritonitis. New Orleans M. & S. J. 87: 32-39 (July) 1934.
12. Richardson, M. H.: Remarks upon Appendicitis. Based Upon a Personal Experience of One Hundred and Eighty-one Cases. Am. J. of the M. Sc. 107: 1-23 (Jan.) 1894.
13. Deaver, J. B.: Appendiceal Peritonitis, Surg., Gynec. & Obst. 47: 401-405 (Sept.) 1928.
14. Sworn, B. R., and Fitzgibbon, G. M.: An Analysis of 2.126 Cases of Acute Appendicitis. Brit. J. Surg. 19: 410-414 (Jan.) 1932.
15. Guerry, Le Grand: A Study of the Mortality in Appendicitis. Ann. Surg. 84: 283-287 (Aug.) 1926.
16. Mattingly, C. W.: Caecostomy in the Treatment of the Ruptured Appendix and Peritonitis. New Orleans M. & S. J. 87: 31-32 (July) 1934.
17. Maes, Urban; Boyce, F. P., and McFetridge, E. M.: Acute Appendicitis Between the Extremes of Life with an Analysis of 910 Cases, New Orleans M. & S. J. 87: 24-30 (July) 1934.
18. Christopher, Frederick, and Jennings, W. K.: Certain Factors in the Operative Mortality of Acute Appendicitis, Am. J. Surg. 18: 16-18 (Oct.) 1932.
19. Coller, F. A., and potter, E. B.: The Treatment of Peritonitis Associated with Appendicitis. J. A. M. A. 103: 1753-1758 (Dec. 8) 1934.
20. Boland, F. K.: Results in the Treatment of Acute Appendicitis: Review of 4,270 Cases in Atlanta. J. A. M. A. 99: 443-448 (Aug. 6) 1932.
21. Deal, Don: When to Interfere in the Acute Abdomen. Internat. J. M. & S. 45: 577-579, 582 (Dec.) 1932.
22. Stanton, E. MacD.: Acute Appendicitis; a Study of the Correlation Between the Time of Operation. the Pathology and the Mortality. Surg., Gynec. & Obst. 59: 738-744 (Nov.) 1934.
23. Gile, J. P., and Bowler, J. P.: The Management of Perforated Appendicitis. J. A. M. A. 103: 1750-1753 (Dec. 3) 1934.
24. Buchbinder, J. R., Droegemueller, W. A., and Heilman, F. R.: Experimental Peritonitis, Surg., Gynec. & Obst. 53: 726-729 (Dec.) 1931.

IRRADIATION VERSUS SURGERY IN BREAST LESIONS*

WM. PERRIN NICOLSON, JR., M.D.

Atlanta

This is not an attempt to champion the cause of either surgery or irradiation to the exclusion of the other. Both are good, and in most cases of breast malignancies should be used in conjunction with each other. Statistics show that the number of cases of cancer are annually increasing. It therefore behooves us to exert every effort to control it. Since every cancer is a local disease at one time, our chief success will lie in diagnosing the cases earlier. This can best be accomplished by further educating the profession and laity.

For many years the American Society for the Control of Cancer has conducted educational campaigns under the slogan "fight cancer with knowledge." Much good has been accomplished, but in some cases cancerphobias have resulted. These are unfortunate, but are not any excuse for discontinuing the work.

Perhaps in an effort to calm excited persons, or for some other equally good reason,

*Read before the Medical Association of Georgia, Atlanta, May 10, 1935.

should like to feel that surgery offered not only the best, but even the only means to reach such an end. It does not. The most enthusiastic surgeon could not feel that way. Nor should the radiologist feel that his is the only good treatment. At one time Lee, in a personal communication, said he was prepared to state that the best treatment for any early operable cancer of the breast was by a combination of interstitial and external irradiation, without surgery. Before his lamented and untimely death he retracted this statement. Time does not allow me to include in this discussion the surgeon who feels that irradiation has no place in any case, nor the radiologist who holds a similar negative opinion of surgery. There are few, if any, such persons.

To the surgeon who uses irradiation, either x-ray or radium, following operation, or in inoperable cases and who does not use preoperative irradiation, I ask the question. "If you feel your patient is benefited by postoperative irradiation, why not have the added protection afforded by preoperative irradiation also?" His most likely response will be that the delay incident to irradiation is too dangerous.

In a recent conversation with Shipley, he said he did not employ preoperative irradiation because he expected to surgically remove all of the initial lesion, and that he reserve his irradiation for the possible metastatic lesions. He said that when anyone would or could convince him that the lymphatics were obliterated following irradiation he would use it preoperatively. I believe in preoperative irradiation, not because I think all of the cancer cells will be killed, but because those that are not killed are at least devitalized, and the likelihood of any cells liberated by the operation successfully implanting themselves in other parts of the body is thus decreased. If one can clinically diagnose a lesion of the breast as a grade I, sclerosing type carcinoma, then I am ready to agree that the delay incident to preoperative irradiation is not justified. In other cases I think it is. In but few cases can such a clinical differentiation be made.

It is not my purpose, nor do I feel qualified, to discuss the technique or dosage of preoperative irradiation, except in so far as our results at Steiner Clinic have indicated an advantage or a disadvantage. I understand that the present tendency of the radiologists in Washington and Baltimore, and perhaps other places, is to treat the entire area to the point of producing desquamation, and then to wait six weeks before operating. We have not been giving such large doses, nor do we wait so long. Our effort is to give a suberythema to an erythema dose through several small ports and to wait ten days to three weeks after the last treatment before operating.

Another objection frequently raised to preoperative irradiation is that it makes the operation more difficult and bloodier. Any increased difficulty produced by the irradiation is usually due to the time at which the operation is performed. I do not recall a single patient on whom I have operated within three weeks after the last x-ray treatment in which I could honestly feel the irradiation had in any way increased the diffciulties of the operation.

The logical question would then seem to be, why wait at all? Several factors are to be considered. Some malignant cells are probably killed at the time of the treatment; others die as a result of cutting off their circulation; others become enmeshed in fibrous tissue resulting from the irradiation. Then, too, if there is an obliteration of the lymphatics, it does not take place until some time after the treatment. If we operate too soon after irradiation, the resulting erythema of the skin may interfere with the healing of the incision. If we wait longer than three weeks there is not only that much more delay, but there is a definite scar tissue formation which renders the operation more difficult.

Another objection that has been raised to preoperative irradiation is the possibility that the patient may refuse operation because of the great improvement, or even the complete disappearance of the tumor mass. One has to use judgment in this respect—being a surgeon, I naturally feel that in the great majority of cases a person is safer with surgery alone than with irradiation alone. If I am dealing with a highly neurotic patient who is inherently opposed to an operation,

concepts of tissue tolerance, and that the results by
which we are now being judged were accomplished
with technics now considered obsolete. It takes more
nerve and equal training to irradiate a patient just up
to the saturation and toleration point, and more per-
suasive powers to keep that patient submitting to
radiation, than it does to perform a radical operation.
At present, average surgery is on a higher plane than
radiology. Nor is our procedure the less disagreeable
of the two methods, for irradiation sickness and
radiodermatitis are very troublesome factors. But in
this disease we are striving to better end results, and
not to placate a patient. We are on the verge of
standardizing our technic. The next decade will answer
this question.

A combination of irradiation and surgery should
be the rule. Preoperative x-radiation is of more
value than postoperative. The loss of time is of no
moment when the improvement in results are noted.
An area larger than that included in the excision
should be x-rayed. The total dosage should be given
within two weeks. Quick advocates 2400 pr, and
deferring the operation six weeks. Auxiliary dissection
will then be slightly more difficult. Healing will not
be impaired. Lee advocated two treatments on each
of two successive days, and operating two to four
days later. While the cancer cells will not show
microscopical changes, they have had a devitalizing
dose, and those spread during the operation are less
likely to live. He said that to operate at two or three
weeks, during the stage of erythema, would delay
normal healing. Postoperative irradiation should follow when primary healing takes place.

If we grant, as we must, that there is virtue in irradiation, that we include areas which cannot possibly be excised, that according to Portmann, of the
Cleveland Clinic, eighty-five per cent of all patients
reporting for operation show axillary involvment,
that according to Lee this axillary involvment reduces
the five year cures forty to fifty per cent, we should
adopt that surgical adjunct which even if it does
not kill all cancer cells, it does cause a degree of
growth restraint which is in favor of the patient.

DR. C. H. RICHARDSON (Macon): I agree with
Dr. Nicolson that the title of his paper should have
been "Irradiation Plus Surgery in Breast Malignancies."
He asked the question whether we can today do much
more for a patient with a breast malignancy and
give her any better outlook than we could ten years
ago. Definitely, I think we can.

I wish to report one case of a white female, aged
30, who weighed 200 pounds, and who came to me
in 1932. She had large pendulous breasts, and a hard
nodular growth in her right breast. She had multiple cystic growths in her left breast. The question
of operability came up, and she was sent to the Steiner
Clinic for an opinion. Their opinion was first adverse. They felt she had an inflammatory type of
carcinoma, which was not amenable to surgery, and
advised irradiation. She came back and was given
an erythema dose of irradiation, and was sent back in

a period of about two weeks for another opinion. At this time, they felt that she should probably have the benefit of surgery. So she came back, and in about four weeks from the time she had the erythema dose of irradiation, she was subjected to radical operation on her right side and a simple mastectomy on the left. The axillary glands were palpable and visible at operation. She was then followed up with a series of deep x-ray therapy, extending over a period of one year, in which she received doses at intervals of about four to six weeks. Her weight was reduced from 200 pounds voluntarily to 160, and she has been back to report every month since the operation in 1932. Three years have elapsed and there is not the slightest evidence of return.

Of course one swallow does not make a summer, but that is such an unusual case in which even the advisability of operation was questioned, and in which the malignancy was verified by a reliable pathologist; and which in three years has had no return. Consequently, I feel that the accepted technic in breast malignancies can be standardized and that it should be preoperative irradiation, radical operation, and postoperative irradiation, and of the three, possibly, or at least of the two types of irradiation, possibly the preoperative irradiation is more important.

DR. WILLIAM P. NICOLSON, JR. (Atlanta). I would like to call Dr. Richardson's attention to the fact that I was careful in specifying the length of time. Ten years ago the patient he reported could have received the same treatment, and I said within the last ten years I did not think there was any definite improvement that we could offer such patients, and I don't think there is, except in getting the patient to you earlier, because ten years ago we had that same technic. I think the statement, if limited to ten years, is true.

Sedimentation Time in Acute Cardiac Infarction. Charles Shookoff, Albert H. Douglas and Meyer A. Rabinowitz. Ann. Int. Med. Feb. 1936.

Using the method of Linzenmeier, the authors studied the red cell sedimentation rate in 26 cases of acute cardiac infarction. They found a very definite increase in every case at some time between the second and eighth day with a gradual return to normal from the thirteenth to thirty-ninth days. The sedimentation rate remained rapid after the fever and leukocytosis had disappeared. They consider this an adjunct to diagnosis when an electrocardiogram cannot be made and also an aid in recognition of subsequent thrombosis or infection—also this method of examination "makes less arbitrary the duration of bed rest.'

Abstract by Wm. R. Minnich, M.D.

The American Public Health Association will hold its sixty-fifth annual meeting in New Orleans, Louisiana, October 20, 21, 22, 23, 1936.

A report on the state of the nation in matters of public health and personal health will be presented.

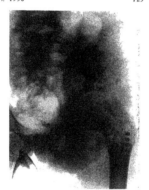

FIG. 1
Endothelial myeloma (Ewing's sarcoma). Proven by biopsy
of metastatic mass fungating through skin.
Note multiple lesions.

tion of the femur, about 9 per cent of tumors of the femur arising in this location and
a few in the midshaft of the humerus. A
striking feature of this disease as will be seen
to some extent in some other bone tumors,
is that the region of the knee is a favorite
location. The lower end of the femur furnishes 52 per cent of all cases of osteogenic
sarcoma and the upper end of the tibia 20
per cent, a total of 72 per cent of all cases
occurring in this region. The upper end of
the humerus accounts for 9 per cent. It is
doubtful if osteogenic sarcoma occurs in the
phalanges, but practically all other bones
have been involved by this tumor.

General Symptoms. The first symptom
is pain and in this respect bone sarcoma differs from other forms of malignancy. Pain
is noted a long time before there is any other
clinical evidence of the disease. The pain
may be intermittent but it gradually increases
in severity. These patients are frequently erroneously treated for rheumatism or growing
pains before the true condition is realized.
The pain is frequently much more severe at
night, causing loss of sleep and rest, thereby
accounting to some extent for loss of weight.

As the disease progresses, there begins a swelling in the region of the tumor, usually a fusiform enlargement of the limb. Local temperature may be elevated and the skin becomes shiny and thin as the tumor enlarges. Veins are dilated. The skin is not involved by the tumor until very late as the capsule of the tumor is usually pushed ahead of the enlarging mass. This again differs from carcinoma where skin invasion takes place rapidly. If the capsule is perforated or bursts, the tumor may fungate through the skin. Rate of growth varies greatly. It depends much upon the type of cell composing the tumor, but frequently this is no criterion for even tumors of marked differentiation may show very rapid growth. Spontaneous fracture frequently accelerates growth in any bone tumor. These fractures may heal under roentgen therapy, the healing taking place by fusion of tumor bone and not through callus formation as in the usual fracture. Some osteogenic sarcomas may pulsate under the hand and this is most frequently seen in the very vascular types or malignant bone aneurysm of older writers. This is a true pulsation of the numerous large vessels and must be differentiated from a transmitted pulsation from some adjacent vessel. Elevation of body temperature is not especially common though it may occur in intermittent attacks. It is much more frequent at the time of generalization of the disease with pulmonary metastases. Usually the blood picture is normal except for an increasing secondary anemia becoming very marked late in the disease. Metastases occur by the blood stream to the lungs, less frequently to the lymph nodes. Blood phosphatase is said to be elevated while the blood calcium and phosphorus remain normal.

X-ray Study. This is of the greatest importance for it is by the x-ray that the early case will be diagnosed and at a time when there will be some hope of cure. One must realize that the diagnosis in any bone tumor is not made upon one single set of findings: complete clinical data must be considered along with the roentgenographic and at times when available, the pathologic. *No one should attempt a diagnosis of any bone lesion without all these data on hand.* The x-ray

produced which deforms the bone but shows little destruction. The cortex is gradually invaded and destroyed and likewise the medullary cavity, and the tumor extends further in the shaft, at the same time extending outward increasing the bulk. In many cases, the outlines of the shaft can still be seen extending through the tumor. In some cases, new bone is laid down at right angles to the shaft, giving a "sunburst" appearance. Many will not make a diagnosis unless such a picture is present, and yet in the Registry of bone sarcoma cases; only 18 per cent show such a picture. One should also remember that this may be present in certain cases of periostitis and in myositis ossificans. Longitudinal striation is of less importance as a diagnostic feature in this particular type. The epiphyseal line is usually a sharp barrier to progress of the tumor, but it may eventually perforate into the epiphysis or may extend outward and invade the joint by way of the surrounding soft tissues. There is no sharp line of demarcation in the shaft, but the tumor gradually fades away into the more healthy portion of the bone. Fracture may occur in any portion. Following radiation there may be increased bone production in a few cases, the tumor is converted into a smooth solid bony mass which is sharply defined, but the great majority of these tumors are highly resistant to any form of radiation, and very little more than palliation can be expected from this form of treatment.

Giant Cell Tumor

Time does not permit us to go into the theories of this interesting type of bone lesion. There are numbers of pathologists who still believe that this is not a true neoplasm, but rather a process of inflammation and repair. On the other hand there are those who recognize certain features which are not present in the ordinary types of inflammatory processes and which seem to indicate that this is a true tumor process. However, it is practically universally agreed that this tumor is primarily benign and therefore does not deserve the designation of "giant cell sarcoma" formerly used. That a few of them may develop malignant characters under certain conditions can hardly be disputed

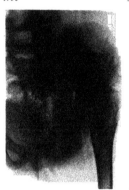

FIG. 3
Osteomyelitis. Multiple inflammatory lesions in other bones and skin.

for we frequently find one which is much more active or more cellular than others, and there has been reported an occasional case which has metastasized. A majority of those which have developed definite malignancy have done so after repeated recurrences, surgical insults and infection, and then there will always remain the question whether they might not have been malignant or atypical osteogenic sarcomas from the start.

Giant cell tumor is most frequently seen between the ages of 30 and 40 though they may appear at any age, a point which helps to separate it from osteogenic sarcoma. When seen in young children, they are very frequently atypical in location and roentgenographic appearance. It seems to affect males and females in equal proportion. As in osteogenic sarcoma, the region of the knee furnishes the greatest number of cases, the lower end of the femur 38 per cent, the upper end of the tibia 14 per cent, the lower end of the radius 8 per cent, and the upper end of the humerus 6 per cent. It is interesting to note its frequency in the lower end of the radius, where osteogenic sarcoma is practically unknown. Giant cell tumors are usually single, very few and somewhat doubtful multiple tumors being reported.

As in the other forms of bone tumors, pain is usually the first symptom, calling attention to the area involved. It is usually not as severe as in osteogenic sarcoma, but is likewise progressive and frequently worse at night or after strain. As the disease progresses, there will appear a globular or swelling which seems to be somewhat more sharply defined at its upper border than does osteogenic sarcoma. The skin will become thin and stretched and there may be local increase in temperature, with distended veins. Constitutional symptoms are usually absent, except, those due to prolonged pain and disability due to the enlarging tumor. Fracture may take place and the bony shell of the tumor may be so thin as to crackle like an egg shell under the fingers.

X-ray Study. This examination shows a tumor of the *epiphysis* if occurring in a long bone, it being unusual to find it in the shaft of the bone. There is a gradual expansion of the bone with bone destruction in areas which are rather well defined and separated by thin bony trabecula giving a multicystic appearance which is characteristic of this type of tumor. The expansion of bone and the multicystic character help to differentiate this from simple bone cysts and abscesses. The outer shell of bone becomes thinner and may eventually break through into the soft tissues but this is not a sign of malignancy but only of progress of the tumor in destroying the bone. The tumor shows a rather marked and sharp line of demarcation where it joins the shaft of the bone which appears normal above the tumor. The periosteum is not elevated beyond the tumor and there is no "reactive triangle."

Following radiation therapy the effect on this tumor is remarkable. There is first a negative phase during which time there seems to have been no effect on the tumor whatsoever, in fact the tumor seems to increase considerably and rapidly in size, although the pain may be relieved in many cases. In others pain persists. The tumor area becomes reddened and more swollen and unless this effect borne in mind, the patient, his family and physicians will believe that there has been

increased activity and that the process is malignant. However, after a varying period of from weeks to several months of this seemingly increased activity, there follows a positive phase of the reaction, characterized by a slowing of the rate of growth, formation of new bone, the tumor becomes denser in the films and some shrinkage takes place. Of course, restoration to the original size of the bone is not to be expected, but useful function is obtained in the majority of cases if taken early.

Endothelial Myeloma

This tumor is primarily one of childhood, 50 per cent occurring before the age of 20 and many of them in the first decade. Occurring as it very frequently does in poorly developed and undernourished children it offers many difficulties in diagnosis. In many cases it simulates osteomyelitis and the clinical evidence is frequently quite similar. It affects males slightly more than females. Pain again is an early and important symptom, but in this disease the pain is more frequently of an intermittent type, occurring at intervals along with definite and sometimes very marked exacerbations of temperature as high as 104°. Pain may be present for a few days and then absent for several days or weeks. Each attack of pain is usually more severe than the preceding one. The febrile attack is frequently accompanied by a leukocytosis as high as 20,000 but the differential count is usually normal. Definite and progressive anemia occurs early. It is easily recognized that every one of these symptoms is that of an inflammatory process except for the normal differential, and may be expected in osteomyelitis. The disease may occur in any bone, long or otherwise, yet it shows a certain predilection for the small bones of the feet, and also the skull and vertebra. When it occurs in a long bone, it involves the midshaft of the bone first extending up and down. The tumor while usually single, is frequently multiple due to multiple foci or origin and not metastases. The second tumor may develop considerably later than the first. The solitary tumors offer the best chance of cure. As in other bone tumors, there is local redness and elevation of temperature, not so marked in contrast with other portions of the body as the entire body is hotter. A diffuse swelling along the bone occurs, of fusiform shape and smooth rounded surface. Lymph nodes may be involved and also internal organs via the blood stream.

X-ray Appearance. The roentgen diagnosis of this tumor presents many difficulties. The disease involves more of the bone than does osteogenic sarcoma, often more than half of the bone being destroyed. The growth is diffuse, probably due to multiple foci of origin in the single bone. The films will show the diaphysis involved with the shaft widening but still intact through the tumor. As the shaft widens, the periosteum lays down longitudinal layers of new bone, a reactive process and not bone formed by the tumor cells, for they are incapable of forming new bone. No "lipping" of the periosteum is noted in this disease. Marked and irregular deformity of the bone is seen, the marked destruction frequently suggesting osteomyelitis.

One very special and important diagnostic sign is the response to radiation therapy. This tumor is the most radiosensitive of any bone tumor, the response to heavy therapy being very prompt and regression may be noted in a very few days. This radiation effect will help to differentiate this tumor from osteogenic sarcoma which is resistant, with delayed reaction if any, and from certain inflammatory lesions of bone.

Multiple Myeloma

This is primarily a tumor of elderly people, occurring as a rule between the ages of 40 and 60. The disease as its name implies is characterized by the formation of multiple tumors in one and many bones, as high as forty having been found in the skull in one individual. On the other hand, there have been a few cases reported in which there was only a single tumor. It affects males slightly more than females and the greatest number of cases occur in the sternum, ribs, skull and vertebra. In long bones, the humerus and femur are more frequently involved. As distinguished from other malignant tumors of bone, in myeloma pain is relatively late, appearing after the bone has been considerably destroyed. Fracture frequently occurs before

the disease is suspected. Secondary anemia develops rather late also in this disease. There is usually less swelling in this tumor than in other forms of bone tumors as the bone is simply destroyed with very little enlargement of the bone or reaction of the surrounding tissues.

In former years, one placed a considerable reliance in the appearance of Bence-Jones proteose in the urine, as almost a pathognomonic sign. On heating the urine, a precipitate appears at about $55°C$ which disappears on boiling, and reappears as the urine cools. While this is found in a certain percentage of cases of multiple myeloma, it is also found in leukemia, metastatic carcinoma involving bone and certain other conditions affecting the bone marrow. Therefore it simply indicates a destruction of the bone marrow and not any specific type of tumor process.

X-ray Appearance. In this disease there are multiple areas of bone destruction, often rather sharply outlined and discrete. There is less of the diffuse bone destruction as seen in endothelial myeloma, and the bone appears to be eaten out in small foci. There is no bone production as the cells of this tumor are not related to osteoblasts and therefore can not produce bone. There is less periosteal reaction so inflammatory bone is likewise absent. Perforation of the cortex and invasion of the surrounding tissue is very seldom seen. The chief difficulty in diagnosis of this tumor is differentiation from osteolytic sarcoma and from metastatic carcinoma. However, the moth-eaten appearance of the bone is usually typical and multiple foci in a single bone more to be expected in myeloma than in metastatic lesions or osteogenic sarcoma.

In regard to biopsy diagnosis of bone tumors, I am firmly of the opinion that this method of diagnosis has no place in the early diagnosis of these conditions and in the majority of cases is not required, the clinical and roentgenographic evidence being sufficiently conclusive. This diagnostic procedure is fraught with much danger to both the patient and to the pathologist. The capsule of any tumor is a strong defensive barrier to its progress and any incision destroys its effectiveness and permits the tumor to grow wild.

Likewise it permits the introduction of infection to stimulate the growth of the tumor and hasten the death of the patient. Especially is this true of tumors located where amputation or resection is impossible. In tumors of long bones, if after all the evidence has been carefully considered, and if radiation has failed to produce sufficient regression, and the diagnosis still remains in doubt, it is then permissable to perform biopsy for immediate diagnosis with the patient. on ·the operating table ready for amputation should the biopsy prove the diagnosis of malignancy. In many instances, the examination of a small piece of tissue fails to give a correct impression of the nature of the tumor. In osteogenic sarcoma, it is not uncommon to find areas which seem to show conclusively that the tumor is one of giant cell character, when other portions are definitely malignant. Giant cells are frequently found in various portions of malignant tumors especially about areas of absorbing bone. These giant· cells are identical with those found in benign giant cell tumors and if too much reliance is placed in the structure of the small piece of tissue removed as a biopsy, the true nature of the tumor may remain in doubt or may be erroneously diagnosed. In endothelial myeloma the diagnosis from a biopsy is much more difficult for the biopsy may show only areas of inflammatory tissue with large number of lymphocytes and leukocytes. again suggesting osteomyelitis. In these cases radiation will do more toward establishing diagnosis than a small piece of tissue removed at random from the tumor. All the difficulties encountered in a well prepared paraffin section, are greatly multiplied when attempting diagnoses of bone tumors by frozen section.

There are many other things which should be considered in a discussion of malignant bone tumors. Time and space do not permit the consideration of the gross and microscopic description of these tumors which·in themselves would permit a lengthy discussion. Likewise the prognosis and treatment of these tumors, which subjects permit much debate and many varied opinions. These will be presented in another article. However, it is hoped that the above dis-

cussion of some of the clinical features of bone tumors will aid in their diagnosis in the early stages of the disease when there is some hope and chance that a cure may be obtained by suitable treatment.

THE PSYCHOLOGY OF PREJUDICE AND MOB ACTION IN TRIBES AND NATIONS

SAMUEL KAHN, M.D.
Atlanta

Prejudices are feelings and beliefs and conclusions which are not based directly on facts. Prejudices may turn favored opinions into facts. A fact to a faithful person, may be a prejudice to a skeptic. Some prejudices are helpful, and some are detrimental. One may be prejudiced for, or against, a person, a thing, an idea, an institution, or even a race or a religion. One man cannot see a homestead as another man who was born in it sees it. We frequently interpret the same facts differently, largely because of prejudice. Even patriotism is a form of prejudice. Prejudice, itself, is an emotion. Prejudice and sentiment are closely related. At times, it is better that a man be ruled by his heart than by his head. That man has become what he is, not so much by his head, but by his heart, is certainly a truism. Frequently, it is the heart which helps the completion of evolutionary needs. It is quite frequent that a woman's intuition is more conducive to progress and results than is man's reason. There is no doubt that intuition is influenced by prejudice and is related to it.

Because of prejudice, there is favoritism and antagonism. Originally, nature endowed her tribes with the spirit of antagonism, which produced good and bad results. This spirit of antagonism is identical with what we now call race prejudice. Tribes finally developed into nations. If one analyzes the dynamics of nations, it can be seen that they are very similar to the dynamics of tribes. Both want, independence. As a result of prejudice, man reasons·thusly: If my fellow tribesman kills an alien tribesman, then, his act is heroic; but if my friend, or tribesman, were to be slain by an alien enemy,

over-confident because of their numbers, and are afraid to remain outside of the mob because of fears and panics. Although some of the individual mob members may be very intelligent, they may be unable to practice and use their intelligence, because of panicky feelings of being left out of the mob and of feelings of helplessness and inadequacy unless they are organized and with the mob. This mob, through prejudice, assumes the attitude that intolerance is praised and guilt feelings are lost. Might is right, and hence group justification, group protection, and group power. Such mobs cannot understand intellectualization, philosophication, true altruism and civilization. They look for applause and approval, which remove their guilt feelings, even though they practice ridiculous intolerance. Through slogans, they abuse facts and disguise truths. Slogans, whether truthful or not, are accepted by the heart first, regardless of whether they are acceptable to the head or not, and even though slogans are usually not scientific and impossible to be carried out. With mobs, there are always associated demagogues, who understand how to use prejudice.

Mobsmen and demagogues who belonged to a mob of olden times were seldom as vicious as new mobsmen, who were originally outside of it, and who have adopted the mob of late. The more the new mobsmen and demagogues fear and doubt their place in the mob, the more vicious they may become. Then, they spread hatreds which may become self-sufficient, resulting in men and nations fighting even after the original cause of the quarrel has long disappeared.

Demagogues then prejudice mobsmen through what they call national pride, and individual love for themselves and their countries; but in reality, they hunger for love of importance and personal publicity for themselves. The greater their own demands for this prestige, the stronger do they force the formation of prejudices; the more these demagogues demand the applause, approval and love of others, the more they hate each other and those who may not believe as they do. The more leaders of mobs love themselves and desire this degree of love, the more

(Continued on Page·135)

THE JOURNAL
OF THE
MEDICAL ASSOCIATION OF GEORGIA
Devoted to the Welfare of the Medical Association of Georgia

478 Peachtree Street, N.E., Atlanta, Ga.

APRIL, 1936

WELCOME TO SAVANNAH

Savannah, the mother city of Georgia and home of the oldest medical organization in the State, extends to you a most hearty welcome to attend the annual session of the Medical Association of Georgia, April 21, 22, 23, 24, 1936.

In Savannah, Oglethorpe established his first colony and made peace with the Yamacraw Indians;. John Wesley preached and taught; Whitfield built the first orphanage in America; the greatest battle of the Revolution was fought and Jasper captured British officers single-handed.

Historical places still standing are: homes that Washington visited; tavern which Aaron Burr visited after his duel with Hamilton; Fort Pulaski as in the sixties; Telfair Art Gallery, the largest in the South.

The golf courses will be open. Excellent opportunities for fishing and swimming are offered.

Bring your family to Savannah and give them a liberal education in the history of Georgia.

JOHN W. DANIEL, M.D.

Savannah   Presdent, 1923-1924.

We have learned that the distance is no greater from Atlanta to Savannah than from Savannah to Atlanta. We, the physicians of Savannah, most earnestly urge you to attend the next session of the Medical Association of Georgia, to be held in Savannah, April 21-24, 1936, and give us an opportunity to shower Savannah's hospitality upon you. We will be happy to entertain the members of the Association and Woman's Auxiliary and will be keenly disappointed if our invitation is not accepted. Hope you will honor us with an unusually large attendance.

In addition to the social features, the officers of the Assocation have put forth great effort to assure you a superior and profitable program.

WILLIAM R. DANCY, M.D.

Savannah.   President, 1929-1930.

TREATMENT OF ECLAMPSIA

Eclampsia takes the lives of approximately 4,500 women in this country each year. Until the etiology is known, the treatment of this condition is empirical. Numerous supposed etiologic factors have been responsible for various lines of treatment, resulting often in methods so extreme as hardly to be considered rational. So great a confusion developed that leading obstetricians have produced a flexible standard outline of treatment, formulated and presented to the medical profession by the "American Committee on Maternal Welfare"[1]. It was not the purpose of this committee to stifle new thought or damper new ideas, but to definitely identify such new ideas or thoughts as experimental until sufficient data have been accumulated to prove their worth and warrant their acceptance.

The question of the exact terminology indicating toxemia of pregnancy is unimportant. The term "pre-eclamptic toxemia" is used chiefly by them because it is probably familiar to more physicians than any other term used to define all toxemias of late pregnancy which may ultimately produce a convulsion.

It is well stated in their report that the toxemia of late pregnancy is a non-surgical condition, which should be treated by medical measures in the majority of cases. Careful investigation has shown that the maternal death rate is more than 20 per cent in many localities following cesarean section, or other operative measures, whereas it is reported to be about 5 per cent in series of cases in which the treatment is primarily by medical measures.

When a pre-eclamptic patient presents herself with such symptoms as a systolic blood pressure of 140, a two plus albuminuria, a marked edema, or severe headache, her diet is limited (often milk only for two days is beneficial), the salt intake eliminated, free saline catharsis instituted, and sedation accomplished by the administration of bromides, chloral or barbiturates to assist in re-

how pregnancy should be conducted in the best interest of mother and fetus. When gestation has reached the period of viability it is safer for both, if pregnancy is terminated. When the period of viability has not been reached, the chance of the fetus surviving is exceedingly remote and the life of the mother is endangered by the continuation of pregnancy.—When the convulsions have been checked, termination of pregnancy should be advised by the method best suited to the obstetric indications and environment."

E. BRYANT WOODS, M.D.

REFERENCES

1. American Committee on Maternal Welfare. (Drs. Fred L. Adair, Chicago, chairman; George W. Kosmak, New York, vice chairman; James R. McCord, Atlanta, Ga., secretary; Frederick H. Falls, Chicago, treasurer; LeRoy A. Calkins, Kansas City, Mo.; Robert L. DeNormandie, Boston; Rudolph W. Holmes, Chicago; Robert D. Mussey, Rochester, Minn.; Everett D. Plass, Iowa City; Arthur J. Skeel, Cleveland, and Philip F. Williams, Philadelphia). Jour. A. Med. Assn. 104: 1703-1705 (May 1935).

2. Sharp, J. C.: "Bromide Intoxication." Jour. A. Med. Assn. 102: 1403 (1934).

3. Bryant, Richard II: "Veratrum Viride in the Treatment of Eclampsia." Am. Journ. Ob. & Gyn. 30: 46-53 (1935).

*Parenthesis supplied by author.

APPENDICITIS

Dr. Robert T. Morris in his recent autobiography "Fifty Years a Surgeon" relates "in Africa, when a lion leaps out upon a herd of zebra and makes a kill, the rest of the herd merely trots off to a distance and goes to grazing again. There is a concensus of opinion that this will happen now and then. They take their death rate for granted. This little study in comparative psychology explains the surgeon's complacence over his appendicitis death rate. We toss appendicitis death rate statistics aside as being impersonal. They are not impersonal. You and I have simply not been included among them as yet. Only when it is your own loved one dead will you realize what death rate means."

In this issue of the JOURNAL are two papers upon this important subject with a review of cases and mortality statistics, taken from the white and colored divisions of Grady Hospital in Atlanta. It is significant that these authors working independently have arrived at the same conclusions, one by the finding of positive evidence and the other supplying negative evidence for comparison. Certainly with a realization of these facts all surgeons should review their results, reconsider their views on therapy, and restudy the literature upon this subject in an effort to reduce their individual mortality and thus collectively reduce this high mortality of the whole.

OFFICIAL CALL

To the Officers, Fellows and Members of the American Medical Association

The eighty-seventh annual session of the American Medical Association will be held in Kansas City, Missouri, from Monday, May the eleventh, to Friday, May the fifteenth, Nineteen hundred and thirty-six.

The House of Delegates will convene on Monday, May the eleventh.

The Scientific Assembly of the Association will open with the General Meeting held on Tuesday, May the twelfth, at 8:30 P.M.

The various sections of the Scientific Assembly will meet Wednesday, May the thirteenth, at 9 A.M. and at 2 P.M. and subsequently according to their respective programs.

JAMES L. MCLESTER, *President*
NATHAN B. VAN ETTEN
Speaker, House of Delegates

Attest: OLIN WEST, *Secretary*
Chicago, Feb. 24th.

HOUSE OF DELEGATES

The House of Delegates will convene at 10:00 a. m. on Monday May 11, 1936, in the Ballroom of the Hotel Muehlebach, Twelfth and Baltimore.

REPRESENTATION

The apportionment of delegates made at the Cleveland Session of 1934 entitles your State Association to three delegates for 1935-36-37.

"A member of the House of Delegates must have been a member of the American Medical Association and a Fellow of the Scientific Assembly for at least two years next preceding the session of the House of Delegates at which he is to serve.

"Delegates and alternates from constituent associations shall be elected for two years. Constituent associations entitled to more than one representative shall elect them so that one-half, as near as may be, shall be elected each year. Delegates and alternates elected by the sections, or delegates appointed from the United States Army, United States Navy and United States Public Health Service shall hold office for two years."—*Chap. 1.Secs. 1 and 2, By-Laws.*

RULES FOR THE GUIDANCE OF THE COMMITTEE ON CREDENTIALS

Adopted by the House of Delegates at Atlantic City, N. J., June 6, 1912

1. Credentials shall be of two parts. The first part shall be sent to the office of the Secretary of the American Medical Association by the secretary of the constituent association, not later than seven days prior to the first day of the first meeting of the House of Delegates, and shall be a list of delegates and alternates for that association. The constituent associations shall designate an alternate for each delegate, who may take the pledge of the delegate when authorized to do so by said delegate in writing. In the absence of such authority, any alternate who has been duly chosen by the constituent association may be seated in place of any delegate who is unable to attend, provided he presents proper official authority from said association. A certificate signed by the president or secretary of the constituent association shall be deemed legal authority (*as amended June 7, 1921*).

2. Each delegate shall be furnished with a credential by the secretary of the association by which he is elected on a prescribed form furnished by the Secretary of the American Medical Association, which shall give the date and term for which he was elected and who was elected to act as alternate for him in case of his inability.

3. A delegate, on presenting himself to the Committee on Credentials, may be seated even though he may not present part 2 of his credential, provided he is properly identified as the delegate who was elected by his association and whose name appears on the Secretary's record.

4. No alternate may be seated unless his credentials meet the same requirements as designated for the delegate and he can show written evidence that he is empowered by his delegate to act for him, except as provided for in Section 1 as amended. (*as amended June 7, 1921*).

5. When a constituent state association reports that one of its elected delegates and his elected alternate are both unable to attend a specified annual session of the American Medical Association, the constituted authority of said constituent state association may fill the vacancies caused by the absence of both an elected delegate and his elected alternate, and such a substitute delegate or his substitute alternate who presents proper credentials signed by the president and secretary of said constituent state association shall be eligible to regular membership in the House of Delegates of the American Medical Association in such a specified session (*as adopted, May 12, 1932*).

Scientific Assembly

The Opening General Meeting, which constitutes the opening exercises of the Scien-

BOOK REVIEWS

Year Book of Obstetrics and Gynecology 1935. By Joseph B. DeLee, A.M., M.D., Professor of Obstetrics, University of Chicago Medical School, and J. P. Greenhill, B.S., M.D., F.A.C.S., Professor of Gynecology, Loyola University Medical School, and Cook County Graduate School of Medicine. Chicago: The Year Book Publishers, 1935. $2.50.

Drs. DeLee and Greenhill have again recorded in this volume of the Year Book series 613 excellent abstracts of recent articles on obstetrics and gynecology which were published in 62 domestic journals and 44 journals of foreign countries. Some illustrations are reproduced. The articles on numerous subjects are well classified, grouped and indexed. The comments of the editors, who are men of experience and sound judgment, are particularly numerous this year and add greatly to the value of this comprehensive review of the literature.

                                        JAS. N. BRAWNER, JR., M.D.

Lobar Pneumonia and Serum Therapy by Frederick T. Lord, Clinical Professor of Medicine, Emeritus, Harvard Medical School; Member of the Board of Consultation, Massachusetts General Hospital; Member of the Massachusetts Advisory Committee on Pneumonia and Roderick Heffron, Field Director, Pneumonia Study and Service Massachusetts Department of Public Health. pp. 91. Price $1.00. Publishers, The Commonwealth Fund, New York. 1936.

This little book should be in the library of every physician who treats pneumonia. It is primarily a report of a study of lobar pneumonia made in Massachusetts from 1931 to 1935.

It is shown that the pneumococcus is the etiologic agent in the majority of cases of lobar pneumonia. More than half of these cases belong to Types I and II for which specific serum is of proved benefit. This serum is available through the drug houses.

Before serum is given the sputum should be typed. The technic for this by the Neufeld method which is simple and rapid is given. Directions are included for making the eye and skin tests which should precede the administration of serum. The precautions to be taken, the contraindications, and the results to be expected are clearly detailed. In this study 60,000 to 100,000 units of serum, the amount depending on the severity of the disease, were given intravenously in divided doses. Deaths were reduced from 25 per cent in cases to whom serum was not given to 11 per cent in those treated with serum in pneumonias of Type I and from 41 to 27 per cent in Type II. It is emphasized that the earlier the diagnosis is made and the serum given the better the result. The authors believe that antipneumococcic serum should be administered to every patient over twelve years of age having Type I or Type II pneumonia unless he is very old, has pulmonary edema, is moribund, or shows by history or test sensitivity to serum.

                                        AMEY CHAPPELL, M.D.

WOMAN'S AUXILIARY

OFFICERS

President—Mrs. Ernest R. Harris, Winder.
President-Elect—Mrs. Wm. R. Dancy, Savannah.
First Vice-President—Mrs. Hulett H. Askew, Atlanta.
Second Vice-President—Mrs. T. J. Ferrell, Waycross.
Recording Secretary—Mrs. W. R. Garner, Gainesville.
Corresponding Secretary—Mrs. S. T. Ross, Winder.
Treasurer—Mrs. W. M. Cason, Sandersville.
Historian—Mrs. Marvin Haygood, Atlanta.

Parliamentarian—Mrs. Ralph H. Chaney, Augusta.

Committee Chairmen

Health Films—Mrs. A. J. Mooney, Statesboro.
Student Loan Fund—Mrs. Benjamin Bashinski, Macon.
Public Relations—Mrs. J. A. Redfearn, Albany.
Press and Publicity—Mrs. J. Harry Rogers, Atlanta.
Jane Todd Crawford Memorial—Mrs. Eustace A. Allen, Atlanta.
Research in Romance of Medicine—Mrs. D. N. Thompson, Elberton.

COUNTY AND DISTRICT MEETINGS

Ninth District

The semi-annual meeting of the Ninth District Auxiliary convened on March 18th at Canton. Mrs. D. H. Garrison, District Chairman, presided.

Mrs. T. J. Vansant gave the message of welcome from the Cherokee-Pickens Counties Auxiliary, and Mrs. C. C. Aven responded.

Dr. J. L. Campbell made an instructive address on the nature of cancer and stressed the importance of early diagnosis and treatment.

Dr. Theodore Toepel spoke for enlistment of more members and urged the cooperation of the Auxiliary in educating laity to the importance of regular physical examinations.

Dr. Edgar D. Shanks suggested a definite program of work as a plan for greater usefulness and stimulation of the units of the Auxiliary.

A short memorial service was devoted to Mrs. M. B. Allen of Hoschton, and Mrs. W. M. Willingham of Canton.

Lovely and appropriate songs were contributed by Mrs. C. J. Roper of Jasper, accompanied by Mrs. Sheppie Hawkins, Canton.

The business session included the election of Mrs. G. C. Brooke, Canton, as Vice-Chairman for the District.

Following adjournment and a social period the Auxiliary joined the members of the Medical Society for lunch in the hotel dining room.

Chatham County

The February meeting of the Georgia Medical Society Auxiliary in Savannah was featured by plans for the entertainment of the State Auxiliary April 21-24. Committee chairmen appointed were: Mrs. Lee Howard, General Chairman of Arrangements with the following chairmen: Mesdames G. Hug Johnson, Publicity; Rufus Graham, Registra tion; Lehman Williams, Hospitality; G. H Lang, Decorations; Luther DeLoach, Trans portation; William Myers, Music; and J. S Howkins, Toastmistress. Delegates to th convention elected were: Mrs. Luther A. De Loach and Mrs. Charles Usher, with Mr. C. G. Redmond and Mrs. R. V. Martin, al ternates.

Mrs. Lehman Williams reported on th meeting of the Woman's Auxiliary to th Southern Medical Association and plans wer made for the observance of Doctors' Day o March 30, with Mrs. William Myers Chair man, assisted by Mrs. Hugo Johnson an Mrs. Lee Howard.

Mrs. A. A. Morrison, Jr., appointed th following committee chairmen: Mesdame Luther DeLoach, Hygeia; J. C. Metts, Healt Education; Lester Neville, Health Films; El liot Wilson, Public Relations; H. H. McGe Scrapbook; C. R. Riner, Organization; Har ry M. Kandel, Press and Publicity; G. Hug Johnson, State Press and Publicity; John L Elliot, House; Lehman Williams, Program Ralston Lattimore, Historian; J. S. Howkin; Parliamentarian; Julian Quattlebaum, Legis lation; Charles Usher, Research and Romance in Medicine; E. N. Maner, Jane Todd Craw ford, Memorial; C. R. Riner, Membershir and Lee Howard and G. H. Lang, members a large.

Tenth District

The Auxiliary to the Tenth District Medi cal Society met February 12, in Augusta, th Augusta Auxiliary was hostess.

The meeting was called to order by th District Manager, Mrs. Ralph H. Chaney. Re ports from several Auxiliaries showed mem bers were co-operating with other civic or ganizations for better health conditions. A report was given by Mrs. H. G. Banister o the consolidation of Oglethorpe-Madison

Franklin counties with Clarke County Auxiliary.

The highlights of the day's program were the informative talks given. Dr. James E. Paullin, President of the Medical Association of Georgia, spoke on "The Place of the Medical Auxiliary as an Aid to the Medical Society"; Dr. Edgar D. Shanks, Secretary-Treasurer, spoke briefly urging Medical Auxiliaries to aid in carrying out the program on Cancer Education; Dr. B. H. Minchew, President-Elect, outlined study on Romance of Medicine as an aid in developing an interest in program making; Mrs. Wm. R. Dancy, President-Elect of State Auxiliary, read an outline of organization work; Mrs. H. R. Creamer, District President of Tenth District P.-T. A., talked on "Better Training for Girls in Mothercraft."

The District Manager, Mrs. Ralph H. Chaney, presented the following distinguished guests: Dr. James E. Paullin, President of the Medical Association of Georgia; Dr. Edgar D. Shanks, Secretary-Treasurer; Dr. B. H. Minchew, President-Elect; Mrs. B. H. Minchew; Mrs. J. E. Penland, Past President of State Medical Auxiliary; Mrs. Wm. R. Dancy, President-Elect.

After the meeting the Auxiliary members were served a delightful luncheon at the Oakdale Tea Room.

Habersham County

The Habersham Medical Society and Auxiliary met on February 13th at the home of Dr. and Mrs. T. H. Brabson. After the business session an interesting lecture and exhibit was given by Dr. Edgar Angel and Dr. Furman, of Franklin, N. C., on "Two Thousand Appendectomies."

During the social hour, Mrs. Brabson, assisted by Mrs. Ella Eberhart, Mrs. Stinewinters and Miss May Warren, served refreshments.

Those present were Dr. and Mrs. Bruce Schaefer, Toccoa; Dr. and Mrs. Rankin, Dr. and Mrs. Whelchel, of Alto; Dr. and Mrs. W. H. Garrison, Dr. and Mrs. D. H. Garrison, Clarkesville; Dr. and Mrs. Robert Lamb, Demorest; Dr. and Mrs. E. H. Lamb, Dr. and Mrs. O. N. Harden, Cornelia; Mrs. Stinewinters, Gainesville; Miss May Warren, Franklin; and Mrs. Ella Eberhart, Cornelia.

Tri-County Organized
(Burke-Jenkins-Screven Counties)

An Auxiliary to the Tri-County Medical Association, composed of Burke-Jenkins-Screven Counties, was organized in Millen on February 14 at the same time the Medical Society was in session there. Mrs. Cleveland Thompson, President of the Auxiliary to the First District Medical Society, invited the doctors' wives to accompany them for the purpose of organizing the Auxiliary and an excellent representation from Savannah, Sylvania, Waynesboro, Sardis, Midville, Vidette and Millen attended the meeting. Mrs. W. R. Dancy, of Savannah, State President-Elect, spoke on the purposes of organization.

Officers were elected as follows: Mrs. L. F. Lanier, of Sylvania, President; Mrs. W. W. Hillis, of Sardis, Vice-President; and Mrs. O. A. Mulkey, of Millen, Secretary-Treasurer. The group will meet in February, June and October each year, and all meetings will be held in Millen, which is centrally located.

Mrs. Thompson entertained the Auxiliary members at a beautifully appointed dinner at her home, the Valentine color scheme being effectively carried out in all appointments.

Fifth District

The Fifth District Auxiliary met at the Academy of Medicine in Atlanta on March 27th, the members enjoyed a buffet dinner as guests of the Fifth District Medical Society prior to the business meeting.

Mrs. Joseph Yampolsky, President, presided. Dr. Frank Boland, of Atlanta, gave an excellent talk on "The Romance of Medicine," and illustrated his talk with pictures of men memorable in the history of medicine. Dr. Benjamin H. Minchew of Waycross, President-Elect of the Medical Association of Georgia, spoke of the work the Auxiliary could accomplish to assist the doctors and gave many helpful suggestions. Dr. James E. Paullin, President of the Medical Association of Georgia; and Dr. James N. Brawner, Chairman of the Advisory Committee to the Auxiliary, both brought inspiring messages.

The meeting was well attended and much enthusiasm manifested.

The effectiveness of the Sippy Regime in Neutralizing the Gastric Juice of Patients if the amount of Alkali is not varied. Paul H. Wosika and Edward S. Emery, Jr. Ann. Int. Med., Feb. 1936.

In an effort to determine how often a patient following the unmodified Sippy regime will have complete neutralization of the stomach contents, the authors studied 45 patients thoroughly during the whole period of hospitalization. The routine on the days of study consisted of examination of the stomach contents every half hour during the day from 7 A.M. to 7 P.M., thirty minutes before taking the powders or the milk. They found that the treatment abolished symptoms in all cases; if free acidity does not rise above 20 after an alcohol test meal, the acidity can be perfectly controlled with the regime. Calculations regarding the theoretical amount of alkali necessary showed that from 25 to 50 times more than was necessary was given.

Abstract by Wm. R. Minnich, M.D.

GEORGIA DEPARTMENT OF PUBLIC HEALTH

T. F. ABERCROMBIE, M.D., *Director*

ACTIVITIES OF THE HEALTH OFFICERS

The special qualifications for public health officers, recently adopted, were outlined in the September 1935 issue of this JOURNAL. It is proposed in this article to give a brief outline of their duties and activities. To give these activities in detail would require volumes so this will not be attempted. Each of the basic activities has its distinct place and value and no attempt will be made to list them in their order of importance.

1. *Vital Statistics.*—To the trained health officer this is a very important function. Apparently, many physicians do not recognize the real value and uses of birth and death certificates to the public health worker. A complete list of all births and data pertaining thereto, properly stated, is necessary if the health department performs its duty in maternal and infant welfare. Properly executed death certificates are of value in many ways. Death certificates, giving tuberculosis as the cause of death, furnish a very important lead for finding contacts. By this means alone, a tuberculosis case rate of more than 40 per 1,000 population was discovered in a Georgia county recently. A majority of the cases found in this way were in the early stages and gave good promise for a cure.

2. *Communicable Disease Control.*—This work requires one or more visits to every case of communicable disease reported, with the exception of a few milder and more common infections.. The purpose of these visits is twofold: (a) to institute precautions for the prevention of spread from the case. These precautionary measures are applied during the acute course of the disease and in many cases, such as typhoid, diphtheria, tuberculosis and others, may require supervision for weeks or. months. Obviously, control measures differ for almost every communicable disease. A regulation of the State Board of Health requires that all cases of typhoid be kept under control until at least two successive negative cultures of stool and urine specimens, collected at intervals of fifteen days, have been secured. It is often necessary to collect fifteen or more specimens from convalescent carriers. From two to four per cent of the cases remain chronic carriers and are to be kept under control indefinitely. Two negative cultures from the throat and nose of convalescent diphtheria cases are required before release. (b) To

investigate and discover the origin of this particular case. This may not always be easy, but in most cases it can be done and other infections prevented. Such investigation often leads to the discovery of a typhoid carrier, a case of chronic fibrosis tuberculosis, etc.

3. *Sanitation.*—The health officer must be familiar with the sanitary conditions in his jurisdiction, with especial reference to the safety of the water supply and the proper disposal of human wastes. It is not necessary to dwell on the importance of this part of his work nor to stress the great need for this work in Georgia, if we are ever to eradicate typhoid, dysentery and hookworm disease.

4. *Food and Milk.*—The health officer is responsible to his people for a safe food and milk supply, with emphasis on the milk and milk products.

5. *Maternal and Child Hygiene.*—The span of human life has been lengthened mainly because of the work done in saving the lives of babies and children. This should still receive a just proportion of the health officer's time. He, of course, realizes that the time to start child hygiene is before birth. Georgia's maternal mortality and morbidity is far from being a cause for pride. It is, therefore, proper that the public health department should make every effort to see that every expectant mother receives adequate prenatal care and that every child visits a physician for regular care.

6. *School Work.*—The health officer is required to give every school child a physical examination each year. If any defects are found, he notifies the teacher and parents, with the advice that the family physician or dentist be consulted. It is the health officer's duty to examine each teacher, janitor or other persons coming in direct contact with school children, as well as to see that the school buildings and grounds are kept in a sanitary condition.

7. *Clinics.*—With the cooperation and assistance of the private physicians, the health officer promotes and organizes clinics for the early diagnosis of tuberculosis, the diagnosis and treatment of venereal disease of the indigents, and for the administration of protective agents against typhoid, diphtheria and smallpox.

8. *Consultation Service.*—The health officer is at all times available to the local physi-

HONOR ROLL FOR 1936

1. Randolph County, Dr. W. G. Elliott, Cuthbert, October 30, 1935.
2. Dougherty County, Dr. I. M. Lucas, Albany, December 27, 1935.
3. Monroe County, Dr. G. H. Alexander, Forsyth, February 14, 1936.
4. Hancock County, Dr. H. L. Earl, Sparta, February 25, 1936.
5. Elbert County, Dr. A. S. Johnson, Elberton, March 6, 1936.
6. Worth County, Dr. G. S. Sumner, Sylvester, March 12, 1936.
7. Rockdale County, Dr. H. E. Griggs, Conyers, March 21, 1936.
8. Morgan County, Dr. W. C. McGeary, Madison, March 30, 1936.
9. Turner County, Dr. J. H. Baxter, Ashburn, March 30, 1936.
10. Ware County, Dr. Kenneth McCullough, Waycross, March 30, 1936.

COUNTIES REPORTING FOR 1936

McDuffie County Medical Society

The McDuffie County Medical Society announces the following officers for 1936:
President—C. W. Churchill, Thomson.
Vice-President—B. F. Riley, Jr., Thomson.
Secretary-Treasurer—J. R. Wilson, Thomson.
Delegate—J. R. Wilson, Thomson.

Worth County Medical Society

The Worth County Medical Society announces the following officers for 1936:
President—H. S. McCoy, Sylvester.
Vice-President—J. L. Tracy, Sylvester.
Secretary-Treasurer—G. S. Sumner, Sylvester.
Delegate—W. C. Tipton, Sylvester.
Alternate Delegate—H. S. McCoy, Sylvester.

Telfair County Medical Society

The Telfair County Medical Society announces the following officers for 1936:
President—S. T. Parkerson, McRae.
Vice-President—W. H. Born, McRae.
Secretary-Treasurer—F. P. Harbin, Lumber City.
Delegate—F. R. Mann, McRae.

Ben Hill County Medical Society

The Ben Hill County Medical Society announces the following officers for 1936:
President—G. W. Willis, Ocilla.
Vice-President—J. E. McMillan, Fitzgerald.
Secretary-Treasurer—L. S. Osborne, Fitzgerald.
Delegate—Lewis Abram, Fitzgerald.
Alternate Delegate—E. J. Dorminy, Fitzgerald.

Elbert County Medical Society

The Elbert County Medical Society announces the following officers for 1936:

President—J. E. Johnson, Sr., Elberton.
Vice-President—W. A. Johnson, Elberton.
Secretary—A. S. Johnson, Elberton.
Delegate—D. N. Thompson, Elberton.
Alternate Delegate—A. C. Smith, Elberton.

Laurens County Medical Society

The Laurens County Medical Society announces the following officers for 1936:
President—O. H. Cheek, Dublin.
Vice-President—A. T. Coleman, Dublin.
Secretary-Treasurer—R. G. Ferrell, Jr., Dublin.
Delegate—C. A. Hodges, Dublin.

Rockdale County Medical Society

The Rockdale County Medical Society announces the following officers for 1936:
President—P. J. Brown, Conyers.
Vice-President—P. S. Smith, Conyers.
Secretary-Treasurer—H. E. Griggs, Conyers.
Delegate—S. A. Ware, Conyers.

Toombs County Medical Society

The Toombs County Medical Society announces the following officers for 1936:
President—J. E. Mercer, Vidalia.
Vice-President—H. D. Youmans, Lyons.
Secretary-Treasurer—W. W. Odom, Lyons.
Delegate—H. D. Youmans, Lyons.

Polk County Medical Society

The Polk County Medical Society announces the following officers for 1936:
President—S. L. Whitley, Cedartown.
Vice-President—Chas. V. Wood, Cedartown.
Secretary-Treasurer—John M. McGehee, Cedartown.
Deelgate—J. W. Good, Cedartown.
Alternate Delegate—Chas. V. Wood, Cedartown.

Dooly County Medical Society

The Dooly County Medical Society announces the following officers for 1936:
President—H. A. Mobley, Vienna.
Secretary-Treasurer—M. L. Malloy, Vienna.
Delegate—E. B. Davis, Byromville.

Terrell County Medical Society

The Terrell County Medical Society announces the following officers for 1936:
President—Guy Chappell, Dawson.
Vice-President—J. H. Lewis, Dawson.
Secretary-Treasurer—Steve P. Kenyon, Dawson.
Delegate—Steve P. Kenyon, Dawson.
Alternate Delegate—J. T. Arnold, Parrott.

Houston-Peach Counties Medical Society

The Houston-Peach Counties Medical Society announce the following officers for 1936:
President—J. W. Story, Perry.
Vice-President—H. E. Evans, Perry.

Secretary-Treasurer—R. L. Cater, Perry.
Delegate—J. W. Story, Perry.

Turner County Medical Society

The Turner County Medical Society announces following officers for 1936:
President—H. M. Belflower, Sycamore.
Vice-President—W. L. Story, Ashburn.
Secretary-Treasurer—J. H. Baxter, Ashburn.

Morgan County Medical Society

The Morgan County Medical Society announces following officers for 1936:
President—W. M. Fambrough, Bostwick.
Vice-President—D. M. Carter, Madison.
Secretary-Treasurer—W. C. McGeary, Madison.
Delegate—J. L. Porter, Rutledge.

Meriwether County Medical Society

The Meriwether County Medical Society announ the following officers for 1936:
President—T. W. Jackson, Manchester.
Vice-President—V. H. Bennett, Gay.
Secretary-Treasurer—R. B. Gilbert, Greenville.
Delegate—R. B. Gilbert, Greenville.
Alternate Delegate—W. P. Allen, Woodbury.

Stephens County Medical Society

The Stephens County Medical Society announces following officers for 1936:
President—J. H. Terrell, Toccoa.
Vice-President—E. F. Chaffin, Toccoa.
Secretary-Treasurer—C. L. Ayers, Toccoa.
Delegate—W. B. Schaeffer, Toccoa.
Alternate Delegate—J. E. D. Isbell, Toccoa.

Coweta County Medical Society

The Coweta County Medical Society announces following officers for 1936:
President—W. H. Tanner, Newnan.
Vice-President—G. W. Hammond, Newnan.
Secretary-Treasurer—M. F. Cochran, Newnan.

Franklin County Medical Society

The Franklin County Medical Society announces following officers for 1936:
President—S. D. Brown, Royston.
Secretary-Treasurer—B. T. Smith, Carnesville.

Greene County Medical Society

The Greene County Medical Society announces following officers for 1936:
President—E. G. Adams, Greensboro.
Secretary-Treasurer—Goodwin Gheesling, Greeboro.

Blue Ridge Medical Society

The Blue Ridge Medical Society announces the lowing officers for 1936:
President—J. M. Daves, Blue Ridge.
Vice-President—E. L. Prince, Morganton.
Secretary-Treasurer—C. B. Crawford, Blue Ridge
Delegate—E. W. Watkins, Ellijay.

pers on the scientific program were: *Diagnosis and Classification of Menstrual Disorders*" by Dr. John C. Burch, Professor of Clinical Gynecology, Vanderbilt University School of Medicine, Nashville, Tenn.; *Carcinoma of the Breast*, Dr. Wm. Perrin Nicolson; *Partial Esophagectomy for Cancer—Presentation of Patient*, Dr. Murdock Equen; *Some Recent Developments in the Problem of Pellagra*, Dr. V. P. Sydenstricker, Augusta, Professor of Medicine, University of Georgia School of Medicine, Augusta. Adresses by Dr. James E. Paullin, Atlanta; Dr. B. H. Minchew, Waycross; and Dr. Edgar D. Shanks, Atlanta, President, President-Elect and Secretary-Treasurer of the Association, respectively.

The Louis A. Dugas Club of the University of Georgia School of Medicine, Augusta, met on March 16th. Dr. Carl G. Hartman of the Carnegie Institute of Embryology, spoke on *Physiology of Menstruation*. Dr. Hartman addressed the student body and faculty of the University on *Physiology of Ovulation* on the morning of the 16th.

Dr. C. L. Allgood, Scottdale, has been reappointed to the DeKalb County Board of Education.

Dr. and Mrs. E. J. Dorminy, Fitzgerald, entertained the members of the Ben Hill County Medical Society to a turkey dinner in their home recently.

Dr. B. T. Beasley, Atlanta, was elected Secretary-Treasurer of the Southeastern Surgical Congress at its annual meting in New Orleans on March 10th.

A statue of Dr. Crawford W. Long was unveiled at Danielsville on March 30th. Dr. L. G. Hardman, Commerce, Ex-Governor of Georgia, introduced Dr. Hugh H. Young of Baltimore, who delivered the unveiling address. Other physicians on the program were: Dr. Jas. E. Paullin, Atlanta, President of the Association; Dr. R. M. Goss, Athens; Dr. W. D. Gholston, Danielsville; Dr. Stewart D. Brown, Royston.

Dr. J. D. Applewhite, Macon, read a paper before the Macon Medical Society of Bibb County entitled *Endemic Fever* on March 17th.

Dr. W. F. Shallenberger, Atlanta, read a paper before a meeting of the Spalding County Medical Society at the Strickland and Son Memorial Hospital, Griffin, on March 17th.

Dr. and Mrs. M. A. Rountree, Reidsville, entertained the members of the Tattnall County Medical Society and Auxiliary in their home on March 11th.

The staff meeting of St. Joseph's Infirmary, Atlanta, was held on March 24th. Dr. Stephen T. Barnett, Jr., reported a case of *Cancer of the Fundus with Uterine Bleeding*; Dr. Wm. O. Martin, Jr., made a clinical talk on *Headache*.

By the will of Mrs. Frederick Pope, the University Hospital, Augusta, has been bequeathed an amount estimated at $265,000.00, though this amount will not be available during the life time of Mrs. Pope's principal legatee.

The Coffee County Medical Society met at Douglas on March 31st. Dr. L. H. Shellhouse, Willacoochee, read a paper entitled *Present Status of Research;* Dr. Sage Harper, Wray, *The Clinical Problem.* The discussion was led by Dr. J. G. Crovatt, Douglas.

The Thomas County Medical Society met at the John D. Archbold Memorial Hospital, Thomasville, March 18th. A symposium on cancer featured the scientific program. *Cancer—Lantern Slide Illustration* by Dr. C. H. Watt; *Early Signs and Symptoms of Cancer of the Cervix,* Dr. Arthur D. Little; *The Need for Early Diagnosis and Treatment of Malignancies,* Dr. Mary J. Erickson.

The Ninth District Medical Society met at Canton on March 18th. Title for papers on the scientific program were: *Diagnosis and Treatment of Early Tuberculosis,* Dr. C. C. Aven, Atlanta; *Surgical Treatment of Pulmonary Tuberculosis,* Dr. F. B. Murphy, Canton; address by Dr. B. H. Minchew, Waycross, President-Elect of the Association; *Puerperal Sepsis,* Dr. Grady N. Coker, Canton. Dinner was served. Doctors from Atlanta who attended the meeting were: Wm. Willis Anderson, C. C. Aven, J. L. Campbell, Edgar D. Shanks and Theodore Toepel.

The Seventh District Medical Society met at Trion on April 1st. Dr. D. B. Douglas, Trion, read a paper entitled *Genito-Urinary Tuberculosis;* Dr. L. B. Marriam, Fort Oglethorpe, and Dr. H. D. Brown, Summerville, led the discussion. Dr. Lester Harbin, Rome, *The Use of Well-Leg Countertraction in the Treatment of Fractures of the Upper End of Femur;* Dr. W. M. Gober, Marietta, and Dr. Lloyd Wood, Dalton, led the discussion. Dr. T. F. Little, Cedartown, *The Arguments for Conservation of the Ovaries;* Dr. J. W. Stanford, Cartersville, and Dr. G. M. White, Rockmart, led the discussion. Dr. C. B. Upshaw, Atlanta, *The Management of Breech Labor;* Dr. W. H. Perkinson, Marietta, and Dr. H. L. Sams, Dalton, led the discussion. Dr. W. H. Lewis, Rome, *Values in Medicine;* Dr. D. S. Middleton, Rising Fawn, and Dr. G. B. Smith, Rome, led the discussion. Dr. J. J. Rodgers, Trion, *Tracheo-Esophageal Fistula of the New-Born;* Dr. Fred Simonton, Chickamauga, and Dr. Inman Smith, Trion, led the discussion.

If interested in a new location to practice, write the Secretary-Treasurer.

The Eighth District Medical Society met at Waycross March 31st. The scientific program consisted of: *Address* by Dr. Jas. E. Paullin, Atlanta, President of the Association; *Osteomyelitis,* Dr. C. A. Witmer, Waycross; *Modern Methods of Tuberculosis Control,* Dr. M. F. Haygood, Atlanta; *Some Observations on Diseases of the Thymus,* Dr. B. G. Owens and Dr. A. M. Johnson, Valdosta; *Neurosurgical Consideration of*

Epilepsy, Dr. J. G. Lyerly, Jacksonville, Fla.; *The Microscopic Diagnosis of Amebiasis,* Dr. G. E. Atwood, Waycross; *The Well, Sick Woman,* Dr. J. B. Oliphant, Sparks. Dinner was served at the Phoenix Hotel.

On Tuesday, March 31st, Dr. A. P. Briggs, Assistant Professor of Internal Medicine, St. Louis University Medical College, addressed the members of the faculty and student body of the University of Georgia School of Medicine, Augusta, on the subject of renal function.

The Georgia Medical Society, Savannah, has held two important and outstanding meetings this year. At its regular meeting on February 25th, Dr. J. C. Patterson, Cuthbert, spoke to a throng of doctors on *Acid Ulcers with Especial Reference to Acute Perforations.* The different phases of his discussion were thoroughly correlated, interesting and of unusual scientific importance. Many members of the Society and Dr. Johnson of New York City, engaged in the discussion of the subject. At the Society's regular meeting on March 24th, Dr. Roy R. Kracke, Emory University, made an extemporaneous address to a packed hall on *Leukopenic Diseases.* Available space for standing was filled. Dr. Kracke's audience were profuse in their compliments on his talk and many expressed the opinion, that they had never heard a lecture in which the speaker exhibited more skill and talent in his discourse.

The First District Medical Society met at Statesboro on March 18th. Titles on the scientific program were: *Case Report* by Dr. S. E. Bray, Savannah; *Sinusitis in Children,* Dr. G. H. Faggart, Savannah; *Tumors of the Bladder,* Dr. H. Y. Righton, Savannah; *Do We Want Health Insurance?* Dr. Wm. H. Myers, Savannah; *The Autonomic Nervous System in Its Relation to Clinical Medicine,* Dr. Cleveland Thompson, Millen; *Bacterial Emergencies,* Dr. Lee Howard, Savannah.

Dr. Philip R. Stewart, Monroe, will have Dr. C. R. Gillespie, formerly of Monticello, associated with him in the practice of medicine at Monroe according to announcement published in the *Walton News.*

The Fulton County Medical Society met at the Academy of Medicine, Atlanta, April 2nd. Dr. N. B. Bateman reported a case of *Partial Intestinal Obstruction Producing Severe Headache.* Dr. C. C. Aven made a clinical talk, *Bronchiectasis—A Diagnostic Problem.* Dr. F. Kells Boland, Jr., read a paper. *Postoperative Evisceration Among the Colored Race.* The discussion was led by Dr. Dan C. Elkin, Dr. A. O. Linch and Dr. Stephen T. Barnett, Jr.

The Randolph County Medical Society met at the Patterson Hospital, Cuthbert, on April 2nd. Dr. T. F. Harper, Coleman, read a paper on *Acute Obstruction of the Bowel.*

Dr. Howard J. Morrison, Savannah, spoke on *Tuberculosis not Inherited* before a meeting of the Junior Auxiliary Board of the Chatham-Savannah Tubercu-

born and reared in Emanuel county and had practiced
in Emanuel and adjoining counties for more than forty
years. Dr. Sample took post-graduate work in New
York City and Baltimore a number of times after he
began the practice of his profession. He was an able
and outstanding physician. He was a member of the
Emanuel County Medical Society, First District Medical Society, Southern Medical Association, American
Medical Association and the Methodist church. Surviving him are three daughters: Mrs. G. C. Rountree, Summit; Mrs. E. F. Applegate, Savannah; Mrs. A. D.
Donehoo, Miami, Fla.; three sons, John and Horace
Sample, Summit; Wm. L. Sample, New York City.
Funeral services were conducted by Rev. L. E. Williams and George R. Martin from the Methodist church.
Members of the Emanuel County Medical Society and
the First District Medical Society formed an honorary
escort.

Dr. *Paul Plez Cooper*, Alma; University of Georgia
School of Medicine, Augusta, 1911; aged 47; died of
heart disease at his home on March 12, 1936. He had
practiced in Alma and vicinity for nine years, moved
there from Thomasville. Dr. Cooper enjoyed an excellent practice and was held in high esteem by many acquaintances. He was a member of the Masonic lodge
and Baptist church. Surviving him are his father, J.
D. Cooper, Thomasville; one brother, Hugh Cooper,
Thomasville; three sisters, Mrs. E. Whitehead, Savannah; Mrs. Jesse Carroll, Thomasville; Mrs. Della
Barnes, Miami, Fla.

Dr. *George W. Ragsdale*, Hiram; University of
Georgia School of Medicine, Augusta, 1902; aged 58;
died suddenly of heart disease at his home on March
25, 1936. He was a leading physician of Paulding
county and had practiced there for thirty-three years.
Dr. Ragsdale was a member of the Masonic lodge,
Shrine and Baptist church. Surviving him are his
widow, three daughters, Mrs. C. R. Hart, Temple;
Misses Lila and Reese Ragsdale, Hiram; one son, Kenneth Ragsdale, Hiram. Rev. E. C. Swetnam conducted
the funeral services from the Poplar Springs Baptist
church. Burial was in the churchyard. The members
of the Masonic lodge and physicians of that section
formed an honorary escort.

Dr. *Alexander Smith Cantrell*, Dahlonega; College
of American Medicine and Surgery, Atlanta, 1883;
aged 73; died at his home on December 26, 1935. He
was a prominent physician of Lumpkin county and
held in high esteem by hundreds of acquaintances.

Dr. *Nicholas Peterson*, Tifton; member; Louisville
Medical College, Louisville, Ky., 1890; aged 67; died
of pneumonia after an illness of short duration at a
private hospital in Tifton on March 13, 1936. He was
born and reared near Tifton and had practiced medicine there for more than forty years. Dr. Peterson
served for a number of years on the State Board of
Medical Examiners and for two terms represented Tift
county in the General Assembly of Georgia. He was
assistant local surgeon for the Southern Railway Com-

pany at Tifton and local surgeon for the A. B. & C. Railroad at the time of his death. Dr. Peterson made many friends by his charitable disposition and striking personality. He was a member of the Tift County Medical Society and the Methodist church. Surviving him are his widow, one son. Malcolm Peterson of Tifton. Funeral services were conducted from the Methodist church and interment was in the city cemetery.

Dr. T. Ellis Drewry, Griffin; member; Emory University School of Medicine, Emory University, 1887; aged 75; died at his home on March 18, 1936. He was born and reared near Jonesboro. After he received· his degree in medicine he moved to Griffin and had practiced there for almost a half century. For many years he had an extensive practice and was one of the foremost physicians in that section. Many people held Dr. Drewry in high esteem. He was a member of the Spalding County Medical Society, Fourth District Medical Society and the Baptist church. Surviving him are one daughter. Miss Anne Drewry, Griffin; one son, Dr. Harris Drewry, New York City. Dr. J. B. Turner and Rev. L. W. Blackwelder conducted the funeral services from the Baptist chnrch. Burial was in Oak Hill cemetery.

BOOK REVIEWS

The Doctor and the Public. A Study of the Sociology, Economics, Ethics and Philosophy of Medicine, Based on Medical History. By Peter Warbasse, M.D. Publishers: Paul ·B. Hoeber, Inc., New York City, Pages 573.

The first few chapters record the names of the outstanding pioneers of their time—Michael Servetus, the martyr; Leonarde De Vinci, handsome as an Adonis, artist, sculptor, architect, anatomist, physician, pioneer in aviation, inventor, author; Sanctorinius, pioneer in metabolism; Sydenham, the physicist; Gottfried Purmann (1649), pioneer in intestinal surgery, blood transfusions and ligations of aneurisms; Lavoissier, founder of biological chemistry, beheaded during the French revolution; Auenbrugger, who developed percussion; Dorothy Linde Dix, who did so much for the institutional care of the insane.

The book is charmingly written and makes historical subjects interesting reading; the sequence of history is accurate and the subject is covered up-to-date. Running through the book is a vein of delightful philosophy. The last chapter deals ably with the question of social medicine and makes the reader think.

The book is deserving of a place in every well rounded medical library.

A. J. MOONEY, M.D.

Clinical Laboratory Methods, W. E. Bray, M.D., Professor of Clinical Pathology, University of Virginia, pp. 324, publishers. C. V. Mosby Company, price $3.75.

. This volume is indeed a synopsis of clinical laboratory methods. The author has borrowed freely from text-books dealing with clinical pathology, but has shown rare judgment in his selection.· To cover· the literature and put into form for use the common laboratory tests and to add many of the uncommon tests, is something achieved by too few authors.

The illustrations are excellent and the type is easy to read.

Common Contagious Diseases by Phillip M. Stimson. Assistant Professor Clinical Pediatrics, Cornell University Medical College; Visiting Physician Willard Parker Hospital; Chief of Staff, The Floating Hospital of St. John's Guild. Price $4.00. Lea and Febiger, Philadelphia.

The author has given undergraduates, nurses, internes, general practitioners, public health officers, and officials, and specialists a very excellent manual on contagious diseases. This book is an enlargement on lectures to the students at Cornell University Medical School on common contagious diseases and the author has drawn vividly and carefully from his wide store of knowledge on these diseases as studied at Willard Parker Contagious Hospital.

The presentation of this work is clear and very concise in style. In treating each disease separately the author takes up in detail, etiology, pathology, immunity, clinical manifestations, complications, differential diagnosis, mortality and prognosis, isolation and quarantine, prophylaxis and treatment.

The first chapter of the book deals with principles of contagion, including differentiation of the different types of immunity and the nature of infection. The second chapter is very good indeed and takes up in detail serum reactions.

Chapters three through fourteen deal with the specific contagious diseases and these are most complete. The last chapter takes up the general management of contagious diseases with special stress on the management of these diseases in schools and in the home.

This book would serve as a very valuable book in the library of all medical men and women.

DON F. CATHCART, M.D.

Diseases of the Thyroid Gland. Edited by Arthur E. Hertzler, M.D., Chief Surgeon, Halstead Hospital; Professor of Surgery, University of Kansas. Price $7.50, pp, 340 with 181 illustrations. St. Louis: The C. V. Mosby Company, 1935.

Characteristically readable, this revised edition again presents the author's views and experiences and is in no way a rehash of other works. He has purposely omitted detailed pathology, though each condition is adequately portrayed by good descriptions. He stressed the necessity of early and more complete operations .in order to prevent what he feels is the "normal termination" of thyroid disease, namely, a cardiac death. He feels that the "basal metabolism has been considerably over-rated and is never safe to use as a deciding factor in determining a patient's operation."

Following a chapter of "general considerations," there is a classification and study of etiology and morphology, followed by a consideration of each type of goiter. The whole work is climaxed by a wonderfully clear and generously illustrated description of the operative procedures.

NEW YORK POLYCLINIC MEDICAL
SCHOOL AND HOSPITAL

At a meeting of the Clinical Society of the New York Polyclinic Medical School and Hospital, New York City, held on February 3rd, the following program was presented:

1. "Some improved methods in plastic reparative surgery—illustrated by cinematograph film in natural color" by J. Eastman Sheehan, M.D. The discussion was opened by Clarence R. Straatsma, M.D. and Arthur J. Barsky, M.D.

2. "Diagnosis and treatment of carcinoma of the colon and rectum" by Richard B. Cattell, M.D., of Lahey Clinic, Boston, Moss. The discussion was opened be Jerome M. Lynch, M.D., and Frank C. Yeomans, M.D.

At the March meeting of the Clinical Society of the New York Polyclinic Medical School and Hospital there were two notable contributions:

1. "The present status of endocrine therapy in gynecology" by Archibald D. Campbell, M.D., of Montreal, Canada. The discussion was opened by Raphael Kurzrok, M.D., Aaron S. Blumbarten, M.D., and Irving Pardee, M.D.

2. "The genesis and surgical treatment of hypertension" by George W. Crile, M.D., of Cleveland Ohio. The discussion was opened by Harlow Brooks, M.D., and J. Murray Steele, M.D.

Dr. Roger Anderson, of Seattle, Washington, gave a special afternoon lecture on March 20th on: 1. "An anatomical or non-operative method of treating fractures of both bones of the forearm." 2. "Ambulatory method of treating fractures of the femur.

SOLUTION LIVER EXTRACT
CONCENTRATED

The constant aim of the Lilly Research Laboratories is not alone to develop new therapeutic products, but to improve methods used in the preparation of medicinal agents already available.

A recent advance of the latter type has been brought about and includes improved methods of conserving the original store of antianemic substances in liver during the process of their extraction. This allows for reduction in the cost of the materials required for adequate parenteral treatment of pernicious anemia. These economies are based on the fact that the new methods allow preparation of effective solutions from surprisingly small amounts of whole liver. That there can be no doubt as to the effectiveness of solutions prepared in this manner has been shown by the clinical testing of the new solution in cases of pernicious anemia.

Solution Liver Extract Concentrated, Lilly, prepared by the new method, when administered parenterally in a 3cc. dose, produces an effect comparable to the ingestion of 1400 to 2100 Gm. of fresh liver. Its cost to the physician is but a fraction of that of the solutions of liver extract hitherto available. This solution produces full therapeutic response (maximal) when injected intramuscularly once a week in a 3 cc. dose; this is the maintenance dose suitable for use in the usual or average case of pernicious anemia after remission has been established. For patients in relapse at the time treatment is instituted, more frequent injections are desirable or may be required until the blood count has been brought to normal.

SUMMER DIARRHEA IN BABIES

Casec (calcium caseinate), which is almost wholly a combination of protein and calcium, offers a quickly effective method of treating all types of diarrhea, both in bottle-fed and breast-fed infants. For the former, the carbohydrate is temporarily omitted from the 24-hour formula and replaced with 8 level tablespoonfuls of Casec. Within a day or two the diarrhea will usually be arrested, and carbohydrate in the form of Dextri-Maltose may safely be added to the formula and the Casec gradually eliminated. Three to six teaspoonfuls of a thin paste of Casec and water, given before each nursing, is well indicated for loose stools in breast-fed babies. Please send· for samples to Mead, Johnson & Company, Evansville, Indiana.

The Twelfth Scientific Session of the American Heart Association will be held on Tuesday, May 12, 1936, from 9:30 to 5:30 P.M., at Hotel Phillips, Kansas City, Missouri. The program will be devoted to Cardiac Insufficiency.

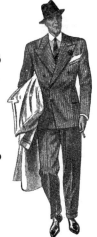

THE DOCTOR
EATS AN APPLE...

Sometimes, to a doctor, home must seem like nothing more than a place from which he is constantly being called away at inconvenient hours. But after all, doctors do have homes and, even as you and I, they have home problems. They, too, or at least some of them, have to tighten the legs on the ironing board, put a piece of paper in the window to stop its rattling, clean their feet before they come into the house, help with their son's arithmetic lessons—and do all the other thousand and sixteen things that an agile-minded female always can find for her husband to do.

●

We happen to know one doctor personally whose persistent (a mild word) wife finally drove him to doing something about his habit of reading under poor light. Eventually he surrendered to the point of calling one of this Company's Home Lighting Advisors and what she did was a caution! Why, at practically no expense, she revised the lighting arrangements in his study to the point where he no longer can find a single place to sit without having adequate, shaded, glareless light fall across his book. And *does* he like it!

●

She told him, too, that while proper lighting will not cure defective eyesight or any other ailment, it most certainly reduces the danger of eye-strain, with its threat of nervous and physical fatigue and the more serious illness which may follow.

●

Now, that same doctor takes advantages of us in a manner we relish very much. He suggests to various and sundry of his patients that some of their ills might be relieved by using the same prescription his wife had forced on him. Our Home Lighting service is available, without charge, to any customer of this Company. Eighty skilled, experienced young ladies, properly equipped, are at your service. If they can help you or any of your patients, we will be very pleased.

GEORGIA POWER CO.
Home Lighting Division

THE JOURNAL
OF THE
MEDICAL ASSOCIATION OF GEORGIA
DEVOTED TO THE WELFARE OF THE MEDICAL ASSOCIATION OF GEORGIA
PUBLISHED MONTHLY under direction of the Council

| Volume XXV | Atlanta, Ga., May, 1936 | Number 5 |

LEARNING BETTER HOW TO LIVE*

JAMES E. PAULLIN, M.D.
Atlanta

It is difficult to find words which will adequately express my thanks and deep appreciation for the honor conferred upon me two years ago when I was made President-Elect of this Association. To occupy this office is to accept the highest honor the members of the Medical Association of Georgia can bestow. For all of this I am deeply grateful and profoundly appreciative. It is to be hoped that the efforts which have been made for the upbuilding of the profession have not betrayed the confidence reposed in me as your chosen representative.

For some reason, best known to the Association, it has been the custom for the President each year to deliver an address, the nature of which is not specified, but by implication, he is supposed to give an account of his stewardship as well as to discuss policies or measures which will be useful in the further advancement of the profession, and of those ideals of medical practice which this Association sponsors. During my term of office it has been my pleasure to be closely and intimately associated with many members of the Association as well as to attend many county and all district medical society meetings. From this contact and intimate relationship I am led to believe that organized medicine, as never before, has its feet planted more firmly on solid ground, and that it cannot either be persuaded or forced to depart from the accepted methods of medical practice which have been our heritage for the past hundreds of years.

*President's Address, read before the Medical Association of Georgia, Savannah, April 23, 1936.

In these rapidly changing times there is so much uncertainty, dissatisfaction, and unrest relating not only to social, religious, and financial problems, it is quite natural that the medical profession and its related branches should also be included among the various organizations needing to be changed; this, despite the fact that today, with our present system of medical care, the people of the United States of America are the recipients of the best medical service of any nation on the globe. This statement is easily verified when one studies the morbidity and mortality statistics of this country in comparison with those of the other countries of the world. The contributions of organized medicine in the United States for the cure of disease and the prevention of sickness are unequaled. Despite these facts, however, efforts are being made by self-appointed reformers to discard what they describe as old, wornout, antiquated methods of rendering medical care to the sick and preventing disease, and to urge in their stead the adoption of newer methods promulgated in sociological laboratories by hired individuals who have no intimate or practical first hand knowledge of the complex problems involved in rendering medical service to the people of a community or state. We are asked and expected to discard those things, which time and experience have shown to be of most value, for other methods which are supposed to be more efficient and more modern, methods which are more easily subjected to either arithmetical, geometrical or political control. The danger from such a course lies in the fact that some few may be enticed, on the spur of the moment, into accepting many of these theoretical considerations; however, if "the considerations" are subjected to thoughtful analysis and sound reasoning, it is soon found that such schemes are filled with glaring imperfections.

Every intelligent physician today willingly and gladly admits that the practice of medicine and the type of medical service which is generally rendered can be improved. We freely admit that the methods now used in rendering medical care can be made more efficient, and we are equally as certain that better facilities can be established for the medical care of the people. We are also cognizant of the fact that in some communities of this State the availability of physicians can be greatly improved. We would also like to point out that from year to year these conditions are improving, as can be seen when one observes the constantly decreasing mortality and morbidity statistics furnished to the people by the State Board of Health. These changes are being brought about surely and gradually by physicians who are the only persons qualified to do this work. The Medical Association of Georgia has been active in attempting to remedy many of these defects for the past eighty-seven years and it will continue to do so as long as time lasts, with increasing benefit to the public and inward satisfaction to the doctors as long as they are left free and unregimented in their endeavors. No one man alone can accomplish a great deal but working together as a unified body, we can do a tremendous amount. There are many difficulties besides those above mentioned which prevent progress in the rendition of adequate medical care. If it were possible to immediately banish ignorance, fear, superstition, doubt and general contrariness among the citizenry of this State, which is manifest in all stratas of society, the problem would become very much easier and simpler to handle.

May I quote to you Article II of The Constitution of this Association which so clearly defines the objects of organized medicine: "The purpose of this Association shall be to federate and bring into one compact organization the entire medical profession of the State of Georgia; to extend medical knowledge and advance medical science; to elevate the standard of medical education and to secure the enactment and enforcement of just medical laws; to guard and foster the material interests of its members and to protect them from imposition; and to enlighten and direct public opinion in regard to the great problems of state and medicine, so that the profession shall become more capable and honorable within itself, and more useful to the public in the prevention and cure of disease and in prolonging and adding comfort to life." For these things every member of this Association stands. In view of this fact, why is it then that well organized and heavily endowed agencies are coming forward with plans and prescriptions which attempt to tear down and destroy all of the things which we have learned by custom and tradition to respect, honor and revere? May it not be worth while for us to consider calmly, placidly, without animosity, and without hate, some of the basic factors responsible for this upheaval?

The present trend of endeavor, whether in industry, the sciences, or what not, is for efficiency. Machines are made to replace human brawn and human brain because they can be made mechanically more efficient. In the sphere of human relationship as well as in the manufacturing plant an attempt is being made to fit everything into a certain mathematical formula. X plus Y must equal Z at all times and on all occasions. If it does not, then the machine, whether made of iron or of human material, must be made to fit this formula. From the mathematical standpoint Z is the desideratum which represents the peak of efficiency. The trouble arises when the human being (man), with all of his different physical, mental, emotional and behavior characteristics is made to fit this formula. He is treated as a machine—the fact is lost sight of that he is human and individual and quite unlike every other individual on earth. It is not realized that he cannot be made to follow at all times a definite formula. Certain changes or adaptations of the formula must be made to suit his individual needs. It is only in this way that it is possible to keep him functioning to the best of his capacity. Failure to appreciate this fact will eventually cause the development of many mental and physical signs of ill health. It therefore behooves us as physicians, by precept and example, to become active participants in a well-rounded program which will demonstrate to our pa-

withstand, without severe damage to body and mind, the constant illogical and strenuous demands of the present day methods of living.

Among the many duties and obligations of the members of this honorable body one cannot find anything greater than that which will guide the rank and file of educated and ignorant people back into a safer method of living and a happier existence than that which is now offered. To do this it requires that the physician must let his good qualities as a capable advisor be known. Unless they are known, very little can be accomplished. A light hidden under a bushel will neither be seen, attract attention or serve any useful purpose. To learn better how to live we must become better students of the humanities, less selfish, and more a part of the world in which we live, move and have our being. There must be the development of a greater interest, not only in the medical but the social, religious and recreational welfare of our fellow men. We must appreciate our responsibility as citizens as well as physicians in seeing that methods for the public good are supported. The people must be protected from the faddist, not only the medical faddist but that other group of ill advised faddists who extract hard earned dollars from the ignorant and unsuspecting by promising unreasonable, impossible and unattainable cures. By precept and example we must demonstrate that work is an excellent tonic for the mind and wholesome for the body; that the responsibility for doing the day's work well is purely individual. Recreation sensibly utilized, relaxation wholesomely employed, and freedom from the stress and strain of life are attainments individually to be acquired, but are necessary for useful and happy living.

What is your State Medical Association doing to help accomplish these things? During the past year in co-operation with the State Board of Health and the United States Public Health Service, an economic and medical survey has been made of sixteen widely scattered counties of this State. Factual data from this study are not as yet at hand which can be utilized for the basis of constructing a definite program of action. However, after this study has been completed, the Medical Association of Georgia will have before it valuable information in which the needs of the people of this State can be definitely determined and appropriate remedies suggested. In other words, a beginning has been made towards the determination of the economic and medical needs of a cross-section of this State and we are prepared as soon as the needs and necessities are known to suggest remedies and begin work. We are certain that when these problems are known they will receive adequate attention from the members of this Association and we believe that in co-operation with the State Board of Health the medical profession will assume responsibility for the suggestions and the promulgation of a program which will result in better health, less disease, and a happier life for those under our care. This can be done and will be done by organized medicine acting with the help and co-operation of other groups of individuals who are interested in the same problems. With this we not only will teach people better how to live in peace, happiness and contentment but there also should be added a greater enjoyment of living in harmony with their fellow men.

EMORY MEDICAL ALUMNI CLINIC WEEK

The fifteenth annual Emory Medical Alumni Clinic Week will be held June 2nd to 5th, inclusive.

The clinics will begin on Tuesday, the 2nd, at 8:00 A.M. with registration at Grady Hospital on Butler Street, Atlanta, and will continue from 8:00 A.M. to 4:00 P.M. daily through Friday.

As is customary, the week will be concluded with the annual Medical Alumni banquet and Alumni Address on Friday evening.

Saturday is Alumni Day. This Centennial Year Homecoming will bring a greater number of alumni to the campus than ever before. Plan to attend and take part in the celebration. This is your best opportunity to get an intimate view of the Emory of today.

Every effort is being put forth to make the Clinic Week of real value to you. The week gives an opportunity for four days of intensive post-graduate study, class reunions, renewing old acquaintances, and the making of many new friends, both in and out of our profession.

A program will be mailed later. Get busy and write your classmates to meet you in Atlanta.

MARION C. PRUITT, M.D., *Secretary.*
Atlanta, May 9, 1936.

Dr. John M. Wheeler, Professor of Ophthalmology, Columbia University, was presented with the Leslie Dana Gold Medal for achievements in the prevention of blindness on May 10th.

total of 85 sacral anaesthesias. In 10 cases,
with a total of 13 injections, the nerve block
was used solely for operative delivery or as
expectant treatment in dystocia, preliminary
to operative intervention. In the remaining
55 cases, with a total of 72 nerve blocks, the
anaesthetic was employed as a routine method
for alleviation of pain in labors that were expected to prove normal.

Toxicity

The safety of sacral anaesthesia has been
so thoroughly demonstrated by its widespread use in other fields, that there is no need
to cite statistics. This, however, does not
mean that toxic effect cannot be observed,
or indeed that fatalities cannot result. Procaine is relatively non-toxic, but alarming
symptoms and even tragedies have resulted
from mistakes in dilution, deteriorated solutions, inadvertent injection into the blood
stream or into the dural sac. Labat[18], has
pointed out that toxicity increases with concentration, but in considerably greater than
direct proportion. In other words, if an individual can well tolerate 400 c.c. of 0.5 per
cent solution, it by no means follows that
he can tolerate 200 c.c. of 1 per cent solution, or 100 c.c. of 2 per cent solution, an
amount which is dangerous.

One should bear in mind when injecting
local or regional anaesthesia, that a safe dosage is not necessarily the average dose, but the
actual amount well tolerated by the individual receiving it. Hence, in using dilutions
of 1 per cent or stronger, one should inject
slowly while observing reactions. Toxic
symptoms due to novocaine in the order of
their occurrence are as follows: 1—Rapid
pulse; 2—Palpitation; 3—Increased respiratory rate; 4—Pallor; 5—Labored breathing;
6—Nausea; 7—Vomiting; 8—Dystal cyanosis; 9—Cold sweats; 10—Haze in front
of the eyes.

The first four symptoms may be due to
adrenalin as well[18].

Of the 85 injections herein reported
only five had obvious symptoms of reaction.
Three complained of moderate palpitation,
one became unduly talkative for 10 minutes,
and one case had palpitation and became so
talkative as to be called drunk. In 18 others
there was a rise of 12-16 in the pulse rate.

Practically everyone using caudal anaesthesia reports these slight reactions in from 25 to 30 per cent of cases, but further symptoms are rare indeed[*][*][*][*]. It is the rule that these manifestations last three to five minutes, and call for no treatment[*]. Observation of the blood pressure at five minute intervals was done in ten consecutive cases, but showed no fluctuation and was discontinued. If due precautions be observed, danger to the parturient, as to serious toxicity is negligible; as to slight transient reactions, more likely than with infiltration anaesthesia, but of no more import. The possibility of remote sequelae, such as neuritis, may be dismissed if no break in asepsis occur nor old, unstable, irritating solutions be used.

As to safety of the foetus, there are no established grounds in theory or practice, for attributing any effect to regional block. Kelso had several instances of impaired children, but could not exclude morphine and rectal ether as causative factors[*]. All other reports unanimously find no embarrassment of the foetus. Of my cases, with 61 viable infants, one had sluggish respirations and was cyanosed for four minutes, responding well to alpha lobelin. This case had shown meconium in amniotic fluid four hours previously, but no other symptoms of distress, and was not interferred with. The remaining 60 infants had immediate spontaneous respirations, sometimes crying before being completely expelled.

Technique

It is unnecessary to go into detail concerning the technique of injecting the sacral canal. Those unfamiliar with this step can find it most adequately covered in Labat's book on Local Anaesthesia[*], and in the chapter written by Farr in Lewis' Surgery[*]. As regards various bony anomalies, Meeker and Scholl have reported at length a study of 100 sacra[*]. There are, however, some points peculiar to the pregnant woman and to the use for which the anaesthesia is intended. It is difficult, even after considerable practice, to enter the sacral canal with the patient lying on her side, particularly with the stout flabby overlying tissues, often edematous, sagging as much as an inch or more and distorting the surface anatomy. This is an obstacle that can be overcome only by individual experience. Certainly obesity and marked edema are factors of technical interference.

It seems practical to make a distinction between high and low sacral infiltration. The average sacral canal in an adult has a capacity in the neighborhood of 15 c.c. or slightly more. It has been proved in the cadaver that solutions of from 90 to 120 c.c. deposited in the sacral canal under pressure, will travel not only laterally, but invariably will extend sub-durally up the vertebral column, sometimes as high as the cervical area[*]. Even when the quantity injected is only 20 c.c., the use of a long needle, placed high, and with rapid injection, will give sub-dural extension to the lower thoracic area and show little effect upon the lowermost sacral nerves[*]. Whether extension be obtained by quantity of solution or by a high deposit of the agent, the effect produced may be termed "high sacral epidural anaesthesia." By "low sacral" we mean the introduction of the needle sufficiently far beyond the sacro-coccygeal membrane as to be certainly in the canal, then withdrawing it almost to the point of puncture of the membrane and injecting 15 c.c. or more into the lowermost portion of the canal. If the "low sacral" injection be used, epidural extension upward may be obtained and accurately controlled in proportion to the amount of solution injected. By "low injection" I have obtained satisfactory pelvic floor anaesthesia with as little as 10 c.c. of 3 per cent procaine. However, a minimum of 15 c.c. is usually required and results are best, in my experience, with 20 to 26 c.c. It is my habit to inject slowly 18 to 20 c.c. and if a slight rise of 10 or 15 occurs in the pulse rate, to wait about five minutes, with the needle in position, before supplementing this amount. It should be emphasized that aspiration be done to exclude the possibility of being within a vein, or an anomalous dural sac.

Solutions

The sheaths covering the nerves within the sacral canal are, perhaps, the least permeable of any nerve sheaths in the body. It is therefore not surprising that the use of one-half to 1 per cent novocaine, should give inconsistent results in caudal anaesthesia.

Prior to this series, I have tried 1 per cent procaine in the sacral canal in obstetrical and gynecological cases. The results were disappointing. In the cases here reported, we have used 25 to 30 c.c. of 2 per cent and 18 to 30 c.c. of 3 per cent solution, the stronger more frequently. The 2 per cent solution acts 60 to 90 minutes, and the 3 per cent solution gives a block lasting nearly two hours. The addition of 3-4 drops of 1-1000 adrenalin, seems to prolong the anaesthesia by perhaps 15 minutes, but also appears to be more associated with the slight reactionary symptoms than the procaine itself. In the hospital we use standard, freshly prepared solutions of procaine without adrenalin. In the home I prefer to make my own solution fresh, from sterile saline and sterile neocaine in individual packages.

Oldham, Meeker and others have not found that the addition of sodium bicarbonate produces any prolongation of anaesthesia[4][5]. Various strengths of quinine urea hydrochloride have been added to secure prolongation. Oldham, in over 500 cases gets anaesthesia in excess of six hours, using 30 c.c. of 2 per cent procaine, to which is added 6 c.c. of 3 per cent quinine urea[4]. However, it is not generally conceded that there is any quinine derivative which, concentrated enough for prolonged anaesthesia, does not cause tissue damage. Nupercaine, in 1-1000 solution, is supposed to give from five to six hours anaesthesia, but so far as I know has not been used in labor[1].

Analgesic Efficiency

For 10 minutes after an injection is completed, the patient notices a gradual lessening in the intensity of her suffering. After this time has elapsed, all painful sensations cease for the duration of the anaesthetic. A few patients perceive a cramping sensation over the fundus, coincident with contractions, but they describe it as a drawing or pulling, and not painful. The terrific tearing pain in the back is entirely abolished, as is the sensation of distention and pressure in vagina and rectum. The majority of patients have to be told when they are having a contraction. The urge to bear down is gone, and this must be combatted by instructing the patient to use her voluntary efforts. Some feel the head slip painlessly over the perineum; others express doubt when told that this has occurred. Unless she has been previously given large sedative doses, the patient is fully awake and oriented, and can cooperate with the accoucheur. Where labor has suddenly become active with stormy pains, before the sacral is given, the patient may receive gas-oxygen with the pains until the injection can be made and the block take effect.

If delivery does not seem imminent after about an hour, preparations are made to repeat the block, and this is done when sensation begins to return. I have given three blocks in seven instances and two injections in thirteen. Just what limit should apply to the number of repetitions is a matter of conjecture.

In our 55 cases of routine labor, the only drug used in addition to the local, was sodium amytal. The barbiturate was usually given just before the sacral, 15 to 30 minutes. In such cases, three grains was given. In a few instances, a previous dose of six grains was given, the medication just before the injection being omitted. Morphine, scopolamine, and magnesium sulphate were not used. This was done, not because of any particular preference or prejudice, but for the sake of consistency, and because a small dose of barbiturate is indicated before the injection of procaine.

Where analgesia is desired for the stage of descent and expulsion only, it should be given about the end of the first stage in primiparae. This is entirely too late for multiparae, in which labors, the second stage must be anticipated by 30 minutes to one hour. If only one block is to be used, the matter of timing is necessarily difficult. If supplementary injections are to be made, timing will afford less concern. In 39 consecutive private cases, 20 primiparae and 19 multiparae, an effort was made to supply analgesia from the time the patient began to complain of the pains. If the labor was apparently well progressed, sacral anaesthesia was induced at this time. Otherwise a moderate dose of barbiturate was given and the injection made later if no relief obtained, or the case advanced. In no case was it necessary to give more than a third block, and in all, the analgesia was sufficiently prolonged for delivery and repair.

Effect Upon Labor

The effect of sacral anaesthesia on the mechanism of labor depends upon just how high an epidural extension is secured. With the smaller quantities where presumably sacral nerves, 2-3-4 and 5 are affected, insensibility and paralytic relaxation of the lower uterine segment, cervix, vagina, perineum and anus, is noted in 10 minutes. Rarely is any lessening in frequency and intensity of the uterine contractions observed. When from 25 to 30 c.c. of solution is injected, there is usually a partial inertia of the uterus, occurring in about 10 minutes and lasting from 10 to 20 minutes'². At the end of this time, contractions are resumed with the same frequency and intensity as before. In 39 consecutive private patients followed personally throughout the labor, appreciable inertia occurred in 20; the longest period was 20 minutes. The smallest amount used in any of these 20 cases was, 24 c.c. in one case; four other cases had about 26 c.c., and the rest 30 c.c. Of the 19 cases who exhibited no inertia, only one had as much as 30 c.c.; one had 28 c.c.; three had 25 c.c., and the remainder less. This is of no great significance, however, since such a short delay is of no consequence.

That the paralyzing effect upon the cervix hastens dilatation and retraction, there can be no doubt. I have frequently given a block with a dilatation of 4 cm. and made a rectal 10 or 15 minutes later, to find the cervix out of the way. When stripping and rupturing the membranes after a sacral, the almost complete lack of resistence on the part of the cervix is striking. In the second stage, anterior rotation often is hastened. I have observed too frequently for it to be a coincidence, that with a posterior occiput and nearly dilated cervix, an examination made as soon as the anaesthesia has taken complete effect shows that within the 15 or 20 minutes since the last examination, the cervix has dilated and the head rotated.

The pain from pressure of the head on the vagina and pelvic floor, is abolished, and with it the impulse to bear down. The patient, feeling no pain or local distention, is apt to lie there and allow the analgesia to wear off without using her voluntary expulsive powers, and must therefore be appraised when she is having a contraction and urged to bear down. By the same effect, precipitate delivery is practically precluded. With little effort, the head will usually descend readily to the perineum, where, in primiparae, it may be delayed as compared to cases receiving no anaesthesia. The incidence of outlet forceps is doubtless increased, as is the case with any method of analgesia carried to the extent of satisfactory relief. In 28 primiparae, 22 delivered spontaneously, five had outlet forceps for perineal delay, and one had rotation and mid-forceps for transverse arrest. An incidence of 21.4 per cent operative delivery. This figure is lower than average for first labor under analgesia by other methods'⁴. If the patient's intelligent co-operation be secured, I am confident that intervention because of expulsive failure, can be further reduced. Of 27 multiparae, none had perineal delay.

In comparison with cases receiving various general anaesthetics or rectal ether, there seems to be a distinctly shorter third stage where regional anaesthesia is employed. Any effect of sacral anaesthesia upon the amount of bleeding has not been apparent to me. In none of our cases did we have post-partum hemorrhage or relaxation bleeding. According to reports bleeding is minimized'¹³.

The incidence and extent of injury to the perineum and vaginal sulci is considerably less under caudal than with other methods of anaesthesia, except spinal. Theoretically, cervical injuries should be lessened. The complete relaxation of the birth canal is of great value for operative obstetrics.

I have used sacral anaesthsia in eight instances of dystocia, most of which were advanced. Six were toxic, four were exhausted, and in two, the foetus had died. In all of these, the patient was as free from pain as with a general surgical anaesthetic, yet the time element, so long as completed within an hour and a half, could be entirely disregarded, and no additional shock was apparent. Except for episiotomies, and one instance where the cervix was incised, there were no injuries to the soft parts. In two instances, with non-viable foetus, surgical induction and rapid accouchement was done because of advanced renal insufficiency.

Summary and Conclusions

The pains of labor may be entirely allayed by a block of the sacral and ano-coccygeal nerves. Low sacral injection with 2 or 3 per cent procaine is probably the most practical method for such a block. The following advantages are suggested:

1—It is quite safe to mother and child, being purely a peripheral nerve block, and having none of the risks inherent to general or spinal anesthesia.

2—Including technical failures, it is dependable for a high degree of efficiency. One block is effective for one and one-half hours or longer, and may be safely and easily repeated.

3—Most operations and manipulations from below may be painlessly performed under regional anaesthesia and the relaxation of the soft parts is of greater aid to the operator than with general anaesthesia.

4—The abdominal muscles and diaphragm are unaffected; the patient is conscious and able to cooperate with expulsive efforts. Precipitate labor is prevented.

5—The higher innervation of the uterus is but little interfered with. The involuntary powers act efficiently and the first stage is apparently shortened.

6—The method is readily available, as much for the home as in a hospital. There is no elaborate or cumbersome equipment, and the material is inexpensive. No trained assistant is required.

There are the following disadvantages:

1—A prejudice may be encountered, due to the fact that the procaine is administered by puncture in the back, and can be confused with spinal anesthesia. This is due to ignorance, and with the intelligent is usually dispelled by simple explanation.

2—In primiparae, the bearing down reflex being absent, perineal delay may occur. The incidence of outlet forceps is increased thereby. However, this is no greater than the average incidence of prophylactic forceps with other analgesias, if as great. If morale

and cooperation be well cultivated, this factor is subject to lessening.

3—The necessary technical skill and likewise knowledge as to timing of the induction, must be developed. This may be acquired at no risk to patients, and more readily than the skill required to administer general anaesthesia safely.

4—The short duration of a single block is a real objection. The quinine derivatives may be the answer, but the possibility of local slough must be eliminated before these products can be advocated without reservation.

5—Obesity or edema may render the method technically inapplicable. Local skin lesions are, of course, a contra-indication.

Sacral anaesthesia has a wider field of application in obstetrics than is generally recognized. It is safe, effective, available, and has a minimum of by-effect on the progress of labor. If a means be devised to prolong the action of a single injection to six hours, with no increase in toxicity, it may become the anaesthetic of choice for normal as well as operative delivery. With this, as with all anaesthetics, results as to both safety and efficiency, are dependent, rather upon the skill with which it is used than upon any virtue inherent to the anaesthetic agent or the method.

BIBLIOGRAPHY

1. Jour. A. M. A., 101: 1019, (Sept. 21) 1933.
2. P. Duhall; Gynec. et Obstet., 26: 260-368, (Sept.) 1932.
3. W. Haupt and R. Krause; Zentralbl. f. Gynak., 57: 129-134, (Jan. 21) 1933.
4. J. R. Henry and L. Jaur; Gynec. et Obstet., 19, (Jan.) 1929.
5. S. P. Oldham; Ky. M. Jour., (July) 1922; page 321-324.
6. S. P. Oldham; Anaesth. & Analg., 6: 192-196, (Aug.) 1927.
7. B. E. Bonar and W. R. Meeker; J. A. M. A., 81: 1079-1083, (Sept. 29) 1923.
8. M. P. Rucker; Anaesth. & Analgesia, 9: 67-70, (Mar.-Apr.) 1930.
9. W. Pickles and S. Jones; New Eng. J. Med., 199: 988-994, Nov. 15, 1928.
10. W. Pickles; R. I. Med. J., 8: 193-197, Dec. 1925.
11. C. H. Knauer; Anaesth. & Analges., 8: 243-249, (July-Aug.) 1929.
12. J. W. Kelso; Am. J. Obs. & Gyn., 18: 416-419, (Sept.) 1929.
13. B. Tucker and H. Benaron; Am. J. Obs. & Gyn., 27: 850-863, (June) 1934.
14. R. D. Mussey; (Editorial) S. G. & O., 59: 112-115, (July) 1934.
15. G. Labat; "Regional Anaesthesia"; W. B. Saunders Co.
16. R. E. Farr; Chapter 4, Vol. 1, "Lewis' Practice of Surgery"; W. F. Prior Co.
17. W. R. Meeker and A. J. Scholl; Ann. of Surg. 80: 739. 772, 1924.

The American Public Health Association will hold its sixty-fifth anual meeting in New Orleans, Louisiana, October 20-23, 1936. Health officials from every state in the U. S., Canada, Cuba and Mexico will be present.

MILIARY SYPHILIS OF THE INTESTINE IN THE NEW-BORN*†

A Discussion of the Pathology of Syphilis of the Gastro-Intestinal Tract in Children

JOSEPH YAMPOLSKY, M.D.
C. D. FOWLER, M.D.
Atlanta

Since the advent of modern antisyphilitic treatment, intestinal manifestations of congenital syphilis have become rare. Holt and McIntosh[1] state that: "in stillborn infants or in those dying within the first few weeks with very extensive lesions, there may be associated changes in the small intestine or colon. These consist of a diffuse thickening and fibrosis of the submucosa with a mononuclear cell infiltration. In the more extensive lesions minute foci of necrosis, the so-called miliary gumma, may be present. In one or two patients whom we have seen, children who have lived for some time, these lesions were associated with diarrhea. At autopsy of these cases they were visible as diffuse yellowish thickenings extending over six to ten centimeters, in quite localized areas in the intestine. These lesions show in sections a marked fibrous thickening and cellular infiltration in the submucosa. In one of them the overlying mucosa was in part destroyed and replaced by granulation tissue."

The pathologic picture of syphilis of the small intestine is well described by McCallum[2], who described the following changes: "Changes in the submucosa of the small intestine and especially of the duodenum have impressed us lately. They have been observed by many others, and consist of a dense infiltration of the submucosa with wandering cells, probably with some new formation of connective tissue; ulcerations and even abscess-like areas of necrosis extending into the submucosa have been found."

Of special interest is the report of D. Y. Ku[3]. He gave a detailed description of four cases of congenital syphilis of the intestine. He referred to Oberndorfer who, in 1900,

compiled all the cases in literature reported up to that time. "In most of his cases a focal involvement of the small intestine was present. The intestinal wall, in places, was thickened by the gummatous infiltration in the submucosa. Terrace-like elevations had formed. The overlying mucosa may be atrophic or may be destroyed by the gummatous infiltrations. The latter may involve all layers of the intestinal wall, according to Mracek. Due to necrosis of such infiltration foci, ulcers of various forms develop. Jurgens and Mracek have observed rupture of such an ulcer with subsequent peritonitis. Birch-Hirschfield observed a diffuse sclerotic form with increasing thickness of the intestinal wall. According to most investigators, the transformations are localized in the small intestine only, namely, in the jejunum. According to Foerster, however, the principal location of the transformation is found in the Peyer's patches. Oberndorfer found gummatous infiltration in the large intestine also. The vessels, especially the small arteries and veins, are regarded as the point of emanation of the disease of the intestine." Spirochetes at the margin of the necrotic foci were first found by Verse and Fraenkel. Simmonds also demonstrated them in the meconium.

Holland[4], in his report on the causation of fetal death, impresses us with the fact that the demonstration of the spirocheta pallida is absolute evidence of syphilis. "There is, however, a great deal of other evidence; some of great and some of small value. This other evidence forms what may be termed the secondary attributes of fetal syphilis. It may be stated that one of these secondary attributes, osteochondritis, may be regarded as pathognomonic; another, typical histologic changes in the placenta, is highly reliable."

In summarizing the histologic examination of the four cases of congenital intestinal syphilis Ku states that three different forms may be distinguished: "(1) A severe atrophy of the mucous membrane with substitution by slightly hemorrhagic granulation tissue, as well as the appearance of miliary syphilomas in the muscular layers. At several sites of the duodenum and ileum formation of nodular thickening in mucosa and submucosa due to granulomas. Acute congenital intes-

*From the Department of Pediatrics, Emory University School of Medicine and the Pediatric Ward of Grady Hospital, Atlanta, Ga.
†Pathology by Dr. J. C. Norris.

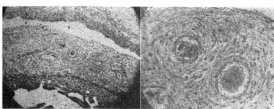

FIGURE 1.
Low power. Disintegration of the mucosa with general inflammation between the mucosa and muscularis and peritoneum. Reaction is one of new forming vessels and fibroblasts with particular thickening of the adventitia of the two vessels in the center. The process of inflammation in general extends through to the peritoneum, a portion of which is seen in the upper right portion of the picture.

FIGURE 2.
High power showing fibroblasts and other cells.

tinal syphilis. (case 1); (2) Fairly uniform thickening of the entire intestinal wall, produced by the proliferation of connective tissue in the mucosa and submucosa with marked recession of lymphocytic and leukocytic aggregations. (case 2); (3) Gummatous transformation, especially of the mucosa and submucosa, with secondary severe focal necroses (case 4) and ulcers (case 3) due to vascular transformations.

"The change of the transformations in the different forms is explainable on the basis of (a) the degree of severity of the infection, (b) differences of time, and (c) different resistance capacity of the infantile organism at different stages. The transformations are especially localized in the small intestine. In two cases they were preponderantly localized in the ileum. All layers of the intestinal wall may be involved, most regularly the mucosa and submucosa. Spirochetes were found only in cases 2 and 3, namely, in the subepithelial layer of the mucosa. The infection of the intestinal wall occurs by way of the blood."

That other organs beside the intestine may be involved in congenital syphilis has been repeatedly proven through pathologic examinations of the stomach. Vebrycke[5] described a case of suspected congenital syphilis of the stomach in a boy of thirteen. This boy was undernourished and all examinations except that of the abdomen were negative. The stomach contents gave the reaction of free hydrochloric acid and there was found con-

siderable mucus and some streaking of blood in the specimen.

"Fluoroscopic studies of the heart, lungs and esophagus were negative. The stomach, however, was found to be of a peculiar boot-shape, of fair tone, but with slight increase in size of the fundus extending down to nearly the distal third. Here the shadow became very narrow, producing almost an hour-glass picture, but with the entire antrum narrow and irregular. It was the sort of appearance that one might expect in advanced malignancy. Emptying occurred within six hours. Because it was thought that the extreme deformity could not be due to anything but syphilis without his general condition being much worse than it was, the tentative diagnosis of syphilis of the stomach was made while he was behind the fluoroscopic screen."

"Active antisyphilitis treatment was started at once with potassium iodide and salvarsan. Subjectively improvement began almost at once. In the first month the boy gained three pounds and the pain almost entirely disappeared. During the next two weeks he had two slight attacks of pain, but no vomiting. Roentgenograms made after the first five salvarsan injections showed no great difference objectively, in spite of the very wonderful subjective improvement. His weight steadily increased. Fluoroscopic examination showed a distinctly favorable change in the outline of the stomach, but there was still a considerable narrowing of the antrum which, I am inclined to think, was fibrotic and permanent."

There is, of course, reasonable doubt at-

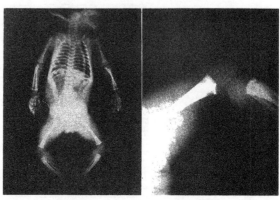

FIGURE 3.
Diaphyses of all long bones showed a moderate disturbance of calcification. **FIGURE 4.** The ends are irregular and moth eaten and very typical of a syphilitic infection.

tached to any diagnosis of syphilis of the stomach. In this case the stomach condition cannot be proved to be due to congenital syphilis or even to the syphilis at all, but the x-ray examination was so typical in appearance and the response to specific therapy so brilliant, that the author was convinced of the correctness of the diagnosis.

According to Gatewood and Kolodny[2]: "A positive Wassermann reaction in conjunction with a gastric lesion does not prove the syphilitic nature of the lesion; syphilitic gastric disease may also exist in the absence of positive blood. findings. Although fibrous changes, contracture, stenosis, and stiffening of the walls are characteristic of syphilis of the stomach, there is no pathognomonic roentgenographic sign. Symptomatic improvement usually follows efficient treatment with intravenous injections of diarsenol, combined with various forms of mercury, and with oral administration of potassium iodide. However, the deformities may increase inasmuch as the gummatous lesions heal by contraction and frequently form a stenosing scar. The effect cannot be roentgenographically distinguished from progressive proliferative lesions, such as

carcinoma. The differentiation lies in the fact that in treated syphilis the disease does not progress rapidly to the fatal termination; cachexia is less common and less marked than in cancer of the stomach. The presence of occult blood in the stools and gastric content is of great value in excluding syphilis. A gumma may bleed, but the hemorrhage is rarely continuous, and usually ceases after specific treatment is instituted."

These two authors state that intestinal syphilis is rare. The disease may take the form of an early catarrhal enteritis, occurring as a part of the secondary exanthema, a general roseola, or of late involvement of tertiary lesions, with symptoms resembling those of other forms of ulcerative enterocolitis. Obstructive and stenotic symptoms may also ensue if large gumma form. The usual sign is severe diarrhea, with colicky pains, tenesmus, with mucus pus and blood in the stools. There may be moderate fever. Loss of weight may be marked, and cachexia is sometimes present. The condition may simulate typhoid fever, tuberculous intestinal ulceration, or idiopathic ulcerative colitis. Profuse hemorrhages may occur, or perforation with peritonitis, as a result of deep ulceration with secondary intestinal infection. Death is usually due to ileus, perforation, or exsanguination.

Roentgenographic evidence is of little value. If syphilis is suspected, antisyphilitic treatment should be begun at once. Obstructive lesions require surgical intervention.

We wish to present at this time a case of miliary syphilis in a new-born child since involvement of the intestine is rare in congenital syphilis.

Mother's History: Colored, aged 22, was admitted to the hospital for delivery January 16, 1934, estimated date of labor February 17, 1934. No toxic symptoms other than dizzy spells were experienced during pregnancy.

Past History: Asthma for two years; three previous pregnancies all full term and born alive; two living children; one child died at the age of one month, cause not known. Patient did not come to clinic for treatment.

Examination: Blood pressure—systolic 126, diastolic 40; temperature, pulse and respiration normal. There was a general dermatitis consisting of small, circumscribed, dark pigmented macules over the abdomen, chest and extremities. There was a diastolic murmur over the aortic valve area. Position of child was a breech, the fundus was at the ensiform process; the fetal heart tones were not heard. Albumen in urine was 2 plus, Wassermann negative, January 17, 1934.

Patient's History: Baby girl: cord Wassermann 4 plus. Patient apparently an eight month baby, delivered by single footling breech mechanism; total labor seven hours. No complications experienced during delivery except fetal heart tones were not heard. The baby did not breathe well and died one hour after delivery. Placenta presented many infarcts.

Autopsy Report: Patient's weight 2,125 grams, length 40 centimenters; abdomen greatly distended. Distension appeared to be due to ascites and not gas. The liver was palpable below the costal margin. On opening the abdominal cavity a large amount of yellow colored fluid was found. Appendix was retrocecal and was bound down by the peritoneum over the posterior abdominal wall. A small adhesion was found between two loops of jejunum.

There were two areas of inflammation in the jejunum. One was at a point about two inches below the upper limit of the jejunum and extended for a distance of about three-fourths of an inch, involving practically all of the gut in this area. The second area was about three inches below the first and involved about the same amount of intestinal surface. There was an adhesion between this second area and a loop of the intestine. A similar area of inflammation was present on the adherent loop, although not so extensive. The adhesion was broken in the removal of the tissue for study. There were scattered areas in the jejunum which were just beneath the peritoneal surface and which did not communicate with the lumen. These areas were slightly elevated and presented a white granular (bumpy) appearance. In some respects they resembled a tubercle of the very earliest type; yet they were not

typical. The inner lumen was moderately red and slightly inflamed. The process seemed in no way to definitely affect the mucosa. The lymphatics of the mesentery were hypertrophied.

MICROSCOPIC EXAMINATION OF THE SECTIONS

Lungs: The lungs were atelectatic. The blood vessels were congested. About some of the vessels there was an early increase in the adventitia.

Heart: There was little interfiber fibrosis. The blood vessels were not thickened. There was slight cloudy swelling.

Spleen: Weighed 23 grams. The spleen presented a chronic and acute congestion. There was a general congestion with red blood cells, so much so that the germinal cells were depressed. In some places there was hemorrhage into the splenic pulp. There was considerable blood pigment present. Wandering lymphocytes and an occasional polymorphonuclear cell were seen, suggesting a chronic splenitis.

Thymus: Weight 8.2 grams. Normal except for a slight inflammatory reaction within the connective tissue stroma which separates the lobules.

Liver: Weight, 123 grams. Normal.

Intestine: The mucosa presented a rather intense chronic inflammation in which there is an increase in fibroblasts and many new forming blood vessels. The submucosa showed the veins to be engorged and the arterioles to have slight thickening of the walls, and there were many new forming capillaries. In this area of fibroblastic tissue there were also infiltrating cells of many varieties such as lymphocytes, occasional plasma cells, very few polymorphonuclears, except about an occasional blood vessel one saw evidence of a subacute and chronic inflammation in which the cells were mostly lymphocytes and a few polymonphonuclear cells, very suggestive of syphilis.

Roentgen-ray Examination: Revealed that the diaphyses of all long bones had a moderate disturbance of calcification. The ends were irregular and moth eaten and very typical of a syphilitic infection.

Discussion

A case has been presented in which the family history demonstrates that the mother is probably syphilitic, although her blood Wassermann is negative. The lesion in the aortic area, especially in the colored race, is diagnostic of syphilis. The baby presented many signs of congenital syphilis. The cord Wassermann was positive, the roentgenograms are definitely diagnostic of syphilis and the pathologic picture at autopsy, especially in the jejunum, is diagnostic of syphilis when the rest of the picture is taken into consideration. Although at the time of autopsy spirochetes were not looked for, and the finding of the latter certainly would demonstrate the diagnosis, yet we feel that this is not always possible to accomplish and taking the picture as a whole, we have a definite case of syphilis of the jejunum in the new-born.

Castro-intestinal symptoms are very common in congenital syphilis, and on many occasions with a negative blood Wassermann in the patient, but with some definite history of the mother having had syphilis, we get excellent results in relieving these symptoms when the patient is put on antisyphilitic treatment. We believe that the spirochetes affect children suffering from congenital syphilis more often so far as the gastro-intestinal tract is concerned. That has been demonstrated in the past and for that reason we feel that cases with autopsy findings presenting these lesions should be reported from time to time.

BIBLIOGRAPHY

1. Holt, L. Emmet, Jr., and McIntosh, Rustin: "Diseases of Infancy and Childhood." Tenth Editor, D. Appleton and Co., page 1096, 1933.

2. McCallum, W. G.: "Textbook of Pathology." W. B. Saunders Co., page 740, 1931.

3. Ku, D. Y.: "On Congenital Syphilis of the Intestine on the Basis of Four Cases." Virchowe Arch. f. path. Anat., 280, 852, 1931.

4. Holland, Eardley: "Report on the Causation of Fetal Death." Ministry of Health, London. Published under authority of His Majesty's Stationary Office. Page 29, 1922.

5. Verbrycke, J. Russell, Jr.: "Congenital Syphilis of the Stomach." The American Journal of Syphilis, 13: 524-526 (October) 1929.

6. Gatewood, E. and Kolodny: "Gastric and Intestinal Syphilis. Report of Case. Clinical Course and Morbid Pathology." American Journal of Syphilis. 7: 648 (October) 1923.

CRAWFORD W. LONG MEMORIAL PRIZE COMMITTEE REPORT

Inasmuch as no essays were submitted to this Committee for consideration during the past year, there will be no award made of the Crawford W. Long Memorial Prize. The committee expresses the hope that there will be a larger number of contestants this coming year.

The committee has decided to consider all essays read at the annual convention of this Association as being in the contest for this prize, unless the author of some particular essay especially desires to withdraw his essay from that contest. The requirements of the contest are that each essayist shall submit five copies of his essay, in order that each member of the Committee may independently pass on the essay. These essays must be submitted by October, first, following the annual convention of the Association. The secretary is requested to communicate by letter with each essayist requesting his five copies and urging him to send them to the Chairman of this Committee by October, first. The secretary is also requested to state these requirements in the JOURNAL, so that the essayists will be doubly reminded.

WM. R. DANCY, M.D., *Chairman.*

The American Medical Association will hold its eighty-eighth annual session in Atlantic City in 1937.

Usually the diagnosis of puerperal infection is easily made from the clinical history. Older observers attributed an elevation of temperature on the third or fourth day to lacteal secretions, but the normal puerperium should be afebrile. A temperature of over 100F. for twenty-four hours should be considered infectious. Typhoid fever and malaria are a common diagnosis of the practitioner who wants to shield himself from neglected aseptic preventions in the conduct of his cases. Occasionally a latent malarial infection does recur, but other factors should be excluded before such a diagnosis is made. Bacteriologic examinations are an aid in the diagnosis, such as blood cultures and examination of the lochia.

During the past five years it has been the privilege of the writer to see four cases of puerperal infection. The case reports are as follows:

Case No. 1—Mrs. A. W., aged 40, was delivered of a female baby August 5, 1930; breech presentation, chloroform anesthesia, easy manual delivery, but dry labor. On the day of delivery the patient's temperature was 102F and the following day her temperature was subnormal and the pulse normal. On the third day her temperature rose to 102F and the pulse rate was 120. At this time she had a slight chilly sensation. The fourth day, following chilly sensation, her temperature rose to 103F and finally to 106F, pulse 130. This patient was seen by me on the fifth day of the illness and at that time was anemic, complaining of slight pain in the lower abdomen and a general weakness.

Physical examination showed the eyes, ears, nose and throat negative; lungs negative to percussion and auscultation; heart normal in size and sounds; pulse 1930, blood pressure 115; abdomen slightly tender, with slight soreness on palpation across lower quadrant. Uterus palpable and slightly enlarged, lochia very scant and little odor. At this time it was thought advisable to give her 20 cc. of anti-streptococcus serum. On the sixth day of her illness she received another 20 cc. of streptococcus serum, following which her temperature rose to 108F and the pulse to 160. The next day her temperature did not rise above 103F or pulse over 110. At that time she was seen by a third physician in consultation who suggested repeated small blood transfusions. On the ninth day of her illness she had a small transfusion by the indirect method, followed by a temperature of 107F and pulse of 155. The second day after that she had another transfusion, following which her temperature did not go over 104 F and the pulse over 110, and she showed her first signs of improvement, continuing to improve gradually until the nineteenth day, when she received another transfusion which seemed to improve her condition still more.

On the twenty-first day she received her last transfusion, following which her temperature for five days did not rise over 101F and her pulse rate not over 100. On the twenty-fifth and twenty-sixth days she had an elevation of temperature of 103F, and her pulse rate was 110, but the following week there was a gradual decline in her pulse rate and temperature, and two weeks later she was able to sit up.

Blood culture made on this patient at the time that she was first seen showed a slow growing streptococcus viridans. This is a representative type of streptococcus infection and one of·the most amazing results I have ever seen. It also demonstrates the value of repeated small blood transfusions in septicemia.

Examination of this patient last year· showed her heart and lungs to be normal, blood pressure normal, hemoglobin 80, weight normal, menstruation normal, and, as far as could be observed, she is well at the present time.

Case No. 2—Mrs. T. P. I., aged 31, was seen by the writer June 2, 1931, in consultation. Her complaint at that time was chilliness and pain across the lower abdomen. The present illness began three weeks ago when the patient was delivered of a normal living baby which was her fourth child. During the first twelve days of the puerperium she had an uneventful recovery, sitting up on the tenth day. On the twelfth day she had a severe chill and elevation of temperature, accompanied by pain and chills intermittently during the next several days, fever ranging from 101F to 105F. She was admitted to the hospital and physical examination at that time showed:

Patient appears very drowsy and anemic. Eyes, ears, nose and throat normal; lungs clear; heart rapid, regular, good volume, no murmurs; abdomen obese, slight tenderness over right upper quadrant and over middle lower quadrant, no rigidity, no masses felt, but slight muscular tenderness over right kidney. Extremities normal. Urine: cloudy, dark brown, slightly acid, specific gravity 1.015, albumin three plus, sugar slight trace, microscopic examination shows large amount of clumped and scattered pus (voided specimen). Catheter specimen showed apparently the same results. Blood examination: hemoglobin 50, white blood count 10,000. A diagnosis of pyelitis was made and the patient was treated accordingly. Her condition improved gradually and she was dismissed from the hospital June 19, 1931, but was again admitted June 26, 1931, following a severe attack of kidney colic, right side, and at this time she had some more trouble with her pyelitis. Since the last admission to the hospital her condition has improved gradually and she is apparently well at the present time.

I report this case because a lot of our apparently puerperal infections, after thorough examination, show some other lesion causing trouble.

. *Case No. 3*—Mrs. T. G. M., aged 22, was admitted to the hospital April 17, 1931, complaining of fever and uterine bleeding. Three weeks before admission the patient was delivered of a normal child, but had a slow delivery of the placenta. Patient had a profuse lochia and a general weakness during first nine days following

her delivery and was unable to stay up any length of time after the tenth and eleventh days, at which time she began to pass a lot of clots and· had a severe pain across lower abdomen.· Her bleeding stoped until three days before admission to the hospital, when she had another uterine hemorrhage accompanied with a profuse vaginal discharge of an unpleasant odor.

Examination upon admission showed her eyes, ears, nose and throat negative: pyorrhea around all teeth: lungs clear, no rales; heart, no· murmurs, pulse rate 110, blood pressure 90/50; abdomen typanitic, slight general tenderness of abdomen, more intense across lower quadrant, no masses were palpable. Pelvic examination showed: slight enlargement of uterus and the pelvis was filled across the culdesac with a soft doughy, tender mass. A diagnosis of pelvic abscess was made following a puerperal infection, which was drained through the vagina and lower abdomen. At the time of the operation the pelvis was found filled with pus. This patient died the third day following her operation of a general peritonitis, probably of the colon bacillus origin.

I report this case because it represents a case of puerperal infection which localized in a pelvic abscess, later rupturing and causing a general peritonitis.

Case No. 4—Mrs. R. T. T., aged 15, was admitted to the hospital October 28, 1935, complaining of being in labor and unable to deliver.

Labor began the previous day, after a normal fullterm prenatal course. Pains came on intermittently and of short duration. · This morning her pains became more severe, every ten minutes, and the doctor was called. On examination he found a mass in the vagina obstructing delivery and sent the patient to the hospital. Patient had a chill last night lasting several minutes. Past history negative; first pregnancy; temperature 102.4F, pulse 110, respiration 30.

Examination: Woman of small stature; weight about 125 pounds. Head normal, heart and lungs normal, B.P. 120/80, heart rapid. Abdomen: enlarged uterus extending to epigastrium. Fetal heart sounds: heart in L.L.Q.; small parts felt; position O.L.A. Pelvic: large soft mass in post-fornix, protruding in front of cervix, which is dilated about three inches. Mass about the size of a medium size orange, not movable. Fetal head felt in cervix. Extremities: normal. Impression: pregnancy and labor. Pelvic abscess (?).

Operation: classical cesarean section. Removal dermoid cyst and right ovary.

Findings: trochar passed ·into dependent portion of mass in back part of vagina. Large amount of white, cheesy material exposed. Ball of hair and bone felt but unable to remove. Patient was prepared for an abdominal operation and through a midline incision an attempt to remove the ovarian dermoid cyst around the pregnant uterus was unsuccessful. The· uterus was incised in anterior midline of fundus and the baby delivered by forceps. After suturing the uterus in layers a large dermoid cyst of the right ovary was removed at the pedicle and the abdomen sewed tight.

Immediate condition: fair. Prognosis, grave.

The patient had a very stormy recovery with very much abdominal distention, with a secondary abscess at the lower end of incision.

A Case of Acute Unilateral Retro-Bulbar Neuritis
Associated with Nasal-Sinus Disease. R. R. James, Sir
St. Clair Thomson, Lionel Colledge and H. Graham
Hodgson, C.V.O. (London). Brit. J. Ophthal., Vol.
XX. p. 164, 1936.

The patient was a medical man, aged 75 years, who
was known to have had normal vision in each eye
with slight hypermetropic correction since 1923. He
called on May 8, 1933, complaining that he had
woken up on May 7 to find the sight of the left eye
blurred. There was also some pain on movement of
the globe.

The right eye was normal in every respect, with
6/6 vision after correction.

The pupil reaction to light on the left side was extremely sluggish; tension was normal; vision, only
hand movements. Visual fields were full save for a
slight contraction, in the upper nasal quadrant, and
there was a large central scotoma. The blood pressure
was 200/110.

Radiograms were taken of the sinuses with the patient in the erect position, on May 11. All sinuses
showed pathologic changes radiologically except the
right antrum. The left sphenoidal sinus and the left
posterior ethmoid cells showed a fluid level.

There was a history of previous antral trouble on
the left side, for which Sir St. Clair Thomson had performed a radical operation a few years before, with
excellent results.

The deterioration of vision was very rapid. On the
morning of May 12 the eye was practically blind. The
pupil hardly acted to light; only bare perception of
light was present and no field could be charted. The
left disc was swollen 1.0 D. and the vessels were tur-
gid. Sir St. Clair Thomson strongly advised immediate operation and that afternoon Mr. Colledge opened
and drained the left sphenoidal and ethmoidal cells.
Under cocaine and adrenalin anaesthesia there was
visible a pulsating spot of light on the purulent discharge in the neighborhood of the ostium of the sphenoidal sinus, resembling the pulsating spot often seen
in the neighborhood of a perforation in the tympanic
membrane when drainage is unsufficient. With Hajek's
forceps the anterior wall of the sphenoidal sinus was
cut away and some posterior ethmoidal cells opened.
Healing was rapid and satisfactory.

Unfortunately, although the operation was done
within five days of first appearance of the symptoms,
there was no improvement in vision. A month and
a half later the fundus examination showed a secondary type of optic atrophy with some narrowing of
the vessels. The right eye was normal throughout
and, when seen in November, 1935, was quite healthy,
with 6/6 vision after correction.

The authors inferred that the massive lesion of the
optic nerve was due to a direct spread of infection from
a focus in the posterior ethmoidal cells and sphenoidal
sinus, and that the patient was fortunate in that the
infection confined itself entirely to the nerve and that
no backward spread into the cavernous sinus took place.

ALTON V. HALLUM, M.D.

FIRST MEETING OF THE HOUSE OF DELE-
GATES OF THE MEDICAL ASSOCIATION
OF GEORGIA, SAVANNAH
April 21, 1936

Abstract

The first meeting of the House of Delegates of the
Medical Association of Georgia convened at Hotel
DeSoto, Savannah, 2:00 P.M., April 21, 1936.

The roll was called and a quorum present.

The President appointed three Reference Committees: No. 1, No. 2, and No. 3, personnel as follows:

No. 1. *Reports of Officers:* C. H. Richardson,
Macon, Chairman; H. C. Sauls, Atlanta, and G. Lombard Kelly, Augusta.

No. 2. *Reports of Committees:* C. W. Roberts,
Atlanta, Chairman; C. W. Strickler, Atlanta, and D.
N. Thompson, Elberton.

No. 3. *Miscellaneous Reports and Recommendations:* T. C. Davison, Atlanta, Chairman; W. G. Elliott, Cuthbert, and J. B. Kay, Byron.

*Reports of the following Officers were read and
submitted:* President, President-Elect, Second Vice-
President, Parliamentarian, Secretary-Treasurer and
Delegates to the American Medical Association.

*Reports of Committees by Chairmen were as fol-
lows:* Economics, Scientific Work, Public Policy and
Legislation, Medical Defense, Hospitals, Cancer Com-
mission, Sub-Committee on Medical History, Abner
Wellborn Calhoun Lectureship, Crawford W. Long
Memorial Prize, L. G. Hardman Loving Cup, Ad-
visory—State Board of Health, Advisory—Woman's
Auxiliary, Crawford W. Long Bronze Statue, Post-
graduate Medical Study, offer of Trophy by Raymond
V. Harris.

Report of the Committee on Scientific Work was
adopted.

Motion carried to authorize the President to appoint
a Sub-Committee of three as an Advisory Committee
to the State Board of Health to work for the benefits
of the Social Security Act which is now a national law.

Report of the Committee for the Study of Maternal Mortality and Infant Deaths.

Report of the President of the Woman's Auxiliary.

Second Meeting of the House of Delegates
April 24, 1936

The L. G. Hardman Loving Cup Committee reported that the name of Dr. Glenville Giddings, Atlanta, had been selected to be engraved on the Cup for
his research and study on the subject of "Sleep".

RECOMMENDATIONS OF THE REFERENCE COMMIT-
TEES ON REPORTS OF OFFICERS AND
COMMITTEES WERE APPROVED
AS FOLLOWS

President: Concern of the medical profession over
the increased number of indigent patients, medical economic survey in cross-section of State, protection of
public from illegal and poorly trained practitioners,
suggested that Councilors be diligent in the organization of county societies, enlighten the lay public
through the press, radio and public meetings, that dues

for 1937 be fixed at $7.00, medical relief committees
to direct emergency work in any section of the State
when and where any disaster occurs, give courses in
public health work in all of the ten districts of the
State.

President-Elect: Medical Economic Survey, amendment of the Workmen's Compensation Act, safeguard
the use of barbiturates, promotion of Social Security
Act, opposition to State Medicine, improvement of
health conditions in industrial plants, sponsor public
health meetings.

Secretary-Treasurer: Report approved.

Delegates to A. M. A.: Report approved.

Parliamentarian: Recommendation in reference to
election of Councilors, incorporation of resolutions
adopted from 1921 to 1935 in Constitution and By-
Laws as far as amenable to such procedure.

Medical Economics: Suggest that members carefully
study report when published; make specific plans to
furnish medical care to the indigent and develop provisions for better medical care for the sub-comfort
group with some form of prepayment plan or smaller
fees, medical care for the indigent should be recognized
by the public and government as charity as much so
as food, clothing and housing and to improve the financial status of physicians, people should be so informed to better care for the indigent and sub-comfort
group, eighteen health districts should be organized
in the State with a health officer in charge of a centrally located clinic for ambulatory patients to be examined and treated, that all physicians in the district be
engaged in the work under a rotating system; group
hospitalization as outlined by the Georgia Hospital
Association is approved; suggest that each county medical society appoint a Committee on Medical Economics
and secure from the Bureau of Economics of the American Medical Association literature on this problem,
acquaint themselves with it and decide on methods for
improvement; that the committees make definite and
persistent efforts to obtain from county commissioners
appropriations to pay fees, even though small, for
medical care of the indigent.

Public Policy and Legislation: That a special fund
be provided to promote favorable legislation in Georgia and to defeat that inimical to public welfare;
amendment of the Workmen's Compensation Act to
insure more adequate compensation for hospitals, nurses
and physicians; sponsor the Basic Science Bill and continue our efforts until it is enacted into law; Group
Hospitalization Bill as introduced in the last legislature; legislation to protect hospitals, nurses and physicians for the care of emergency accident cases; cooperation with other organizations in the State to secure the benefits of the Social Security Act.

Medical Defense: Commend the Committee and attorneys for their excellent success; advise all members
threatened with suits for alleged malpractice to refer
everything to the Secretary-Treasurer, make no oral or
written statement to any one else until you get the
advice of the Association's attorneys; ask members to
read the "Pink Slip", entitled "Malpractice Suits", reprint from the JOURNAL, July, 1935.

Hospitals: A lien law for the protection of hospitals: amendment to the Workmen's Compensation Act to increase the liability of companies from $100.00 to $300.00 or such part as may be necessary; legislation to enable county governments to pay hospital expenses for the indigent regardless of the location of the hospital and to permit counties to contract with hospitals for the care of the indigent sick: proper inspection and standardization of all hospitals with 25 beds or less.

Resolutions: Memorialize all radio broadcasting stations in Georgia to restrict facilities to ethical and approved organizations to disseminate public health information; and sponsor statewide move to control tuberculosis.

History: Accept report and file.

Calhoun Lectureship Fund: Accept report and file.

Crawford W. Long Memorial Prize: Accept report and file.

Advisory—Woman's Auxiliary: Accept report and file.

Crawford W. Long Bronze Statue: Accept report and file.

Advisory—State Board of Health: Approve and recommend report.

Cancer Commission: Program approved.

Postgraduate Study: Recommendations approved.

Raymond Benjamin Harris Trophy: Recommend that trophy offered by R. V. Harris, Savannah. in memory of his father, be accepted.

Council: Report by Chairman and recommendation that dues for 1937 be fixed at $7.00 approved.

CONSTITUTION AND BY-LAWS AMENDMENTS

Article VII, Section 1. Amended to read as follows:

"The annual session shall take place on the second Wednesday in May at such place as shall be designated by the Association, provided that in case of conflict with the annual session of the American Medical Association or on petition of the county society of the host city made at least six months before the fixed dates for the annual session, the Council may change the dates by publishing a notice in the JOURNAL OF THE MEDICAL ASSOCIATION OF GEORGIA three months before the session.

Article IX, Section 3. Part of lines 5, 6, 7, 8, 9, changed to read as follows:

"The Councilors shall be elected at the same time on nomination by their respective district societies at the annual meetings of such societies preceding the annual session of the Association at which the vacancies occur, but if no nomination from a district society is brought before the Association, the nomination for Councilor may be presented from the floor."

The American Association for the Study of Goiter will hold its annual meeting in Chicago, Illinois, June 8, 9, 10. Dr. T. C. Davison and Dr. D. Henry Poer are on the program to read a paper, entitled *Goiter in Georgia—A Statistical Study of 500 Consecutive Cases.*

CANCER COMMISSION*

I submit herewith the annual report of your Cancer Commission for the year 1935-1936.

We have been able to reach a greater number of people with our educational messages than for several years. We hope that we will be able to carry on until the doctors and people of the State become "cancer minded."

Besides many other activities we furnished the Woman's Auxiliary with 12,000 leaflets entitled "Cancer in Woman." . In these leaflets we continued to feature cancer of the cervix and uterus, breast, stomach. and rectum. The leaflets were widely and wisely distributed. We believe that it was well received, for the *Atlanta Constitution* published the entire text on the "feature page" of their Sunday paper and wrote an editorial commending it and the work of the Association. A few weeks ago the *Constitution* also published another of our articles with editorial comment. For this good work we wish to express our appreciation.

A set of charts and placards has been prepared for public and professional meetings. We are now using several of them in our exhibit. These charts with a number of lantern slides are available for meetings of the district and county medical societies or for public meetings. We have had under consideration the purchase of a moving picture film, but we fear that it would soon be destroyed unless some one thoroughly competent to manipulate it could carry it to the meetings. Therefore, no purchase has yet been made.

Mr. Butler Toombs. of the Department of Public Health prepared a review of the cancer mortality in Georgia for a recent issue of the Association's JOURNAL. In it he estimated that there are 5,000 cancer patients in Georgia at any given time. This review, with an editorial published in the same issue, has been reprinted and distributed to the presidents and secretaries of the district and county medical societies and to a select group interested in cancer control.

A series of one-page articles by some of our best known cancer students is now being published by the JOURNAL under the title "Early Signs and Symptoms of Cancer." If we can secure the necessary funds we will have these reprinted in attractive form and sent to all the doctors in the State. By constant pursuance of this policy we hope in a few years to have the entire profession sufficiently "cancer conscious" to recognize early cancer and pre-cancer.

A survey of the hospitals in Georgia was attempted in 1932. It revealed that very little interest was being taken in the treatment of cancer. Many hospitals had admitted no cancer patients during 1931. Twenty of them, representing 1,177 beds, reported 534 patients treated during the year. Little effort had been made to tabulate the cases. so we considered the survey a failure so far as revealing the cancer situation was concerned.

Last year another hospital survey was made, the results of which indicate a greatly increased interest

*Report of the Cancer Commission of the Medical Association of Georgia to the House of Delegates at the Savannah session, April 21, 1936.

in the treatment of cancer throughout the State. We sent questionnaires to all general hospitals in Georgia where it was indicated that cancer patients might be treated. Our list was compiled from the Journal of the American Medical Association or the American and Canadian Hospital Directory, and represented 3,998 beds. Replies have been received from 49 hospitals. Seven, totaling 174 beds, had no cancer patients during 1934 or had kept no record of having any; 42 hospitals, totalling 3,183 beds—79.6 per cent of the general hospital bed-capacity—had admitted 1,565 cancer patients. Of these hospitals, 40 classified their patients as to sex. There were 379 men and 878 women. Classification according to race showed 1,056 white and 374 colored. Below is a tabulation of cancer patients and their distribution among the hospitals reporting:

17 hospitals reported 126 cancers of the breast.
18 hospitals reported 397 cancers of the female genital organs.
14 hospitals reported 71 cancers of the colon and rectum.
15 hospitals reported 77 cancers of the stomach, liver, pancreas.
11 hospitals reported 60 cancers of the mouth.
9 hospitals reported 48 cancers of the bladder and prostate.
11 hospitals reported 109 cancers of the skin.
5 hospitals reported 28 cancers of the bone.
11 hospitals reported 82 cancers of the other organs and parts of body.

A graphic chart has been made showing the percentage of patients in each group. Wherever possible sex has been indicated. Figures from the hospitals reporting ages showed that by far the largest number of cancers occurred between the ages of 40 and 60.

Several noteworthy facts are revealed from a comparative study of these hospital reports and the report of the Bureau of Vital Statistics for the same period. The percentage of female patients with cancer of the genital organs who were admitted to hospitals was nearly triple the percentage of deaths reported for lesions of these organs. Thirty-six per cent more patients with breast cancer were treated in our hospitals than died during 1934. We cannot account for this variation except by a belief that our campaign of education and the increased interest in the treatment of cancer are beginning to bear fruit. We hope that we may be able to continue our work with renewed interest. Therefore, we urge the Association to appropriate sufficient funds for the Cancer Commission to carry out the following program:

(a)—To have the cancer articles now appearing in the JOURNAL reprinted and sent to every doctor in the State.

(b)—To circularize the state and county officials with popularly written material at least twice during the year.

(c)—To encourage public meetings to which the school officials, teachers and older students shall be invited. (This may be done through our already strong ally, the Parent-Teacher Association.)

(d)—To co-operate with the State Board of Health in urging the general hospitals at

the accompanying symptoms of fever, leukocytosis, pain and other evidence of inflammation make the differentiation from osteomyelitis very difficult. Even the x-ray appearance
of the lesion is frequently atypical. One
should not lose sight of the fact that this disease frequently occurs as a multiple primary
tumor.

Numerous other forms of cancer which are
common to middle and old age may be seen in
young individuals. Cancer of the rectum is
by no means unknown in children and cancer
of the stomach in young patients is usually
overlooked until too late. Melanoma, or the
"malignant mole," is by no means uncommon in children and even cancer of the larynx
and of the tongue have been reported. Even
the common skin cancer of epidermoid carcinoma of the basal cell type which is so common in elderly patients must not be overlooked in patients under twenty.

The diagnosis of cancer in children probably offers more difficulty than in adults.
However, the same methods of diagnosis
must be employed and the diagnosis must be
established by means of clinical, x-ray and
biopsy, or operative findings. As a general
rule, cancer in children is probably more
malignant and the course more rapid than in
adults, but, of course, there are numerous and
marked exceptions. Treatment is the same
as a rule, but it should be remembered that
many of the malignant tumors of children are
of embryonal and anaplastic type, highly
malignant and very sensitive to radiation.
Different types of tumors in the same location
respond differently to radiation therapy.
Osteogenic sarcoma is notoriously resistent to
any form of radiation while Ewing's sarcoma
is one of the most sensitive. In lymph nodes,
lymphosarcoma is probably the most sensitive of all malignant tumors, while endothel-
ioma and Hodgkin's disease are distinctly less
so. The resistance may increase as the disease progresses or after repeated insufficient
treatment. On account of the marked radiosensitivity of many of these tumors in children, this form of therapy is frequently indicated in preference to surgery in dealing
with cancer in the young individual, at the
same time remembering that the prognosis is
grave in spite of any type of treatment.

THE JOURNAL
OF THE
MEDICAL ASSOCIATION OF GEORGIA
Devoted to the Welfare of the Medical Association of Georgia

478 Peachtree Street, N.E., Atlanta, Ga.

MAY, 1936

OUR PROBLEMS

In assuming the office to which I have been elected to serve the coming year, I am not unmindful of the great honor which the membership of the Medical Association of Georgia has paid me. I want to express my sincere appreciation of this high honor, and I trust my conduct in this office will be in keeping with the high standard set by my predecessors. I have kept in close touch with the administration just closed and have watched with keen interest, the able and resourceful manner in which our retiring President has conducted the affairs of the office. He has given us the benefit of his splendid leadership into a program outstanding in its fine results toward the problems with which we have to deal as a profession.

I want to pay tribute to our Secretary-Treasurer for the splendid manner in which the affairs of this office have been conducted. Every detail of this office has had his careful and immediate attention, and I am looking forward to the very great help which he will render during the current year in the problems which will come before us during our administration.

I want to promise the membership it will be my purpose and desire to carry on from this administration the usual problems of the organization. We will, on the other hand, have to assume some current problems on account of the meeting of the General Assembly.

The Committee on Public Policy and Legislation presented a program of needed legislation to the House of Delegates for their endorsement. When this is printed and distributed, we trust each member of the Association will study the needs of this program and enlist the support of his representatives in the coming session of the General Assembly. The results of previous efforts to pass beneficial legislation is not encouraging, but this report contains so many matters of value

to the physician, as well as to the lay peopl we trust it will be received with more conce than heretofore.

We should like to see an increase in t maximum fee for compensation in the trea ment of accident cases, coming under t Compensation Act and Industrial Commi sion of Georgia. This fee at present is i adequate. Any case which requires hospita ization for two weeks or longer, the fee consumed in hospitalization and very little no balance is left for the physician.

We are fully aware of the danger of t promiscuous sale and use of the barbitui acid derivities as sedatives. A great mar deaths, more than most of us know, have o curred within the past few years as a dire cause of the free use of this dangerous dru We hope to have some measure passed by t coming session of the Legislature which w prohibit the sale of any of these preparatio without the prescription of a registered phy cian. Such legislation and the safegua would be a fitting tribute to Dr. Roy] Kracke, one of our own group, for his scie tific and comprehensive study of this dr and its effect upon the human body.

The Social Security Act has placed befo us some very important measures which t lay people must look to the Medical Ass ciation of Georgia for direction. The provi ions of this Act, if passed or adopted at t next session of the General Assembly, course can be followed in a large measure l the original Social Security Act. Other ben fits of this measure must be anticipated by o own group and applied to the peculiar nee of our own State. We have in mind a M ternal Welfare Committee from our organiz tion which should work in cooperation wi the Department of Public Health in the a ministration of the provision of the Feder Act. Maternal welfare is an important ma ter, and one which our State is sadly lackii in interest, as well as application.

We trust that the Department of Publ Health will receive more adequate financi assistance from the Appropriations Commi tee of the next General Assembly than heret fore. The record of this department, wi the meagre appropriations, is one of the ou standing achievements of the program of t

physicians of Georgia, and it is due in a large measure to the resourcefulness of Dr. T. F. Abercrombie, Commissioner of Health. In this connection, I should like to emphasize the need of a Health Education Program conducted, if possible, through the Department of Public Health and its chairman, Mr. Robert F. Maddox. If it were possible for us to give, in some degree, his interest and knowledge of the needs of the people to the average layman, our difficulties in the matter of health education and preventative medicine would be solved. Is it not a good time for us to give to the people of Georgia the economic value of improved health conditions while we have this great business leader serving in the capacity as chairman of this department?

The Bureau of Vital Statistics report shows that during 1935, there were 898 deaths from accidents involving motor vehicles, as compared with 564 in 1930, 348 in 1925, and only 140 in 1920. This information concerns the physician possibly more than it does the lay people, and yet some of the provisions that we have attempted heretofore, to prevent this wanton waste of life, as well as the protection of those dependent on persons killed in these accidents, by compulsory liability insurance, has met with most stubborn opposition when presented as legislation sponsored by the Medical Association of Georgia.

The pioneer work by the past administration in obtaining information through the Economic Survey of the conditions under which the average physician in Georgia has to work, and the service he is rendering, is an unfinished project which we shall undertake to carry on during our term of office. The information gained through this survey will be the means of creating a better understanding between layman and physician when it can be given as information of a general nature. This survey will undoubtedly give us the information needed in overcoming some of the misguided and misdirected efforts to place the practice of medicine under federal and state control. Some of the remedies promised by the advocates of "state medicine" can be entirely met with the information we will have from this survey. Much has been learned already from preliminary reports.

It will be shown that there has been little, if any, neglect in the treatment of the sick among the indigent poor of our State. It may be admitted that we must have a more intelligent method of treating all classes of individuals during their periods of illness, but this "better method" will not be by regimentation of the physicians. The experience of Germany over a period of fifty years, as well as many other countries of Europe over shorter periods, has shown that "state medicine" does not meet the measure. America today is treating all classes of individuals with more efficiency than many of those countries which adopted some form of state or provincial control.

The fine ideals which have made the practice of medicine more than a vocation with the physician, more than a means of earning a living, have met the problems found in the homes of our poor by the physicians, and has been a voluntary and frequently a sacrificial act, which created the service which no government control can apply or maintain. The sacred relationship between physician and patient existing through centuries is something which employment or control by federal and state agencies cannot improve, or even maintain. The social, moral and frequently the business relationship assumed by the physician in his community, would be lost within a generation or two, and any other method than that which inspires him to live nobly and serve his people under all conditions, as one apart from the ordinary man. The desire to practice medicine does not come from the hope that one will gain employment, or develop through seniority but that his talents and his abilities may be used in voluntary service to suffering humanity. The solving of the problems of medical care will not come through any political creed or the selfish ambitions of anyone who would like to prey upon the ignorance of any group, but through the best minds of those whose sincerity is based upon intelligent information.

BENJAMIN HARVEY MINCHEW, M. D.
President.

The Medical Association of Georgia will hold its eighty-eighth annual session in Macon, May 11, 12, 13, 14, 1937.

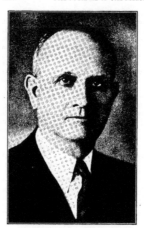

GEORGE ALBERT TRAYLOR, M.D., Augusta
President-Elect, 1936-37

GEORGE ALBERT TRAYLOR, M.D.

Dr. George Albert Traylor, President-Elect of the Medical Association of Georgia, was born in Abbeville County, South Carolina, October 7, 1879. His parents were Dr. Oliver Alexander Traylor and Mary Patterson Traylor.

After attending the public schools at McCormick, S. C., Dr. Traylor studied at Furman University, from which institute he graduated with the degree of Bachelor of Science in 1900. The following year he devoted to teaching school, but soon decided upon a medical career and entered the Medical College of Georgia, now the Medical Department of the University of Georgia. In 1904, he was awarded his degree of Doctor of Medicine and an honorary certificate. Another year and a half was occupied as an intern at the Augusta City Hospital after which time he located in Augusta to practice his profession, serving as the surgical assistant of the late Dr. Thomas R. Wright. He was married to Louise Bothwell of Augusta in 1912.

Dr. Traylor has long been identified with medical education and has held numerous

and assure the patient that she "may live a long time without food by mouth," but that when her stomach has rested sufficiently for her to desire food, you will try and have her appetite appeased. Let the needles used in parenteral therapy be rather large, and the technic a bit rough. The more disgusted a patient becomes with the treatment, the sooner she will find her "stomach sufficiently rested" to assume its normal function. Allow no company, least of all her husband, and remove the patient to a hospital, or to the home of a kind, understanding, but firm relative or friend in case the home environment cannot be controlled. Endocrine therapy has not yet demonstrated its efficacy although doubtless many good results have come from suggestive therapy accompanying such treatments. Progesterone (corporin) from the corpus luteum has been administered with some reported success and rationale, as it supposedly allays smooth muscle contractions.

If complications are carefully watched for and physiologic balances restored, one need not be too alarmed about the case. "With rectal, duodenal and nasal feedings, also parenteral, together with blood transfusions one can usually carry the patient along until her own powers counteract the 'toxemia' or bring her psychoneural system into equilibrium or until it is demonstrated to our satisfaction that the 'X quantity,' or toxemia is too much for her and, therefore, we must disgracefully empty the uterus to save the mother's life. No test can tell us when to do this. Clinical observation must elicit the signal."[5]

E. BRYANT WOODS, M.D.

BIOGRAPHY.

1. Atlee, H. B. J. Ob. & Gyn. Brit. Emp. 41:750 (1934).
2. Plass, E. D. & Meugert, W. F. Jour. Am. Med. Assn. 101:2020 (1933).
3. Gerstle, M. and Lucia, S. P. California and West Med. 40:167 (1934).
4. Tillman, A. J. B. Am. J. Ob. and Gyn. 27:240 (1934).
5. DeLee, J. B. Year Book of Obstetrics & Gynecology (1934). (Editor's note, p. 140.)

The Medical News Service of the Medical Society of the State of N. Y., says that the "Mandelbaum Health Insurance Act now pending in the State Legislature (N. Y.) is one of the worst specimens of medical legislation proposed in many years. The Mandelbaum bill combines cash benefits with medical service."

THE EIGHTY-SEVENTH ANNUAL SESSION

The medical profession of Savannah, the Woman's Auxiliary, the First District Nurses' Association, the hospitals, hotels and civic leaders are entitled to hearty congratulations from the medical profession of the State for their excellent entertainment of the Medical Association of Georgia and Woman's Auxiliary in annual session April 21-24.

Savannah, old and beautiful, graciously entertained the five hundred thirty-one physicians registered for the session. While the various scientific and business meetings consumed much time, many of the visiting physicians and their wives enjoyed sojourns to homes and gardens, boat trips, fishing, golf and skeet shooting.

The scientific program met with general approval as evidenced by the large attendance at the meetings. Our guest speakers brought messages of good will in addition to their excellent scientific papers. The House of Delegates and Council held their regular meetings and transacted a large volume of business important to the welfare of every physician in Georgia. Exhibits, both scientific and commercial, were unusually attractive.

Macon was selected for the 1937 annual session.

DON'T ANSWER THREATENING LETTERS

One of the most important matters brought out in the report of the Committee on Medical Defense at the Savannah meeting, in April, was the advice given by the attorneys of the Medical Association of Georgia, urging the members not to attempt to answer letters containing threats to sue for alleged malpractice. Our attorneys have had a large amount of experience in handling these suits and threats to sue, and have achieved marked success in the work. They are much better qualified to reply to these letters than almost any member of our Association. In replying to such a letter most of our members will give a long detailed account of the case and is liable to make statements which may cause trouble if the case comes to trial. Our lawyers know best how to answer these letters so as to leave no loopholes for future trouble. No matter how innocent of neglect a doctor may be he

may so word a letter as to give an opposing lawyer good material for damaging the doctor's case. Our members are advised to turn threatening letters over to our attorneys or to the Committee on Medical Defense.

Concerning Fractures

Another significant thing which appears every year in the report of the Committee on Medical Defense is that about 75 per cent, of damage suits are based on some alleged neglect in the treatment of fractures. Although many of our predecessors obtained excellent results in the treatment of fractures without the use of the x-ray, it now becomes absolutely necessary to use the x-ray if for no other purpose, to combat damage suits. No doubt many fractures could be handled satisfactorily without resorting to the x-ray, but if no x-ray is used and there is the slightest trouble about the case, failure to employ, x-ray examination before and after treatment often is given as the cause of a suit for damages. Therefore, our members are urged to treat every fracture as a potential case for a damage suit and be sure to utilize the roentgen ray whether it is considered to be necessary or not.

Through its Fracture Committee the American College of Surgeons is now putting on a campaign in Georgia to secure better diagnosis and treatment of fractures. This applies not only to more careful and improved methods of handling by doctors, but also the more efficient first aid management of fractures by laymen. The latter applies especially to the treatment of fractures of the long bones where early traction is so important. Attempts are now being made to have Thomas splints and other apparatus placed in ambulances and at convenient points throughout the State, where they will be readily available to laymen who will be taught to put them on until the patient can reach a doctor or a hospital. The earlier traction is applied in the fracture of extremities the better the end result will be and the less suffering the patient will have to undergo.

The Georgia Fracture Committee intends to urge the officers of various medical organizations of the State to include fracture demonstrations, papers and clinics on their programs to a greater extent than has been done in the past. A fracture is one of the most

Medical Defense

Frank K. Boland, Chairman (1938) ....Atlanta
Wm. A. Mulherin (1939) ....Augusta
A. R. Rozar (1941) ....Macon
J. A. Redfearn, Chairman of Council........Albany
Edgar D. Shanks, Secretary-Treasurer.......Atlanta

Hospitals

R. H. Oppenheimer, Chairman (1937).....Atlanta
Arthur D. Little (1941), ...Thomasville
D. Henry Poer (1938) ....Atlanta
C. D. Whelchel (1939) ....Gainesville
L. P. Holmes (1940) ....Augusta

Abner Wellborn Calhoun Lectureship

Jas. E. Paullin, Chairman (1938) ....Atlanta
H. I. Reynolds (1939) ....Athens
Eugene E. Murphey (1940) . . . . Atlanta
J. M. Smith (1941) ....Valdosta
Frank K. Boland (1937) ....Atlanta

Economics

Lewis M. Gaines, Chairman (1940) ....Atlanta
C. W. Roberts (1938) ....Atlanta
C. L. Ridley (1941) ....Macon
Dan Y. Sage (1937) ....Atlanta
J. H. Downey (1939) ....Gainesville

Sub-Committee on Compilation
Medical Economics

Jas. E. Paullin, Chairman ....Atlanta
C. W. Roberts ....Atlanta
L. M. Gaines ....Atlanta
T. F. Abercrombie ....Atlanta
Edgar D. Shanks, Secretary-Treasurer.......Atlanta

Necrology

A. J. Mooney, Chairman ....Statesboro
Thos. J. McArthur...................Cordele
C. K. Sharp........................Arlington

Medical History of Georgia
Sub-Committee

Frank K. Boland, Chairman...........Atlanta
William R. Dancy....................Savanah
Arthur G. Fort......................Atlanta
V. H. Bassett......................Savannah
Allen H. Bunce....................Atlanta

Crawford W. Long Memorial Prize

William R. Dancy, Chairman...........Savannah
Stewart R. Roberts..................Atlanta
V. P. Syndenstricker ....Augusta
George Bachmann ....Atlanta
Edgar R. Pund ....Augusta

Cancer Commission

Jas. L. Campbell, Chairman.............Atlanta
William H. Myers...................Savannah
Charles H. Watt...................Thomasville
J. C. Patterson.....................Cuthbert
Kenneth S. Hunt....................Griffin
Charles C. Harrold..................Macon
W. P. Harbin, Jr......................Rome
Kenneth McCullough ....Waycross
Grady N. Coker.....................Canton
Ralph H. Chaney...................Augusta

Advisory—State Board of Health

C. W. Roberts, Chairman..............Atlanta
Craig Barrow ....Savannah
M. E. Winchester...................Brunswick
M. M. McCord.........................Rome

Marvin H. Head...................Zebulon
A. H. Hilsman......................Albany
T. F. Abercrombie..................Atlanta

Sub-Committee
Advisory—State Board of Health
Social Security Act
J. R. McCord, Chairman.............Atlanta
O. R. Thompson.....................Macon
Joseph Akerman ....Augusta

Advisory—Woman's Auxiliary
Jas. N. Brawner, Chairman..........Atlanta
Wm. R. Dancy.....................Savannah
W. A. Selman.......................Atlanta
W. R. Garner....................Gainesville
Benjamin Bashinski ....Macon

L. G. Hardman Loving Cup
W. A. Selman, Chairman.............Atlanta
Wm. A. Mulherin...................Augusta
Chas. H. Watt...................Thomasville
M. M. McCord........................Rome

Post-Graduate Study
G. Lombard Kelly, Chairman.........Augusta
Russell H. Oppenheimer.......Emory University
Chas. H. Watt...................Thomasville
W. W. Chrisman.....................Macon

Scientific Exhibit ..
Mark S. Dougherty, General Chairman......Atlanta
Thomas Harrold, Local Chairman.........Macon
Lee Howard ....Savannah
Everett L. Bishop..................Atlanta
J. L. Campbell.....................Atlanta
W. L. Pomeroy.....................Waycross
Wm. P. Harbin, Jr...................Rome
Wm. F. Jenkins...................Columbus
Roy R. Kracke.............Emory University
Fred A. Mettler....................Augusta
J. A. Redfearn.....................Albany
T. F. Sellers......................Atlanta
Ernest F. Wahl.................Thomasville

Prize for Hookworm Control*
W. F. Reavis, Chairman............Waycross
E. F. Wahl....................Thomasville
H. M. Tolleson....................Eastman
*Award by the Ware County Medical Society.

Study of Maternal Mortality and Infant Deaths
H. F. Shapley, Jr., Chairman..........Savanah

First District
A. J. Mooney....................Statesboro
A. J. Waring.....................Savannah

Second District
W. L. Wilkinson..................Bainbridge
W. W. Jarrell...................Thomasville

Third District
Herschel A. Smith.................Americus
J. C. Patterson...................Cuthbert

Fourth District
H. J. Copeland.....................Griffin
Emory R. Park....................LaGrange

Fifth District
E. D. Colvin.......................Atlanta
J. R. McCord.......................Atlanta

Sixth District
Otis R. Thompson...................Macon
T. C. Clodfelter..................Eatonton

Seventh District
P. O. Chaudron..................Cedartown
W. Mayes Gober....................Marietta

Eighth District
M. E. Winchester.................Brunswick
C. M. Stephens....................Waycross

Ninth District
Pratt Cheek ....Gainesville
Geo. C. Brooke.....................Canton

Tenth District
S. S. Smith........................Athens
John W. Thurmond, Jr..............Augusta

ex officio
T. F. Abercrombie, Director, Department of
Public Health for Georgia.............Atlanta

Fraternal Delegate to the
Georgia Dental Association
R. Hugh Wood......................Atlanta

Fraternal Delegate to the
Georgia Pharmaceutical Association
Glenville Giddings ....Atlanta

Fraternal Delegates to Other State Meetings
To VISIT ALABAMA: Wallace H. Clark, LaGrange,
and C. K. Sharp, Arlington.
To VISIT FLORIDA: Wm. S. Goldsmith, Atlanta,
and Arthur G. Fort, Atlanta.
To VISIT NORTH CAROLINA: Clarence L. Ayers,
Toccoa, and Grady N. Coker, Canton.
To VISIT SOUTH CAROLINA: Wm. A. Mulherin,
Augusta, and H. M. Michel, Augusta.

State Board of Health
First District—Cleveland Thompson, Millen, Sept. 1,
1939.
Second District—C. K. Sharp, Arlington, Sept. 1,
1939.
Third District—Mr. R. C. Ellis, Americus, Sept. 1,
1936.
Fourth District—Marvin M. Head, Zebulon, Sept. 1,
1937.
Fifth District—Mr. Robert F. Maddox, Atlanta, Sept.
1, 1936.
Sixth District—A. R. Rozar, Macon, Sept. 1, 1938.
Seventh District—Mather M. McCord, Rome, Sept.
1, 1938.
Eighth District—Henry W. Clements, Adel, Sept. 1,
1938.
Ninth District—L. C. Allen, Hoschton, Sept. 1, 1939.
Tenth District—Wm. A. Mulherin, Augusta, Sept.
1, 1937.

State of Georgia at Large
Pharmaceutical Association
T. C. Marshall, Atlanta, Sept. 1, 1941.
W. T. Edwards, Augusta, Sept. 1, 1941.

Georgia Dental Association
J. G. Williams, D.D.S., Atlanta, 1940.
Paul McGee, D.D.S., Waycross, Sept. 1, 1940.

WOMAN'S AUXILIARY

OFFICERS, 1936-1937

President—Mrs. Wm. R. Dancy, Savannah.
President-Elect—Mrs. Ralph H. Chaney, Augusta.
First Vice-President—Mrs. B. H. Minchew, Waycross.
Second Vice-President—Mrs. Clarence L. Ayers, Toccoa.
Third Vice-President—Mrs. J. A. Redfearn, Albany.

Recording Secretary—Mrs. Warren A. Coleman, Eastman.
Corresponding Secretary—Mrs. Lee Howard, Savannah.
Treasurer—Mrs. W. A. Selman, Atlanta.
Historian—Mrs. Grady N. Coker, Canton.
Parliamentarian—Mrs. John E. Penland, Waycross.

PRESIDENT'S REPORT

Nine students have been helped through medical schools since the organization of the Student Loan Fund. One will graduate at the University of Georgia School of Medicine, Augusta, this year.

Members reported to date by twenty-two Auxiliaries are 339. Ten other counties have not been heard from. Two members at large from unorganized counties have been reported. Toombs and Troup County Auxiliaries have been organized. Auxiliaries in Burke, Jenkins and Screven counties have been consolidated into one organization.

The Advisory Committee of the Association outlined our program for the year on heart disease and child psychology and supplied health material on the following subjects: Suggestions for New Mothers, Lighting the Home, Whooping Cough, Glasses We Wear, Georgia Mothers, Help to Health, Posture Fever, Pneumonia, How to Care for the Heart, Skin Diseases of Children, Parents Responsibility in Disease Control and Cancer in Women.

A total of 32,000 pamphlets have been distributed.

Contact with every civic organization in Georgia was made by our Public Relations Chairman.

Health Films have been shown by practically all Auxiliaries.

Histories of the county organizations and of the State have been written. District and State scrapbooks have been kept.

Doctors Day was observed. Its observance demands some act of kindness, gift or tribute. The resolution to observe "Doctors Day" was submitted by our Auxiliary and adopted by the Auxiliary to the American Medical Association in June, 1935.

Mrs. J. Harry Rogers, Press and Publicity Chairman, Atlanta, has obtained space in the Atlanta Constitution for reports of the Auxiliary.

Names of members who have died during the year are: Mrs. M. B. Allen, Hoschton; Mrs. T. J. Charlton, Sr., Savannah; Mrs. H. H. McGee, Savannah; Mrs. J. A. Selden,

Macon; Mrs. J. H. Terrell, Toccoa; and Mrs. Willingham, Canton.

The Auxiliary studied health conditions in various counties and cooperated with health officers in their work to prevent diphtheria, smallpox, tuberculosis and typhoid fever.

Obtained subscriptions to Hygiea.

Contributed to the Romance in Medicine Library and used its facilities for our enlightenment.

Programs were sponsored on Jane Todd Crawford, other heroes and heroines.

Clarke County

Mrs. G. O. Whelchel was hostess to the members of the Auxiliary at the home of Mrs. H. H. Cobb on Milledge Avenue, Athens, on May 1st. Mrs. W. H. Cabaniss was in charge of the program. Mrs. Chas. Brightwell gave a sketch of the "Life of Jane Todd," who submitted to an abdominal operation without an anesthetic, recovered and lived for several years. Mrs. S. S. Smith gave a brief history of the life and work of "Louis Pasteur," who discovered a treatment for the prevention of rabies.

Miss Mary Sue Oliver sang, "If God Left Only You," accompanied by Miss Wynelle Johnson, pianist.

Mrs. H. W. Birdsong, President, called the meeting to order and offered the opening prayer.

The Treasurer's report showed that $5.00 had been sent to the storm sufferers at Gainesville.

Plans were made for the picnic for the husbands and children of members in May.

Annual report to the State convention was read.

Most of the members present paid dues for the fiscal year to April, 1937.

Officers elected for the ensuing year were: Mrs. H. G. Banister, Ila, President; Mrs. S. S. Smith, Athens, Vice-President; Mrs. G. L. Loden, Colbert, Secretary; and Mrs. H. M. Fullilove, Athens, Treasurer.

Habersham County

The Woman's Auxiliary entertained the members of the Habersham County Medical Society in the home of Dr. and Mrs. T. H.

Brabson, Cornelia, March 30th, "Doctor's Day."

Miss Ramona Garrison, daughter of Dr. and Mrs. D. H. Garrison, Clarkesville, read "Menagerie Diet;" Miss Hazel Addison, Piedmont College, sang "Alice Blue Gown" and "Smoke Gets in Your Eyes," accompanied by Miss Betty Boling, Piedmont College, pianist. Mr. G. C. Jackson, son of Dr. and Mrs. J. B. Jackson, Clarkesville, read "Kep' In;" Miss Doris Brabson, daughter of Dr. and Mrs. T. H. Brabson, read "Morning Dale;" piano solo, "Manhattan Serenade" by Miss Addison. Refreshments were served. Dr. D. H. Garrison read one of his own compositions in response to requests.

Clarke County

The members of the Clarke County Medical Society were entertained Monday evening, March 31st, by the members of the Auxiliary, at the home of Dr. and Mrs. H. W. Birdsong, Athens.

Upon arrival the guests were served a course dinner at small tables grouped around. The place cards were tiny telephones. The guests found their places at the tables by finding their own telephone numbers. As they were seated each guest was given two sheets of paper and a few pins, and while they were waiting to be served they made hats of this paper. Mrs. Paul Holliday received a lovely garden hat and a flower sprinkler as the ladies' prize for the best hat. Dr. Stewart Brown, Royston, was the winner of the contest for the men, and received a set of garden tools.

A wealth of golden and pink shaded flowers decorated the rooms very beautifully in artistic arrangement.

Mrs. Birdsong, the President of the Auxiliary, told the object of the meeting—that it was "Doctor's Day," a day the Auxiliary had set aside to honor the doctors past and present. She also announced that a committee headed by Mrs. G. O. Whelchel that morning placed flowers on the graves of twenty-three of the doctors who in the past have practiced medicine here—among the list was the name of Dr. Crawford W. Long. A tribute to the medical profession written by Mrs. J. Bonar White was read.

Mrs. H. G. Banister, Ila, the Vice-President of the Auxiliary, directed the program. Miss Evelyn Christian of Elberton, delighted the members with her tap dancing. Miss Caroline Vance gave a reading. Mrs. Thomas Seymour, of Elberton, sang, "Sylvia." She was accompanied on the piano by Mrs. D. N. Thomson, of Elberton.

John Hudson and William Hammack gave a radio program. They delighted their audience for several minutes pulling jokes on almost every doctor present.

Those assisting Mrs. Birdsong in entertaining were her daughter, Miss Elizabeth Birdsong, Miss Cornelia Smith, Mrs. G. L. Loden, and Mrs. H. G. Banister.

Among the out of town guests were Dr. and Mrs. Stewart Brown, of Royston; Dr. and Mrs. D. N. Thompson, and Dr. and Mrs. D. V. Bailey, of Elberton; Dr. and Mrs. W. D. Gholston, of Danielsville, and Dr. and Mrs. L. L. Whitley, of Crawford.

HISTORY

A MESSAGE FROM THE HISTORY COMMITTEE

It will be impossible for the Committee on History to prepare a satisfactory account of medicine in Georgia without assistance from many sources. To publish a history giving mainly dates and statistics would be most uninteresting. In order to write a history which will be interesting, as well as full of facts, the Committee very much desires to secure any ancedotes and stories concerning Georgia doctors and medicine in the Empire State.

When attending a state medical meeting one constantly hears various members tell what this or that doctor said or did, or what one of their old professors had stated. To catch incidents of this kind and put them into print will give the history a human touch, or in other words give it some of the color which is spoken of so much today.

The members of the Medical Association of Georgia are urged to send the Committee material of this kind. It is true that some of the matter might not be available for publication, but the Committee feels that through this means important data may be obtained for publication in the Medical History of Georgia.

COMMITTEE ON THE HISTORY OF MEDICINE IN GEORGIA.

COUNTY REPORTING FOR 1936

Grady County Medical Society

The Grady County Medical Society announces the following officers for 1936:

President—A. B. Reynolds, Cairo.
Secretary-Treasurer—J. V. Rogers, Cairo.
Delegate—J. V. Rogers, Cairo.

The Julius Rosenwald Fund, 4901 Ellis Avenue, Chicago, has just published a booklet entitled "New Plans of Medical Service."

GEORGIA DEPARTMENT OF PUBLIC HEALTH

T. F. ABERCROMBIE, M.D., *Director*

SOME OBSERVATIONS ON MORBIDITY AND THE REQUIREMENTS OF ENTRANCE INTO THE MORBIDITY REPORTING AREA

"Morbidity statistics had their origin in the requirement of the notification of cases of certain dreaded diseases, notably, smallpox." With the appointment of health officers and the establishment of health departments, the reporting of other diseases has been requird. As the knowledge of the cause, source, and transmission of disease has become available, health authorities have become charged with an ever-increasing responsibility for the control of preventable disease. The list of notifiable diseases has continued to grow, and rightfully so, since the demand for accurate data concerning the causative agent, incubation period, length of illness, means of transmission, proper methods of prevention and control, are most useful weapons in the hands of practitioners as well as health authorities. It is impossible to effectually control any disease without first knowing when, where, and under what conditions that disease is occurring. No one would think of attempting control of an outbreak without first making provision for the prompt and accurate reporting of data regarding the occurrence of cases. Further, it is necessary that accurate and complete morbidity reports be obtained from cities, counties and states in order that we may know what is happening in the United States, in any state, or in any community. The correlation of these reports by the epidemiological section of the League of Nations gives us knowledge of the entire world at any given period, or over periods of years. Comparisons, trends, and incidence of diseases certainly can be made on this large scale which are not applicable to smaller communities.

We have a law in Georgia comparable to the law of most states, which requires either physicians or laymen, having knowledge of communicable disease, to report to the proper health authority. Unfortunately, we have not progressed to the point where reporting of communicable disease is as important as condemning an unsafe building. If a school building were condemned, it would be vacated and a new one built. If communicable disease occurs, it is taken as a matter of course. Yet which is the greatest cause of death?

What is wrong with our conception of values?

The Health Department, or no other governmental agency for that matter, has the intimate contact with the general population necessary for the collection of cases of reportable diseases; our chief reliance must be placed in the practicing physician. It is he who has first hand information of what is occurring among his clientele. Here again our sense of values has become onesided. We have had the idea of strict professional ethics drilled into us from the time of our entrance into medical college. We have been taught that each case of illness was our sacred trust and warned against the consequences of divulging its nature. Has our education included that, as physicians, we are primarily charged with the health and protection of our communities? By protecting our ethics don't we frequently break a legal obligation to the state, and what is more important a moral one to our clientele and respective communities? Certainly the failure to report communicable disease may lead to its spread among others whose rights we have ignored.

The question can be asked, what is the need of reporting? Prompt, accurate, and complete reporting gives the health ocffier as well as the physician:

1. The color, sex, and age distribution of disease.
2. The geographical distribution and seasonal occurrence of diseases.
3. The location of cases which constitute foci.
4. The source of occupational diseases and often their remedy.
5. The need of sanitation, pure water, drainage, sanitaria, immunizations, etc.
6. Knowledge of incidence, virulence and trends over periods of time.
7. Knowledge of other cases which may require immediate attention as in ophthalmia neonatorium and diphtheria.
8. An accurate picture of what may be accomplished by good health work.
9. Many other factors which may lead to a better understanding and better methods of treatment and prevention.

The chief source of error in morbidity statistics is failure of reporting. The U. S. Public Health Service has set up a standard by which reporting may be judged. Quoting from reprint No. 1478 of Public Health Reports, Vol. 46: 22, we find that: "This plan is based (a) on the facilities of the health department for collecting reports of cases of notifiable diseases and (b) on the case fatality rates for five diseases for three years. The requirements are as follows: (1) Inclusion in the registration areas for deaths and births; (2) adequate legislation to enforce reporting; (3) machinery for securing reports and keeping records; (4) a clerical force sufficient to do the work required; and (5) a willingness to cooperate in efforts to secure more nearly complete reports of morbidity." The State Department of Health can comply with all of the above requirements except the last. "Consideration is given to the results of the survey of the completeness of morbidity reporting which was conducted during 1930 in all states where this survey was made. In addition, the reports to the Public Health Service for the years 1927, 1928, and 1929 have been examined and an analysis of these reports on the basis of case fatality rates (number of cases per death) has been made. The diseases used in the analysis were diphtheria, measles, scarlet fever, typhoid fever and whooping cough.

"For each year for each disease we calculated a fatality rate (cases per death) based on all cases and deaths reported to the Public Health Service by all states which were in the registration area for deaths. This gave 15 standards, each of which was practically the average fatality rate for one year for one disease in the entire death registration area.

"The reciprocal of each fatality rate for each state was divided by the reciprocal of the proper standard fatality rate, and the resulting percentages were tabulated. The percentages for each state for the three years were averaged, and then these separate averages for the five diseases were again averaged. This gave a single percentage for each state, which percentage was based on the fatality rate for three years for the five diseases. States showing a general average of more than 100 per cent (that is, having better reporting than the average as indicated by the fatality rates) were graded "Standard,' while those states falling below the average of 100 per cent were classed as "Below Standard." Equal weight was given to the fatality rates for each of the five diseases." Let us now look at Table I where we can compare the standing of the various states since the inauguration of this plan.

Looking over the results since the inauguration of this plan we find that twenty-four states were admitted in 1931, two in 1932, four in 1933, two in 1934, and five in 1935. Georgia lies fifth from the bottom of the list of those remaining twelve states rated as "Below Standard."

I do not believe that it is the desire of the physicians of Georgia that our State shall remain among the few states that have not complied with the regulations for admission to the morbidity reporting area. All of the re-

at Eighty-Seventh Annual Session of the Medical
eorgia, Savannah, April 21, 22, 23, 24, 1936

Calhoun, F. P., Atlanta.
Campbell, J. L., Atlanta.
Cason, H. B., Jr., Warrenton.
Carpenter, Geo. L., Wrens.
Cathcart, Don F., Atlanta.
Chandler, J. H., Swainsboro.
Chaney, Ralph H., Augusta.
Cheney, G. W. Holmes, Brunswick.
Charlton, Thos. J., Savannah.
Cheek, O. H., Dublin.
Chisholm, Julian F., Savannah.
Chisholm, Julian F., Jr., Savannah.
Chrisman, W. W., Macon.
Clark, Jas. J., Atlanta.
Clifton, Ben H., Atlanta.
Coker, Grady N., Canton.
Cole, W. A., Savannah.
Coleman, Warren A., Eastman.
Coleman, Y. R., Macon.
Collier, Thos. W., Atlanta.
Colvin, E. D., Atlanta.
Colvin, E. G., Locust Grove.
Colvin, J. T., Jesup.
Cone, R. L., Statesboro.
Conn, Webb, Brunswick.
Cook, Wm. C., Columbus.
Corry, J. A., Barnesville.
Cousins, M. L., Atlanta.
Cranston, W. J., Augusta.
Crawford, W. B., Savannah.
Crawley, Walter G., Acworth.
Crovatt, J. G., Douglas.

Dancy, Wm. R., Savannah.
Darden, Horace, Sparta.
Davis, E. B., Byromville.
Davidson, A. A., Augusta.
Daniel, Jno. W., Savannah.
Daniel, Jno. W., Jr., Savannah.
Daniel, J. Wallace, Claxton.
Davison, Hal M., Atlanta.
Davison, T. C., Atlanta.
Deal, B. A., Statesboro.
Dean, J. G., Dawson.
deCaradeuc, St. J. R., Savannah.
Demmond, E. C., Savannah.
Derrick, H. C., Oglethorpe.
Dew, J. Harris, Atlanta.
Dickens, C. H., Madison.
Dismuke, H. L., Ocilla.
Dozier, H. W., Rocky Ford.
Dougherty, Mark S., Atlanta.
Downing, E. E., Newington.
Drane, Robert L., Savannah.
Dunn, L. B., Savannah.

Echols, Geo. L., Milledgeville.
Edmondson, H. T., Moultrie.
Edwards, D. B., Savannah.
Egan, M. J., Savannah.
Egloff, G. E., Savannah.
Ehrlich, M. A., Bainbridge.
Emery, W. B., Atlanta.
Elliott, W. G., Cuthbert.
Elrod, J. O., Forsyth.
Epting, M. J., Savannah.
Equeen, Murdock, Atlanta.
Eubanks, Geo. F., Atlanta.
Evans, E. L., Tifton.
Exley, Howard T., Savannah.

Faggart, Geo. H., Savannah.
Fancher, J. K., Atlanta.
Farmer, C. Hall, Macon.

Ferrell, R. G., Jr., Dublin.
Ferrell, Thomas J., Waycross.
Fincher, E. F., Jr., Atlanta.
Findley, C. W., Vidalia.
Fitts, Jno. B., Atlanta.
Fleming, Carlton A., Tifton.
Floyd, Earl, Atlanta.
Floyd, Waldo E., Statesboro.
Folk, Jno. J., Augusta.
Fort, Arthur G., Atlanta.
Fountain, Jas. A., Macon.
Fowler, A. H., Marietta.
Fowler, Major F., Atlanta.
Fowler, R. W., Marietta.
Franklin, R. C., Swainsboro.
Freedman, L. M., Savannah.
Fuller, Geo. W., Atlanta.
Funderburke, N. A., Trion.

Gaines, Lewis M., Atlanta.
Garner, J. R., Atlanta.
Gardner, W. A., Stone Mountain.
Garver, C. C., Atlanta.
Garrard, J. L., Rome.
Gary, Loren, Jr., Shellman.
Gay, Clifford J., Augusta.
Gay, J. Gaston, Atlanta.
Gay, T. Bolling, Atlanta.
Gholston, W. D., Danielsville.
Giddings, Glenville, Atlanta.
Gibson, B. Harrison, Allenhurst.
Gilbert, R. B., Greenville.
Gleaton, E. N., Savannah.
Goldsmith, Wm. S., Atlanta.
Goodwyn, Thos. P., Atlanta.
Goolsby, R. Cullen, Macon.
Graham, Rufus E., Savannah.
Gray, J. D., Augusta.
Greene, Ed H., Atlanta.
Greer, Chas. A., Oglethorpe.
Greer, C. B., Brunswick.
Greenblatt, Robt. B., Augusta.
Griggs, H. E., Conyers.
Gross, O. S., Vidalia.

Hall, J. I., Macon.
Hamm, W. G., Atlanta.
Harbin, W. P., Sr., Rome.
Harper, Harry T., Augusta.
Harper, Sage, Wray.
Harrell, H. P., Augusta.
Harris, E. R., Winder.
Harris, R. V., Savannah.
Harris, Wendel P., Augusta.
Harrold, Chas. C., Macon.
Head, M. M., Zebulon.
Henry, C. G., Augusta.
Hesse, Herman W., Savannah.
Hicks, Chas. L., Dublin.
Hill, Roy A., Thomasville.
Hillis, W. W., Sardis.
Hilsman, A. H., Albany.
Howard, H. L., Springfield.
Howard, Lee, Savannah.
Holliday, J. C., Athens.
Holmes, L. P., Augusta.
Holt, J. T., Baxley.
Holton, C. F., Savannah.
Hubert, M. A., Athens.
Hughes, J. M., Glennville.
Hunt, Kenneth S., Griffin.

Johnson, A. M., Valdosta.
Johnson, G. H., Savannah.
Johnson, Raymond L., Waycross.

Johnson, Ralph N., Rome.
Johnston, Z. V., Calhoun.
Jones, Jabez, Savannah.
Jones, John Paul, Savannah.

Kandel, H. M., Savannah.
Kay, Jas. B., Byron.
Keaton, J. C., Albany.
Keen, O. F., Macon.
Kelley, D. C., Lawrenceville.
Kelley, L. H., Atlanta.
Kelly, G. L., Augusta.
Kendrick, D. B., Atlanta.
Kilpatrick, A. J., Augusta.
King, Ruskin, Savannah.
Kirkland, Spencer A., Atlanta.
Kicklighter, R. B., Glennville.
Kiser, William, Jr., Atlanta.
Kitchens, S. B., LaFayette.
Kite, J. H., Atlanta.
Klugh, Geo. F., Atlanta.

Lancaster, E. M., Shady Dale.
Lancaster, H. H., Clermont.
Lang, G. H., Savannah.
Lang, J. Harry, Jr., Atlanta.
Lanier, L. I., Soperton.
Laws, Clarence, Atlanta.
Leadingham, Roy S., Atlanta.
Lee, Lawrence, Savannah.
Leslie, J. T., Augusta.
Levington, H. L., Savannah.
Levy, M. S., Augusta.
Little, Arthur D., Thomasville.
Long, W. V., Savannah.
Longino, L. P., Milledgeville.
Lowry, T., Cartersville.
Lunsford, Guy G., Savannah.

Maner, Edwin N., Savannah.
Mann, F. R., McRae.
Martin, J. D., Jr., Atlanta.
Martin, R. V., Savannah.
Martin, Wm. O., Jr., Atlanta.
Massey, W. F., Chester.
Massoud, M. A., Pineora.
McAllister, J. M. C., Rochelle.
McArthur, Thos. J., Cordele.
McCarver, W. C., Vidette.
McCollum, R. Roy, Kingsland.
McCord, Jas. R., Atlanta.
McCord, M. M., Rome.
McCord, Ralph B., Rome.
McCollough, K., Waycross.
McDaniel, J. G., Atlanta.
McDonald, Harold P., Atlanta.
McElveen, J. M., Brooklet.
McGahee, R. C., Augusta.
McGeary, W. C., Madison.
McGee, H. H., Savannah.
McGehee, Henry M., Moultrie.
McLaughlin, C. K., Savannah.
Mercer, J. E., Vidalia.
Mestre, Ricardo, Atlanta.
Metts, J. C., Savannah.
Michel, Henry M., Augusta.
Miles, W. G., Milledgeville.
Miller, Clifford, Portal.
Minchew, B. H., Waycross.
Mixson, W. D., Waycross.
Mobley, J. W., Jr., Pelham.
Monfort, J. M., Atlanta.
Montgomery, R. C., Butler.
Mooney, A. J., Statesboro.
Morrison, A. A., Savannah.
Morrison, Howard J., Savannah
Mulherin, Wm. A., Augusta.
Mulkey, O. A., Millen.
Mull, J. H., Rome.
Murphey, Eugene E., Augusta.

Muse, L. H., Atlanta.
Myers, Martin T., Atlanta.
Myers, Wm. H., Savannah.

Neal, L. G., Cleveland.
Neville, R. L., Savannah.
New, J. E., Dexter.
Newman, W. A., Macon.
Nicolson, W. P., Atlanta.
Norris, Jack C., Atlanta.
Norvell, John T., Augusta.
Nutt, J. J., Bowdon.

Oden, Thos. E., Blackshear.
Oliver, Robt. Lee, Savannah.
Olmstead, G. T., Savannah.
O'Neal, R. S., LaGrange.
O'Neill, J. C., Savannah.
Oppenheimer, R. H., Emory University.
Osborne, V. W., Atlanta.
Owens, J. D., Rochelle.
Owensby, N. M., Atlanta.

Palmer, J. W., Ailey.
Parkerson, I. J., Eastman.
Patterson, J. C., Cuthbert.
Paullin, Jas. E., Atlanta.
Pendergrass, R. C., Americus.
Penland, J. E., Waycross.
Penington, C. L., Macon.
Peterson, T. A., Savannah.
Phillips, A. M., Macon.
Philpot, W. K., Augusta.
Pinholster, J. H., Savannah.
Poer, D. Henry, Atlanta.
Pomeroy, W. L., Waycross.
Porter, J. L., Rutledge.
Price, W. T., Augusta.
Primrose, A. C., Americus.
Pruitt, M. C., Atlanta.
Pund, Edgar R., Augusta.

Quattlebaum, Julin K., Savannah.

Rabhan, L. J., Savannah.
Rawls, L. L., Macon.
Redfearn, J. A., Albany.
Redmond, C. G., Savannah.
Reid, C. W., Pelham.
Rhodes, R. I., Augusta.
Rhyne, W. P., Warm Springs.
Richards, W. R., Calhoun.
Richardson, Chas. H., Macon.
Righton, H. Y., Savannah.
Riner, C. R., Savannah.
Ritch, Thos. G., Jesup.
Rogers, F. D., Coleman.
Rogers, Harry, Atlanta.
Rogers, J. V., Cairo.
Roberts, C. W., Atlanta.
Roberts, H. Hines, Atlanta.
Robertson, J. Righton, Augusta.
Roles, C. J., Camilla.
Roper, C. J., Jasper.
Rosen, E. F., Waycross.
Rosen, S. F., Savannah.
Ross, Thos. L., Macon.
Roule, J. Victor, Augusta.
Rudder, Fred F., Atlanta.
Rushin, C. E., Atlanta.
Rushing, W. E., Millhaven.
Roy, Dunbar, Atlanta.
Rozar, A. R., Macon.

Sage, Dan Y., Atlanta.
Sand, Harry H., Savannah.
Sanderson, E. S., Augusta.
Sandison, J. Calvin, Atlanta.

Sanford, S. P., Savannah.
Sauls, H. C., Atlanta.
Saunders, Albert F., Valdosta.
Schaefer, W. B., Toccoa.
Schley, F. B., Columbus.
Schmidt, H. T., Augusta.
Schwalb, O. W., Savannah.
Sellers, T. F., Atlanta.
Selman, W. A., Atlanta.
Shallenberger, W. F., Atlanta.
Shanks, Edgar D., Atlanta.
Sharp, C. K., Arlington.
Sharpley, H. F., Savannah.
Sharpley, J. G., Savannah.
Shaw, L. W., Savannah.
Shepard, W. O., Bluffton.
Sherman, J. H., Augusta.
Simmons, Jno. W., Brunswick.
Simmons, Walter E., Metter.
Simonton, Fred H., Chickamaug
Simpson, J. A., Athens.
Smisson, R. C., Fort Valley.
Smith, A. C., Elberton.
Smith, Geo. B., Rome.
Smith, Horace D., Macon.
Smith, Leo, Homerville.
Smith, J. M., Valdosta.
Smith, R. H., Lincolnton.
Smith, S. S., Athens.
Smith, Wm. A., Atlanta.
Stapleton, C. E., Statesboro.
Stephenson, Frank, Savannah.
Steward, W. Dean, Augusta.
Stewart, J. A., Portal.
Stewart, Philip R., Monroe.
Storey, W. Edward, Savannah.
Strickland, L. V., Cobbtown.
Strickler, C. W., Atlanta.
Stultz, Walter A., Augusta.
Swanson, Cosby, Atlanta.
Sydenstricker, V. P., Augusta.

Taylor, R. L., Davisboro.
Tessier, L. P., Augusta.
Thomas, D. R., Jr., Atlanta.
Thomas, Frank E., Albany.
Thomas, J. W., Augusta.
Thomas, M. R., Savannah.
Thompson, Cleveland, Millen.
Thompson, D. N., Elberton.
Thompson, O. R., Macon.
Thompson, W. C., Dublin.
Tidmore, J. C., Atlanta.
Tidmore, T. L., Atlanta.
Tolleson, H. M., Eastman.
Touchton, Geo. L., Savannah.
Train, Jno. K., Savannah.
Traylor, Geo. A., Augusta.
Travis, W. D., Covington.
Trimble, W. H., Atlanta.
Turner, W. W., Maxwell.
Tyre, J. Lawton, Screven.
Tye, J. P., Albany.

Upchurch, W. E., Atlanta.
Usher, Chas., Savannah.

Wahl, Ernest F., Thomasville.
Waites, S. L., Covington.
Walker, D. D., Macon.
Walker, Geo. L., Griffin.
Wall, C. K., Thomasville.
Wall, J. Cox, Eastman.
Wall, W. H., Blakely.
Wallis, J. R., Lovejoy.
Ware, D. B., Fitzgerald.
Ware, R. M., Fitzgerald.
Waring, A. J., Savannah.
Waring, T. P., Savannah.
Wasden, C. N., Macon.

Watson, O. O., Macon.
Weaver, H. G., Macon.
Weaver, O. H., Macon.
Weaver, J. Calvin, Atlanta.
Welborn, T. W., Hinesville.
West, C. M., Atlanta.
Whelan, E. J., Savannah.
Williams, A. F., Collins.
Williams, L. A., Abbeville.
Williams, L. W., Savannah.
Williams, M. W., Savannah.
Williams, W. J., Augusta.
Willis, C. H., Barnesville.
Willis, T. V., Brunswick.
Wilson, Pleas, Newborn.
Wilson, R. B., Atlanta.
Wilson, S. E., Savannah.

Winchester, M. E., Brunswick.
Wise, B. T., Americus.
Wood, D. L., Dalton.
Woods, E. B., Augusta.
Wright, Edward S., Atlanta.
Wright, Geo. W., Augusta.
Wright, Peter W., Augusta.

Yampolsky, Jos., Atlanta.
Yarbrough, Y. H., Milledgeville.
Youmans, H. D., Lyons.
Youmans, J. R., Columbus.

GUESTS

Castle, Wm. Bosworth, Boston, Mass.
McLester, Jas. S., Birmingham, Ala.

Meakins, Jonathan C., Montreal, Quebec, Canada.
Shipley, Arthur M., Baltimore, Md.

VISITORS

Davis, T. H., Green Cove Springs, Fla.
Gray, F. D., Orlando, Fla.
Harrell, C. B., Rock Hill, S. C.
Johnston, B. R., Estill, S. C.
Mathis, W. H., North Augusta, S. C.
Morgan, Hugh J., Nashville, Tenn.
Pearson, Homer L., Miami, Fla.
Quillan, Warren W., Miami, Fla.
Warwick, H. L., Fort Worth, Tex.
White, E. P., Columbia, S. C.

NEWS ITEMS

Dr. W. L. Ballenger, Atlanta, was elected President of the Garden Hills Civic League at its annual meeting on April 13th.

Dr. R. B. Gilbert, Greenville, recently entertained the members of the Meriwether County Medical Society at dinner in the Manchester Hotel.

Dr. Harry Ainsworth, Thomasville, was elected Secretary of the Atlantic Coast Line Surgeon's Association at its annual meeting in Charleston, S. C., April 8th.

Dr. Hulett H. Askew announces that he has returned to his former practice of general medicine and surgery. His offices are located in the Candler Building, Atlanta.

Dr. Jack W. Jones has resumed his practice at Suite 711, Medical Arts Building, Atlanta, after being out of his office for several months.

Dr. Clarence B. Palmer, formerly of Rutledge, announces his removal to Suite 16, Star Building, Covington.

Dr. J. D. Gray, Augusta, spoke at the monthly meeting of the nurses' staff of the Richmond County Department of Health on *The Treatment of Diabetes* on April 16th.

Dr. T. M. Ezzard, Roswell, and Dr. John R. Walker, Atlanta, have installed equipment and opened a clinic in North Roswell in the Weaver Building.

The Second District Medical Society met at Quitman on April 10th. Titles of papers on the scientific program were: *The Diagnosis and Treatment of Hay Fever and Asthma*, by Dr. Hal M. Davison, Atlanta; *Transurethral Prostatic Resection*, Dr. J. C. Keaton, Albany; *Harelips and Cleft Palates*, Dr. Wm. G. Hamm, Atlanta; *Tobacco Amblyopia*, Dr. H. M. Moore, Thomasville; *Irregular Signs and Symptoms in Surgical Conditions*, Dr. C. S. Pittman, Tifton.

The Georgia Medical Society, Savannah, met on April 14th. Dr. H. J. Morrison read a paper entitled, *Antitoxin Treatment of Meningococcus Infection and Meningitis*; the discussion was led by Dr. A.

J. Waring and Dr. J. C. Metts. Dr. T. J. Charlton reported a case of *Acromegaly*. Refreshments were served.

The staff meeting of St. Joseph's Infirmary was held on April 28th. Dr. John W. Turner reported cases of *Primary Syphilis* and *Adenocarcinoma*; Dr. Randolph Smith, *Review of the Cases Injured in the Gainesville Storm*.

The Colquitt County Medical Society met at Hotel Colquitt, Moultrie, on April 7th. Dr. J. A. Redfearn, Albany, discussed the *Electrocardiograph and Its Use in the Diagnosis of Various Heart Conditions*; Dr. T. H. Chesnutt, Moultrie, read a paper on *Diphtheria*.

Dr. Chas. A. Greer, Oglethorpe, a former member of the lower house of the General Assembly of Georgia, announces his candidacy for State Senator to represent the Thirteenth District.

Dr. Evert A. Bancker, Jr., announces the removal of his offices to Suite 919, Doctors Building, 478 Peachtree Street, N.E., Atlanta.

The Macon Medical Society of Bibb County met in Ridley Hall, Macon, April 7th. Dr. Everett L. Bishop, Atlanta, gave a lecture on *Bone Tumors and Their Treatment by Radiation or Surgery*. Dr. Chas. C. Harrold, Dr. G. Y. Massenburg, Dr. A. R. Rozar and Dr. Thomas Harrold, all of Macon, reported cases.

Dr. C. C. Aven, Atlanta, spoke before a meeting of the Fifth District Nurses' Association, held in Atlanta on April 1st.

The officers of the medical staff of the Warren A. Candler Hospital, Savannah, were re-elected on April 3rd, as follows: Dr. W. A. Cole, President; Dr. D. B. Edwards, Vice-President; Dr. J. L. Elliott, Secretary-Treasurer.

The members of the Habersham County Medical Society were entertained in the home of Dr. and Mrs. T. H. Brabson, Cornelia, on March 30th, by members of the Woman's Auxiliary to the Society.

Dr. T. C. Davison, Dr. Hal M. Davison, Dr. Mason I. Lowance, Dr. Crawford F. Barnett and Dr. Marvin A. Mitchell announce the removal of their offices to Suite 207, Doctors' Building, 478 Peachtree Street, N.E., Atlanta. The offices were open to visitors on Tuesday afternoon, April 28th.

The Southeastern Surgical Congress will meet in Louisville, Ky., in 1937. The last assembly was held in New Orleans.

Dr. Calhoun McDougall, Atlanta, was elected to the Board of Directors of the Fulton National Bank at the April meeting of the Board.

The Sixteenth Annual Meeting of the Medical and Surgical Section of the Association of American Railroads was held at the Stevens Hotel, Chicago, Ill., May 11, 12. Surgeons on the program and titles of scientific papers were: Dr. J. R. Garner, Atlanta, *The Proper Study of Mankind is Man;* Dr. R. C. Webb, Minneapolis, Minn., Chief Surgeon of the Great Northern Railway, submitted report as Chairman of the Committee on Fractures; Dr. N. C. Gilbert, Chicago. *Predictable Causes of Sudden Disability;* Dr. Geo. G. Davis, Chicago, *Diagnosis and Treatment of Gas Bacillus Infection;* Dr. S. C. Plummer, Chicago, report as Chairman of the Committee on Developments Resulting from Physical Examinations; Dr. J. D. Collins, Detroit, report as Chairman of the Committee on Disability and Rehabilitation; Dr. Roland P. Mackay, Chicago, *Vascular Changes, Their Hazards Among Railway Employees;* Dr. T. R. Crowder, Chicago, report as Chairman of the Special Committee on Medical Aspects of Air Conditioning of Cars. Officers of the Association are: Dr. J. R. Garner, Atlanta, Chief Surgeon of the Atlanta and West Point Railroad Company, The Western Railway of Alabama and the Georgia Railroad, Chairman; Dr. D. B. Moss, Chicago, First Vice-Chairman; Mr. J. C. Caviston, New York City, Secretary.

The First District Medical Society will meet at Hotel DeSoto, Savannah, July 15th.

The Fulton County Medical Society met at the Academy of Medicine, Atlanta, on April 16th. The program consisted of a *Symposium on Obstructive Lesions of the Genito-Urinary Tract.* Dr. Montague L. Boyd read a paper entitled *Obstructive Lesions of the Kidney and Ureter;* discussed by Dr. Stephen T. Brown and Earl H. Floyd. Dr. E. G. Ballenger, Dr. O. F. Elder and Dr. H. P. McDonald, *Obstructive Lesions Involving the Bladder and Vesical Neck;* discussed by Dr. W. B. Emery, Dr. Major Fowler and Dr. M. K. Bailey. Dr. W. L. Champion, *Obstructive Lesions Involving the Urethra;* discussed by Dr. F. C. Nesbit and Dr. W. E. Upchurch. Dr. S. J. Sinkoe, *Mechanical Obstruction, An Important Factor in Urological Diagnosis and Therapy;* discussed by Dr. S. A. Kirkland and Dr. Clinton Reed.

The Coffee County Medical Society met in Douglas on April 28th. The scientific program consisted of a symposium on *Infections of the Genito-Urinary Tract.* Dr. B. O. Quillian, Douglas, read a paper entitled *Anatomy as Related to Symptoms;* Dr. T. H. Clark, Douglas, *Diagnosis and Treatment.* Dr. Sage Harper, Ambrose, led the discussion.

Dr. E. C. Harris, formerly of Hawkinsville, has removed to Macon and opened offices in the Bibb Building.

The regular staff meeting of the Macon Hospital, Macon, was held on April 28th. Members of the staff and visitors discussed case histories and unusual cases. The program was arranged by Dr. O. R. Thompson.

Dr. R. S. O'Neal, LaGrange, was elected President of the Alumni Association of the University of Georgia School of Medicine.

The Fulton County Medical Society met at the Academy of Medicine, Atlanta, May 7th. Dr. W. L. Cousins reported a case, *Type Four Pneumonia;* Dr. Stewart R. Roberts, *The Hemorrhagic Disease—Two Cases of Leukemia;* Dr. Everett L. Bishop made a clinical talk, *Some Observations on Melanoma—Lantern Slides;* Dr. Walter W. Daniel, *Influence of Pregnancy on Tuberculosis;* Dr. Linton Smith read a paper entitled *Prenatal Use of Quinine with Report of Sixty Cases.* Dr. W. A. Selman, Dr. Jno. C. Ivey and Dr. Jane Grezda led the discussion.

Dr. Dan C. Elkin, Atlanta, reported to the American Association of Thoracic Surgeons at Rochester, Minnesota, on May 4th, the success of *Surgical Treatment of Thirteen Persons with Stab Wounds in Their Hearts.*

Conferences on public health, sponsored by the Medical Association of Georgia, State Board of Health and the United States Public Health Service, have been scheduled for the dates and places mentioned: Seventh District, Rome, Monday, June 15th; Fifth District, Atlanta, Tuesday, June 16th; Ninth District, Cornelia, Wednesday, June 17th; Tenth District, Athens, Thursday, June 18th; Sixth District, Milledgeville, Friday, June 19th; Fourth District, Warm Springs, Monday, June 22nd; Third District, Americus, Tuesday, June 23rd; Second District, Albany, Wednesday, June 24th; Eighth District, Waycross, Thursday, June 25th; First District, Savanah, Friday, June 26th. Two teams will direct the conferences. The first team will discuss pediatrics, obstetrics and venereal diseases; the second team, heart disease, cancer and preventive inoculations. The second team will begin on Monday, June 22nd at Rome and follow the same hours and itinerary as the first team.

Dr. J. R. Garner, Atlanta, on invitation from the North Carolina Industrial Commission, spoke on *Proper Seating Increases Industrial Efficiency* before the seventh annual State-Wide Industrial Safety Conference at Charlotte, N. C., held on May 14-15.

At the time of his death, he was a member of the Carroll County Medical Society, American Medical Association, F. & A. M., Shrine, and the First Presbyterian church of Atlanta. Surviving him are his widow and one brother, Chas. A. Lyle, Cedartown. Funeral services were conducted from the First Baptist church at Carrollton by Rev. H. P. Bell, Rev. E. A. Kilgore and Rev. H. C. Emory. Burial was in the city cemetery. Members of the Carroll County Medical Society formed an honorary escort.

Dr. *James Meriweather Hull*, Augusta; member: University of Georgia School of Medicine, Augusta, 1879; aged 77; died at his home after a long illness on April 13, 1936. He was born in Athens and moved with his mother to Augusta when quite young. His father was killed in the Confederate Army during the Civil War. Dr. Hull received his literary education at Georgetown University. After graduating in medicine, he spent three years at Vienna and Berlin under professors of universities in those cities. Immediately after completing his studies in Europe, he returned to Augusta, began practice and was appointed on the faculty of the University of Georgia School of Medicine. For more than a half century, Dr. Hull had been engaged in the practice of medicine and an instructor in medicine, and was regarded as the dean of the profession in Augusta. Surviving him are three sons, J. M. Hull, Jr., and Frank L. Hull, both of Augusta, and Lamar Hull, of New York City; two daughters, Mrs. Earl M. Kaminer and Mrs. R. Beverly Herbert, both of Columbia, S. C. Funeral services were conducted from the residence of his son by Rev. John A. Wright, Rector of the St. Paul's Episcopal church. Interment was in Magnolia cemetery.

Dr. *Charles Williams Crane*, Augusta; member: University of Georgia School of Medicine, Augusta, 1898; aged 61; died at his home on April 1, 1936. He was a skilled surgeon and gained wide recognition for his unusual ability and thoroughness. Dr. Crane was for a number of years Clinical Professor of Surgery at the University of Georgia School of Medicine. He was active in civic affairs and had many close personal friends. Surviving him are his widow and one sister, Miss Caroline B. Crane. Private funeral services were conducted from the residence by Rev. E. C. Lucas, Pastor of the First Christian church. The body was transferred to Macon for cremation.

Dr. *John Monroe Sigman*, Macon; member: University of Georgia School of Medicine, Augusta, 1904; aged 56; died in the United States Veterans' Hospital, Atlanta, April 10, 1936. He was born at Social Circle, moved to Hancock County with his parents while a youth, and after he received his degree in medicine, he moved to Macon and began practice. For many years before his death Dr. Sigman limited his practice to dermatology. He served as Major in the medical corps of the United States Army during the World War. Dr. Sigman was charitable, as shown by his act in writing off about fifty thousand dollars of accounts during the recent depression and mailed receipts to his patients and clientele. He was a prominent physician, held in high esteem by many acquaintances and one of the State's best citizens. Dr. Sigman was a member of the American Legion, Macon Medical Society of Bibb County and the American Medical Association. Surviving him are his widow, two daughters, Misses Mary Shaw Sigman and Margaret Sigman, of Macon; his mother, Mrs. Fanny Cheney Sigman, Sparta. Funeral services were conducted from the Burghard-Connally Funeral Home, Macon, by Dr. J. P. Boone, Pastor of the First Baptist church. Burial was in the family burial lot in the Sparta city cemetery. Members of the American Legion and the Macon Medical Society formed an honorary escort.

Dr. *William Eugene Worsham*, Macon; Louisville Medical College, Louisville, Ky., 1891; aged 71; died of pneumonia in a private hospital at Macon on April 14, 1936. He was born in Crawford County and moved with his parents to Macon while an infant. Dr. Worsham attended the public schools of Macon, then Mercer University, later the Louisville Medical College. After he served his internship, he returned to Macon and began practice with his father, Dr. J. H. D. Worsham. He was a prominent physician and practiced in Macon for more than forty years. Surviving him are one daughter, Mrs. C. T. Hodges, Macon; two sons, D. W. Worsham, Macon, and Jas. A. Worsham, Portland, Oregon. Funeral services were conducted by Dr. Ellis Sammons, Pastor of the Vineville Baptist church, from the Burghard-Connally Funeral Home. Burial was in Riverside cemetery.

Dr. *William Henry Estes*, Lincolnton; University of Georgia School of Medicine, Augusta, 1900; aged 59; died at his home on April 21, 1936. He was widely known as a physician and had many friends throughout the State. Dr. Estes served two terms in the lower house of the General Assembly of Georgia. He was a good citizen and philanthropist.

Dr. *Robert Lee Miller*, Waynesboro; member; University of Georgia School of Medicine, Augusta, 1891; aged 66; died at his home on March 31, 1936. He was born at Hephzibah, Richmond County, and received his high school education there and later attended Mercer University, Macon. Dr. Miller practiced for more than forty years and won hundreds of friends by his kind and skilled treatment of patients. He was favorably known by the medical profession of the State through his loyalty to the Association and attendance at many of its annual sessions. Dr. Miller was a member of the Burke County Medical Society and the Waynesboro Baptist church. Surviving him, are his widow, two sisters, Mrs. Ruth Miller Thomas, Waynesboro, and Mrs. Lula Miller Frost, Hephzibah. Rev. Walter L. Moore conducted the funeral services from the Waynesboro Baptist church. Interment was in Magnolia cemetery. Members of the Burke County Medical Society and many from the Richmond County Medical Society, formed an honorary escort.

Dr. *Jesse P. Prescott*, Lake Park; member; Emory University School of Medicine, Emory University, 1890; aged 70; died at his home after a short illness

the book with interest and ease. In all, this is a
very interesting and instructive book.

JOSEPH C. MASSEE, M.D.

The Paratyphoids in Health and in Disease. By Dr.
David H. Shelling, B.Sc., M.D., John Hokins Hospital, Baltimore, Maryland. 335 pages. St. Louis,
Missouri: The C. V. Mosby Company, 1935. Cloth.
$5.00. This volume is most timely. The parathyroids
were first described in 1860, but their importance was
not understood until the last twenty-five years.

Dr. Shelling has given us a very comprehensive study
of the subject, including the anatomy, physiology and
pathology of the parathyroids. He has given full details of the most recent investigations on the effects
of parathyroid tumors on calcium metabolism, which
has so radically changed our views on certain bone
pathology.

This book will be of special interest to the various
specialties as well as to the surgeon and the internist.
There is attached an exhaustive bibliography for the
benefit of those who wish to investigate the subject
further. This volume should be in every medical library.

T. C. DAVISON, M.D.

ELEVENTH REVISION OF THE UNITED STATES PHARMACOPEIA

On June 1 of this year, the eleventh revision of
the United States Pharmacopeia becomes official. In
general style and method of presentation the new revision follows closely the old one. The degree of
progress achieved in this new revision can perhaps
be better measured by examining the deletions and
admissions.

In all there are 119 deleted products in the new
Pharmacopeia. The most common reason for these
deletions is that these products have become obsolete
in usage or have been superceded by pharmaceutically
and medicinally better products.

The new additions to the Pharmacopeia, although
only 58 in number, are examples of very careful and
conservative selection by the Committee of Revision.
Many of these additions are already familiar to the
physician in new and non-official remedies. They now
achieve the distinction of being officially recognized.
The official biologicals have been increased from three
in the Tenth Revision to thirteen in the present one.
Their nomenclature and standardization are controlled
and regulated by the National Institute of Health. A
sub-committee on Vitamins will supervise the standardization of vitamins A and D in Cod Liver Oil
Preparations. Liver and stomach preparations will be
controlled by the U. S. P. Anti-anemia Preparations
Board.

There has been various changes in pharmaceutical
products too numerous to mention in detail. These
revisions were effected with the view in mind to
provide greater uniformity in strength, stability, quality and purity. Among the minor changes are several on nomenclature and spelling. While not vitally
important, it is well to be informed of these changes

even at the risk of being considered meticulous.

In practice initiated within the past two years of issuing an Interim Revision will become an established policy in the new Pharmacopeia. This should tend to keep the Pharmacopeia up-to-date as it will no longer be necessary to wait several years to introduce products of established value.

The Committee of Revisions and publishers are to be congratulated and thanked for their altruistic and untiring efforts; and although this is not the type of book that will be read "from cover to cover" it should be included in the library of every physician and druggist, and it is hoped that they will soon acquaint themselves with this worth while work.

J. D. KITCHENS, PH.G.

RAYMOND HERTWIG, FORMER SECRETARY OF THE COMMITTEE ON FOODS OF THE A. M. A., ASSOCIATED WITH BORDEN CO.

Raymond Hertwig, Secretary of the Committee on Foods of the American Medical Association since the committee's organization in 1930, has become associated with The Borden Company.

Mr. Hertwig's services were available in consequence of the recent decision of the Board of Trustees of the American Medical Association to combine the work of its various Councils under one directorship and to largely restrict the work of the Committee on Foods.

Coming to the Committee on Foods when it had just been organized, Mr. Hertwig developed its program, the purpose of which was to prevent or discourage unwarranted, incorrect or false advertising claims in the promotion and merchandising of food products. This pioneer work is declared to have had a strong influence on food advertising and to have raised general advertising standards.

Officials of the Borden Company expressed great satisfaction over Mr. Hertwig's availability to their organization because the ideals of food quality and advertising ethics of The Borden Company have coincided so closely with those of the Committee on Foods. To date, 45 products of The Borden Company have been granted the Seal of Acceptance by the Committee.

Mr. Hertwig spent 12 years with the Bureau of Chemistry of the United States Department of Agriculture from which he gained an intimate knowledge of the manufacture, analysis, composition, adulteration and misbranding of foods and of the enforcement of the Federal Foods and Drugs Act.

THE TRUE ECONOMY OF DEXTRI-MALTOSE

It is interesting to note that a fair average of the length of time an infant receives Dextri-Maltose is five months: That these five months are the most critical of the baby's life: That the difference in cost to the mother between Dextri-Maltose and the very cheapest carbohydrate, at most is only $6 for this entire period—a few cents a day: That, in the end, it costs the mother less to employ regular medical attendance for the baby than to attempt to do her own feeding, which in numerous cases leads to a seriously sick baby eventually requiring the most costly medical attendance.

AN IMPROVED ANESTHETIC TECHNIQUE FOR GENERAL SURGERY

Fraser, W. A., and Gwathmey, J. T. (Surgery, Gynecology and Obstetrics, 62: 236-237, (Feb. 1), 1936)

In this study, various combinations of analgesic and anesthetic drugs were used with a view of attempting to improve on the present surgical technique, first, by abolishing psychic influence before operation; second, by securing a better brain block and greater relaxation during operation; and third, by diminishing gas and wound pain after operation. The procedure as evolved was carried on more or less completely in over 300 patients.

The final technique is to give a dose of a barbiturate about two hours before the operation, then one hour before the operation inject intramuscularly 1/48 grain of Dilaudid in 2 cc. of a 25 per cent solution of magnesium sulphate, repeating in 15 minutes. After the second dose the patient is turned on the left side and a retention enema of ether 2½ ounces, olive oil 1½ ounces, and chlorbutanol 10 grains is given. Up until this time no expert attention is necessary and this quiet sleep is converted into surgical anesthesia and relaxation, with an open mask, nitrous oxide (or ethylene) and oxygen being used—15 per cent to 50 per cent to which 5 per cent vapor of ether may be added, if necessary.

The physiological balance between respiration and circulation is retained, with respiratory and circulatory rate normal. The patient is in good condition at all times and relaxation is only second to that obtained by spinal and, in some cases, was equally as good. The long, quiet sleep after the operation is restful and life-saving, enabling the tissues to resume their normal relationship without painful reaction. With this method and technique, the convalescence of the patient starts on the operating table and this is as it should be.

The synergism of magnesium sulphate with dilaudid is even more striking than with morphine. The dosage of dilaudid was decreased and its effect was prolonged and in a vast majority of cases patients awoke without pain, nausea or vomiting. Ether vomiting is a thing of the past.

In conclusion, the authors state:

1. "A definite prolongation of the effect of dilaudid is made by the addition of a 25 per cent solution of magnesium sulphate.

2. The small amount of ether counteracts the depressing effect of dilaudid magnesium solution on the respiratory center.

3. A comfortable relaxation with less shock and greater postoperative comfort occurs with this technique than with any procedure heretofore used."

Complete information on dilaudid can be obtained

m the Bilhuber-Knoll Corporation, Jersey City, J.

GOLF, AND INFANT FEEDING

t is possible to play over the entire course with a le club and bring in a fair score. But playing n only one club is a handicap. The best scores made when the player carefully studies each shot, ermining in advance how he is going to make it, selecting from his bag the particular club best pted to execute that shot.

'or many years, Mead Johnson & Company have red "matched clubs," so to speak, best adapted to t the individual requirements of the individual y.

We believe this to be a more intelligent approach n the use of a single "baby food" to meet the ny situations presented by many babies. "There is average baby."

BOVINE AMNIOTIC FLUID

One of the remarkable immunologic mechanisms the human body is the defense of the abdominal itoneum against infection. This is almost certain be overcome, however, if pathogenic bacteria escape m the intestinal tract and contaminate the peritoneal faces.

Of the various methods of increasing the immunity the peritoneum to inflammation (peritonitis), in-

cluding the use of vaccines, possibly the most promising has been developed quite recently and consists of introducing a purified fraction of bovine amniotic fluid into the peritoneal cavity either before or during any abdominal operation. Even where contamination of the peritoneum is only a remote contingency, the use of amniotic fluid excites a defense mechanism, characterized by the production of a serofibrinous plastic exudate which is rich in leukocytes, lytic ferments, and various antibodies, and healing of the peritoneal surfaces is stimulated.

Not alone does the use of "Amfetin" (Amniotic Fluid Concentrate, Lilly) provide a very considerable factor of safety in abdominal surgery, but the postoperative course of the patient is much smoother and more comfortable.

If you are a surgeon in your "thirties" and interested in a position as "Surgical Adviser" with one of the old established insurance companies, write the Association's office.

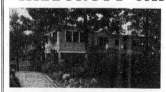

THE JOURNAL
OF THE
MEDICAL ASSOCIATION OF GEORGIA
DEVOTED TO THE WELFARE OF THE MEDICAL ASSOCIATION OF GEORGIA
PUBLISHED MONTHLY under direction of the Council

| Volume XXV | Atlanta, Ga., June, 1936 | Number 6 |

THE FIFTH LUMBAR VERTEBRA AS A CAUSE OF LOW BACK PAIN*

THOMAS P. GOODWYN, M.D.
H. WALKER JERNIGAN, M.D.

Atlanta

Low back pain is a condition encountered frequently in orthopedic practice. The disability varies from mild pain in the low back to severe pain which completely incapacitates the patient. Goldthwait[1] in 1905, and again in 1907, was the first to attribute pain in the low back to faulty mechanics of the skeletal system. It was his belief that the condition was located in the sacro-iliac joints. Assuming that the motion in the sacro-iliac joint was responsible for the pain several operations were devised for ankylosing this joint. The most widely accepted are the Smith-Peterson intra-articular bone-block and the extra-articular fusion by Dr. Willis Campbell. In the last decade it has been shown that many patients suffering with low back pain were found to have anomalies of the fifth lumbar vertebra. Von Lackum[2], in 1924, made an amatomic study of the lumbosacral region, and since that time much valuable work on this subject has been contributed from the New York Orthopedic Hospital and Dispensary. At the present time this group is responsible for much of the teaching that the majority of patients suffering from low back pain have symptoms originating in faulty mechanics of the lumbosacral junction.

In former years we have seen a number of patients with low back pain which was thought to be of sacro-iliac origin. We now believe that many of these were due to anomalies of the fifth lumbar vertebra or lum-

*Read before the Medical Association of Georgia, Atlanta, May 8, 1935.

bosacral junction. It has been found that patients who were operated upon for fusion of the sacro-iliac alone, had recurrence of symptoms on the same side or the opposite side, while patients on which the lumbosacral joint was included in the fusion did not have a recurrence of pain.

Anatomy of the Fifth Lumbar Vertebra

Most textbooks of anatomy give the variations of the fifth from the other lumbar vertebrae as follows: "The fifth lumbar is characterized by its body being much deeper in front than behind. The transverse processes arise from the bodies as well as the roots of the pedicles and are thicker and shorter[3]." The inferior articular facets are described as facing forward and slightly laterally and are set wider apart than the other lumbar vertebrae. The ligaments are the same in this region as in the remainder of the lumbar spine and in addition, there is the iliolumbar ligament which passes from the transverse process of the fifth laterally to the ilium. Gray[3], Morris[4], and Cunningham[5] mention variations in the fifth lumbar as failure of fusion of the laminae and spondylolithesis or failure of fusion of the pedicles with slipping forward of the body. Cunningham[5] mentions sacralization of the transverse process on one or both sides. No mention is made of variations in the articular facets. This region is supplied with strong muscles posteriorly and on both sides, though in front there is no muscle support. The muscles assist in taking the strain off of the ligaments. Danforth and Wilson[6] have shown that the intervertebral foramen between the fifth lumbar and sacrum is smaller than between any of the other lumbar vertebrae and also that the fifth lumbar nerve is the largest of the spinal nerves in this region. This is an important point in the consideration of the anomalies to be described later.

Mechanics

The lumbosacral junction is relatively a weak joint. This is due to a number of causes.

1. It is the most mobile of the lumbar vertebrae. The motions are flexion, extension, lateral mobility, and to a slight degree rotation.

2. It is the junction of a mobile and a relatively immobile part of the spine.

3. It rests on the sacrum at an angle. This angle is the one formed by a line drawn parallel to the superior surface of the sacrum with the horizontal. From anatomic measurements von Lackum[2] has obtained an average in 30 specimens of 42.6 degrees. Whitman[7], from roentgenogram measurements, has obtained an average of 45 degrees.

4. von Lackum[2], Mitchell[8], and others have conceded that much of the weakness of this joint is due to the skeletal modification made necessary in the evolutionary change from the quadripedal to the bipedal state.

5. This joint is the site of many anatomic variations that contribute to instability.

We then have the entire weight of the upper part of the body transmitted to this joint which rests on a tilted platform and has no muscular support anteriorly. The articular facets, ligaments and muscles are the binders that prevent the fifth lumbar from slipping forward into the pelvis. Therefore any loss of muscle tone or injury to the ligaments may allow the fifth lumbar nerve to be encroached upon causing pain.

Anatomic Variations

The anatomic variations as described by Ferguson[9] were followed in making the diagnosis on the patients to be presented here. He gives the following as constituting a mechanically weak back:

1. Anomalies of the articular facets of which the most important is asymmetry. An example of this is one in which the articular facets are of the internal-external type on one side and of the anterior-posterior type on the other.

2. Spondylolisthesis or anterior displacement of the body of the vertebra due to failure of fusion of the pedicles.

3. Prespondylolisthesis or failure of fusion

We frequently learn more from our poor results than from the good so we will consider the former first. The two patients who had fair results were much better off than before operation and were well pleased. In three of the patients the failure can be attributed to arthritis. In one of these the arthritis progressed rapidly and when last seen in October, 1934, this patient had practically complete ankylosis of the entire spine. The only motions visible were slight rotation of the head on the neck and slight motion of the cervical spine. The other two patients had abscessed teeth which were removed after operation; one also had the tonsils removed. Both patients had partial relief following this; however, both continued to have pain in the back as well as in other joints. One patient had failure of fusion with return of symptoms. One patient had prespondylolithesis, his fusion extending from the fourth lumbar vertebra to the sacrum. The fusion in this type of anomaly does not give complete stability of this region as the pedicles are not united to the body of the vertebra. This patient was able to resume his former occupation of painter with the aid of a brace. One of the patients who died had lobar pneumonia and subsequently an empyema. He lived about three months after the operation. The second patient who died developed pleurisy on the seventeenth postoperative day followed by bronchopneumonia, circulatory collapse and death on the twentieth day.

The remaining eighteen patients were all symptom free and able to return to their former occupations.

Summary

1. The anatomy of the lumbosacral junction is briefly described.

2. The mechanics and reasons for instability are enumerated.

3. The anatomic variations are listed.

4. The results obtained in twenty-seven patients who had the fifth lumbar fused to the sacrum are presented.

5. Patients with generalized arthritis are not, as a rule, relieved.

6. Patients with spondylolithesis and prespondylolithesis do not give as satisfactory results as in the other anomalies.

478 Peachtree Street, N. E.

BIBLIOGRAPHY

1. Goldthwait, Joe E.: The Pelvic Articulations, J.A.M.A. 49:678-774 (Aug. 31, 1907).
2. von Lackum, H. L.: The Lumbosacral Region, J.A.M.A. 82:1109-1114 (Apr. 5, 1924).
3. Gray' Anatomy ed. 21, Lea & Febiger, 1924, p. 306.
4. Morris, Henry: Human Anatomy, ed. 8, P. Blakiston Son's & Co. 1925 p. 92.
5. Cunningham: Textbook Anatomy, ed. 5, William Wood & Co., 1923 p. 112 and 1436.
6. Danforth, M. S.: Wilson, P. D.: The Anatomy of the Lumbosacral Region in relation to Sciatic Pain, J. Bone & Joint Surgery, vol. 7 number 1, p. 109, January, 1925.
7. Whitman, Armitage: Observations Upon an Anatomical Variation of the Lumbo-Sacral Joint: Its Diagnosis and Treatment, J. Bone & Joint Surgery, vol. 6 number 4, p. 808 October, 1924.
8. Mitchell, G. A. B.: The Lumbosacral Junction, J. Bone & Joint Surgery, vol. 16 number 2, p. 233 April, 1934.
9. Ferguson, Albert B.: The Clinical and Roentgenographic Interpretation of Lumbosacral Anomalies. Radiology, vol. 22 number 5, p. 548-558, May, 1934.

THE DILUTION AND CONCENTRATION TESTS OF KIDNEY FUNCTION*

W. EDWARD STOREY, M.D.

Columbus

The physician who treats various types of nephritis is confronted with the questions of how much permanent or temporary damage has been done by the disease process and to what extent the functional capacity of the kidneys has been reduced, and furthermore, what steps he should take to safeguard the remaining healthy renal tissue. The answer to these questions can usually be obtained by performing one or more of the tests of renal function and it is the purpose of this discussion to enlarge upon the dilution and concentration tests as examples of these. The presence of albumin, blood and casts in the urine certainly indicate the existence of kidney disease and the relative proportions of these elements often point clearly to the type of underlying pathologic process, i.e., inflammatory, vascular, or nephrotic. Conversely the relative amounts of these give no reliable indication of the extent or the permanence of impairment[1] and for this information one resorts to kidney function tests. It is important to bear this in mind and not confuse the *type of underlying pathologic process* with *extent of damage*. It will be apparent, therefore, that just as in heart disease it is really more important to know what a given heart can do in the way of performing its natural function than it is to know the exact nature of valvular or myocardial lesions, so in kidney disease it is equally if not more important to know how well the organs can perform their functions of water and solid elimination than it is to classify the pathologic process.

Renal function is usually estimated in one or more ways. The amount of phenolsulphonphthalein excreted within a given time is probably the most common test. Performed in the usual manner, this test has fallen into disrepute in some quarters. Van Slyke and his collaborators[2] have shown that often the extent of renal damage must be severe before the two-hour phenolsulphonphthalein test will indicate it; Christian[3] and others[4] have been

unable to obtain results consistent with the known pathologic findings. A second test is the determination of the fasting blood nonprotein or urea nitrogen. While an increase above normal indicates impaired renal function, unfortunately it occurs too late to serve as a timely warning to the physician. The determination of the rate of glomerular filtration by the use of such substances as urea[5] or creatinine[6][7] is perhaps the most accurate and precise method available at present but unless the patient is hospitalized or reliable laboratory facilities are convenient the test is impractical. For adaptability, ease of performance and accurracy the dilution and concentration tests promise to become invaluable in the early detection of impaired kidney function. These tests have the further advantage that they express the total functional capacity to excrete all substances met with under ordinary circumstances and are not dependent upon the excretion of a single substance.

The physiologic facts upon which the dilution and concentration tests are based are: (a) that urine is a solution of solids in water, (b) that in health the relative concentration of solids in water varies within wide limits according to the demands upon the kidney to eliminate water or solids, and (c) that in certain diseased states of the kidney the variation in concentration under test conditions is restricted to distinctly narrower limits. These are demonstrated truths and their acceptance does not depend upon a belief in any particular theory of urine formation. The difficulties lie in the proper interpretation to be set upon variations from the normal because the concentration of the urine may vary with the amount of solid or water and this admits of the effect of certain extrarenal factors which will be mentioned later. That disease of the kidney may bring about a reduction in its functional capacity was first accurately demonstrated by von Korányi of Budapest[8]. He measured the freezing point of urine from patients with and without kidney disease and found that the greater the degree of destruction the less the freezing point depression. In extreme cases the freezing point of the urine was found to coincide with that of deproteinized blood and was to be interpreted as meaning such kidneys are no longer able to with-

*Read before the Medical Association of Georgia, Savannah, April 22, 1936.

to be taken during twenty-four hours. Hourly specimens are collected beginning at 10 A. M., specimens every two hours beginning at 1 P. M. and one 12 hour specimen from 9 P. M. to 9 A .M. Lunch, supper, and break-fast may be chosen from meat, potatoes, cheese, rolls, toast, and eggs; these are to be eaten "dry." The quantity and specific grav-ity of each specimen is measured and a simple heat test for albumin is done on the most concentrated specimens. Kidneys not harbor-ing disease sufficient to impair their function will respond as follows: (a) during the first four hours the total amount of urine passed should equal or nearly equal the amount of fluid ingested i.e. 1000 cc., (b) the lowest specific gravity encountered should not exceed 1005; these items compose the dilution test. During the remainder of the twenty-four hours the volume of each specimen should gradually diminsh and the specific gravity should gradually rise until (c) the lowest figure encountered should not be less than 1025. These items compose the concentra-tion test.

As with many clinical laboratory proced-ures there are certain difficulties to be borne in mind during interpretation of the results. For example, there are the technical points of the temperature at which the specific gravity is measured and the accuracy of the mano-meter used. For practical purposes ordinary room temperature (20 to 25 degrees C.) and a manometer of good make will suffice but in studying results it is well to bear in mind that these factors can account for differences of .001 to .003. Furthermore, the factor of albuminuria, when present, exerts some in-fluence though, according to Fishberg[16], not sufficient to make allowance for unless it is massive. The common disturbing factors are, as might be imagined, dehydration, edema, and states of diuresis. A dehydrated patient will naturally retain that portion of the orig-inal 1000 cc. which he needs and thereby fail to dilute his urine properly and likewise a cardiac patient who is edematous will fail to excrete water by virtue of his crippled circu-lation. Contrariwise patients in a state of diuresis due to drugs or to an improving cir-culation will fail to concentrate properly be-cause of an excess of fluid escaping at the time. Other conditions tending to invalidate results have been pointed out by Addis and Shevsky[17], and Mosenthal[18]. Among these are various nervous, metabolic, and endocrine disturbances, such as neurasthenia, anemias, bladder paralysis, prostatic hypertrophy and diabetes insipidus. Usually, however, when one of these latter conditions is sufficiently marked to interfere with the tests it will be apparent and allowance can be made for it. Most cases will not involve these difficulties but many will require careful exclusion of the effects of paucity or excess of tissue fluid and of circulatory disturbances.

Regardless of extensive studies of the dilution and concentration tests in various types of kidney disease there have been surprisingly few reports of results in normal individuals. Thus, in 1926, Pratt[14] could find no larger series than seven, a report by Schon from Strauss's clinic. Recently Ellis and Weiss[19] have made a more extensive study. On the whole, however, investigators are in agreement with the general findings in pathologic states, where the tests have been studied in comparison with clinical and necropsy findings and with other tests of renal function. In a careful study of patients with various grades of glomerulonephritis, Alving and Van Slyke[20] conclude that both concentration and dilution tests yield results paralleling the urea clearance test though the dilution test was less sensitive and therefore, they consider, superfluous. If the kidney is able to produce urine with a specific gravity of 1026 or over, they regard function as in nowise impaired and accept this in lieu of the urea clearance test, a significant statement when it is remembered that the urea clearance test is the most precise method available. In individual instances there are differences in favor of the urea clearance test but in view of its practicability the maximum specific gravity is an adequate indicator of renal function. Ellis and Weiss[21] in studying renal function by means of the urea creatinine clearance and the dilution and concentration tests found in a group of twenty-four patients with arterial hypertension but without clinical signs of cardiac or renal failure and in a group of eight cases of glomerulonephritis that, for practical purposes, the maximum specific gravity was as reliable an indicator of impaired renal function as the urea and creatinine clearance tests.

urine. The procedure as outlined is simple and practical and easy of performance, and while personally I have not used the dilution test. I have found the concentration test most valuable and I shall add the dilution test in the future.

DR. GEORGE L. WALKER (Griffin) : I have enjoyed Dr. Storey's paper very much. I think it is a very timely subject that he has taken up, and I think he has covered it in a very thorough, practical sort of way.

This is not a new test, and it seems rather strange that a test as old, as practical, as easily performed and as accurate as this test is, is not in more general use. There are several things I should like to emphasize in relation to Dr. Storey's paper, the first being the simplicity of the test, and the fact that one needs only to control the patient for twenty-four hours. The specific gravity of the urine must be measured, and complicated laboratory procedures are not required.

Another beautiful thing about this test is the fact that it is so very sensitive. As a matter of fact, the concentration test is probably the most delicate method we have of measuring the earliest impairment of renal function. The phenol-red test, or so-called phenolsulphonphthalein has been used very much, and I think all of us will agree that it is not very accurate. As Dr. Storey mentioned, it is valuable only in the latest stages of kidney impairment. He has also mentioned the fact that blood chemistry determinations do not give us what we want. In any condition in which we think kidney function might be affected, the concentration test gives our first and most sensitive way of demonstrating impairment in kidney function. Unfortunately, in later stages of nephritis, where the kidneys are severely damaged, we cannot follow the progress with concentration tests as well as with other tests. If impairment is moderate or severe, and the conditions progresses to uremia, we find that changes in the concentration test do not coincide with the progress of the disease, and we have to resort to other methods. The fact remains that it is the most practical, most easily used and most sensitive test for early kidney impairment that we have.

DR. W. EDWARD STOREY (Columbus) : Dr. Metts mentioned that he had used the concentration test but not the dilution test. I think that for practical purposes, unless he is interested in studying the dilution test, there is no practical advantage in using it, because the more reliable data regarding kidney function is to be had from the concentration test. Dr. Arthur Fishberg told me in June, 1934, that he had practically eliminated the dilution test in studying kidney function and relied almost entirely on the concentration test. The phenolsulphonphthalein test has had widespread use, but there is today considerable disagreement as to its value. In the past year results have been published in the American Journal of Medical Sciences on a modified phenolsulphonphthalein test, and I wish to refer you to it for further information on the subject of that test. Thank you.

FUSOSPIROCHETAL DISEASES OF THE LUNG*

JAMES P. TYE, M.D.

Albany

The ever increasing interest in the study of fusospirochetal diseases of the lung dates back to 1906, when Castellani[1] first recognized this pathologic condition. Although Leyden and Jaffe[2] had observed spirochetes in sputum as early as 1867, it was Castellani who described the pathogenicity of these organisms and their causal relationship to the production of bronchopulmonary lesions. The disease was thought to be restricted to the tropics until it was discovered in the civilian population of France in 1918. This discovery, of course, precipitated a world-wide search for these cases. The first case reported in the United States is credited to Johnson[3], of Mississippi, in 1909. It is interesting to note that Rothwell[4] of Missouri reported two cases one year later and designated the condition bronchial Vincent's angina since the sputum contained the spirochetes as well as the fusiform bacilli originally described by Vincent in 1896[5]. Castellani did not mention the presence of the fusiform bacillus in the sputum of his cases. The spirochete and fusiform bacillus as described by Vincent are found normally in the buccal cavity and the ability of these organisms to produce pathologic changes was described by the same author.

Vincent's organisms attack the respiratory system through three avenues of approach: (1) The most common mode of infection is by aspiration of the organisms into the bronchi. This condition may occur at any time but most often it occurs during general anesthesia, especially when surgery of the mouth or throat is being done; (2) The attack may be embolic in nature. This condition occurs infrequently but has been proved by Hedbloom[6]; (3) Jackson[7] proved that we have infection of the bronchi by direct extensions from lesions in the throat.

When these organisms reach the lung in sufficient numbers, they may either become the sole agents or contributors to the patho-

*Read before the Medical Association of Georgia, Savannah, April 22, 1936.

an attempt to locate this therapeutic note, and today, we are still in doubt as to its origin. The small number of cases that we have had the opportunity to use this drug with, have shown striking beneficial results and in further defense of its specific reaction we wish to call attention to the results that two of our friends in the dental profession have had with its use. Before the use of bismuth had been called to their attention, they, in the more extensive Vincent's infections of the mouth, had been resorting to the intravenous administration of neosalvarsan. During the past six years, they have used bismuth in several hundred such cases with, so they tell me, very excellent results.

The fundamental principle in the treatment of the more extensive lesions of the lung tissue, such as abscess and gangrene, is drainage. The simplest, safest method which fulfills this requirement is the best. Postural drainage should certainly be given a trial before more radical procedures are resorted to. In certain cases bronchoscopic lavage has been indicated and yielded excellent results. Pneumothorax has its advocates and in many instances has proven of great value. Tewksbury[12] reports thirty-five cases of lung abscess treated by means of pneumothorax with recovery in twenty-eight cases. Whitmore and Balboni[13] collected one hundred twenty-seven (127) cases treated with pneumothorax with sixty-eight reported cured.

Abscess formation in the apices and in the periphery of the lung must be dealt with surgically, thoracotomy drainage and cautery extirpation usually being the procedure of choice. In gangrene of the lung, Hedbloom[14] resects the infected area by means of the cautery.

Our first patient to receive bismuth had a fusospirochetal bronchiectasis of over twelve months standing. He had been treated spasmodically during the time with large doses of neosalvarsan and on several occasions he was considered completely recovered. However, the cough and expectoration of large quantities of foul-smelling sputum soon reappeared after the drug had been discontinued. He was given eighteen injections of neosalvarsan during the twelve-month period. His condition at the end of this time was not as good as it was before the drug was administered regardless of the fact that he apparently fully recovered after each series of injections. He lost thirty pounds during the year and, in April, 1930, he was very much discouraged. He was expectorating about 500 cc. of foul, purulent, and blood-tinged sputum, and was unable to eat on account of the foul odor that was ever present on his breath. The food that he did take was most always vomited during a coughing paroxysm. He was given bismuth intramuscularly at intervals of every three days without any further injections of neosalvarsan. After two weeks, he was able to take his food without nausea, his cough was considerably improved, and the amount of sputum expectorated was materially reduced. The bismuth was continued for a period of eight weeks at which time he was dismissed as fully recovered. He has been observed over a period of almost six years and has at no time had any symptoms of recurrence.

The second case treated was begun in 1930. This patient had been sick about three months when I first saw him. He had a temperature of 100° F., and his pulse rate was 120 to 130. He was coughing quite persistently and expectorating a very foul, offensive sputum. Microscopic examination showed large numbers of spirochetes associated with numerous fusiform bacilli. He was given 0.6 gram of neosalvarsan and 0.05 gram of bismuth sodium tartrate on his first visit to the office. The neosalvarsan produced quite an unpleasant reaction. He was nauseated and vomited for a period of six to eight hours; his coughing was exaggerated and the sputum definitely more blood-stained than before. It was decided to omit further doses of neosalvarsan and to continue with the bismuth. His condition rapidly improved and he was dismissed after five weeks completely recovered.

Since 1930, we have treated three patients with bronchiectasis whose sputums were loaded with spirochetes and fusiform bacilli. Bismuth alone was used in these cases and in each patient the recovery was remarkable.

The only instance of recurrence was noted in a young woman who had a bronchiectasis associated with asthma. Our treatment consisted of six doses of neosalvarsan and fourteen doses of bismuth. She made a remarkable recovery, gaining about fifteen pounds, but

one year later she returned to the office with a condition about the same as when she first came. She was given another series of bismuth injections in the fall of 1935, and her sputum is now free of spirochetes and fusiform bacilli.

The most remarkable favorable recovery was a young man who had multiple abscess formation in his left lung following the extraction of a tooth. Several attempts were made to administer neosalvarsan in small doses, but the reaction was so severe that it had to be discontinued. One-tenth gram doses caused him to vomit for forty-eight hours and invariably his condition was made worse after four attempts were made to administer this drug. Even though he was sick for a period of eight months and it was necessary to drain one of the localized abscess cavities surgically, we feel that bismuth had a large part in his eventual recovery.

BIBLIOGRAPHY

1. Castellani, A.: Note on a Peculiar Form of Haemoptysis with Presence of Spirochaetae in Expectoration, Lancet, 1: 1384, 1906.
2. Leyden, E., and Jaffe, M.: Deutsche Arch f. Klinische, Med., 2: 488, 1867.
3. Johnson, W. B.: A Case of Spirillosis of the Lungs, Memphis M. Mouth., 29: 183-184, (April), 1909.
4. Rothwell, J. H.: Bronchial Vincent's Angina, J. A. M. A., 54: 1867, 1910.
5. Vincent, M. H.: Sur l'Etiologie et sur les Lesions Anatomo–, Pathologiques de la Pourriture D' Hospital, Ann de 1. inst. Pasteur, 12: 488, 1896.
6. Hedbloom, C. A.: Lewis' Surgery, Vol. Five, Chapter One, Page 60.
7. Jackson, C.: Post-tonsillectomic pulmonary abscess, Atlantic M. J., Harrisburg, 29: 309-315, 1926.
8. Herman, W. G.: J. Med. Society, New Jersey, Nov., 1931, 28: 836.
9. Kline, B. S., and Berger, S. S.: Spirochaetal Pulmonary Gangrene Treated with Araphenamines, J. A. M. A., 85: 1452, 1925.
10. Smith, D. T.: Fuso-Spirochaetal Disease of the Lungs, Its Bacteriology, Pathology, and Experimental Reproduction, Am. Rev. Tuberc., 16: 584.
11. Spector, H. I.: Bronchopulmonary Fuso-Spirochaetosis with a Note on Treatment with Small Doses of Neo-Salvarsan, The Journal Lancet, 54: 572-575, 1932.
12. Tewksbury, W. B.: Acoute Pulmonary Abscess Following Tonsillectomy Treated with Artificial Pneumothorax, Ann. Clin. Med., Balk, 4: 347-349, 1925.
13. Whitemore, W., and Balboni, Gerardo, M.: Nontubercular Bronchopulmonary Suppurative Lesions. Result of Treatment with Artificial Pneumothorax, Archives of Surgery, 16: 228-278, 1928.
14. Hedbloom, C. A.: Lewis' Surgery, Vol. 5, Chap. 1, Page 2.

Discussion on Paper by Dr. J. P. Tye

DR. HENRY M. McGEHEE (Moultrie): Dr. David T. Smith of Duke University has done a wonderful piece of work on this subject of fusospirochetal disease. Dr. Smith makes a statement in his monograph that, excluding the tubercle bacillus, these organisms are responsible for more chronic infections in the lung than any we encounter. Also he states that the pathology of this infection is more widespread than the pathology caused by any organisms other than that caused by treponema pallidum. These two statements by such an authority impress us with the fact that this is a disease we have overlooked in the past, and a

mouth thoroughly and then washing the mouth with sterile water for a period of ten or fifteen minutes before the specimen is obtained. Then these specimens should be examined, whether by smear or dark-field examination, within two to three hours, because of the fact that these spirochetes seem to disintegrate after that period. It is known that in these conditions the fusiform bacilli are found in many cases, and not the spirochetes. I think that is the reason for that.

Experimentally, none of these lesions have been produced in the presence of merely the spirochete and the fusiform bacillus. They have been injected in animals intratracheally, without infection in the lung. It has been found that it is always necessary that some pathogenic bacillus be present, at the same time. These are most frequently found to be hemolytic streptococci and sometimes staphylococci.

Then I think that certainly the most common lesion we find in fusospirochetal diseases of the lung are the later lesions; lung abscess, gangrene, and certain cases of unresolved pneumonia. However, last year in April Dr. Field and Dr. Pierce of the University of Michigan reported eleven cases of a new type of pneumonia which is lobular in character, and which they thought was due to the fusiform bacillus. These have a very characteristic symptomatology, the onset being with a dry cough, later pain in the chest, fever, some hemoptysis, but in the later stages none whatever. The duration of these symptoms was from nine days to a matter of weeks.

The initial bacteria in these conditions were found to be pyogenic. Later, as the disease progressed, the organisms were found to be the spirochete and fusiform bacillus.

The x-ray findings were rather characteristic, and began with initial bronchitis, bronchial pneumonia, and edema, like many pneumonias. Resolution of these processes left no appreciable scar in the lung. They did not go on to abscess formation, atelectasis or gangrene, as most of them do. The elapsed time from the onset of illness, that is from the appearance of the dry cough and fever, was anywhere from twenty-four days to nine months, and that shows us how much we must be on guard in looking for these infections.

I should like to emphasize also that when neoarsphenamine is used, the smaller doses seem to give more beneficial results, doses from 0.15 to 0.3 gram. In looking up these subjects in the literature, I was unable to find any reference to the use of bismuth.

I think Dr. Tye can certainly be complimented for bringing us this added treatment for such a widespread condition.

DR. GEORGE L. ECHOLS (Milledgeville): I wish to thank the writer for bringing this subject to our attention, and also thank the gentlemen for their discussions. This is a problem that is met in state hospitals rather frequently, though not quite as much now as formerly.

When our patients are admitted, one of the first proceedings is to have the dentist make a careful examination of the mouth, one of the points in mind being this particular disease. There occurred just a few months ago an article in Dental Cosmos that our dentist wanted to have me study. If you get hold of that article you will find that it will throw quite a bit of light on the mouth. I have been hoping since then that some other laboratories and research workers would do similar studies of the other parts involved than the mouth.

One of the things I want to call your attention to is that you are liable to get delirious states and excitement along with this disease, as with other sicknesses. Ten weeks ago I saw a lady who was very restless, excited, talkative, very confused, with partial delirium. The dentist told me promptly what my diagnosis was, and after he and some of the other physicians had done their work I had the pleasure of sending this lady back home last week restored mentally. It was purely a psychosis, associated with this particular disease.

There is another thing I want to call to your attention. I have had a great deal of experience with these conditions at the Milledgeville State Hospital, and the more experience I have the more I am impressed with the necessity of careful isolation of these cases. I may be all wrong about it, but it seems to me that the more we isolate this type of disease, the less of it we have, and I should like to stress that point.

DR. HAL M. DAVISON (Atlanta): About two years ago, Dr. Crowe, of the State Sanatorium at Alto, came down to Atlanta, and gave a paper at the meeting of the Atlanta Tuberculosis Association. Dr. Crowe reported a rather large number of cases at Alto with fusospiracheal disease of the lungs. These cases were sent in with typical symptoms of tuberculosis, typical findings on x-ray, large amounts of sputum, but no tubercle bacilli were found in the putum. These cases did not improve after the usual therapy for pulmonary tuberculosis, and puzzled the doctors considerably for a time.

Up to that time we had identified practically none of such cases. Now we attempt to have the sputum from every case voided in the laboratory, and since this has been done, we are finding the organisms more often. It is usually easy to obtain fresh specimens, because practically all of these cases have a lot of sputum.

I think it should also be emphasized here that we do not find in most of these cases the typical symptoms laid down by Dr. Tye. The organisms may be found in the sputum of any patient who suffers from chronic bronchitis. We have also found this condition in a fair percentage of our cases of asthma, and it is possible that some of the relief resulting after our administration of sodium iodide with sodium cacodylate has been due to the effect of these drugs on an undetected fusospirochetal complication.

We have also observed in the past cases who had large amounts of sputum, hemoptysis, fever, that is, giving the appearance of a tuberculosis, yet in whom we could not obtain a positive reaction to the tuberculin skin test, and in whose sputum we could find no tubercle bacilli. These cases cleared up after a course

of small doses of sodium cacodylate, administered in some of the cases for a period of two or three years, and I suspect that they were cases of fusospirochetal disease that we had not discovered.

We now believe it important to investigate every case of chronic bronchitis, particularly if bronchiectasis is present, for fusospirochetes in the sputum.

As a routine treatment we give six small doses of neoarsphenamine, follow this with six doses of bismuth, allow the patient to rest for two weeks to a month. Then we repeat the same course twice more, three times in all. Most of the cases yield very readily to treatment. To promote drainage we have found useful the intratracheal administration of iodized oil. The oil loosens up mucus plugs, displaces sputum in the more distal bronchioles, and allows the patient to cough up the waste matter with more ease.

DR. A. A. DAVIDSON (Augusta): The part of the subject on which I care to address a few remarks may be without real point, since the organisms may be found in a normal mouth, but a few years ago I treated a young lady with an ulcerated tonsil, she got well and about a year from that time she went to her dentist and he told her he thought she had trench mouth. She came back to me. I made a smear from the gums, which were spongy, and got a positive report for the spirochete and fusiform bacillus.

After observing this young lady's gums I began to make smears from all spongy gums which came my way, and since that time I think of very few exceptions to the fact of a positive report when these smears on the slide were submitted to the Board of Health.

I wondered if such uniform returns of Vincent's positive reports were not because the organisms inhere in the mouth, sometimes normally, and I began to take smears from normal gums, not spongy gums, and uniformly I got negative reports.

When I took the smear from the spongy gum I would take pains to roll the swab from below upward, and then take the smear. Only yesterday I got three positive reports from the Board of Health. Coming in a minute ago and hearing this paper, it occurred to me to stress the fact that nearly all spongy gums, particularly at the base of the incisor teeth, carry this fusiform bacillus and the spirochete of Vincent. They have to begin in the mouth before they get in the lungs.

DR. J. P. TYE (Albany): I want to thank the gentlemen for their discussions.

Dr. McGehee made the statement that Castellani failed to recognize the fusiform bacillus due to the fact that he made all of his studies by means of the dark-field, and, due to the motility of the bacillus, it was confused with the spirochete. I do not wish to take issue with Dr. McGehee, but I have been under the impression that the fusiform bacillus is nonmotile.

Again, to answer Dr. McGehee as to clearing up the infections in the mouth before the lung infection can be properly treated: If this could be done satisfactorily, it would be fine. However, it is a well-known fact that to rid the mouth of the infection.

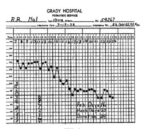

FIG. 1.
Temperature chart in Case No. 1. Note the fall in temperature 3 days after 25 cc. of 1:5000 merthiolate intravenously.

Ayers[2] found complete inhibition of growth at dilution of 1:1,000,000 for the 24 hour period.

Powell and Jamieson[1] state that it has an extremely low toxicity to animals and animal tissue; is non-irritating, and is strikingly non-hemolytic in isotonic solutions of 1:-1000 or less. They quote Smithburn as having injected 22 persons in doses up to 50 c.c. of a 1 per cent solution of merthiolate. As many as five intravenous doses, or a total of 180 c.c. of 1 per cent merthiolate, have been given to one individual. These large doses did not produce any anaphylactoid or shock symptoms. Neither did these quantities in the repeated doses bring about any demonstrable later toxic effects.

An ideal antiseptic is one which kills the bacteria without harming the tissue cells, and methods of comparing the toxic effects of antiseptics upon bacteria and tissue cells in vitro have been devised. German (cited by Buchsbaum and Bloom[3]) believes the "efficiency" of an antiseptic to be directly proportional to its bacteriostatic effect, and inversely to its harmful action on the tissues. Against a theoretical ideal rating of 1.0, merthiolate was given a rating of 0.9, iodine 0.5 and phenol 0.2.

Obviously, there is a marked difference in the action of any bacteriocidal agent or any specific organism in a test tube and in vitro, but anything that claims such high efficiency with low toxicity and virtually no irritating effect, should have beneficial results on actual cases of typhoid fever. Although the inci-

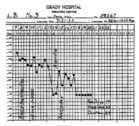

FIG. 2.
Temperature chart in Case 3. Note the normal temperature on the 8th day after 15 cc. 1:3000 merthiolate intravenously.

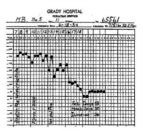

FIG. 3.
Temperature chart in Case 5. Note the increased dosage. 70 cc. of 1:2000 merthiolate intravenously.

dence of typhoid fever has been reduced by improvement in sanitary conditions and by prophylaxis, there is still an average of more than four hundred deaths a year reported in Georgia for the past fifteen years[4]. As the occurrence in negro children is not sufficient to permit using alternate cases, the average febrile duration of the cases treated on the Pediatric Ward of the Colored Division of Grady Hospital from 1924 through 1933 was used as a check. This was 29.4 days for 170 patients. Norris[5], in a study of 100 cases of all ages at the same hospital, found an average duration of 31 days.

Having all the cases from the same social strata, there should be the same possibility of variation in the accuracy of the duration of illness. These were used in all computations, as well as the discharge diagnosis on the hospital record.

In this series of cases, the intravenous dose of merthiolate was the only variation from the regular routine treatment. At first, 0.5 c.c. of 1:5000 solution per pound of body weight was given, which should produce approximately 1:500,000 concentration in the blood. The amount and concentration were later changed in an attempt to determine the optimal dosage. All the temperatures listed were taken rectally at 8 a. m. and 8 p. m. which times were selected beforehand, and the figure at the top indicates the duration. The recording of all blood work is listed on the day it was taken, and not on the day it was reported.

Case Reports

Case 1. R. R. had been ill for one week with headache, fever, abdominal pain and vomiting. His drinking water came from a well. On the 11th day of illness, he received 28 c.c. of 1:5000 merthiolate, and he was afebrile six days later.

Case 2. M. C. had had headache and abdominal symptoms; drinking water came from a well. On the 11th day she received 23 c.c. of 1:2500 solution: she was afebrile on the 23rd day.

This child's mother and uncle, who lived in the same house with her and who drank water from the same well, also developed typhoid fever about the same time. They did not receive merthiolate. They died on the 15th and 22nd day of their illness.

Case 3. For seven days L. B. had been ill with drowsiness and fever. This child, from the country like the first two, had several neighbors ill with typhoid fever. On the 10th day of her illness, she received 15 c.c. of 1:3000 merthiolate and was afebrile on the 18th day. The last few days of fever may have been due to cervical adenitis.

Case 4. M. M. was admitted on the 6th day of an illness characterized by violent headache, nausea and abdominal pain. She received 17 c.c. of 1:3000 solution on the 10th day, and as the blood culture was positive six days later without improvement clinically, she was given 20 c.c. of 1:4000 on the 18th day. The merthiolate did not seem to have any effect on the convalescence.

As only four cases were treated in 1933, due to waiting for positive reports of the blood culture and Widal, the following summer it was decided to inject without waiting. Consequently it was given sooner and, as all cases of typhoid fever that received merthiolate are included in this series, some did not have a positive blood culture.

Case 5. M. B. had had headache, fever, abdominal pain and nausea for one week. She received 70 c.c of 1:2000 merthiolate on the 10th day, and 9 days later was afebrile. This was nearly 1 c.c. per pound of

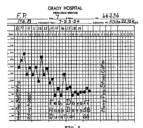

FIG. 5.
Temperature chart in Case 8. Note the fall in temperature 3 days after 25 cc. of 1:3000 merthiolate
intravenously.

W. K., Jr., who did not receive merthiolate, was
febrile for 44 days.

Case 11. D. L. S. was admitted on the 8th day
for fever, headache and abdominal pain. This girl was
another victim to a contaminated well. She received
30 cc. of 1:2000 merthiolate, and her recovery was
the most dramatic of the entire series. She may have
been ill more than eight days before admission, having
a negative blood culture, but the picket fence temperature and leukopenia were typical.

Case 12. H. J. had only diarrhea and fever. As
other cases of dysentery were admitted at the same
time, typhoid fever was not suspected at first. When
positive blood culture and Widal tests were reported,
he received 15 cc. of 1:2000 merthiolate and he was
well 8 days later.

Case 13. R. A., Jr., was admitted on the 14th
day with headache, abdominal pain and epistaxis. On
the 16th and 17th days, he received 30 cc. of 1:3000
solution and gave almost immediate response.

Case 14. W. H. was admitted on the 7th day
with headache, abdominal pain and vomiting. Like
the previous patient she received 25 cc. of 1:3000
merthiolate on the 8th and 9th days. While the
response was not as marked, her improvement was
definite, having only one time, on the 21st day, a
higher temperature than the previous day.

Case 15. V. L. L. had complained of headache,
chills, fever and anorexia when admitted on the 6th
day. From the time of admission, it was evident that
the toxemia was most severe. She received 35 cc. of
1:3000 solution for 3 consecutive days. There was
no response or change in the general condition. Death
was on the 26th day, and the necropsy report confirmed the diagnosis.

Case 16. I. L., the brother of V. L. L., was
admitted four days after her, on his 7th day, complaining of fever, malaise and diarrhea. He received
20 cc. of 1:3000 solution on the 8th, 9th and 10th
days, and his response was rapid, becoming afebrile
on the 15th day. He probably had the same infection
as his sister, but evidently he had more resistance.

Case 17. J. R. was admitted on the 15th day

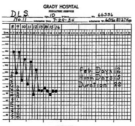

FIG. 6.
Temperature chart in Case 11. Note the normal temperature 4 days after 30 cc. of 1:2000 merthiolate intravenously.

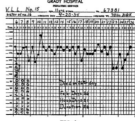

FIG. 8.
Temperature chart in Case 15. Showing no response to 3 injections of 35 cc. 1:3000 merthiolate intravenously.

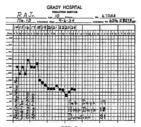

FIG. 7.
Temperature chart in Case 13. Note the fall in temperature the day after the 2nd injection of 30 cc. of 1:3000 merthiolate intravenously.

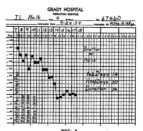

FIG. 9.
Temperature chart in Case 16, brother of the patient in Case 15. Note the fall in temperature by crisis after the 3rd injection of 20 cc. of 1:3000 merthiolate intravenously.

complaining of abdominal pain and headache. He received 20 cc. of 1:3000 merthiolate on the three following days. The convalescence was uneventful, after a febrile duration of 23 days.

Case 18. J. H. lived in a typhoid neighborhood. He was admitted in December, on the 6th day of his illness. His chief complaints were headache, abdominal pain and anorexia. The blood culture and Widal test were both negative on admission but later the Widal became positive. He received 25 cc. of 1:3000 solution on the 7th and 8th days. Due to an infectious parotitis, he was transferred to the Contagious Hospital on his 13th day and 10 days later returned to develop pyelitis and run a prolonged febrile course. The entire febrile course was 38 days.

Case 19. G. B. was the final and only patient of the 1935 period. This was due to using only the cases that had positive blood findings and giving 4 cc. per pound body weight of 1:4000 solution over a four hour period. If given slowly for four hours, there should be a greater concentration of merthiolate for several hours and an increased prolonged bactericidal action.

G. B. had a typical history of short duration.

Shortly after 2 P. M. of the 7th day, she received continuous administration of 1:4000 solution at a rate of about 50 cc. an hour. At the end of two hours, she complained of being thirsty, was restless and irritable. The treatment was discontinued. There was a gradual steady increase in the temperature, although only 103 degrees on the chart at the 8 P. M. reading, it was over 107 degrees rectally, later that night. This was followed by drenching sweats and chills with a gradual decline to 103 degrees the following morning.

Before giving merthiolate, the blood culture was positive, while immediately afterwards the culture was negative. The reaction was similar to that obtained by giving typhoid vaccine intravenously. The improvement was gradual with 26 febrile days.

The death rate for the State, while still high, shows a steady downward trend. Most of these deaths are probably from the rural sections where well water is used. As the febrile duration was the main point of comparison, the proportion of deaths in the check group period and this series, has not been attempted.

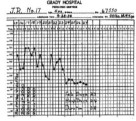

GRADY HOSPITAL
J.R. No.17   _No._ 67550

FIG. 10.
Temperature chart in Case 17. This shows the response after the 3rd injection of 20 cc. of 1:3000 merthiolate intravenously.

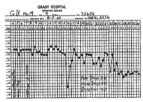

GRADY HOSPITAL
G.B. No.19   _No._ 73636

FIG. 11.
Temperature chart in Case 19. The blood culture taken immediately before 105 cc. of 1:4000 merthiolate intravenously was positive, while that taken immediately after was negative.

as cases of long duration were not considered a fair test for the use of merthiolate.

Summary

On account of the low toxicity and irritability of merthiolate, with the high bactericidal efficiency, it was used in treating typhoid fever by intravenous injections. Nineteen cases are reported, fourteen had a shorter febrile duration than the ten year average of children in the same hospital.

Twelve of the fourteen who received merthiolate recovered from their fever in much less than the average time in our experience at Grady Hospital. Five cases showed no beneficial results: only one failed to recover. There were no deleterious effects from the injections.

At least seven had a water supply from an infected well. Fourteen had a white count of 9000 or less.

Patient	Age	Sex	Bld.Clt.	Widal	W.B.C.	Feb.Dur.
D.L.S.	11	10	F	—	+	3950	12
I.L.	16	4	M	+	+	8500	14
A.C.R.	7	2	M	+	+	4100	15
R.R.	1	10	M	+	+	19000	16
F.P.	8	7	F	+	+	4900	17
L.B.	3	3	F	+	+	2900	17
M.B.	5	11	F	+	+	12800	18
R.A.	13	10	M	—	+	7000	19
M.C.	2	9	F	+	+	9000	22
H.J.	12	2	M	+	+	5300	22
J.R.	17	4	M	—	+	9200	23
W.H.	14	8	F	+	+	9850	23
G.B.	19	9	F	+	+	11000	26
M.K.	10	11	M	—	+	8800	29
M.M.	4	6	F	+	+	8600	31
J.H.	18	7	M	—	+	8300	38
W.M.	6	9	M	—	+	6400	44
S.B.	9	10	M	+	+	8350	49
V.L.L.	15	11	F	+	+	7100	Died

FIG. 12.
Chart to show the results in this series. The cases above the blank space had a shorter febrile duration than the hospital average. The cases are numbered in chronologic order, but are listed in order of the febrile duration.

The first cases received only one intravenous injection of varying concentrations. This was later changed to two injections on consecutive days. As there seemed to be better results from a standpoint of clinical improvement, this was increased to three injections. In one case the continuous drip method was tried and while this patient showed the only pronounced reaction, it may be the most effective method of administration. This method will be used on subsequent cases with a weaker dilution and a longer length of time for the injection, but only cases with positive blood culture and preferably a negative Widal test, will be used.

Conclusions

When merthiolate is given early, there may be a shortening of the febrile duration. After extensive involvement of Peyers patches, there is only slight hope of beneficial results. A consideration of complications has not been attempted, as the series is too small for a fair comparison.

1208 Medical Arts Building.

REFERENCES

1. Powell, H. M., and Jamieson, W. A.: Merthiolate as a Germicide, Am. J. Hyg. 13: 296 (Jan.) 1931.
2. Ayers, A. J.: Personal communication to the author.
3. Buchsbaum, R. and Bloom, W.: Relative Toxicity of Antiseptics or Bacteria and Tissues in Cultures, Proc. Soc. Exper. Biol. and Med. 28: 1060, 1931.
4. Official Bulletin, State Board of Health, Biennial Report, Department of Public Health, 1933-34, 166.
5. Norris, J. C.: Typhoid Fever in the Negro, Report from the Dept. of Public Health, 1933-34, 166.

MYOSARCOMA OF ROUND LIGAMENT·

Report of Case

J. D. MARTIN, JR., M.D.
FRED F. RUDDER, M.D.
Atlanta

There have been several reviews of the cases of tumors of the round ligament. The most recent was that by Horine in reporting one case along with a pathological grouping of thirty-six cases reported since 1914. Although this as a very small group, many more probably occurred but were never reported.

These conditions have long been recognized. According to Horine, Saenger reported twelve cases of fibromyomas together with one case of his own. Emanuel reported eighty cases in 1903 and Taussing found sixty-one cases from 1903 to 1914.

The more common of these tumors were fibromas, fibroleiomyomas, or adenomyomas. There were only a few cases of sarcoma of the round ligament.

The following case is reported since it comes under that class:

A. S., colored, aged 50, was admitted to the Emory University Division of the Grady Hospital with a mass in the left inguinal region. About five and a half years before she noticed that the menstrual periods had increased from three to five days. There was also an increase in the amount of bleeding. One year later there was felt a small swelling in the left inguinal region. The mass at this time was freely movable but not tender and measured about two inches in length. The growth was gradual until about one year before admission when it grew very rapidly. At this time the patient stopped menstruating. During the six months before admission to the hospital there had been sharp stabbing pains in the inguinal region while working. At no time had the mass ever been reduced.

Physical examination: There was a symmetrical enlargement of the thyroid gland. The blood pressure was 230/136 with marked tortuosity, and hardening of the peripheral arteries. The abdomen was pendulous. There was a marked diastasis of the recti muscles. A mass was seen just above and parallel to the left inguinal canal. It was smooth, of firm consistency, not attached to the skin, and measured 18 by 8 cm. No bulging on coughing could be elicited, nor could the mass be replaced in the abdominal cavity. Vaginal examination was negative except for a relaxed perineum.

region, but it is not always easy to differentiate it from the more common lesions, the
most frequent of which are inguinal hernias,
cysts of the canal of Nuck, lipomas in the
inguinal canal, and enlarged lymph nodes.

INFLUENCE OF PREGNANCY ON
TUBERCULOSIS*

WALTER W. DANIEL, M.D.
Atlanta

Casual study of a group of cases of pulmonary tuberculosis complicated by pregnancy leads one to conclude that pregnancy
has a deleterious effect on the disease. The
first three months following delivery is a
precarious time in the woman's life as a
latent tuberculous infection is likely to become active. Contrariwise definite improvement is noted in tuberculous women during
the last trimester of pregnancy, probably due
to relative fixation of the diaphragm by the
pressure of the enlarging uterus.

American writers generally are of the
opinion that an early therapeutic abortion is
advisable for all pregnant women with tuberculosis whether or not the disease is active.
French writers believe that pregnancy is beneficial to tuberculosis and in most instances
they do not consider seriously therapeutic
abortions. English writers are more conservative in their opinions and avoid extreme
views. The French viewpoint may be modified by religious beliefs.

The literature indicates a diversity of
opinion depending on whether a practitioner
is an internist or an obstetrician. It appears
that the internists are a little more liberal in
their attitude, whereas the obstetricians seem
skeptical of all tuberculous conditions complicated by pregnancy. De Lee[1] in a recent
editiorial says that every year he has to comment on the subject and decide anew whether
the radical action he recommended in his
earlier life is justified by his later experience.
His answers generally are affirmative. Only
the exceptional case of tuberculosis in pregnancy is permitted to go through to term, and
he would extend a safe period for abortion to
sixteen weeks. Performed under morphine,

*Read before the Fulton County Medical Society, Atlanta,
May 7, 1936.

scopolomine and local (procaine) anesthesia
he thinks the operation is safe and should not
be followed by shock or pulmonary complications. He recommends that the woman be
relieved of the drain on her strength, that she
be given intensive treatment and states that
when cured she can have babies. The earlier
writers held to the opinion that pregnancy
was actually beneficial to tuberculous women.
More recent authors hold that pregnancy in
tuberculous patients is as a general rule disastrous. All are agreed that lactation and
breast feeding are detrimental to the health
of a tuberculous mother.

Marshall[2] states that all women may be
considered tuberculous as practically every
adult harbors the tubercle bacillus, more or
less shut off from the circulating fluids.
Hiley[3] believes that pregnancy aggravates
tuberculosis and weakens the patient to the
extent of permitting the appearance of fresh
lesions.

Bourne (2) reports 599 cases of tuberculosis in
women—396 non-pregnant, 203 pregnant. Two per
cent of the non-pregnant women died within one year
whereas only 1 per cent of those pregnant died in the
same period. In the moderately active cases, the mortality was 6 per cent for both classes. In the advanced
cases, 37 per cent of the non-pregnant women died
within a year as compared to 46 per cent of those
pregnant.

Rivett (2) reports 423 pregnancies in 237 tuberculous women. He observed that the pregnancy had
no effect on the tuberculous condition in 53 per cent
of the cases, that 16 per cent showed improvement and
31 per cent were made worse. In another series of 422
pregnant women, he reports the tuberculous condition
unchanged in 32 per cent while 19 per cent were improved and 49 per cent were aggravated.

Ornstein and Kovnat (3) compared a series of tuberculous pregnant women with a group of non-pregnant
females and were surprised to find the death rate about
the same. The death rate in the pregnant group was
36 per cent and 33 per cent for the non-pregnant
group. However, in comparing the two groups for
improvement in health it was found that among those
who lived only 18 per cent of the pregnant women
showed unimprovement while 31 per cent of the non-
pregnant group did not improve.

These authors explain their data: They
found that a bad prognosis did not depend
on the pregnancy but on the character of the
pulmonary tuberculosis. All deaths in the
pregnant group were in the caseous pneumonic group. In the resolving exudative and
chronic productive groups, in which the prognosis is generally better, there were no deaths;

thirty-four of these patients were in the hospital and most of them were discharged improved. Pregnancy had no material effect on the prognosis of the disease in the caseous pneumonic group, although it did seem to shorten the span of life to a slight degree as compared to the non-pregnant group. The other two groups (the resolving exudative and chronic productive) were not affected by the pregnancy.

Nearly all authors writing on this subject may be criticised for not classifying their cases of tuberculosis. They should be classified as latent, or active, and the active cases should be further classified as to type and extent; then the percentages given would be informative. To simply state that so many pregnant women who have tuberculosis, or who have had it, died within a year from the disease does not give worthwhile information. Ornstein and Kovnat[3] attempted a classification of tuberculous types and have written an informative paper as did Bourne[2]. Other writers have classified tuberculosis as a group condition.

Conclusions

This review has prompted the following impressions:

1. Tuberculous women should practice contraception.

2. If a tuberculous woman becomes pregnant the advice given her should be individual, depending on her physical condition and not a dogmatic dictum based on facts from groups of cases of this disease. If the patient has been free of clinical manifestations of tuberculosis for a sufficient time (say two years) it may be safe to permit her to have a child, provided she is well off economically and is kept under constant observation.

3. Consultation frequently with a tuberculosis specialist is more valuable than consultation with an obstetrician. The type and development of the tuberculous condition of the patient is an index to the proper procedure to follow; that is, whether or not she should be aborted.

4. If a therapeutic abortion is indicated, it should be done early in pregnancy. DeLee[1] says it should be accomplished before the 16th week.

tainly seems to have a definite place in treatment of blood stream infections and as soon as its action can be explained scientifically, and enough cases obtained to verify the results already obtained, a complete report of its use, with the best combination and strength, will be reported in detail.

MATERNAL MORTALITY IN GEORGIA DURING THE YEAR 1935

We report a survey and analysis of maternal mortality in Georgia, made by your Committee on Maternal Mortality:

The report considers the 438 maternal deaths during the year 1935. It is an analysis of questionnaires returned by attending physicians of 356 or 81.3 per cent of the 438 women who died during pregnancy, labor or the puerperium.

During the year, 60,424 live births were reported. Of these, 35,634 were whites and 24,790 were negroes. Physicians attended 35,701 and midwives attended 24,482 of the births. Of the 35,634 whites, 30,322 were attended by physicians and 5,201 were attended by midwives. Of the 24,790 colored births, 19,281 were attended by midwives and 5,379 by physicians. Of 241 women attended by others than a midwife or physician, 111 were whites and 130 were negroes.

A total of 3,968 stillbirths occurred during this same period. Of these, 1,524 were whites and 2,444 were negroes.

Method of Survey

A copy was made of the certificates of deaths assignable to puerperal causes as reported to the Bureau of Vital Statistics. At the end of each month these copies were turned over to the Committee, which immediately filled in the identifying data and mailed it to the attending physician or midwife. In many instances it was necessary to send several additional forms to the attendants before receiving the desired information.

The maternal death rate for the State was 7.1 per 1,000 live births. The infant mortality was 69.0 per 1,000 live births.

Geographic Distribution of Deaths

Time will not permit a detailed report of the maternal mortality rate for each individual county. The counties in which the maternal death rate was above that of the State as a whole were as follows: Bacon, Baldwin, Bartow, Ben Hill, Bibb, Brantley, Brooks, Burke, Candler, Charlton, Chatham, Clarke, Clinch, Coffee, Colquitt, Cook, Crawford, Dougherty, Douglas, Effingham, Evans, Franklin, Glynn, Gordon, Grady, Haralson, Harris, Henry, Irwin, Jackson, Jeff Davis, Lamar, Laurens, Lee, Liberty, Long, Lowndes, McDuffie, McIntosh, Muscogee, Newton, Oconee, Paulding, Polk, Richmond, Rockdale, Schley, Seminole, Spalding, Stephens, Stewart, Taliaferro, Taylor, Telfair, Thomas, Tift, Toombs, Troup, Ware, Washington, Wilcox and Worth.

*Report to the House of Delegates of the Medical Association of Georgia at its eighty-seventh annual session, Savannah, April 21, 1936.

Causes of Death

Abortion was given as the cause of 53 or 14.9 per cent of the mortalities; sepsis caused 93 or 26.1 per cent; albuminuria and eclampsia, 123 or 34.5 per cent; accidents of labor, 10 or 2.8 per cent; hemorrhage, including placenta previa, premature separation and postpartum hemorrhage, 53 or 14.9 per cent; ectopic gestation, 7 or 1.9 per cent; hyperemesis, 4 or 1.2 per cent and 13 or 3.7 per cent of the deaths were among pregnant women dying of diseases incidental to pregnancy.

Distribution of Deaths Among Whites and Negroes

Of the 356 deaths studied, 188 or 52.8 per cent were whites and 168 or 47.2 per cent were negroes.

Deaths following abortion were higher among negroes than among whites; the percentage of deaths due to hemorrhage was twice as high among whites as in negroes; the percentage of deaths due to sepsis, eclampsia and other causes was approximately equally divided between the two races.

Deaths According to Race and Marital Status

Of the 188 deaths among white women, 13 or 3.5 per cent of them were illegitimately pregnant. Of the 168 deaths among negroes, 40 or 11.6 per cent were illegitimately pregnant. Abortion was the cause of 33 or 62.2 per cent of the deaths of those who were illegitimately pregnant. Nineteen of the abortions were credited with having been criminally induced.

Prenatal Care

After excluding 60 women whose deaths were due to abortions and ectopic pregnancies, there remained 294 who could have received prenatal care. Of these 202 or 63.3 per cent had received no prenatal care from a physician. Forty-two or 14.2 per cent had received inadequate care and 52 or 17.5 per cent were credited with having had adequate care.

The survey made last year revealed that 81.1 per cent of the deaths occurred among women who had had no prenatal care or advice from a physician. This year, as previously stated, the number was reduced to 68.3 per cent.

Parity

Primigravidas made up 173 or 48.6 per cent of the deaths. The percentage of deaths due to abortions, ectopics and to hemorrhages was more than twice as great among multiparous women as in those pregnant for the first time. Sepsis deaths were 9 per cent higher among multiparas. Albuminuria and eclampsia caused 52.5 per cent of the deaths in primigravidas and 17.5 per cent of the multigravidas deaths.

Period of Gestation

Thirty or 8.4 per cent of the women died during pregnancy; 17 or 4.8 per cent during labor, and 309 or 86.8 per cent died during puerperium. Seventy-four died during the first two trimesters and 282 or 76 per cent died after the seventh month of pregnancy.

Operative Deliveries

Of the 282 women who died in the third trimester of pregnancy, 108 or 34.7 per cent had some form of operative procedure directed toward delivery before death. There were 25 deaths following, and due to cesarean section. Forty-four deaths followed forceps deliveries; 29 died following versions; 5 died following breech extractions; 2 died after hysterectomies and 3 women were delivered by some form of operative procedure following a failure of another method. It was found that 40 or 32.5 per cent of the 123 cases of albuminuria and eclampsia were delivered by operative procedures.

Anesthesia

Of the 282 pregnancies reaching the third trimester of pregnancy, 101 or 41.0 per cent were delivered without the use of anesthesia. Chloroform was the anesthetic used in 18.7 per cent; ether in 28.5 per cent; nitrous oxide or ethylene in 9.8 per cent; spinal in 1.6 per cent and local infiltration in 0.4 per cent. Three women died prior to or during operation, under spinal anesthesia, as a result of the injection. Chloroform, although today considered contraindicated in the presence of eclampsia, was administered to 7 women dying of eclampsia.

Method of Onset of Labor

The onset of labor was spontaneous in 255 or 89.9 per cent of women who were in labor during the third trimester. Of the cases induced, the catheter method was most often employed, being used in 3.6 per cent of the cases. In only 37.1 per cent of the 116 women dying of eclampsia was labor induced; the remaining 73 or 62.9 per cent developed convulsions prior to or after labor started spontaneously.

Cesarean Section

Included in the survey are 25 deaths following cesarean section performed on living women. Several other deaths were due to cesarean section but the Committee was unable to obtain answers to the questionnaires sent regarding these deaths. Of the 25 women subjected to cesarean section, eclampsia was the indication in 14, placenta previa in 4, obstructed labor in 5, abnormal position in 1, and premature separation of the placenta in 1. Nineteen or 76.0 per cent of the deaths following section were attributed to sepsis.

Place of Delivery and Place of Death

Of the total 356 deaths, 193 or 54.2 per cent occurred in the home. The remaining 163 or 45.8 per cent occurred in hospitals. One hundred thirty-nine or 39.1 per cent of the hospital deaths were admitted as emergencies or were in a moribund condition.

Infants

From the 282 women reaching the third trimester of pregnancy, there were 187 infants delivered alive. Seven sets of twins and one set of triplets were included in the series.

Attendant at Delivery

Of the 282 women reaching the third trimester of pregnancy, 14 or 4.9 per cent of the deaths were attended by others than midwives and physicians; midwives alone attended 55 or 19.3 per cent; midwives were replaced by physicians in 71 or 25.3 per cent; and 142 or 50.5 per cent of the women were attended by physicians alone.

During the year covered in this survey, midwives attended 24,482 or 40.5 per cent of the 60,424 reported live births.

A question included in the questionnaire was: Do you have any suggestions that you feel would tend to lessen maternal mortality in this State? Eighty-seven physicians did not reply, or answered "no." Of the remaining 269 answers, 166 or 61.7 per cent of the physicians disapproved or were critical of the midwives' presence in their community.

The Chairman, through personal communication with members of the Committee, found that 81 per cent of the members answering his letter considered the midwife an asset to his community. The majority of these based their opinion on the fact that the midwife is usually called upon to shoulder the burden in attending obstetric cases not desired by the physician.

In conclusion, after reviewing the records of 356 maternal deaths, we cannot deny that maternal mortality should be materially reduced in this State. It is a mutual problem of the combined laity and the medical profession. Until organized medicine appreciates the importance of maternal mortality, and until we realize its cause, it is of little use to appeal to the public for its cooperation. Too often we physicians are unwilling to accept the blame for a large number of maternal deaths that studies show to have been preventable. An example of this is the frequency of failure to appreciate the signs, delay in reaching a diagnosis and postponement of definite measures in terminating pregnancy among patients suffering with the toxemias of pregnancy. In many instances preeclampsia treated expectantly was permitted to develop into eclampsia. In contrast to this there exists a number of physicians who believe in radical procedures, and continue to treat extremely ill toxic patients by operative procedures—illustrated by cesarean section on women in eclampsia.

Too often there is a lack of understanding of just what is meant by prenatal care. To be able to render prenatal care, a physician must not only understand it, but he must be willing to render it conscientiously.

Much blame can be placed on the public for its failure to apply for and cooperate in prenatal care. The profession must be willing to instruct and guide the public by continuously and persistently giving advice in all matters pertaining to pregnancy. This advice will be especially valuable in controlling deaths due to abortions and toxemia.

The profession alone without the cooperation of the laity, can make little progress in decreasing maternal mortality. The public must be advised and it must be strongly urged to cooperate in this problem of such vital interest. If we can reduce the number of deaths due to abortions, improperly handled toxic conditions, wrongly managed hemorrhages and poorly selected emergency cesarean sections, the death rate will be greatly reduced.

Physicians cannot undertake to change the economic system, nor are they in a position to bring about a change in the general level of intelligence throughout the State. Superstitions, ignorance and illiteracy continue to handicap scientific efforts. However, in the interest of the advancement of preventive medicine it is the duty of organized medicine to undertake to eliminate those factors not of a medical character which increase maternal mortality. Once the cooperation of the public is obtained and a system of prenatal care instituted, the death rate from eclampsia alone should be reduced 50 per cent. It is alarming to think of this almost preventable disease as causing 30 per cent of the deaths last year.

No matter what interpretation may be given the statistics in this and the preceding report, they indicate that the maternal mortality in this State is entirely too high.

The Committee wishes to express its thanks and appreciation to the members of the Bureau of Vital Statistics for their splendid aid during this survey. It especially appreciates and thanks many members of the Medical Association of Georgia for their whole-hearted cooperation and the valuable information given to the Committee in supplying the statistical data in its questionnaires.

A. J. Mooney, M.D.
A. J. Waring, M.D.
W. L. Wilkinson, M.D.
W. W. Jarrell, M.D.
Herschel A. Smith, M.D.
J. C. Patterson, M.D.
H. J. Copeland, M.D.
Emory R. Park, M.D.
J. R. McCord, M.D.
Otis R. Thompson, M.D.
T. C. Clodfelter, M.D.
P. O. Chaudron, M.D.
W. Mayes Gober, M.D.
M. E. Winchester, M.D.
E. J. Overstreet, M.D.
Pratt Cheek, M.D.
Geo. C. Brooke, M.D.
S. S. Smith, M.D.
John W. Thurmond, Jr., M.D.
T. F. Abercrombie, M.D.
EMMETT D. COLVIN, M.D., *Chairman,*
Committee for the Study of Maternal Mortality.

HONOR ROLL FOR 1936

1. Randolph County, Dr. W. G. Elliott, Cuthbert, October 30, 1935.
2. Dougherty County, Dr. I. M. Lucas, Albany, December 27, 1935.
3. Monroe County, Dr. G. H. Alexander, Forsyth, February 14, 1936.
4. Hancock County, Dr. H. L. Earl, Sparta, February 25, 1936.
5. Elbert County, Dr. A. S. Johnson, Elberton, March 6, 1936.
6. Worth County, Dr. G. S. Sumner, Sylvester, March 12, 1936.
7. Rockdale County, Dr. H. E. Griggs, Conyers, March 21, 1936.
8. Morgan County, Dr. W. C. McGeary, Madison, March 30, 1936.
9. Turner County, Dr. J. H. Baxter, Ashburn, March 30, 1936.
10. Ware County, Dr. Kenneth McCullough, Waycross, March 30, 1936.
11. Georgia Medical Society (Chatham County), Dr. Otto W. Schwalb, Savannah, April 17, 1936.

MEDICAL ECONOMICS*

The subject of medical economics is more and more demanding the thoughtful attention of the organized medical profession. Within the last few years nearly all of the state medical associations have appointed committees to study the problem. In many of the states regular bulletins are issued once a month to keep the membership of the different associations abreast with the progress of the economic situation as it affects the medical profession.

State and national medical journals are constantly presenting various phases of the economic problem. Lay magazines and newspapers are filled with discussions, many of which are fantastic and ill-considered. The so-called Foundations are in many instances sponsoring movements to revolutionize the methods of medical practice which have been in vogue from time immemorial. The agitation for change has extended to the federal government and under the "New Deal," plans of considerable magnitude are afoot which, if carried out, would shake the very foundation of our medical structure. These plans are at present lying dormant, partially for the reason that the American Medical Association has been able to exert sufficient pressure to temporarily halt them. Be not deceived however. Such plans have not been abandoned. The medical profession is being given time to develop for themselves constructive and adequate methods of dealing with this problem and for this reason it behooves us to make every effort to measure up to our responsibilities.

Not only have those interested in bringing about a change in the methods of providing medical care filled newspapers and magazines but many books are appearing and still another movement of profound implications has arisen. I refer to the thousands of high-school students who for the past year or two have been debating over the United States the question: *"Resolved, That the several states should enact legislation providing for a system of complete medical service available to all citizens at public expense."* Certain foundations have issued extensive hand-books providing debators with every conceivable argument pro and con. This adroit method with its implications whereby the rising generation is being subtly taught what kind of opinion to have about this subject, should not be taken too lightly. In a word, the medical profession as never before is threatened with socialized medicine or if you prefer the term, "state medicine." This cry of "wolf" has sounded in our ears for many years and many no doubt are of the opinion that the wolf will not come. But, never before has such concerted and unrelenting action been taken by those who wish to bring about revolutionary methods of medical care.

In a very recent book by E. C. Buehler of the University of Kansas entitled "Free Medical Care," this paragraph may be quoted from his preface:

"The problem of medical care is woven in the fabric of our economic and social life. Medical service, like a commodity, has its purchase price. Each year the

*Report by the Committee on Medical Economics to the House of Delegates of the Medical Association of Georgia, Savannah, April 21, 1936.

people of the United States spend three and one-half billion dollars for medical service and medical goods. The hospitals in the United States represent a capital investment of three billion dollars and the education, training and physical equipment of the medical practitioners represent three billion more. The profession of medical care has become one of the largest industries in the country."

Considered from a financial and commercial point of view, this is a different viewpoint from the one we are accustomed to look at in the past. It is evident that very serious thought, consideration and watchful care, are essential to our best interests as a profession. Your Committee on Medical Economics has undertaken with the invaluable assistance of the President and Secretary of the Association during the past year, and with the collaboration of other interested persons, to make as far as we were able to do so a survey of certain phases of the economic situation in our State.

There was mailed to twenty-six hundred and sixteen white and to one hundred and ninety-five colored physicians in Georgia a questionnaire which no doubt all of you have seen. The object of this questionnaire was to secure first hand information regarding the income of doctors, membership in organized medical societies, whether the profession was availing itself of postgraduate medical instruction, how available were hospitals and laboratory facilities throughout the State, what percentage of general medical practice during the previous year was charity and to what extent drugs were furnished free to charity patients, whether the various counties made any provision for payment to physicians for the care of charity patients and finally, an effort was made to secure an expression of opinion directly from the physicians of the State regarding suggestions they might offer for the improvement of the health of their communities and for increase in financial returns from medical practice.

Five hundred and ninety-seven questionnaires from the white physicians were returned (22.44%) and from the colored 23 (11.79%). While the Committee would have been much pleased to receive a larger percentage of replies, particularly as they were not requested to sign their names, nevertheless, the Committee was grateful to have received as large a percentage as they did and the information below given, it must be understood, is based upon the questionnaires received from a total of six hundred and twenty physicians scattered throughout the State of whom twenty-three were colored.

Unfortunately there evidently arose confusion in reports regarding gross and net income from medical practice so that the Committee was obliged to discard this information as it was felt it was not reliable. However, a good deal of valuable information was obtained to other questions.

Taking first the average of the State-at-large it was found that 93.8 per cent were members of county medical societies leaving 6.2 per cent not members. Eighty-seven per cent stated that they had regularly attended during the past three years meetings of their county, district and state medical societies; 96.6 per cent reported regular attendance of county medical

society meetings: 88.7 per cent regularly attended district meetings; 87 per cent were regular attendants at state meetings and 39 per cent at national meetings; 38 per cent reported that during the past five years they had availed themselves of postgraduate medical instruction; and 81 per cent reported that laboratory and hospital facilities were available in their county.

From the State-at-large the report was that 32 per cent of practice during the past year was charity; 43 per cent of the physicians stated that they furnished drugs to charity patients; 21 per cent reported that the county made some provision for payment to physicians for charity patients while 79 per cent reported that no such provision was made.

It was felt by the Committee that some additional valuable information could be obtained by considering the size of the communities in which those who answered lived for the reason that conditions of medical practice vary. Thus it was ascertained that the towns with a population under one thousand only 39 per cent reported that laboratory and hospital facilities were available to them, that 35 per cent of their practice was charity and that 82 per cent of the physicians furnished drugs free to charity patients while only 14 per cent reported that the county made any provision for payment to the physician for the care of charity patients. As the population of towns increases there is a considerable rise in the availability of laboratory and hospital facilities and in the other figures which have just been given of the small community.

The Committee feels that the suggestions which have been received are of interest as indicating how over six hundred physicians in widely scattered areas of our State feel regarding efforts to improve the health of their communities and to increase physicians' incomes. The following is a tabulation of the outstanding suggestions which are grouped according to the size of the towns from which the replies came:

Under 1,000

Better cooperation among physicians	27%
Payment to physicians by Government, State or County for charity patients	40%
Abolish crop control	8%
Free postgraduate courses	1%
Recognition of ethics	1%
Exemption from professional taxation	1%
Taxation and insurance laws	1%
Visiting nurses and midwives are a menace	2%
Education of the public	5%
Better conditions for the poor, drainage, etc.	14%

1,000—5,000

Better cooperation among physicians	14%
Payment of physicians by Government, State or County for charity patients	40%
Eliminate quack hospitals and laboratories	3%
Better hospital facilities	13%
Ellis health law	4%
Better economic conditions	10%
Malarial and hookworm survey	9%
Better medical ethics	2%
Credit bureau	5%

5,000—10,000

Better cooperation among physicians	9%
Payment to physicians by Government, State or County for charity patients	39%
Education of rural sections	9%
Investigate financial status of charity patients	2%
Better hospital facilities	12%
Better conditions for poor	11%

Credit bureau 7%
Some form of taxation.................... 6%
Elect more physicians to legislative, executive
  and judicial bodies 2%
Stop county nurses and midwives from practic-
  ing medicine 3%
          10,000—25,000
Better cooperation among physicians......... 23%
Payment to physicians by Government, State or
  County for charity patients.............. 46%
Education of people to meet their obligations.. 5%
Investigate financial status of charity patients.. 9%
Abolish free hospitals 1%
Keep Government out of business 1%
Better sanitary conditions................. 5%
Establish credit bureau.................... 9%
Insurance 1%
          25,000—50,000
Better cooperation among physicians......... 42%
Payment to physicians by Government, State or
  County for charity patients.............. 17%
Education of public 9%
Credit bureau 16%
Investigate financial status of charity patients.. 8%
Better hospital facilities 8%
          50,000—100,000
Better cooperation among physicians......... 9%
Payment to physicians by Government, State or
  County for charity patients.............. 40%
Stop health officers from practicing medicine... 3%
Better economic conditions................. 7%
Abolish free hospitalization 2%
Educate people against quacks.............. 3%
Investigate financial status of charity patients.. 15%
Increase public health work................ 8%
Stronger county medical society............. 2%
Better hospital facilities 8%
Hospital for scientific development of colored
  physicians 3%
          100,000—300,000
Better cooperation among physicians......... 14%
Payment to physicians by Government, State or
  County for charity patients 30%
Investigate financial status of charity patients.. 23%
Educate people to meet their obligations...... 12%
Educate people against quacks.............. 5%
Insurance by clinics....................... 4%
Abolition of Veterans' hospital and other
  charity hospitals 5%
Support for Medical Service Bureau......... 5%
Curtail contract practice.................. 1%
Better conditions for the poor 1%

    In addition to the medical survey which your Asso-
ciation has attempted it has been possible through the
United States Public Health Service and the hearty
cooperation of Dr. T. F. Abercrombie, Secretary of
the Board of Health, as well as Miss Gay Shepperson,
W. P. A. Director for Georgia, and many others, to
secure funds obtained from the Federal Government to
the amount of over $20,000 for a medical survey of
sixteen widely scattered counties throughout the State.
Schedules have been obtained from over 12,000 families, rural and urban, black and white. We expect to
obtain from this source information of great value.
Complete tabulation of information derived from these
schedules will not be completed for some months but
the results will be reported by your Committee as soon
as they are available.

    A very large number of plans for furnishing medical
care have been devised and promoted in almost every
state in the union. Many of these plans have been
found unethical, have tended to exploit physicians and
have in one way or another violated the principles laid

down by the American Medical Association as a guide
to be followed in the formation of any plan. Time
will, of course, not permit an enumeration of these
various plans. It might be said that the so-called
Washington Plan, has created a good deal of interest,
is in operation in Washington, D. C., St. Louis, Missouri, and Newark, New Jersey, and has been recommended for state-wide adaptation in the state of Missouri by representatives of the Missouri State Medical
Association.

Conclusions

1. It appears to the Committee that the threat of
socialized or state medicine is definitely greater at
the present time than it has ever been in the past
and that the best method to avert such a catastro-
phic change would be the adoption of certain definite and specific plans to furnish the people with
more adequate medical care and at the same time
provide physicians with an adequate income.

2. The burden of the care of indigent patients has
become unbearable. Our survey indicates that practically one-third of the patients served by the physicians of Georgia belong in this indigent group.
Not only were the physicians expected to donate
their services but also at the expense of time, gaso-
line, and often of the drugs prescribed. It is felt
by many physicians that a certain proportion of
these so-called charity patients could arrange payment on a lower than the standard charge and that
some method of educating them to meet their obligations for medical services and some method of
investigating the financial status would be of considerable aid.

3. The Committee has been impressed by the considerable percentage of physicians who have felt
that an important method of improvement is by
better cooperation among physicians. This should
give us serious thought. Unless at a time like this
there is cooperation we may be ultimately forced
to cooperation under a political bureaucracy. How
much better it would be to have control of this
situation ourselves.

4. The Committee feels that a more adequate plan for
rendering service to the indigent of the State is of
the greatest importance. Under an ideal plan there
would be formed in the State eighteen Health Districts. In the center of such a district, under the
superivision of the district officer connected with
the Public Health Service there would be established a clinic to which ambulatory patients could
come for examination and treatment. The physicians of the district could rotate in attendance at
the clinic for the purpose of rendering medical service and should be paid at least a nominal fee for
such service. This fee should be paid from county
funds by the taxpayers through the County Commissioners. Included also should be dental services,
the dentists likewise to rotate in their attendance
and also be paid. A district nurse should give her
full time to such a clinic, making necessary home
visits outside of clinic hours in her district. Such
a plan would greatly improve the health of the
(Continued on page 214)

THE JOURNAL
OF THE
MEDICAL ASSOCIATION OF GEORGIA
Devoted to the Welfare of the Medical Association of Georgia

478 Peachtree Street, N.E., Atlanta, Ga.

JUNE, 1936

THE KANSAS CITY SESSION OF THE AMERICAN MEDICAL ASSOCIATION

The A. M. A. has just concluded one of the most successful sessions in its history. The Kansas City profession lived up to their promise made to the House of Delegates last year and provided every facility needed for the expeditious conduct of a great convention. The hospitality of this unique midwestern city can not be surpassed. The gods favored the occasion by a season of superb weather. The magnificent new city auditorium, costing several millions of dollars, gave ample room for section meetings, social gatherings and for the showing of the scientific and commercial exhibits. The session was formally launched in this great auditorium on Tuesday evening. There was some 15,000 in attendance.

Among others the governors of Missouri and Kansas spoke—interest appearing to center in the address of Governor Landon.

Kansas City is near the geographic center of the United States and in easy reach of a large per cent of our population. It is not surprising that 6824 doctors registered—a most pleasing attendance for a meeting away from the Atlantic Seaboard.

The Council on Scientific Assembly had arranged, through some fifteen sections into which the proceedings are divided, a program of unusual merit. Few members of the A. M. A. realize the voluminous correspondence required and the fine sense of discretion exercised in the building of these annual programs. The two days preceding the opening of the scientific session were devoted to the presentation of thirteen outstanding clinical papers. This innovation of the past few years has proved of significant interest as is evidenced by the large attendance and the careful attention accorded the essayists by their listeners.

The section meetings followed the usual plan and were so well staggered that those doing work in allied specialties could attend both morning and afternoon sessions. The scientific exhibits, as before, made up one of the most instructive features of the program. There were 170 exhibits presented offering a wealth of easily available information, capable of review within a brief space of time. This feature taken with the scientific program of the various sections constituted a combination which for its interest could not be rivaled anywhere in the world, a veritable week of postgraduate instruction of surpassing excellence. Physicians can not well afford to deny themselves the privilege of attendance on these annual meetings.

Lack of space, as well as the volume of work done by the House of Delegates precludes a recording here of even a resume of its proceedings. Suffice to say, that the House this year was concerned primarily with the relationship of physicians to hospitals, with the new experiments that are being tried for the furnishing of medical care to the low income group, with the status of contraceptive methods and with the bolstering of standards of medical education and ethical practices. Contrary to the sessions of the past two years, the deliberations of the House were harmonious. Perhaps harmony was contributed to by two factors. There was evidence everywhere of a heightened sense of economic security. Fear of bureaucratic medicine seems to have abated. Another factor was, the unanimous desire in the House to find a way to install Dr. J. Tate Mason as President. His serious illness threw a pall over the sessions of the House in the proceedings of which he partook through written messages presented by proxy as well as through telegraphic direction. At the opening meeting of the scientific assembly by unanimous resolution of the House of Delegates he was duly installed in absentia. Interest was complemented by the presence of the following distinguished guests: Lord Horder, physician of King Edward VIII of London, Leon Ascher of Switzerland and Wolfgang Heuber of Berlin. Lord Horder proved to be a great story teller as well as an erudite clinician. He was interested in many features of the meeting, both scientific and social, but none more than the recipe for the making of a mint julep a la southern style.

TUBERCULOSIS IN ADOLESCENTS

As more than two thousand years ago the Father of Medicine noted, consumption takes its heaviest toll between the ages of 15 and 30. Adolescence, the beginning of this period, is then the most critical age. By the early diagnosis of tuberculosis during this time it is possible to diminish the ravages of the disease and to lower its mortality.

Hardly ten years ago it was generally held that most persons were infected with the tubercle bacillus in early life; later on, the clinical manifestations of tuberculosis developed if the tubercle bacilli became active as the result of lowered resistance on the part of host, in turn the result of an intercurrent illness, insufficient food, "too rapid growth," over-work or dissipation. In recent years, however, it seems to have been established that the primary tuberculous infection is a rather mild affair; that it is a reinfection which causes real trouble. The widespread childhood type of tuberculosis, that is to say, is of importance chiefly as a signal of warning. Expressed in another way, a person, particularly a young person, who harbors no tubercle bacilli is in little or no immediate danger of developing the disease tuberculosis; on the other hand, one who does harbor the bacilli, even though apparently in good health, is in real danger of a second infection, often from the same source as the first one, and subsequently of clinical tuberculosis.

The universal application of the present knowledge of tuberculosis would probably wipe out the disease in a single generation. It may be that some physicians can apply in their private practice principles taken from the program of the Atlanta Tuberculosis Association, an affiliate of the Georgia and National Tuberculosis Associations, so it is offered:

Its program is not only to examine everyone who thinks he may have tuberculosis but also to examine all of the members of a household in which a case is discovered. It has a highly developed social service so that not only is a most successful effort made to keep out persons who could afford to pay a physician but also to keep under observation all eligible persons suspected of tuberculosis. It is essential to reexamine suspects repeatedly not only in the hope of detecting the early positive signs, but also because it is so easy to overlook them on one examination only.

When the boy or girl comes in, a detailed history, temperature and pulse are taken by a nurse, and the height and weight are recorded, compared with a normal for that age. Unless the physical examination reveals obvious pulmonary tuberculosis, a dilute solution of the purified protein derivative of tuberculin is injected *intra*cutaneously. If the first test is negative, the test is repeated with a stronger solution. If either test is positive, an x-ray is ordered. If both are negative, there is no exposure and the child is in good shape, he may be dismissed at once.

The Staff tries just as hard, particularly when there is not manifest exposure, to prove that the patient is not tuberculous as to establish that he is.

Their primary object is to make a diagnosis: Insufficient food, intestinal parasites, and chronic disease of the sinuses or tonsils are frequent simulators of tuberculosis, and attention to the real cause of the trouble often restores health. And an adolescent already handicapped by a tuberculous infection needs care of other diseases ever more urgently than one without tuberculosis.

Those who show a positive reaction to the tuberculin tests or who live in the house with a tuberculous patient are kept under observation. The frequency of the observation is of course determined in each individual case. It may be every two weeks or, rarely, every year—more often from three to six months. A nurse visits each home about midway between the patient's visits to the Clinic. Once the diagnosis of tuberculosis is made, the nurses lend what aid they can, not only in the care of the patient but also in the protection of the rest of the family. Meanwhile, every effort is made to get the patient into Alto or Battle Hill. When the patient is discharged from the sanatorium he is referred back to the Clinic and is again instructed to report for periodic observation.

With this program many cases of tuberculosis are detected in the minimal stages that otherwise would probably have gone on to chronic invalidism and death. From the most purely cold-blooded viewpoint the Associa-

tion has more than justified to the taxpayer the amount of money spent on it.

In the past seven years about five hundred patients have gone through the adolescent department. A definite diagnosis of clinical tuberculosis of the adult type has been made in seventy-seven cases. Only nine of the patients have died of the disease and more than twenty seem to have fully recovered. Thirty-five have received sanatorium care, the others have been cared for entirely at home.

It is not a confession of lack of skill to be uncertain from physical examination as to the presence of minimal tuberculosis. We know now that the x-ray will show a tuberculous lesion long before it can be picked up on physical examination. An x-ray is always desirable when the symptoms suggest the possibility of tuberculosis, but a negative response to purified protein derivatives will save many unnecessary ones. At the same time it should be remembered that a patient who is able to offer no fight against the rapid inroads of the disease may give a negative reaction to purified protein derivatives.

L.M.B.

OLEOTHORAX

The introduction of oil into the pleural cavity, a procedure called oleothorax, merits the attention and consideration of all physicians engaged in diseases of the chest. This method is one of the several that comprise that important group we know as collapse therapy and is inaugurated only in connection with an existing pneumothorax. Oleothorax, in the properly selected case, has considerable virtue and it is regrettable that it has remained behind a veil of obscurity and indifference. A few comments on oleothorax would therefore seem to be both justified and timely.

The method had its genesis in Europe, and today its most enthusiastic advocates and supporters are probably the French. One explanation given for this is that chest surgery has not made the strides in this country, thus leading more to the adoption of the non-surgical methods. It is very probably true that oleothorax cannot, in the end result, accomplish what cannot be so accomplished by some surgical pro-

making up the latter the mixture should stand for at least two weeks before using.

It is hoped that this short discussion will reflect a muchly deserved credit upon a procedure that has not taken its proper place in the sun.

.CHAMP H. HOLMES, M.D.

_____

THE SCIENTIFIC PROGRAM FOR 1937

Realizing that the preparation of a paper on a medical subject is not an easy task when undertaken in the desire to add to the sumtotal of medical knowledge it is not too early for those who contemplate seeking places on the scientific program at the next annual session of the Association in Macon to give thoughtful consideration to the subject, and to submit titles to the President or any member of the Scientific Committee. . It is believed that it would be to the best interest of all concerned if, when sending in your request, a brief outline of what you expect to say could be included. Matters of general interest to the profession as a whole, and those conditions which are encountered in the general routine of daily practice should be chosen rather than the rare and unusual. However, it is not desired to in the least minimize the importance of the latter.

It is unfortunate that so often members write such lengthy articles that the time alloted does not permit the complete reading of all that had been so painstakingly prepared. It should be remembered that the By-Laws of the Association, over which the Scientific Committee has no control, limits the time of any one speaker to fifteen minutes. It is believed that a careful revision and rewriting can encompass what is to be said on the average medical topic in this time. Ephraim McDowell's paper on "Ovariotomy" can be read in ten or twelve minutes, and Louis A. Dugas' article "Penetrating Wounds of the Abdomen" could be read without hurry in fifteen minutes. It is embarrassing for the presiding officer to have to interrupt a speaker with the admonition that he has consumed his allotted time, but he has no alternative.

It is most desirable that members in those portions of the State who have not in recent years favored the Association with contributions to its Scientific Sessions send in requests for places on the program.

The members of the Scientific Committee will be glad to aid any member in any way possible.

> Committee on Scientific Work
> GEO. A. TRAYLOR, M.D., *Chairman*.
> H. C. SAULS, M.D.
> CHAS. H. RICHARDSON, M.D.
> EDGAR D. SHANKS, M.D., Sec'y-Treas.

MEDICAL ECONOMICS REPORT OF COMMITTEE
(Continued from page 209)

State and at the same time lessen the burden of the care of the indigent on the physicians of the State. Lack of funds at present makes it probable that not over six districts could be so established, too large in area to carry out the health center plan and limited in their scope to fully preventive measures such as hookworm eradication, preventive inoculations, and the like.

It is the conclusion of the Committee that all physicians, particularly officers of county medical societies should unceasingly work for the establishment of such a plan as is here briefly indicated.

5. It is the conclusion of the Committee that insufficient publicity has been given to the constructive efforts of the organized medical profession to improve the public health and render adequate medical service. This is particularly true in view of the fact that unceasing propaganda is being constantly spread that the medical profession is failing in its efforts.

6. It is the final conclusion of the Committee that prepayment group hospitalization plans should be further studied in cooperation with the Georgia State Hospital Association. There is by no means unanimity of opinion regarding the wisdom of such plans but the trend of opinion is favorable in many of the states.

Recommendations

1. That each county medical society appoint a Committee on Medical Economics. Such a committee should make a careful and painstaking study of this great problem of medical care as it applies to its individual and separate communities. The first requisite would be that such a committee should secure from the Bureau of Economics of the American Medical Association and from other sources, literature dealing with this problem and thoroughly acquaint themselves with the situation. They should report at intervals to their medical societies the result of their investigation, decide for themselves on methods for improvement, subject to the ethical rules of organized medicine, and maintain contact with the State committee. Such a plan would mean a definite organization and integration of effort throughout the State which it seems should be productive of definite value not only to the public

but to every physician who thus lends his co-operation.

2. That county committees on Medical Economics or constituted officers of county medical societies, make in their respective communities definite and persistent efforts to secure from County Commissioners an appropriation of funds to pay at least some type of fee, even though small, for the medical care of indigent persons.

3. That the State Committee of this Association on Public Policy and Legislation be requested to give as wide publicity as possible to the efforts which the Medical Association of Georgia is making to improve the public health and to render adequate medical service to the people of this State.

> COMMITTEE ON MEDICAL ECONOMICS
> LEWIS M. GAINES, M.D., Atlanta, *Chairman*
> C. W. ROBERTS, M.D., Atlanta
> C. L. RIDLEY, M.D., Macon
> DAN Y. SAGE, M.D., Atlanta
> J. H. DOWNEY, M.D., Gainesville.

Auricular Fibrillation. Auricular fibrillation is so common in the terminal stages of rheumatic heart disease and, indeed, in other types of heart disease, that we are only too apt to consider it one of the very gravest prognostic omens. Orgain, Wolff and White (Arch. Int. Med. *57*: 493, March, 1936) have rendered a real service in reporting in considerable detail 47 patients with auricular fibrillation alone, 5 with auricular flutter alone, and 2 with both, without other evidence of heart disease. They have followed these patients along for a significant number of years and have found a low mortality rate, little important cardiac disease, and only one patient has developed hyperthyroidism. They conclude that such conditions are not infrequent and that the prognosis for life and for the maintenance of adequate cardiac function is good. The outlook for future improvement, manifested by a decrease in frequency or complete cessation of paroxysms, is frequently good. Thus, auricular fibrillation and auricular flutter are in some persons merely exaggerated functional disorders of the heart, no more indicative of cardic disease or of a poor prognosis than are premature beats or auricular paroxysmal tachycardia.

Friedlander and Levine (New England J. Med. *211*: 624, 1934) and W. A. Evans (Ann. Int. Med. *9*: 1171, March, 1936) have reported similar series, which overlapped that referred to above, and have come to the same conclusions.

Cobb County Medical Society

The Cobb County Medical Society announces the following officers for 1936:

President—W. G. Crawley, Jr., Acworth.
Vice-President—W. C. Mitchell, Smyrna.
Secretary-Treasurer, H. B. Terry, Acworth.
Delegate—W. H. Perkinson, Marietta.
Alternate Delegate—W. M. Gober, Marietta.

WOMAN'S AUXILIARY

OFFICERS. 1936-1937.

President—Mrs. Wm. R. Dancy, Savannah.
President-Elect—Mrs. Ralph H. Chaney, Augusta.
First Vice-President—Mrs. B. H. Minchew,
  Waycross.
Second Vice-President—Mrs. Clarence L. Ayers,
  Toccoa.
Third Vice-President—Mrs. J. A. Redfearn,
  Albany.

Recording Secretary—Mrs. Warren A. Coleman.
  Eastman.
Corresponding Secretary—Mrs. Lee Howard,
  Savannah.
Treasurer—Mrs. W. A. Selman, Atlanta.
Historian—Mrs. Grady N. Coker, Canton.
Parliamentarian—Mrs. John E. Penland, Waycross.

COMMITTEE CHAIRMEN

Student Loan Fund
Mrs. Robert C. Pendergrass, Americus
Health Films
Mrs. A. J. Mooney, Statesboro
Legislation
Mrs. Dan Y. Sage, 47 Inman Circle, Atlanta
Press and Publicity
Mrs. J. Harry Rogers, 134 Huntington Road, Atlanta
Research in Romance of Medicine
Mrs. D. N. Thompson, Elberton
Jane Todd Crawford Memorial
Mrs. Eustace A. Allen, 18 Collier Road, Atlanta
Doctors' Day
Mrs. Ernest R. Harris, Winder

TRANSACTIONS OF STATE CONVENTION

The preconvention meeting of the Executive Board met at Hotel DeSoto, Savannah, Wednesday morning, April 22, 1936. Mrs. E. R. Harris, President, presided.

The Lord's prayer was repeated in concert. Minutes of the postconvention meeting were read and approved. Minutes of the summer meeting of the Executive Board were read and adopted.

Nominating Committee: Mrs. D. N. Thompson, Elberton; Mrs. J. E. Penland, Waycross; Mrs. J. A. Redfearn, Albany; Mrs. Ed H. Greene, Atlanta; Mrs. Julian Quattlebaum, Savannah; Mrs. J. Victor Roule, Augusta; and Mrs. Clarence L. Ayers, Toccoa.

Auditing Committee: Mrs. Joseph Yampolsky, Atlanta; Mrs. B. H. Minchew, Waycross; and Mrs. Hugo Johnson, Savannah.

Mrs. D. N. Thompson, Elberton, read the report from the Executive Board.

The sum of $25.00 was appropriated for the President-Elect to cover part of her traveling expenses.

Motion carried for the President to appoint a Committee to ascertain the expense which might be incurred to publish the convention proceedings.

MRS. CLEVELAND THOMPSON,
Secretary Pro tem.

MEETING OF THE EXECUTIVE BOARD AND DELEGATES

The meeting of the Executive Board and delegates was called to order by the President, Mrs. E. R. Harris, at Hotel DeSoto, Savannah, April 22, 1936.

Invocation was offered by Rev. Geoffrey Horsfield, Rector of St. Paul's Episcopal church, Savannah.

The address of welcome was by Mrs. A. A. Morrison, President of the Auxiliary to the Georgia Medical Society, Savannah. Response was by Mrs. J. Wallace Daniel, Claxton.

Presentation of distinguished members by Mrs. J. S. Howkins was as follows: Mrs. A. A. Morrison, Savannah; Mrs. J. A. Redfearn, Albany; Mrs. Wm. R. Dancy, Atlanta; Mrs. C. W. Roberts, Atlanta; Mrs. J. E. Penland, Waycross; Mrs. B. H. Minchew, Waycross; and Mrs. Wm. H. Myers, Savannah.

The nurses of the First District presented the Auxiliary with a beautiful basket of flowers.

Mrs. Ralph H. Chaney, Augusta, read the rules governing the business session.

Minutes of the Eleventh Annual Business Session were read and approved.

Dr. Jas. E. Paullin, Atlanta, retiring President of the Association, spoke encouragingly of our work and future possibilities.

Mrs. L. W. Williams, Savannah, Chairman of the Entertainment Committee, made its report which was accepted with thanks.

Reports from districts were as follows: First District by Mrs. Cleveland Thompson, Millen; Third District, Mrs. E. B. Davis, Byromville; Fourth District, Mrs. R. S. O'Neal, LaGrange; Fifth District, Mrs. Joseph Yampolsky, Atlanta; Tenth District, Mrs. Ralph H. Chaney, Augusta.

Dr. Jas. N. Brawner, Atlanta, Chairman of the Advisory Committee to the Auxiliary, submitted his report which was accepted and filed.

Reports from county Auxiliaries were submitted as follows: Baldwin, Bibb, Bulloch-

Candler-Evans, Chatham, Clarke, E l b e r t, Fulton, Richmond, Stephens, Ware a n d Toombs.

Report of the Executive Board meeting was read by Mrs. D. N. Thompson, Elberton. Recommendations were made as follows: That the name of the Woman's Auxiliary to the Medical Association of Georgia be changed to "Georgia Woman's Auxiliary." Motion carried to defer action and authorize the postconvention session to pass on the recommendation.

Motion carried for the President to appoint a Committee to investigate the feasibility and ascertain the expense which might be incurred to publish the convention proceedings.

Motion carried to appropriate $25.00 to defray part of the traveling expenses of the President-Elect.

Mrs. R. E. Graham, Savannah, Chairman of the Credentials Committee, reported the registration as follows: Guests registered 113; distinguished guests 14, delegates 27, guests 26, local members 46.

Personnel of the Resolutions Committee appointed by the President were: Mrs. H. G. Banister, Ila; Mrs. J. L. Nevil, Metter; Mrs. E. B. Davis, Byromville; and Mrs. R. S. O'Neal, LaGrange.

Courtesy Committee: Mrs. H. D. Allen, Jr., Milledgeville; Mrs. J. J. Anderson, Savannah; and Mrs. J. E. Mercer, Vidalia.

Adjourned.

MRS. CLEVELAND THOMPSON,
Secretary Pro tem.

MINUTES OF TWELFTH ANNUAL SESSION

The Twelfth Annual Session of the Woman's Auxiliary to the Medical Association of Georgia convened on Thursday, April 23, 1936 at 10 o'clock at the Hotel DeSoto, Savannah. The meeting was called to order by the President, Mrs. E. R. Harris, followed by invocation by the Rev. Samuel McP. Glasgow, pastor of the Independent Presbyterian church, Savannah.

The address of welcome was made by Mrs. G. Hugo Johnson of Savannah, to which Mrs. Joseph Yampolsky of Atlanta responded.

The presentation by Mrs. L. W. Williams of the following distinguished guests was made: Mrs. McLester, Birmingham, Ala.; Mrs. C. W. Roberts, Atlanta.

Minutes of the Executive Board and House of Delegates were read and approved.

Address was heard on "The Auxiliary as a Unit in Community Activities" by President-Elect, Dr. B. H. Minchew, of Waycross.

Reports of officers were next order of business.

Mrs. W. A. Coleman took the chair while Mrs. E. R. Harris made a full report of her year's work. It was accepted with a rising vote of thanks.

Mrs. Wm. R. Dancy, President-Elect, read her report which was accepted with thanks.

Dr. J. L. Campbell, Chairman of the Cancer Commission of the Association, spoke of the vital necessity of educational work which should be done.

Mrs. J. Bonar White, Vice-President of the Auxiliary to the American Medical Association, addressed the meeting.

Mrs. W. A. Coleman, Chairman of Hygeia Committee, submitted report which was accepted.

Mrs. Ralph H. Chaney, Parliamentarian, read and submitted a report.

Reports by chairmen of standing committees were read and submitted as follows:

Mrs. Benjamin Bashinski, Macon, Student Loan Fund.

Mrs. T. J. Ferrell, Waycross, Scrapbook.

Mrs. D. N. Thompson, Elberton, Research in Romance of Medicine.

Mrs. J. A. Redfearn, Albany, Public Relations.

Mrs. A. J. Mooney, Statesboro, Health Films.

Mrs. Joseph Yampolsky, A t l a n t a, as Chairman for the Auditing Committee, that the Committee found all records of the Treasurer accurately kept and all funds properly accounted for.

Mrs. J. C. Metts and Mrs. A. A. Morrison, Savannah, report as delegates to the Auxiliary to the A. M. A. for the Atlantic City session in 1935.

Mrs. L. W. Williams, Savannah, delegate to the Auxiliary to the S. M. A., St. Louis meeting, 1935.

The Resolutions Committee submitted and recommended for adoption the following resolutions:

1. WHEREAS, The individual Woman's Auxiliaries have contributed financially to the storm stricken areas of Cordele and Gainesville:

THEREFORE BE IT RESOLVED, That as a State organization, our Secretary be authorized to write letters of sympathy to the Auxiliary at Gainesville and to the wives of doctors at Cordele.

2. WHEREAS, The presidents of county auxiliaries have not been included as members of the Executive Board;

THEREFORE BE IT RESOLVED, That presidents of county auxiliaries be made ex-officio members of the Executive Board.

Motion carried to adopt resolution No. 1.

Under a ruling of the Parliamentarian, resolution No. 2 could not be voted upon at the meeting in which it was submitted.

Motion to adjourn for five minutes carried.
Auxiliary reconvened and called to order by the President.

Motion to adopt resolution No. 2 carried.

Mrs. J. J. Anderson, Chairman of Courtesy Committee, reported. A rising vote of thanks was given the Auxiliary to the Georgia Medical Society for its charming hospitality and excellent programs.

Mrs. H. W. Birdsong, Athens, conducted memorial services for members who died during the fiscal year as follows:

Mrs. M. B. Allen, Hoschton.
Mrs. T. J. Charlton, Sr., Savannah.
Mrs. H. H. McGee, Sr., Savannah.
Mrs. J. A. Selden, Macon.
Mrs. Willingham, Canton.

Unfinished Business

The President appointed M r s. Joseph Yampolsky, Atlanta, to obtain designs and ascertain the cost of an Auxiliary pin.

Officers elected were those whose names were submitted by the Nominating Committee and are shown in the heading of this department.

The new officers were escorted to the platform and installed.

The Chairman of the Credentials Committee reported that 162 had registered; 52 local members; and 18 State officers and guests.

The Chairman of the Entertainment Committee announced that a Dutch dinner would be served at Hotel DeSoto.

Motion carried to direct the Secretary to send letters of sympathy to the following:

Mrs. Allen H. Bunce, Atlanta.
Mrs. Jas. N. Brawner, Atlanta.
Mrs. Ralston Lattimore, Savannah.
Mrs. Dan Y. Sage, Atlanta.
Mrs. Chas. C. Hinton, Macon.

Motion carried to send note of thanks to the First District Nurses' Association for complimentary basket of flowers.

A rising vote of thanks was extended Mrs. E. R. Harris, retiring President, for her efficient and loyal service.

The local Auxiliary presented corsages to the following: Mrs. J. Bonar White, Mrs. E. R. Harris, Mrs. Wm. R. Dancy and Mrs. A. A. Morrison, Jr. The Auxiliary to the Richmond County Medical Society presented a corsage to Mrs. Ralph H. Chaney, President-Elect of the State Auxiliary.

Adjourned.

MRS. CLEVELAND THOMPSON,
Secretary Pro tem.

POST CONVENTION BOARD MEETING

The Executive Board met at Hotel Savannah, April 23, 1936.

Mrs. Wm. R. Dancy, President, called the meeting to order.

Mrs. J. Bonar White made the following suggestions: that the program for work be more diversified; that all local Auxiliaries be asked to study the doctors in literature and art; establish a doctors' shop for the purpose of collecting and preserving relics and antiques pertaining to the practice of medicine; and medical research among early American Indians.

Motion by Mrs. White carried for the president of each county auxiliary to instruct her members in the "Aims and Objectives of the Auxiliary."

The President, Mrs. Dancy, announced that the appointment of members of standing committees would' be made later.

Motion to change the name of the Auxiliary was tabled.

Motion carried to send a letter of thanks to Mrs. Rex Stafford, Society and News Editor of the Atlanta Constitution, for articles published in her department.

Personnel of the Committee appointed to correct the minutes of the Twelfth Annual Session was as follows:

Mrs. Ralph H. Chaney, Augusta.
Mrs. J. E. Penland, Waycross.
Mrs. A. A. Morrison, Savannah.

Adjourned.

MRS. WARREN A. COLEMAN,
Recording Secretary.

SOCIAL FEATURES

The many delightful social affairs arranged by the Savannah women in honor of the visitors added greatly to the success of the convention.

Dr. and Mrs. William H. Myers entertained on Tuesday evening at a reception in their home on Jones Street honoring the officers of the Association and Auxiliary. Receiving with Dr. and Mrs. Myers were Dr. James E. Paullin, of Atlanta, President of the Association; Mrs. Paullin; Mrs. Ernest Harris, of Winder, President of the Auxiliary; Dr. B. H. Minchew, of Waycross, President-Elect of the Association; Mrs. W. R. Dancy, of Savannah, President-Elect of the Auxiliary; Dr. C. F. Holton, President of the Georgia Medical Society; Mrs. A. A. Morrison, President of the local Auxiliary; and Mrs. Lee Howard, Chairman for the convention.

A luncheon was given on Wednesday at the General Oglethorpe Hotel, during which Mrs. J. E. Penland, of Waycross, sang a number of songs, accompanied by Mrs. Cleveland Thompson, of Millen. Following the luncheon a trip was made to historic Fort Pulaski.

Wednesday evening an informal reception, featured by a fashion show, was held at the
(Continued on page 220)

GEORGIA DEPARTMENT OF PUBLIC HEALTH

T. F. ABERCROMBIE, M.D., *Director*

THE PREVENTION, DIAGNOSIS, AND TREATMENT OF CHILDHOOD TUBERCULOSIS

Prevention

In order to prevent tuberculosis, a knowledge of the sources of infection as well as the modes of entry of tubercle bacilli into the body is necessary. Since the discovery of the tubercle bacillus by Koch in 1882, a gradual increase of information regarding both of these factors has been given to us by competent investigators all over the civilized world. It is the consensus of opinion of all modern investigators that practically all of the pulmonary tuberculosis and 80 per cent of all types of tuberculosis are due to infection from human carriers. Bovine tuberculosis, while it accounts for many cases of extrapulmonary tuberculosis, has been greatly diminished through control of dairy herds by means of the tuberculin test. It is not usual for human beings to develop tuberculosis from avian sources, although it has been thought that Hodgkin's disease may result from this type of tuberculous infection and, so far as we know, tuberculosis of cold-blooded animals is not transmitted to human beings.

The entry of tubercle bacilli into the body is varied. They may be introduced directly through inspired air, they may be swallowed with saliva, or food, and gain entrance through the intestinal walls, or they may enter through other mucous membranes, through the tonsils and the skin. No matter how tubercle bacilli enter the body, it is possible for them to reach the lung. It is believed that tubercle bacilli may be taken directly from the gastro-intestinal tract with the chyle through the lymphatics into the thoracic duct to be carried through the subclavian vein to the right heart, and from there directly into the pulmonary circulation so that the first place they may be stopped is in the tissues of the lung. No matter in what tissue the primary focus may be, what is known as a primary complex is developed. This was dicovered by Parrott in 1876 before the tubercle bacillus was discovered, and at that time he made a statement which is known as Parrott's Law which established the fact that when first tubercle bacilli find lodgment in any partcular tissue, they quickly find their way into the lymphatic vessels

draining the area and thence to the glands into which these lymphatics enter.

The reaction that occurs at the focal point is not a specific one for tubercle bacilli but resembles that which occurs when any particulate foreign body enters the tissues and it is not until sensitiveness or allergy is produced by the tuberculo-protein that specific inflammatory reactions occur. This primary complex is not always formed in the lung but may develop in any organ. In the case of entry of tubercle bacilli through the wall of the intestine, the primary focus may develop there and bacilli passing from it through the lymphatics draining the area finally reach the mesenteric glands of the area involved. If the infection has not been too severe, and the natural immunity of the child or person who has this first infection is sufficient no ill effects are produced. So far as clinical signs and discomfort to the patient are manifested, such infections may be entirely unrecognized and fortunately this is found to be true in the majority of primary infections. Often there is extension of these primary infections from the primary focus itself or from the infected gland either through contiguous spread or by means of bacilli being carried to other tissues or organs through the lymphatics or the blood stream. Whether or not immunity develops as a result of this first infection has been discussed pro and con but one thing is certain; practically always an allergy is developed which makes subsequent infections, whether exogenous or endogenous, considerably more dangerous than the first infection because of this increased sensitiveness.

J. Arthur Myers and Francis E. Harrington in an article of the Journal of the American Medical Association of November 17, 1934, bring out some very interesting points. In studies of children, beginning in 1921 and carried through the years, they showed that five times as many children who were tuberculin positive at that time have developed tuberculosis as those who were tuberculin negative at that time. The study was made on two groups of children beginning in 1921 and 1922 respectively and carried up to 1934. If this proves anything at all, it would seem to prove that the first infection should be postponed as long as possible, and that immunity of any consequence is not developed through tuberculous infection but that it

be made. When there is cough, the sputum
if it is obtainable should be examined; if not,
smears made from swabbings from the
pharynx or examination of the gastric contents, and of specimens from the intestinal
tract may disclose the presence of tubercle
bacilli. By such means open and communicable tuberculosis may be definitely established
occasionally.

Treatment

The child that acts normally, plays and
studies and acts well, even though he may
have a slight temperature, a positive tuberculin test, and calcified glands, requires no
special treatment. Attention should be directed in these instances toward establishing
a proper diet, a reasonable amount of open air
activities, regulation of sleeping and eating
habits, and occasional observation by the
physician and usually this is all that is necessary. However, the child that is definitely
toxic should be put to bed and kept there
twenty-four hours a day as long as is necessary to rid him of the symptoms definitely
due to toxemia. The extent of the lesions
and the time required for the symptoms to
disappear, which may be a few days or a few
weeks or even many months of strict bed
care, will determine the amount of rest that
is necessary following it. Ordinarily the
child with either no noticeable lesions or
small ones may be adequately taken care of
merely by correction in diet in which there
should be a pint to a quart of milk daily and
in some cases increased rest which may be obtained easily and adequately by requiring the
child to retire earlier in the evening and get
up later in the morning.

It is not necessary to stuff these children
with milk and eggs or any other particular
kind of food and to do so usually results
disastrously. Neither should a child be
nagged about taking more food than he wants
to take, but he should be encouraged and required within reasonable limits to eat what
is known to be desirable for him to eat. It
is usually sufficient merely to have the food
supply well balanced. Milk is valuable because it affords a natural and rich supply of
calcium. Cod liver oil is valuable and children can usually accustom themselves to its
use easily. Viosterol may be added as the
judgment of the physician dictates. Direct
sunshine should not be used in active tuberculosis. It may be used, however, to advantage in tuberculin positive children in the
absence of symptoms of toxemia. In those
cases where extensive and destructive pulmonary tuberculosis of the reinfection type is
present, treatment should be the same as in
the adult. Strict bed care for as long as may
be necessary is imperative. Many cases can

be benefited by artificial pneumothorax, and it may be used in very young children advantageously.

Conclusions

1. The chief source of tuberculosis in human beings is tuberculosis in other human beings who have it in communicable form.
2. The earliest information that we may have of tuberculous infection in an individual is evidently through the tuberculin test.
3. Because of the development of allergy which is responsible for the disastrous effects of reinfections, the primary infection should be postponed as long as possible. .
4. Every child with a positive tuberculin reaction should be under the close supervision of the family physician to the end that his resistance might be kept by proper dietary and hygienic measures at the highest level and so that, when symptoms of disease develop, early and adequate treatment may be instituted.

H. C. SCHENCK, M.D., Chief,
Division of Tuberculosis Control.

WOMAN'S AUXILIARY SAVANNAH CONVENTION

(Continued from page 219)

Hotel DeSoto. In the receiving line were Mrs. Harris, Mrs. Dancy, Mrs. Morrison, Mrs. Paullin, Mrs. R. H. Chaney, of Augusta, and Mrs. J. S. McLester, of Birmingham. An orchestra played throughout the evening and special musical numbers were given by Mrs. William H. Myers and Hugh Taylor, accompanied by Mrs. Addie May Jackson.

A get-together luncheon at the Hotel Savannah and the annual banquet at the DeSoto Hotel, for the Association and the Auxiliary, followed by a dance, featured Thursday's calendar of social events.

NEWS ITEMS

Dr. Chas. W. Daniels, Atlanta, entertained members of the visiting staff of Grady Hospital and others at the country home of Dr. Frank L. Eskridge, near Jonesboro, on May 9th.

Dr. W. C. McGeary, Madison, spoke at a meeting of the Surgical Association of the Atlanta and West Point Railroad, Western Railway of Alabama and Georgia Railroad at the Ansley Hotel, Atlanta, May 5th, on *Fractures of the Backbone*. He is local surgeon for the Georgia Railroad at Madison.

Dr. Guy G. Lunsford, Atlanta, Director of County Health Work for the State Department of Public Health, addressed the Kiwanis Club at Columbus on the *Ellis Health Law* on May 12th. Among the guests at the

Club were: Dr. Guy J. Dillard, Dr. John E. Walker, Dr. Albert N. Dykes, Dr. I. C. Evans and Dr. Willis P. Jordan, all of Columbus.

The State Child Health and Welfare Council held its second annual meeting at the Biltmore Hotel, Atlanta, May 29th. Dr. B. H. Minchew, Waycross, President of the Association, spoke on *Our Obligation to the Child of Today;* others speakers on the program were: Dr. Mercer Blanchard, Columbus; Dr. T. F. Abercrombie, Atlanta, Director of the State Department of Public Health; Dr. H. C. Schenck, Dr. J. H. Kite, Dr. R. A. Bartholomew, Dr. E. D. Colvin, Dr. L. D. Hoppe and Dr. W. L. Funkhouser, all of Atlanta.

Dr. M. M. Burns, Pelham, was elected Secretary-Treasurer of the Mitchell County Medical Society at a re-organization meeting held on May 8th at Pelham. Members of the Society will be guests of Dr. F. L. Lewis, Camilla, at the next meeting.

Dr. Marion C. Pruitt, Atlanta, was elected President of the National Proctologic Society of America at its annual meeting held in Kansas City, Missouri, May 11-15.

The Fulton County Medical Society met at the Academy of Medicine, Atlanta, May 21st. Dr. John Funke reported a case. *Substitution Therapy Where Drugs Have Failed;* Col. Arthur N. Tasker, M.D., Fort McPherson, made a clinical talk, *The Flagellate Diarrheas;* Dr. Wm. M. Dunn read a paper, *Postoperative Treatment—The Abdomen.* The discussion was led by Dr. J. T. Floyd, Dr. Frank K. Boland and Dr. Edgar Boling.

The staff meeting of St. Joseph's Infirmary, Atlanta, was held on May 26th. Dr. Wm. P. Nicolson reported a case, *Carcinoma of the Uterus;* Dr. Grady N. Coker, Canton, *Rare Surgical Findings.*

The Georgia Medical Society, Savannah, met on May 26th. Dr. A. J. Waring read a paper entitled *Is This Child Nervous?;* the discussion was led by Dr. J. C. Metts and Dr. H. J. Morrison. Dr. M. J. Epting reported a case *Tuberculosis of the Kidney.* Refreshments were served.

The staff meeting of the Macon Hospital was held at Ridley Hall, Macon, on May 26th. Dr. Benjamin Bashinski spoke on *Intracranial Injuries of the New-Born and Differential Diagnosis of Vomiting in the New-Born.*

The Chattahoochee Valley Medical Association will hold its next annual meeting at Radium Springs, near Albany, on July 14-15.

The Coffee County Medical Society met at Douglas on May 26th. Dr. Sage Harper, Ambrose, gave a review of the proceedings of the House of Delegates during the recent Savannah session. Dr. J. G. Crovatt and G. W. Shirley, D.V.M., both of Douglas, spoke

Dr. M. Hines Roberts, Atlanta, was re-elected Chairman of the State Child Health and Welfare Council at the close of its second annual meeting at the Biltmore Hotel, Atlanta, on May 29th. Dr. J. P. Bowdoin, Atlanta, Secretary-Treasurer; Dr. T. F. Abercrombie, Atlanta, Chairman Public Health Section; Dr. W. L. Funkhouser, Atlanta, Chairman Medical Section.

NOTICE! We are just in receipt of a letter from a member of the Association written as follows: "Please note the enclosed. (Copy of order attached). This man got our instruments to repair. Not hearing from him I wrote to the address and the P. M. at Nashville (Tennessee) returned, saying no such address. Nothing has been heard from him since. I hope you will make mention of this crook in the JOURNAL so others will not get stung." The order to repair instruments was dated "12-20-1935."

The Fulton County Medical Society met at the Academy of Medicine, Atlanta, June 18th. Dr. Gerry R. Holden, Jacksonville, Fla., spoke on *The Treatment of Uterine Hemorrhage;* Dr. John Darrington, Yazoo City, Miss., *A Medical and Surgical Potpourri.* The program was sponsored by the Executive Council of the Southeastern Surgical Congress.

The Atlanta Cancer Clinic held its annual meeting on June 5th. Officers elected were: Dr. J. L. Campbell, Director; Dr. Rufus T. Dorsey, President of the Staff; Dr. Cosby Swanson and Dr. Chas. Rushin, Vice-Presidents; Dr. J. G. McDaniel, Secretary-Treasurer; Dr. O. D. Hall, Resident Radiologist; Dr. W. F. Lake, Resident Roentgenologist; Dr. A. J. Ayers, Résident Pathologist; Dr. George F. Klugh, Visiting Pathologist; and Dr. Chas. G. Boland, Photographer.

The State Board of Medical Examiners met for the annual examination of applicants at the State Capitol, on June 10th. Members of the Board are: Dr. J. M. Baird, Columbus, President; Dr. J. L. Howell, Atlanta, Vice-President; Dr. Frank M. Ridley, LaGrange, Secretary; Dr. H. G. Huey, Homerville; Dr. Luke Robinson, Covington; Dr. J. O. Elrod, Forsyth; Dr. C. F. Griffith, Griffin; Dr. O. B. Walker, Bowman; Dr. J. W. Palmer, Ailey; Dr. D. T. Rankin, Alto.

OBITUARY

Dr. Harry Bell Nunnally, Monroe; member; Atlanta College of Physicians and Surgeons, Atlanta, 1906; aged 53; died at a private hospital in Atlanta on May 13, 1936. He was born at Good Hope and moved with his parents to Monroe when only an infant. Dr. Nunnally received his literary education in Monroe and Mercer University, Macon, and made an enviable record as a medical student. After he graduated in medicine, he served as an intern and house physician at Grady Hospital, Atlanta, for three years; then did post-graduate work in New York City. Later Dr. Nunnally was associated in practice with Dr. Guy D. Ayer and Dr. J. D. Manget, in Atlanta. In 1911 he returned to Monroe and in a comparatively short time enjoyed an extensive practice in Monroe and Walton County where he continued until his health failed. Dr. Nunnally was one of the organizers of the Walton County hospital, located at Monroe, and its most valuable supporter. He held the confidence and esteem of the people of his home town and county and it is doubtful if any man in Walton county had more warm personal friends. Dr. Nunnally was a member of the Walton County Medical Society, American Medical Association and the First Baptist Church of Monroe. Surviving him are his widow; his mother, Mrs. W. H. Nunnally, Monroe; two sons, Harry B. Nunnally, Jr., student at Emory University, and George B. Nunnally, Monroe; one brother, J. Roy Nunnally, Monroe; one sister, Mrs. Geo. M. Napier, Athens. Funeral services were conducted from the First Baptist Church of Monroe by Dr. James A. Clarke, assisted by Rev. Frank Quillian. Burial was in the city cemetery. A number of physicians from Atlanta and members of the Walton County Medical Society formed an honorary escort.

Dr. *Lovick Thomas Pattillo*, Atlanta; Atlanta College of Physicians and Surgeons, Atlanta, 1904; aged 61; died at his home on May 12, 1936. He was a native of Buford and moved with his family to Florida when a youth. Dr. Pattillo graduated from the University of Florida at Lake City in 1901, then came to Atlanta to study medicine. After he graduated in medicine, he served as an intern at Grady Hospital, Atlanta, then began the private practice of medicine and was one of the leading physicians of the city. Surviving him are his widow, one daughter, Miss Martha Pattillo; his mother, Mrs. Alfred Pattillo, New Smyrna, Florida; two sisters, Misses Anne Pattillo, New Smyrna, Florida, and Miss Nell Pattillo, Asheville, N. C.; three brothers, Millard Pattillo, Atlanta; Geo. A. Pattillo, Little Rock, Ark., and Lewis Pattillo, Jacksonville, Florida. Rev. O. G. Jones and Rev. Luther Bridges conducted the funeral services from Spring Hill Chapel, Atlanta. Burial was in Rock Springs Cemetery, near Buford.

Dr. *James Lewis Lee*, Pinehurst; University of Georgia School of Medicine, Augusta, 1899; aged 58; died at the U. S. Veterans' Administration Facility (Hospital), Atlanta, on May 16, 1936. He was born in Wilkinson County. Dr. Lee practiced medicine in Dooly and adjoining counties for more than thirty years. He was a sucessful physician, had an extensive practice and held in high esteem by hundreds of acquaintances. Surviving him are his widow, two daughters, Mrs. James M. Coil, Pinehurst, and Mrs. Edward Lowe, Macon; three sons, Robert Lee, Savannah; Dan Lee, Macon; and Watt Lee, Albany. Funeral services were conducted by Rev. Edgar Martin and Rev. James Ivey from the residence. Interment was in Pinehurst Cemetery.

Dr. *James M. Freeman*, Lavonia; member; Georgia College of Eclectic Medicine and Surgery, Atlanta, 1893; aged 67; died at a private hospital in Royston on May 16, 1936. He was born in Tupelo, Mississippi, moved with his parents to Madison County, Georgia, when a youth. After he graduated in medicine, he began practice at Red Hill and after two years

Jubilee edition by the publishers. The new book contains 67 more pages and 70 new illustrations. A 134 page section on the nervous system has been included which presents the newer ideas and technical problems concerned with neurophysiology and neruosurgery. The chapters dealing with muscles, bones and joints have also been revised.

One of the finest things about the book is the simple manner in which it is written. It is not given to lengthy discussion nor is brevity over emphasized, therefore it is good for the students use and it enables the practitioner to obtain essential information without reading through a great mass of data.

The section on tumors covers 96 pages, and is perhaps, the best part of the book. It is natural that such should be the case as Dr. Wood is essentially interested in tumors and is a world-wide authority on this subject.

JACK C. NORRIS, M.D.

Your Hay Fever. By Oren C. Burham, Chief Botanist, Abbott Laboratories. With an Introduction by Morris Fishbein, M.D., and a Chapter on Treatment, by Samuel M. Feinberg, M.D., F.A.C.P. Bobbs-Merrill Company, New York. 250 page. Index, 12 pages. Price, $2.00.

Since one person in every fifty has hay fever, a clear presentation is of vital interest to both the physician and his patient. Mr. Durham accomplishes this adequately. He traces allergic phenomena from antiquity to the present.

His investigations include a study and description of the distribution of hay-fever producing pollens throughout the country. For Atlanta, Georgia, his slides indicate at the height of the ragweed season that the air contains one hundred thirty-one pollen granules per cubic foot. The inhalation of twenty-five granules in a day is sufficient to cause discomfort in an allergically sensitive individual.

Dr. Feinberg's chapter on treatment presents the era of modern allergy, which began in 1910 with the hyposensitization of atopic individuals with pollen extract injections.

This book is a distinct addition to that small group of publications presenting the subject on a basis interesting to both physician and patient.

CRAWFORD F. BARNETT, M.D.

Infant Nutrition—A Textbook of Infant Feeding for Students and Practitioners of Medicine. By Williams McKim Marriott. Second Edition. The C. V. Mosby Company, St. Louis, Mo. Price, $4.50. This is the second edition of Marriott's interesting book on "Nutrition." This book has been completely revised and special attention has been paid to the question of vitamins as they affect nutrition in infancy. Marriott again emphasizes the value of the use of lactic acid and evaporated milk formulas. He apparently relies on this method of feeding and naturally some writers will disagree with him on this question. The chapters on Acidosis, Alkalosis, and Anhydremia have been given special attention. The making of formulas has been simplified and the many difficulties that the average practitioner has in making them have been avoided. The studies of Hartmann and Hempelmann have been incorporated and an additional chapter details such diseases as rickets, scurvy, and tetany. This book is of value both to the general practitioner and pediatrician, and although we may not agree with all the views as expounded by Marriott, we believe that this book will find a valuable space in the physician's library on the problems of nutrition.

J. YAMPOLSKY, M.D.

Textbook of Surgery. By Frederick Christopher. Pages, 1567, with 1349 illustrations. W. B. Saunders Co., Philadelphia, 1936. Price, $10.00.

The author intends to present a cross-section of the teachings of the American schools. He has, therefore, selected as contributors several hundred teachers of surgery, each presenting one or more subjects in which the writer is particularly interested.

This method of presenting the textbook may at first appear erroneous. However, with the rapidly changing surgical opinions, the most authoritative information can be obtained in this manner.

Most of the illustrations are well chosen but much of their value is lost in an attempt to present a composite picture by including too many views on one page. Many captions, therefore, are required to interpret the diagrams.

It is doubted whether much detailed attention to surgical technic should be given to medical students. In some instances the authors have sacrificed technic at the expense of basic principles. This is not generally true throughout the text. The divisions have been carefully planned and the subjects are well presented. The book should, therefore, serve a very useful purpose both to the student and to the practitioner of surgery.

J. D. MARTIN, JR.

EMERGENCY TREATMENT OF WOUNDS

When an individual is wounded, two things that demand prompt attention are pain and the danger of infection. If at that time one could apply locally a preparation that is both anesthetic and antiseptic, these needs would be met. It is desirable that the local anesthetic and the antiseptic both be incorporated in the same vehicle because the contaminated tissue is likely to be included in the painful area. It is also desirable that the vehicle be water-soluble so that it may be washed away easily in case the surgeon desires to use some other local application which might be incompatible. For this purpose a water-soluble jelly would seem preferable to an ointment base.

'Metycaine' (Gamma-(2-methyl-piperidino)-propyl Benzoate Hydrochloride, Lilly) is stated to belong to the group of substituted piperidino-alkyl benzoates prepared by Dr. S. M. McElvain. Its anesthetic effects are obtained, according to Eli Lilly and Company, either by infiltration or by topical application to mucous surfaces. In painful ulcerations of the skin and in some open wounds, the pain may be locally controlled by

duce it by feeding the virus to the monkey even in very large doses. As was brought out in the discussion there is no absolute proof of either theory and at the present writing this question is a debatable one.

Dr. Lucchesi presented the topic, "The Use of Vaccine in the Prevention of Poliomyelitis." In his discussion he told of the fine work done by Drs. Brodie and Kolmer, working independently. This work on prevention in monkeys is not new, but in its application to man it is new and deserves careful consideration.

The vaccine, as prepared by Dr. Brodie, contains poliomyelitis monkey passage virus inactivated by the addition of formalin and incubated from twelve to forty-eight hours. This vaccine was used on six laboratory workers and twelve children and it is interesting to note that all of these had evidence of a small amount of antiviral substance present in the blood prior to injection of the vaccine. Dr. Park, in a recent article, has given statistics in 1300 children innoculated with Brodie's virus during the California epidemic and not one of these children developed the disease. It is interesting to surmise whether these children would have developed the disease if not inoculated.

Dr. Kolmer, with many others, believes that a dead virus vaccine is weaker than a living or attenuated one, and therefore has produced an attenuated vaccine of poliomyelitis virus containing a 4 per cent suspension of monkey spinal cord. This vaccine was given to twenty-five children. Ten of these children had small amounts of antiviral substance present prior to inoculation whereas fifteen of the children had absolutely no protective substances in their blood. After the complete inoculation the fifteen children mentioned had definite evidence of antiviral substance present and the ten children with substance present before inoculation showed a marked increase in this substance. At this writing Dr. Kolmer has inoculated about 350 children without any serious local or general reactions.

This work is still more or less in the experimental stage and naturally many questions arise. Dr. Kolmer believes that, although an attenuated virus tends to become more virulent within the human body, his vaccine is perfectly safe. No exact data as to the duration of immunity has been brought forward, especially with relation to the human. Kolmer has eighteen monkeys that have retained their immunity for three years, but this does not have any bearing on the human immunity possibilities.

Dr. Kramer closed the discussion by stating, "It is unfortunate that the practicing physician is now placed in the same position with the proposed vaccines as he was a few years ago when human convalescent serum was recommended for therapeutic use. The pressure of publicity compelled him, often enough to use convalescent serum, even though he lacked adequate corroborative experimental evidence to justify its use."

Abstract from: Round Table Discussion on Poliomyelitis at Fifth Annual Meeting of the American Academy of Pediatrics. Journal of Pediatrics, August, 1935. Abstract by Don F. Cathcart, M.D., Atlanta.

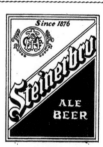
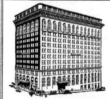
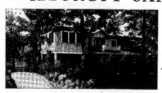

THE JOURNAL
OF THE
MEDICAL ASSOCIATION OF GEORGIA
DEVOTED TO THE WELFARE OF THE MEDICAL ASSOCIATION OF GEORGIA
PUBLISHED MONTHLY under direction of the Council

| Volume XXV | Atlanta, Ga., July, 1936 | Number 7 |

SYMPOSIUM ON THYROID AND PARATHYROID PROBLEMS
Doctors Davison, Gay, Clifton and Broderick

CHRONIC HYPERTHYROIDISM WITH A PERSISTENT LOW BASAL METABOLIC RATE*

T. C. DAVISON, M.D.
Atlanta

The basal metabolic rate is supposedly an accurate measurement of the degree of toxicity in any given patient with goiter and it has been generally accepted that "if hyperthyroidism is present the basal metabolic rate is above normal, and if the basal metabolic rate is normal then no hyperthyroidism exists." In most instances this rule can be depended upon, provided the test has been made in a carefully conducted laboratory by an experienced technician. Very often the test must be repeated before the true basal metabolic rate can be determined. One must not accept either a single high or a normal basal metabolism test as proof of the presence or absence of toxicity when it does not agree with clinical data. Normal basal metabolic tests in truly toxic patients are not common, but they do occur. When the clinical picture is typical of hyperthyroidism and the basal metabolic rate is normal, the test should be ignored and the diagnosis made entirely from the clinical picture.

As diagnosticians, we have become more and more dependent upon laboratory tests, and at times are inclined to overlook the clinical picture that makes the diagnosis evident. I do not wish to underestimate the value of the laboratory and I think it should be utilized to the fullest, but we should be clinicians and not robots. In the study of thyroid

*Read before the Medical Association of Georgia, Savannah, April 22, 1936.

diseases, as in other conditions, we should remember not to use the terms "always" and "never."

Clute[1] in 1928, called attention to a small group of borderline cases of hyperthyroidism with normal or subnormal basal metabolic rates. Troell in 1932, reported fourteen similar cases and Plummer[2] in 1931, reported a case of hyperthyroidism with a basal metabolic rate of minus nine. Lahey[3] emphasizes the clinical importance of the "apathetic type of hyperthyroidism with its relatively low basal metabolism rate and its great tendency to terminate fatally." In 1934, Gordon and Graham[4] reported in detail two groups, one of 17 cases of diffuse toxic goiter and another of 54 cases of nodular toxic goiter in which the basal metabolic rate was consistently low or even subnormal at times. As a rule the toxic symptoms appear after the goiter has been present several years. These patients frequently have consulted several doctors and some have been told that they have no goiter, because the basal metabolic rate is normal or subnormal in spite of a visible enlargement of the thyroid gland and definite symptoms of hyperthyroidism.

The history is usually vague. The onset of symptoms is insiduous and the exact time that illness began frequently cannot be determined. In some cases the symptoms may date back several years with a history of poor health, and at times one or more so-called "nervous breakdowns." The usual symptoms of these patients are nervousness, palpitation, choking sensation, tremor, dyspnea, sweating, fatigue, irritability, emotionalism, insomnia and at times loss in weight. Exophthalmos which occurs in only 45 per cent of exophthalmic goiter and in only 3 per cent of toxic adenomas, rarely occurs in this type of patient; however, the eyes of several patients in this group had a peculiar stare. There is usually a moderate increase in pulse rate, 90 to 110, and a slight rise in the blood pressure above the normal. Miller[a] reports: "tachycardia on excitement and moderate exertion, nervousness without cause and beyond the patients control, and tremor on excitement or exertion are the outstanding diagnostic points in these cases." An individual patient may have two or more of the above symptoms or findings. The patient with true hyperthyroidism is usually optimistic and hopeful of the future, and often shows a mental attitude of marked instability in which the patient passes frequently from laughter into tears without adequate cause.

I am reporting a series of 37 patients, including both diffuse and nodular goiters, in which every patient has some indication of hyperthyroidism, and in no instance was the basal metabolic rate above normal. All of these patients were operated upon with relief of symptoms in the majority of instances. There were 2 men and 35 women in the group. The average age was 32.8 years, the duration of the goiter was 7.3 years and the duration of symptoms 1.1 years. The average basal metabolic rate was plus 2.5 per cent, though it varied from minus 37 to plus 12. The pulse rate was often normal, but averaged 88 and the myocardium in some cases had become permanently damaged.

I have classified this condition "chronic hyperthyroidism" as compared to the more acute type which is usually seen in diffuse toxic goiter with exophthalmos, and in which there is usually a high basal metabolic rate, and which most often has been present only a few months and frequently has developed suddenly. The terms "acute" and "chronic" are not usually used in discussing thyroid toxemias, but I consider them applicable in this discussion.

Why these patients should have a persistent low basal metabolic rate is not entirely clear. There are persons who have normally a lower rate and, therefore, a rate that would be considered normal to one individual might indicate thyrotoxicosis in another. Theoretically, it might be suggested that certain individuals with "chronic hyperthyroidism" have "a low

aid in differentiating a typical hyperthyroidism from conditions simulating it.

The study of this series of patients shows that clinical hyperthyroidism often occurs in the presence of a persistent low basal metabolic rate. We should be very careful about accepting laboratory reports at face value when they do not agree with our clinical diagnosis. The majority of these patients were restored to normalcy by subtotal thyroidectomy. This operation in the hands of a surgeon experienced in thyroid surgery offers a cure to these patients with no risk to life and without danger of their condition being made worse.

Conclusions

1. The interpretation of clinical data should not be based on any one laboratory test.
2. The basal metabolic rate while very helpful when it is elevated should be ignored when normal or subnormal, in the presence of unmistakable evidence of hyperthyroidism.
3. An important fact to bear in mind in connection with the thyroid heart, is that it is one type of heart disease which is preventable, provided the thyrotoxicosis is recognized early and subtotal thyroidectomy is performed before the heart becomes permanently affected.
4. Because of the great frequency of cardiac disease in patients with adenoma of the thyroid, particularly in patients of middle age or beyond, removal of all adenomas, before cardiac symptoms develop, is indicated as an important means of prevention of heart disease.

478 Peachtree Street., N. E.

REFERENCES

1. Clute, H. M.: Borderline Hyperthyroidism. Amer. J. Surg. 1929, 6, 11-16.
2. Plummer, W. A.: Adenomatous Goiter with Hyperthyroidism Accompanied by an Unusually Low Metabolic Rate. Proc. of Staff Meet of Mayo Clinic, 1931, 6:329.
3. Lahey, Frank H.: Apathetic Hyperthyroidism. Annals of Surgery 1931, 93: p-1026-1030.
4. Gordon, Stuart, and Graham, Roscoe, R.: Clinical Hyperthyroidism Associated with a Normal Basal Metabolic Rate. Trans. of Amer. Assoc. for the Study of Goiter. 1924, p-192-199.
5. Morris, Roger B.: The "Thyroid Heart" with Low Basal Metabolism Reading. Am. J. Med. Sciences. 1931, March.
6. Levine Samuel A.: Unrecognized Hyperthyroidism Masked as Heart Disease. Ann. Int. Med. 1930, 4, 67.
7. Strouse, Solomon and Binswanger, H. F.: The Symptom Complex Resembling Hyperthyroidism Without Increased Metabolism. J. Am. Med. Assn. 1927, Jan. 88, 161-164.
8. Miller, J. L. and Raulston, B. O.: The Recognition of Mild Hyperthyroidism. J. Am. Med. Assn. 1922, Oct. 79, -1509-1511.
9. Wohl, M. G.: Atypical Hyperthyroidism and the Significance of the Basal Metabolic Rate. M. Rec. 1934, 140, 372-375.
10. Hamburger, W. W. and Lev, M. W.: Masked Hyperthyroidism. J. Am. Med. Assn. 1930, 94, 2050.
11. Davison, T. C.: Thyroid Disease or Thyrotoxicosis. Interstate P. G. Assembly of N. Amer. 1928. p. 424-428.
12. Davison, T. C.: Thyroid Surgery in Cardiac Patients. Sou. Surgeon. 1934, June. 3, 101-111.

GOITER IN CHILDREN*

J. GASTON GAY, M.D.
Atlanta

Goiter in childhood is not common and relatively little is known about it. This is largely because our diagnostic methods in children are unsatisfactory, and clinical criteria are different from those in adults. Three phases of the subject will be discussed here:

1. Thyrotoxicosis (which includes both exophthalmic goiter and other types of hyperthyroidism).
2. Tumors of the thyroid.
3. A group of cases, which, for want of a better term, may be called adenopathies of the thyroid.

1. *Thyrotoxicosis*

Statistics show that thyrotoxicosis in children accounts for about 2 per cent of all goiters. It may be seen at any age, but most frequently from the seventh to the tenth year. It is overwhelmingly more common in girls than in boys, and is seen as often on the seaboard as in the goiter belt. The etiologic factor or exciting cause is apparently related to infection in the teeth or tonsils, or in both, in 50 per cent of cases; in 22 per cent general infections were of seeming importance. The physical findings differ from those in adults. An irregular enlargement of the gland rather than a diffuse symmetrical one is noted. Exophthalmos is the rule, though in my case it was not marked. Tachycardia out of all proportion to the severity of the disease is constant. Tremor is exaggerated and purposeless movements are more pronounced than in adults. Gastro-intestinal upsets are much more frequent but loss of weight and strength is less marked. Great increase in height is interesting.

At the Good Samaritan Clinic out of 59 cases of goiter in children, we have seen one proved case of exophthalmic goiter and two other cases of definite hyperthyroidism. All three of these patients were girls.

When we consider the importance of the thyroid gland in growth and development, we realize the value of conservatism in treat-

*Read before the Medical Association of Georgia, Savannah, April 22, 1936.

ment. Bloom has reported 40 cases, including twelve of true exophthalmic goiter, in which only medical treatment was used with apparently good results. In our group also we treated the patient with iodine, mild sedatives, gradual clearing up of focal infection, proper periods of rest, a regular routine of living, a diet high in calcium and low in protein and protection from psychic trauma. Although this regime may be followed for a long period with only slight results at first, in time many of these young patients will get well. Let me emphasize, however, that while it is right and proper to prepare an adult for operation with iodine, it is only in children that the careful use of iodine may be tried in the hope of curing goiter. In spite of such measures operation may still prove necessary in some cases. Treatment of thyrotoxicosis in children is still unsatisfactory and there is much to be learned about it.

2. *Tumors*

Tumors of the thyroid in children are rare except when arising from aberrant thyroid tissue. This term includes all tissue not connected with the gland, namely:

1. Lingual thyroid and thyroid tissue found along the thyroglossal tract.
2. Lateral aberrant thyroids or those lateral to the jugular vein.
3. The extremely rare intrathoracic goiter that is not connected with the main thyroid body.

About 60 cases of tumor of the thyroid in children have been reported. The tumor may be noted at any age from birth on. They occur about three times more often in girls than in boys. They vary in size and may be multiple. In the two cases of tumor in the midline, the second my own, the tumor was single. The usual history is that a mass was noted in the neck from one to twenty years earlier, and it has remained stationary in size and has caused no symptoms.

The history is probably the most important point in differential diagnosis. The diagnosis, however, is rarely made preoperatively. The tumor is frequently confused with Hodgkin's disease, branchial cyst, dermoid, carotid body tumor and enlarged lymph nodes. The midline tumor is frequently mis-

to retrograde infection from the deep cervical glands, and this may be the explanation of these tumors. On the other hand, if we accept the work of Womack and Cole, the masses may be the forerunners of the true adenomas of adult life or of the so-called adenomas of Rienhoff.

As regards treatment, the administration of iodine seems to be of no value, or perhaps even harmful. Thyroid extract in small doses at intervals may cause a slight decrease in the size of the tumor. At times moreover the gland may fill up with colloid, thus obscuring the mass. Thyroid extract dissipates the colloid quickly revealing the tumors again. The cleaning-up of foci and general measures for the upbuilding of the patient, such as a high caloric diet, fresh air and exercise seem to be of value.

I have observed about 40 cases of this type, of which only four cases were boys. One patient was 12 years old when first seen eight years ago. Since then she has married and she now has two children. She came back to see me in March, 1936, complaining of a rather rapid increase in the size of the thyroid and also an enlargement in the left lower lobe. She had no symptoms of hyperthyroidism and her basal metabolic rate was minus 15. She was given thyroid extract on the assumption that the enlargement was due to an accumulation of colloid. At the end of about two weeks the gland had decreased in size but two rounded masses simulating adenomas, one in the original location in the isthmus and one at the left lower pole, became evident.

Conclusions

Goiter is relatively uncommon in children and deserves much further study. Let me plead for conservatism in treatment.

Dr. Emanuel Krimsky, Brooklyn, N. Y., speaking for the National Society for the Prevention of Blindness, states that as a rule, "neither tobacco nor alcohol directly affect the eyes, unless they have at first attacked the general health.

Dr. Dean H. Affleck advocates removal of brown or reddish moles on the skin to avoid the possibility of cancer.—Pub. R. Bureau, Medical Society of the State of New York.

The Medical Association of Georgia will hold its eighty-eighth annual session at Macon, May 11-14, 1937.

GOITER AND IODINE*

BEN HILL CLIFTON, M.D.
Atlanta

The literature is replete with evidence that the beneficial effect of iodine on certain goitrous conditions has been known for many centuries. It was known to the ancient Greeks that preparations made from seaweed and sponges had a beneficial effect on certain goiters. Following the discovery of iodine in 1811, Davey, in 1815, found that these natural substances, sponges and seaweed, were rich in iodine and in 1820 Coindet suggested that the beneficial effect was due to the iodine. This suggestion was further substantiated by Cantu, in 1825, who found that certain spring water noted for its power to cure goiter was rich in iodine and as still further proof it was noted, in 1831, by Boussingault that certain sea salt rich in iodine had a good effect on goiter in the Andes and where it was generally used goiter was notably absent.

As early as 1849, Prevost theorized that goiter was a deficiency disease due to water poor in iodine and Kostl, in 1855, advised the use of iodine for all goitrous persons between certain age limits. In 1860 Boussingault experimented on a large scale by giving iodized salt and potassium iodide daily to school children but many developed toxic symptoms and the method was soon abandoned.

The relationship between iodine and goiter was revived by Baumann's discovery of iodine in the thyroid gland in 1895. Since then much experimental work and clinical investigation have been done, notably by Kocher, Marine and Kimball, McGarrison, Kendall and Curtis.

The per cent of iodine in the thyroid gland has been determined to be the highest of any tissue in the body: the thyroid is undoubtedly the principal storehouse for iodine in the body. The per cent has been determined in normal and abnormal glands. In hypothyroidism the iodine content of the gland is increased, in hyperthyroidism the iodine content of the gland is decreased. The iodine content of the blood has been determined in

*Read before the Medical Association of Georgia, Savannah, April 23, 1936.

tion, etc., are prone to precipitate an acute hyperthyroidism which is a serious emergency and should be dealt with just as a postoperative hyperthyroidism.

Iodine Before and After Operations for Hyperthyroidism

This is the most important place for iodine at present in non-endemic areas. H. S. Plummer, in 1923, showed the marked clinical improvement in patients with exophthalmic goiter following the administration of Lugol's solution. At first it was thought that exophthalmic goiter was due to an incompletely iodized molecule and that the iodine completed the product. Since then many reports indicate that it is just as effective in the so-called toxic adenoma as it is in the exophthalmic cases except to a less degree. The custom is to give 10 drops (small doses are just as useful) of Lugol's solution to an adult, three times daily, and with few exceptions marked clinical improvement is noticed within from 6 to 12 days. The pulse will slow, restlessness improves, sleep is better and the patient gains weight. As a rule the patient is transformed into another individual following the administration of iodine preoperatively except in those cases in which iodine has been administered over a long period. The mortality has been markedly lowered, the necessity for multiple stage operations has been reduced and the stay in the hospital has been shortened. However, the administration of iodine must not be depended upon altogether. Proper rest and other safety measures and in some cases multiple stage operations must still be practiced according to the judgment of the surgeon. In other words, iodine is only another adjunct in the handling of the serious cases. Immediately following the operation iodine should be given, the amount varying according to the severity of the case. It can be given per rectum, subcutaneously or even intravenously. Small amounts, say 5 drops three times daily of Lugol's solution should be continued for several weeks following the operation because as Else has shown the remaining thyroid tissue is adjusted more rapidly and recurrences are less apt to occur if iodine is given a few weeks postoperatively.

It is my belief that if this simple plan of using iodine in goiter is adhered to there will be little mischief done and it will keep many patients out of the hands of the ignorant. The maximum benefit from iodine in the treatment of toxic goiter can be expected only when it is not instituted until operation has been scheduled.

REFERENCES

Boothby, Walter M.: Use of Iodine in Exophthalmic Goiter. Mayo Clinic Vol. XVI: page 421, 1924.
Joll: Diseases of the Thyroid Gland. C. V. Mosby Co. 1932.
Crile and Associates: Diagnosis and Treatment of Diseases of Thyroid Gland. W. B. Saunders Co. 1932.
Else, J. Earl: Regeneration of the Thyroid Gland and the Prevention of Recurrent Goiters. J. A. M. A. Vol. 89: page 2153-2158, Dec. 24, 1927.
Graham, Allen: Exophthalmic Goiter and Toxic Adenoma, J. A. M. A. Vol. 87: page 628, Aug. 28, 1926.
Plummer, H. S.: Results of Administering Iodine to Patients Having Exophthalmic Goiter. J. A. M. A. Vol. 80: page 1955, June 30, 1923.
Blanck, E. E.: Preoperative Iodine Therapy in Hyperthyroidism. Surg. Gyn. Obst. Vol. 62: No. 2. page 213, Feb. 1, 1936.
Curtis, George M.: The Iodine Relationships of Thyroid Disease. Surg. Gyn. Obst. Vol. 62: No. 2A. page 365, Feb. 1936.

HYPERPARATHYROIDISM*

J. REID BRODERICK, M.D.
Savannah

Introduction

A relatively new clinical entity has come to recognition in the past several years. This disease is now frequently considered in differential diagnosis, and perhaps when not to make the diagnosis, is the most important feature. With only two probable cases to report, my remarks are based largely on related cases I have studied, from which the disease has been excluded, and on bibliography, which contains the excellent work of Allbright, his associates, and other investigators. Much has been said about the hyposecretion of parathyroid glands with the resulting tetany, etc., and not until in recent years has a clinical syndrome been described which fits in with hyperactivity of these glands.

History

In 1904, Askanazy found a tumor of the parathyroid gland in a case of generalized fibrous osteitis. Later Erdheim remarked about the frequent occurrence of parathyroid hypertrophy in rickets and osteomalacia. The general feeling in the profession at that time was that the hypertrophy of the parathyroids represented an attempt to compensate for the excessive loss of calcium from the body. This hypothesis was adhered to until the work of Hoffheinz in 1925. He noted an associated

*Read before the Medical Association of Georgia, Savannah, April 22, 1936.

are replaced by that from the bones. Serum calcium values have been noted to range from 12.1 to 23.6 mg. in hyperactivity of these glands. Calcium is taken into the system through the gastro-intestinal tract and excreted not only by this tract but also by the kidneys, the placenta and the lactating breasts. If no calcium is ingested, it is probable that small amounts taken from the bones still appear in the urine. When the serum calcium falls to 7 or 8 mg., tetany may develop. "The dentine and enamel of the teeth have nearly the same composition as the bones, and yet they do not seem to act as a reserve supply of the body calcium metabolism. While the teeth are being laid down, faults in the body metabolism at that time may be reflected in the teeth forever after, but there it ends." As Allbright has put it, "the teeth can be acalcified, but not decalcified." "The much quoted 'a-tooth-a-child,' argument of the opponents of this belief have other interpretations than that minerals are taken from the tooth via the blood stream to the child." The teeth generally are not affected, but the jaw is decalcified and in this way the teeth may fall out. In hyperparathyroidism, the serum calcium usually rises higher than 11.5 mg. per 100 cc. blood and the serum phosphorus usually becomes less than 3.8 or 3.5 mg. This is not always consistently found. The urinary calcium and phosphorus increases. The findings regarding phosphorus metabolism are not as definite as those concerning calcium. Serum phosphatase (an enzyme present in calcified cartilage) in early cases is normal, while in later stages with skeletal changes, it is increased. The normal serum phosphatase is two Bodansky units. With this process established, there results a general osteoporosis with possible local secondary changes as deformity, cysts, tumors, and fractures. Cataracts and tetany result when there is a deficiency of parathyroid secretion. This might explain why in race cases, 'it has been possible to help a patient with a cataract without surgery.

Clinical Types of the Diesase

1. Classic hyperparathyrodism — Osteitis fibrosa cystica of von Recklinghausen. Skeletal symptoms predominate and decalcification, multiple cysts, and fractures occur. The x-ray shows the typical diffuse granular osteoporo-

sis. The teeth may become loose and fall out.

2. Osteoporotic form of hyperparathyroidism. Early stage of the classic type. The symptoms are due largely to decalcification— There are no cysts—no tumors. Often diagnosed rheumatism.

3. Hyperparathyroidism with renal disease. Due to precipitation of calcium phosphate, which is the significant finding, Allbright and his associates have subdivided this group as follows:

(a) Calculi in the renal pelvis with resulting pyelonephritis. The classic symptoms are associated with renal stones. In cases where stones occur, and especially those that recur and are bilateral, the possibility of hyperparathyroidism should be called to mind. Hence, renal colic may conceivably be an early symptom of this disease. I am now running routinely, on my cases of renal calculi, blood caₗcₗums and blood phosphates, but so far all have been normal.

(b) Calculi in the renal tubules with resulting renal sclerotic contraction and insufficiency, which simulate Bright's disease. Allbright reports a 13 year old girl with nocturia, albuminuria, and white blood cells but no casts. Renal function tests were low and blood n.-p. n. was 55. Serum calcium 12, and serum phosphorus 4.7. A tumor was removed. She had no increase in calcium or phosphorus in the urine, as is generally the case in hyperparathyroidism. In this type case urinary excretions are not elevated. Excretions of calcium and phosphorus in the feces are elevated. Bones are demineralized and cystic. The kidneys seem to be plugged, and there is a backing up of phosphate leading to a normal rather than a decreased value in the blood.

(c) Precipitation of calcium phosphate in the kidney as one of several organs with acute renal failure and death of undetermined cause in a few hours or days. Renal changes may occur without evidence of changes in the skeleton. The renal changes are an index of the severity of the disease while the skeletal changes are an index of its duration.

4. Acute parathyroid poisoning.

5. Hyperparathyroidism simulating or complicated by Paget's disease.

General Symptomatology

In a general way, the symptoms may be referred to the part of the body especially diseased, depending on the way the kidneys, bones, etc., receive the brunt of the attack.

The disease occurs more frequently in females between the ages of 30 and 50, and the course is usually in years not months.

The symptoms are referred mainly to the skeleton. There are generalized aches and pains over the body. In 72 per cent of cases pain in the back or in the extremities is the chief early symptom. The possibility of this disease must be considered in patients who complain of generalized "neuritic" or " arthritic" pains, and where there is bone tenderness and history of a pathologic fracture. Hypotonia of the muscles occurs, and in 22 per cent the primary complaint is muscular weakness. Frequent falls without good reason and muscular weakness should suggest the possibility of this disease. The patients are often asthenic and easily fatigued. Gastric crises may occur. The circulatory system is often disturbed because of arterial calcification. On palpation, no mass can usually be felt, but in a rare case the finding of an ovoid mass next to the thyroid gland when the patient swallows is significant. Disturbances of gait and the limping and waddling type may develop early. A cyst or tumor of the jaw may be the first symptom and it will not be for several years before the actual diagnosis is made. The teeth may fall or become loose because of mandibular decalcification. There is sometimes polydipsia and polyuria. Genitourinary calculi may occur. The complexion may be pale, while the hemoglobin and red blood cell count are normal. However, there may be a secondary anemia. Roentgenograms may visualize a parathyroid tumor. This can be done in an occasional instance by using barium to visualize the esophagus. The tumors are apt to be near the esophagus and displace it.

Blood will disclose an increase in serum calcium and a decrease in serum phosphorus. The urine shows an increase in both calcium and phosphorus. The x-ray shows a rarefraction of the bones as a result of demineralization. In the skull the calvarium exhibits a finely granular appearance, the bones may become thickened and the tables indistinct, the external and internal layers may disappear, and the skull become soft. Small cysts may be present. Fractures to the skeleton often follow slight injury. The lower extremities may become bowed. Lordosis or kyphosis of the vertebral column may appear and decrease in stature may be noted by the patient. Tumefaction may involve the whole bone or appear only on the surface. Skeletal deformities of all types occur, and may simulate Paget's disease or osteomalacia.

Differential Diagnosis

1. Paget's disease (Osteitis deformans). X-rays do not reveal a generalized skeletal involvement. Normal or only very slightly elevated blood calcium and phosphorus. Clinically, the picture is different from that presented in hyperparathyroid disease.

2. Senile osteoporosis (Very difficult to differentiate). Serum calcium normal. Serum phosphorus normal or slightly reduced. Repeated blood studies.

3. Osteomalacia (Adult rickets). Associated fatty diarrhea. There is a bowing rather than fracture of bones. History of lack of vitamin D. Rapid therapeutic response to vitamin D. Serum phosphorus low. Serum calcium low or normal.

4. Solitary cysts. Normal skeleton in other parts of body. Normal serum calcium and normal serum phosphorus.

5. Solitary benign giant sell tumor. Blood values normal. Remaining skeleton normal. Bone biopsy.

6. Multiple myeloma. Serum phosphorus never low. Blood calcium rarely elevated. Bence Jones protein often present in urine. Bone biopsy.

7. Metastatic malignancy. Often evidence of primary disease. Blood values generally normal. Bone biopsy.

8. Adenoma of pituitary gland. The obesity, hirsuitism, amenorrhea, and hypertension in Cushing's syndrome are not features of simple hyperparathyroidism. Sometimes associated with this disease there is hyperplasia of the parathyroids.

9. Chondrosarcoma. Bone biopsy—Blood values often normal. X-ray findings different.

Report of Cases Under Study

Case 1.—M. P., an invalid, confined to bed, gives the following history of fractures:

Fracture of right humerus at 9 months; fracture of left wrist, at 3 years; fracture of left leg, at 4 years; fracture of right leg at 4 years; at about 5 years of age she fell on a baby carriage and broke the left wrist again; a short while later, she developed whooping cough and fractured a rib; fracture of right femur; she jumped in sleep one night and fractured the left hip; one year later, the wheel chair fell down the steps and both legs were broken again; sitting up in bed one night propped up on arm, it snapped in the left shoulder; while out automobile riding one day, she slipped from automobile seat and fractured right tibia again; she dropped a small weight on the right great toe and fractured it; in peeling sugar cane with her teeth, she fractured jaw; and a few years later had automobile accident resulting in five fractures, two in the left shoulder joint, right wrist, two in the left femur and two months later fell from bed and fractured left hip.

Last fracture occurred in 1926. The patient states that when these fractures occur, the snap can be heard some distance away, and has often startled her before she realized what had happened. In addition to this, in a note to me she says:

"There were other cracked bones besides the bones above mentioned, such as broken and misplaced ribs and collar bone, but, of course, these seemed of minor importance, because of more serious mishaps, so that these are only dimly remembered. I believe these breaks healed in a reasonable length of time, except in the case of a re-break, in which case a large lump formed, which was never absorbed."

Blood calcium on this patient is 12.3.

Blood phosphorus is 2.7.

This patient was kindly referred to me for calcium studies by Dr. Metts and Dr. Williams.

X-rays made by Dr. Drane, whose report is as follows:

"The bone changes are not typical of hyperparathyroidism. There is decalcification but not the marked decalcification and not the granular appearance which one expects. I feel the condition represents osteomalacia with multiple fractures. There are those who feel that these diseases are very similar."

In spite of the x-ray findings, I lean strongly to the diagnosis of hyperparathyroid disease. The advanced skeletal deformities, and very poor physical condition, preclude surgery here at this advanced stage.

Case 2.—Mrs. D.D., aged 22, was referred by Dr. M. J. Epting. She complained of shortening of left leg of 14 years' duration. At 8 years of age, this patient fell and injured the upper part of her left femur. The same injury occurred three years later. X-rays made at that time showed old united fractures. From time to time, she has complained of aches and pains in her bones, resembling rheumatism. X-ray report of the pelvis and hips made by Dr. Drane is as follows:

"Anteriorposterior stereoscopic films of the pelvis show a marked deformity of the pelvis and marked thickening and bowing of the femurs. There is no evidence of a fracture. Films of the skull and chest show nothing abnormal. Films of the right forearm and hand show marked thickening of the radius, first and second metacarpal bones and first and second phalanges of the index finger. Films of the left leg and foot show the same changes in the tibia, fibula, first, third, fourth, and fifth metatarsal bones and in the phalanges. I feel that this condition is osteitis fibrosa cystica of parathyroid origin, which has undergone spontaneous healing."

This x-ray film was sent by Dr. Drane to Philadelphia, where it was studied at a conference there, and the diagnosis was confirmed that the bone changes were the result of hyperactivity of the parathyroid glands.

Blood calcium on this patient is 12.9.

Blood phosphorus is 2.9.

Provisional Diagnosis

Hyperparathyroidism, not as yet confirmed by operative procedures.

Case 3.—J. C., a white boy of 16, veritable pathologic museum, was seen by me with Dr. Holton. The case is reported here because of his pathologic fracture, which aroused the suspicion of overactivity of the parathyroids. He was markedly emaciated, infected with malaria and hookworm, which conditions were complicated with pellagra. He had never seen a moving picture or a train, and had never ridden on a street car. While walking one day, he was taken with an excruciating pain in the right hip. X-ray showed that the head of the right femur was projected through the acetabulum and rested against the sacrum. I made a serum calcium, which was 8.07 and 9.2 mg. and serum phosphorus, which was 5 mg. The urine was negative for Bence-Jones protein and no calcium phosphate crystals were noted. The remainder of the skeleton in the x-ray showed no typical demineralization. Our diagnosis at this time is localized osteomalacia of the hip, due to malnutrition, and lack of Vitamin D.

Case 4.—Mrs. C., housewife, was seen by me through the courtesy of Dr. Egan. For some months, she had suffered with what she thought was arthritis. Dr. Egan had an x-ray made of the hip, and a large cyst discovered. Blood serum phosphorus and calcium were normal here, and parathyroid disease ruled out. Bone biopsy proved it to be a sarcoma.

Case 5.—W. G., a white boy of 16, complained of pain in the left arm. X-ray showed a single bone cyst. Blood calcium and phosphorus were normal. This bone lesion was due to nutritional disturbances, as the lad was markedly malnourished and anemic, and there was a history of lack of Vitamin D. The condition cleared up under correct diet and altered routine of life.

In conclusion, I would say that our diagnostic troubles are increased. "The old lady with her vague aches and pains, and the patient with his attack of renal colic or early bone cyst, may eventually prove to be a parathyroid disturbance." We can not close our eyes to this possibility, because 23 cases have been diagnosed, and the diagnosis corroborated by operation at the Massachusetts General Hospital alone, and in many others.

In all our cases of bone cysts, demineralization of bones, and tumors of the bone, and even bilateral recurring renal calculi, it is imperative that calcium and phosphorus determination be made. It is important that the diagnosis of this disease be made early, for the patient in the course of months and years eventually becomes completely invalided, harassed with pain, deformed, and faced with the ever present danger of recurring fractures.

BIBLIOGRAPHY

1. Allbright, Fuller: Hyperparathyroidism, Its Diagnosis and Exclusion, New England J. Med. 209: 476 (Sept. 7) 1933.
2. Allbright, Fuller: Hyperthyroidism: A case with Several Unusual Features Including a Probably Non-Related Chondrosarcoma, Bence-Jones Proteinuria, and Hyperplasia of all Parathyroid Tissue, M. Clin. N. America 18: 1109 (Jan.) 1935.
3. Allbright, Fuller; Baird, P. C.; Cope, Oliver and Bloomberg, Esther: Studies on the Physiology of the Parathyroid Glands. IV. Renal Complications of Hyperparathyroidism, Am. J. M. Sc. 187: 49 (Jan.) 1934.
4. Allbright, Fuller; Bloomberg, E.; Castleman, B. and Churchill, E. D.: Hyperparathyroidism Due to Diffuse Hyperplasia of all Parathyroid Glands Rather Than Adenoma of One, Arch. Int. Med. 54: 315 (Sept.) 1934.
5. Ballin, Max: Parathyroidism, Ann. Surg. 96: 649-665 (Oct.) 1932.
6. Ballin, Max: Technique of Parathyroidectomy, Surg. Gynec. & Obst. 54: 806-808 (May) 1932.
7. Ballin, Max: Parathyroidism, Am. J. Surg. 24: 36 (April) 1934.
8. Barlaro, P. M.: Hyperparathyroidism, Presna med. argent. 19: 760 (Sept. 30) 1932.
9. Bauer, Walter: Hyperparathyroidism. A distinct Disease Entity, J. Bone & Joint Surg. 15: 135 (Jan.) 1935.
10. Boothby, W. M.: A Case of Parathyroid Insufficiency. Proc. Staff Meet. Mayo Clinic 7: 361 (June 22) 1932.
11. Boothby, W. M.: Treatment of Postoperative Parathyroid Insufficiency, Proc. Staff Meet. Mayo Clinic 10: 87 (Feb. 6) 1935.
12. Churchill, E. D.: The Operative Treatment of Hyperparathyroidism, Ann. Surg. 100: 606 (Oct.) 1934.
13. Churchill, E. D. and Cope, Oliver: Parathyroid Tumors Associated with Hyperparathyroidism: Eleven Cases Treated by Operation, Surg. Gynec. & Obst. 58: 255 (Feb. 15) 1934.
14. Chute, Richard: The Vital Importance of the Relation of Hyperparathyroidism to the Formation of Certain Urinary Calculi—And Its Remedy, New England J. Med. 210: 1251 (June 14) 1934.
15. Compere, E. L.: Bone Changes in Hyperparathyroidism. Surg. Gynec. & Obst. 50: 783-794 (May) 1930.
16. Cope, Oliver: Surgery of Subtotal Parathyroidectomy, New England J. Med. 213: 470 (Sept. 5) 1935.
17. Cutler, Max, and Owen, S. E.: Irradiation of the Parathyroids in Generalized Osteitis Fibrosis Cystica: Report of a Case, Surg. Gynec. & Obst. 59: 81 (July) 1934.
18. Elmslie, R. C.; Fraser, F. R.; Dunhill, T. P.; Vick, R. M., and Harris, C. F., and Dauphinee, J. A.: The Diagnosis and Treatment of Generalized Osteitis Fibrosa with Hyperparathyroidism, Brit. J. Surg. 20: 479 (Jan.) 1933.
19. Gates, Nathaniel: Hyperparathyroidism, J. Michigan Med Soc. 31: 121 (Feb.) 1932.
20. Gutman, A. B.; Swenson, P. C., and Parsons, W. B.: The Differential Diagnosis of Hyperparathyroidism, J. A. M. A. 103: 87 (July 14) 1934.
21. Jaffe, H. L.: Hyperparathyroidism and Its Relationship to Diseases of Bone. Bull. New York Acad. Med. 10: 539 (Sept.) 1934.
22. Labey, F. H., and Haggart, G. E.: Hyperparathyroidism, Clinical Diagnosis and Operative Technic of Parathyroidectomy, Surg. Gynec. & Obst. 60: 1033 (June) 1935.
23. LeRiche, Rene: The Future and Significance of Surgery of the Parathyroids, Presse med. 58: 1133 (July 20) 1932.
24. Merritt, E. A., and McPeak, E. M.: Roentgen Therapy of Hyperparathyroidism, Am. J. of Roentgenol. 32: 72 (July 1934).
25. Pemberton, J. DeJ.: Hyperparathyroidism, Minnesota Med. 15: 729-734 (Nov.) 1932.
26. Sainton, P.: Hyperparathyroidism and the Osseous Syndrome, J. med. franc. 21: 3, 1932.
27. Stone, H. B.; Owings, J. C., and Gey, O.: Transplantation of Living Grafts of Thyroid and Parathyroid Glands, Ann. Surg. 10: 262 (Oct.) 1934.
28. Walton, A.: The Surgical Treatment of Parathyroid Tumors, Brit. J. Surg. 19: 285-291 (Oct.) 1931.

Discussion on Papers by Doctors T. C. Davison, J. Gaston Gay, Ben Hill Clifton and J. Reid Broderick

DR. ROBERT L. RHODES (Augusta): Dr. Clifton has covered his subject admirably in a very short paper and I can only agree with what he said.

His reference to pregnancy suggests three thoughts which were expressed in a paper by me in 1924 and from which I abstract as follows: We believe that some miscarriages at least are due to failure of the thyroid to promptly meet the extra demand thrown upon it by pregnancy and this may be averted by the administration of iodine. In conjunction with obstetricians we have had quite a few such cases who have been carried to term. Upon withdrawal of the iodine, threatening symptoms (flowing) promptly recurred—among them were several who had previously miscarried one to five times and had lost hope of ever having a child. Incidentally in these cases, as well as others, iodine proved a wonderful panacea for the nausea and vomiting of pregnancy. Thyroid disturbance accounts for many of the nervous and mental symptoms during pregnancy and patients showing these symptoms occasionally develop acute hyperthyroidism postpartum which yields readily to Lugol's solution if promptly recognized and treatment instituted.

Again I plead that iodine not be given to the toxic goitre by the medical man—leave it for the surgeon as a part of his preoperative preparation and postoperative treatment.

Discussion of Chronic Hyperthyroidism

In 1920 before this society I presented a paper which subsequently appeared in the JOURNAL, on the diagnosis of toxic goitre and in which I undertook to explain much of the variegated-symptomatology of these cases by analyzing and classifying certain symptoms as to which phaze of the autonomic nervous system they involved—the sympathicotonic or the vagotonic (Cranio-sacral). At that time the use of Basal Metabolism had just begun and we knew but little about it. Since, we have learned to regard it most highly but, as Dr. Davison has suggested, it is by no means a sine qua non.

If we recall that the action of the sympathicotonic nervous system may be summed up in the word action and the cranio sacral or vagal preparedness, their response to stimuli must necessarily vary widely—the latter digs the trenches and holds the supplies, the former goes over the top.

Exophthalmic goitre is certainly one of action and its symptoms are always predominantly sympathicotonic—may be ushered in suddenly, certainly develop rather rapidly as a rule to a certain point, which it maintains, a picture familiar to all—nodular or adenomatous (toxic) goitre on the contrary develops insidiously, until the patient awakens to the fact that something is very definitely wrong and the disease is very well entrenched. Many of the so called minor symptoms, yet equally as diagnostic, appear in this group—cycles of gradual loss of weight followed by gradual gain, or loss of hair and a new growth, irritability, nervousness subjective rather than objective, tachycardia of low grade (80 to 100), slight febrile reaction, 1 to 2 degrees variation morning and afternoon, such a picture as to suggest tuberculosis and many are so diagnosed. Infrequency of winking, giving an appearance of staring, often attracts the doctor's attention—exophthalmus is never present but von Graefe's sign is—and the eyes are moist even to the point of epiphora—salivary flow is increased and the skin is quite active, sweating profusely, especially upon very little effort—gastric acidity is increased, there may be occasionally diarrhoea but more frequently spastic constipation (not atonic) is present. The blood shows a leucopenia with a lymphocytosis and an eosinophilia up to 6-8 per cent. Carbohydrate tolerance is unlessened. A pulsus irregularis respiratorius is practically always noted.

Basal metabolism is after all a measure of the activity of the autonomic nervous system and since the sympathicotonic phase is concerned mostly with action it is a measure of this. The vagotonic, operating much more quietly and subtly, is not so prone to show itself or be capable of measurement. A well defined case of hyperthyroidism with predominantly vagotonic manifestations and a normal basal metabolism is a surgical risk on a parity about equal to that of an Exophthalmic goitre showing a basal metabolism of plus 25 to 40, and far more treacherous in that because of the subtle symptomatology, we are apt to fail to properly evaluate the risk. Iodine or Lugol's solution has a very doubtful place in this group since it frequently aggravates rather than improves.

DR. D. HENRY POER (Atlanta): I will try to show what few cases we have.

(Slide) This represents the type of case Dr. Davison spoke to you of. It is chronic thyroiditis, a definite clinical entity which has not been stressed in the literature, as those of you who have had occasion to look it over have found out. We wish to stress the point, because we find more cases of this type perhaps in the South than we did at one time in the Middle West.

(Slide) Hyperthyroidism in children is a very serious condition to deal with. Here are cases of goiter in a family of four girls. There is the point that Dr. Gay has so well made, not to operate on these cases until all other methods of treatment have been exhausted.

(Slide) Here is a girl with a more marked goiter, fourteen years of age, who is now being treated by conservative measures.

(Slide) Occasionally children do have to be operated upon, and here is a twelve-year-old case in the Good Samaritan Clinic, Atlanta, who came to us for surgery in the thyroid clinic at the Grady Hospital.

There is one point which may be of some value, and that is the value of the blood iodine determinations in the diagnosis of hyperthyroidism. We are running routinely on all cases that determination, the same as you would a blood sugar in diabetes. That has proven

to be of immense value, especially in borderline cases, and I pass it on to you for consideration.

I was anxious to say a few words about experimental work we are doing with parathyroids, removing thyroids and parathyroids, but time will not permit.

DR. J. C. METTS (Savannah): Dr. Clifton's paper devoted entirely to treatment was extremely practical; and I am very sorry that he did not have time to read it in detail. Too often I think we are accurate in our description and vague in our prescription.

He has reminded us of the incidence and the relation between iodine and goiter, pointing out its frequency in those areas in which they have a poor iodine content of the soil and water. In this particular area, we have the very opposite of that condition, in that our soil and vegetables carry a higher iodine content than any other section in the country; so much so, that our neighbors across the river rather proudly call themselves "The Iodine State." As a result, goiter is extremely rare, except for the adenomatous type.

I do not think I can add anything to what Dr. Clifton said. His paper was very interesting, beautifully presented, and extremely practical.

DR. OLIN H. WEAVER (Macon): The limited time in which to discuss these splendid papers makes it possible for only a brief comment on the subjects presented.

The parathyroid glands were formerly of importance to us only as organs to be avoided in operations on the thyroid. Since Mandl in 1925 operated upon an adenomatous parathyroid, thereby relieving a case of generalized fibrosa cystica, has the relationship of disturbances of these glands to certain lesions of bone been firmly established. Since that time much study has been devoted to the subject and a number of cases reported. It is still an infrequent trouble. Less than 200 cases having been recorded. Drs. Wilder and Howell report that only 5 cases have been observed at the Mayo Clinic.

The influence of a lack of Vitamin D and ultra violet irradiation is regarded as a causative factor. Changes in the metabolism of calcium and phosphates, their disappearance from the bones and an increase in the blood and urine are characteristic of hyperparathyroidism. Besides the bony defects there may be calcification of the structure of the kidneys with defective function, also the formation of calculi in the pelvis, these changes may precede changes in the bones.

The genito-urinary specialists should bear this fact in mind. Other symptoms may be changes in the urinary output, pains in joints, and muscles, loss of weight and strength with anemia. A more frequent laboratory estimation of the blood calcium would probably discover more incipient cases. Wilder and Howell call attention to the fact that there appears to be a greater development of cases in certain geographical areas than in others. Being analogous in this respect to thyroid disturbances. They offer as a probable explanation difference of atmospheric conditions, variance in percentage of sunshine, etc. And the additional explanation that in adenomatous development there must be embryonic cells that retain proliferating capacity into adult life. Without these cells no tumor will occur regardless of the amount of stimulus the glands receive. It is likely that an equal number of people in various sections have this potentiality to adenomatous formation, but there must be sufficient stimulus to cause a development of the tumor. This stimulus is a deficiency of vitamin D. These authors are unwilling to accept the diagnosis of hyperparathyroidism in cases of senile osteoporosis, hypertrophic arthritis, Paget's disease and other bone lesions, which some investigators, without good reason, have attributed to hyperfunctions of the parathyroids. They require a minimum criteria for the establishment of an authenticated case. These are that the skeletal abnormality be consistent with that of generalized osteitis fibrosa, or, in the absence of skeletal changes, there be abnormality of calcium metabolism, characteristic of hyperparathyroidism demonstrated in the blood and urine; that a tumorous enlargement either an adenoma or diffuse hypertrophy and hyperplasia of one or more parathyroids be found by operation or autopsy. Cases which do not meet these criteria, with few exceptions, are not this disease.

Medical, surgical and irradiation methods have been employed for the relief of this disease. Surgery has been most successful method in cases of adenoma. Treatment of diffuse hyperplastic cases is not so well established. The difficulties and dangers, immediate and remote, of these operations is much greater than in operations on the thyroid and require the skill of the best trained surgeon.

As to Dr. Clifton's paper, iodine therapy has proven to be of greatest benefit in thyroid disorders. Multiple step operations being practically eliminated thereby, operations made safer and convalescence smoother. The long debated question as to whether preoperative iodine therapy is proper in other than hyperplastic goiter has been affirmatively decided and practiced by a majority of those men who are entitled to an opinion.

The claim that iodine preoperatively will cause toxic adenoma to be aggravated does not hold true in a large percentage of cases. The opinion of many is that toxic adenoma and hyperplastic goitre are clinical variations of one morbid process and that the careful administration of iodine may be given with practically the same benefits in either case. Like most good things, iodine is likewise capable of doing great harm if not given with careful observation and this applies to its use in any thyroid disturbance. I agree with the essayist in the other indications mentioned for the use of iodine. There is a class of cases of goitre, especially of large size, in which there are present many of the general physical discomforts of hyperthyroidism, such as palpitation, rapid pulse, nervousness and irritability in which the metabolism is normal or below that are relieved by thyroidectomy. The strain on the myocardium, from the increased vascular bed in the thyroid, a disturbance of cerebral circulation from pressure on cervical vessels causing anoxemia have been suggested by Dr. Dinsmore as a cause of these symptoms. It seems paradoxical to speak of hyperthyroidism without an increased metabolic rate—as well speak of

symptom and usually precedes all cervical cancers; its significance should be appreciated more fully. Cervicitis is the most frequent cause of leukorrhea. Cervicitis and erosions follow injuries and lacerations incidental to childbirth. It is generally believed that it is not the laceration per se that causes cancer but the consequental inflammation and chronic irritation with their resulting by-products.

The external os and portio vaginalis are lined with squamous epithelium. The mucus membrane of the cervical canal is lined with a single layer cylindric type of epithelium. The normal cervical canal is lined with race-mose type of mucus glands that are embed-ded in the connective tissue and muscle of the cervix. When cervicitis occurs a muco-purulent discharge is produced by the cervical glands that destroy or macerate the epithelial cells leaving a denuded area. This stage is called erosion. If healing is normal the cer-vical lesion disappears, but if the healing is interfered with by changes brought about by lacerations and chronic infection, it predis-poses to malignant growth.

In the treatment of chronic cervicitis and erosion more stress should be laid on curing the cervicitis. The methods generally used in treating cervicitis are electric coagulation, cautery, amputation of the cervix and tra-chelorraphy. The latter is the least successful, for I have three cases that developed cancer following trachelorraphy. At the Women's Free Hospital in Boston where a total of 5,962 cervical patients were treated, covering a period of 52 years, only five cases of cancer of the cervix are known to have developed. They developed in the trachelorraphy group which consisted of 3,814 of the cases. Am-putations were performed in 740 and coagu-lation in 1,408 of the cases.

We have learned from experimental re-search that rats can be bred so that one strain will not have artificial cancer, but certain strains can be selected which will grow arti-ficial cancer with varying degrees of suscepti-bility. From a theoretical standpoint, and from the results of artificial cancer production, one can confidently say that it is not the initial laceration that causes the cancer, but the result of irritants and inherited tendencies.

If this is true of the lower vertebral animal why should it not be true in human beings? That women possess an inherited susceptibil-ity is supported by the fact that you see can-cer develop a few months after childbirth, and in nulliparous women as the result of an ordinary cervicitis. Until we know the specific cause of cancer it behooves us to treat lesions of the cervix which predispose to the development of cancer.

Schiller's test is one of the refinements in early diagnosis. The test is simple. Paint the entire surface with Lugol's solution; wipe off the excess immediately. The normal cervix takes on a deep, smooth, dark-brown color. The reaction depends on the glycogen content on the surface layers of the normal epithelium covering the cervix. If the surface epithelium is destroyed or has lost its glycogen content (or granules) it does not take the dark-brown color. If one or more of the un-stained areas are visible it should be investi-gated further. The unstained areas usually suggest leukoplakia or early carcinoma with-out ulceration. It is impossible to make a positive diagnosis on the unstained areas without histologic study by a competent pathologist. A negative test does not rule out the possibility of a cancer in the deeper por-tion of the cervix not involving the surface epithelium. I think the greatest application of this test is in periodic health examinations and routine physical examinations where no objective or subjective signs have developed. As Schiller says, the object of the iodine test is to call attention to the suspicious areas. If cancer is suspected, excision of the lesion well out into the normal tissue for microscopic ex-amination should be done, for it is generally conceded that proper excision of a section does not predispose to metastasis. The classifica-tion of the growth to different groups has not proved to be as helpful as it was thought to be. In reporting clinical cases I think they should be classed according to the League of Nations' classification so that end results of cases for groups may be compared. As soon as a uniform standard can be had, the more reliable will be our statistics.

It is generally conceded that x-ray and radium are the best treatment for all types of cervical cancer, but cancer of the body of the uterus is best treated by surgical removal. If the growth is large and papular, or if there is infection present, the best results are obtained by giving preliminary x-ray treatment, for most frequently this causes the growth to decrease and helps clear up the infection so that the radium can be used more advantageously. One of the worst complications is radiation slough with infection. The technic of radium treatment of cervical cancer depends on the location and size of the growth, but the amount that I usually give is around 3,500 to 4,000 milligrams hours in and around the cervix, and about 1,500 milligram hours in the uterus, using platinum filter, giving the dose in 48 to 96 hours. I prefer this treatment to the spread-out dose method as advocated by Regaud. X-ray therapy is very important for it is designed to kill the cells which have spread to the adjacent tissues. In recent years it has been found that larger doses give the best results. To quote Healey: "Under the new treatment, or multiple dose plan, the pelvis is divided into a right and a left half and each half into an anterior and a posterior field. The two fields in one half of the pelvis are treated one day 200 R. units to each field at 70 cm. and the two fields in the other half the following day. In this way the patient receives daily treatments to one half of the pelvis, 200 R. at each exposure until each field has received 1000 R. units; then the dosage for each exposure is increased to 300 R. Treatments are continued daily until additional 1,500 R. has been given to each four pelvic fields, making a final total of 2,500 R. to each quadrant as against the former total 750 R. .It takes from 23 to 25 days to give the treatment." This technic, I think, will give the best results in advanced cases. By giving large doses one will get more skin reaction or burns, but the results are better. Formerly an x-ray reaction or burn was considered a reflection on the one giving the treatment, but since the end results are better and more lives are saved by giving large doses even though the patients have scars or burns, it is better to give the required dose. Adverse criticism by doctors and frequent suits for malpractice have been factors in keeping roentgenologists from giving large doses.

TABLE I.
CANCER OF CERVIX FROM STEINER CLINIC
ATLANTA, GA.

Class	Cases	Number Controlled	Per Cent 5 Yrs. or More
I	65	33	50.77
II	35	10	27.
III	108	8	7.
IV	125	0	0
TOTALS	333	51	15.31

The treatment has been by radiation differing very little from that described by Dr. Fountain, except that the cervix and each lateral fornix are treated by the Bailey bomb, and in the bulky growths gold seed are implanted and the growth allowed to regress until the cervical canal can be easily entered. The amount of radium given varies from 5,000 to 8,000 m. c. h. In addition deep therapy x-ray is used.

Our results are as follows:

In class one there were 65 cases, about 20 per cent of the total, and of this group 49 per cent are living without evidence of disease for five years of more.

In class two there were only 35 cases, of which 10, or 27 per cent, are without evidence of disease at the end of five years.

In class three there were 108, of which only 8, or 7 per cent, were salvaged.

In class four there were 125 cases, none being salvaged.

These statistics are not very encouraging, but our follow up has not been as good as we would like and all cases that could not be traced were counted as dead from cancer.

DR. CALVIN B. STEWART (Atlanta): This is a continuation of Dr. Denton's discussion, and will be statistical only.

We are showing this slide (See Fig. 1) to demonstrate that still there is hope for patients who have carcinoma of the cervix. These figures are not good, and we are not proud of them, but they show that there is hope for the early cases, but practically none for the advanced one.

In class one, as Dr. Denton just described, we have had 65 cases, with a little better than half well after five years. In the next class there are 35 cases, with 27 per cent of them well. In group three, there are 108 cases, and only 7 per cent well. In group four none of the 125 cases are well. This gives a grand total of 333 cases, but only 185 were traced.

We are very much ashamed of losing trace of so many. Only 15.3 per cent of this grand total are well and just to show how figures can be manipulated, if we had left out the untraced cases, our results would almost have been double in their optimistic appearance.

I can not help but emphasize very strongly the necessity of preventing cancer of the cervix. It is a great reflection on us here today, that nearly half of the women in Georgia in 1933, were delivered outside of the medical profession. I know it is hard to believe me, but you can find these figures at the state capitol.

If we, the medical profession, were delivering the

other 40 per cent and following them until the cervix healed. I think we would not have half the present cancers of the cervix; perhaps not a fourth. If we could examine all our people every six months to a year, we would not have any Class 3 and 4. This would be a step forward for cancer control as well as other health problems.

DR. E. B. WOODS (Augusta): I should like to call your attention to the importance of having adequate accurate pathologic diagnoses in the treatments of these cases. Not only should the diagnosis of malignancy be made, but the pathologist or the surgeon should attempt to determine the degree of malignancy and degree of radiosensitivity as evidenced by the maturity of the malignant cells. Complete treatment by radiation in many clinics is not the universal rule, the treatment being dependent upon the pathologic findings. When one has embryonal cells which are the most radiosensitive and most frequently found in the epithelial type of tumor, one will have excellent results with radiation. However, if one finds the adenomatous type of tumor in which the cells are usually of the more mature type, consequently less radiosensitive, and finds that this tumor has not extended further than the International type two, it is probable that surgery will be the most beneficial to the patient. Data from many clinics show that the adenomatous type of cervical cancer which has not extended into the pelvic lymph channels is much better handled by surgery than by radiation, because of its lack of radiosensitivity.

May I make a plea also to you gentlemen for the contemplation, at least, of the total hysterectomy. When we found in the University of Iowa Hospital 8.3 per cent of the 257 cases of cervical cancer were in stumps, or cervices which had been left following subtotal hysterectomy, we feel that we have figures that are worth your consideration. In other words, one out of every twelve cases of cervical cancer is going to occur after the subtotal hysterectomy, or the first operation. Frequently carcinoma of the cervical stump is far advanced when found, because the woman does not feel that any thing can be the matter with her, and does not heed little warnings which otherwise would send her to the physician.

Dr. Erwin von Graff reported in the American Journal of Obstetrics and Gynecology in 1934, the aforementioned figures, together with the data compiled from the literature and from information received in some five hundred questionnaires sent to gynecologists throughout the country, showing that the incidence of stump cancer in carcinoma of the cervix varies from six to eleven per cent. Stump cancer, then, is an important classification in cervical carcinoma, and of course, total hysterectomy is the one way we can prevent having stump cancers.

DR. JAS. A. FOUNTAIN (Macon): I appreciate the discussions and I agree with Dr. Denton and Dr. Stewart. I cannot agree, however, with Dr. Wood in doing a complete hysterectomy for non-cancerous conditions, for the mortality rate in doing a total hysterectomy is greater than is the occurrence of cancer in cervical stumps.

been shown to slow the rate of tumor growth.[2] Hypophysectomy has a greater effect than x-ray to the gland in retarding the growth.[3] "The internal secretion of the parathyroid gland stimulates the development of rat carcinoma, but decrease of its internal secretion interferes with the development of such a carcinoma."[4] Prolan experimentally has been found to "check tumor growth to a great degree . . . The administration of prolan so reduces the energy of tumor growth that it flourishes little or not at all upon secondary inoculation (during the second animal residence)."[5]

But to what reach in the whole scale of malignant tumors may the hope of endocrine therapy be applied? Some tumors suggest not at all an induction by recurrent, accruing stimuli, but burst into existence upon the field of tranquil cellular processes.[10] Does such spontaneity derive from regulatory imbalance, or from factors resident in the cell? The fact is forced upon us that the disease called cancer can not be satisfactorily illumined or confined by a stationary, standardized concept. The disease is protean in its manifestations; we must think of a graded series[6] of tissue susceptibilities to autonymous cell growth, ranging from spontaneous predetermined effulgence to that appearing only after long hyperplastic activity. Loeb[7] has given the formula $H + S$ (or $H \times S$)$=C$ to indicate the interrelation of hereditary influence and stimulation to cellular multiplication in the develepoment of cancer. Since H and S must vary reciprocally to give the product C, it is evident that the importance of any stimulation factor, such as hormonal catalysis, is dependent on the assertiveness (value) of the hereditary factor.

The question of the carcinogenicity of hormones has been enlivened by recent investigation[8] of the molecular configuration of principles of the glands of internal secretion as compared to known cancer-producing compounds. By fractionating the tar which had been seen to cause epithelioma, presumably by irritation, principles were isolated that possessed decided carcinogenic ability, and these were found to be closely related in structure to the estrus-producing hormone, theelin (folliculin). Moreover, these tar compounds themselves exhibited a certain degree of estrus-

inducing capacity. It was found that "all the synthetic estrus-producing substances appear to belong to the condensed carbon ring system, and that the most powerful possess the phenanthrene nucleus."[9] To such a ring system belong not only theelin and these tar compounds, but also cholesterol, ergosterol, vitamin D. It was therefore suggested that the native sterols of the body—modified by reduction, dehydration, dehydrogenation—might evolve as carcinogenetic products.[9] In such a manner it may be supposed that a hormone as well could be so altered that in its pharmacologic action estrogenesis (or proper physiologic effect) might be supplanted by carcinogenesis. Or, as Jaisohn[10] would have it, perhaps the highly alkaline serum of cancer patients (from K and Ca abnormalities)—due to hormonal imbalance —could supply a *milieu* for changing sterols to carcinogens.

The carcinogenic effect of h o r m o n e s, whether it thus appears possibly in one way direct, in another circuitous, is after all only indirect so far as can be proved. For the excessive proliferation in the early stages of estrus, or on the skin, bears only a superficial resemblance to carcinoma; "the definite cancerous transformation is preceded by a preparatory period."[7] The hormone has been active during this preliminary period. There is no proof that it was directly responsible for the change to actual malignant growth. When this change has occurred the hormone "no longer needs to be applied; the carcinogenic effect follows spontaneously in the course of time."[7] Apparently internal secretory principles, were it not for their special tissue affinity, deserve only to be classed along with the other factors which instigate proliferative processes.

It is interesting to inquire into the nature of the change which differentiates the hyperplastic prelude from invasive malignancy. Does, at one point, the balance[11,12] between growth stimulating and inhibiting (humoral) substances become so strained as to eventuate in a "cancerous equilibrium,"[7] or is there perhaps a sudden innovation in cellular constitution? The suggestion has been made that cancer may be a cellular mutation, "*brusque et discontinue*,"[13] for such a phenomenon "has the greatest chance of occurring when cells are in division under abnormal environmental conditions unfavorable to the cell."[13] This cellular modification might take place by chance, or be inclined by local influences. Mottram[14] last year reported chromosomal disturbances due to radiation; there was "fragmentation . . . [with] delayed migration to the poles of the spindle." He assumes that the cancer cell may differ from the normal tissue unit in its content of genes.

It seems logical to suspect the chromosomes as probable sites for the residence of factors determining susceptibility to m a l i g n a n t growth, since they are so intimately involved in cell-division. To apply our earlier scope of cancer here, we may consider that the genetic propensity of malignancy varies from the one extreme of predestination to tumor as early as oval division, where the stimulation factor is negligible; to the other extreme of mild chromosomal instability, where the cell schema may be converted fortuitously by preceding hyperplasia to an autonymous organization.

Considerable orientation in the problem of carcinogenesis may be gained from the review of the significance of ovarian hormones in the development of mammary carcinoma in mice. Leo Loeb[7] found in breeding experiments that there is a constant cancer rate for each strain of mice, indicating that such a rate is determined by genetic factors. As an additional predetermined factor Loeb found the age of appearance constant in certain strains. Here was the chance to estimate accurately the influence of altered gonadal function in these animals. When ovaries were extirpated at a sufficiently early age, the cancer incidence fell to zero; it rose progressively and parallel with the length of delay in ovariectomy. The average age at which cancer appeared was increased in proportion to the earliness of spaying. Therefore the conclusion is clear here that ovarian stimulation, if acting upon tissues of known hereditary susceptibility, may be considered causal in the development of malignant tumors in organs specifically responsive to such stimulation.

In the human breast it is estimated that abnormal involution or chronic cystic mastitis (Reclus' disease)—now admitted to be due to endocrine dysfunction—is associated with carcinoma in from 15 per cent to 20 per cent of cases,[15] but those who are most familiar with mammary cancer are hesitant in pronouncing this concurrence incidental or causal. The suggestion is present, at least, that such a large percentage of women sustaining the remittent insult of this *maladie de Reclus* without developing autonymous cell multiplication in their breasts must presumably be, by great good fortune, without a heritage of mammary diathesis to malignant tumor.

An argument to second this view may be found in a survey of the incidence of cancer for the purpose of checking actual against theoretical data.[16] After the probability of the chance occurrence of multiple malignant neoplasms had been calculated, the known ratio for such cases as reported in medical literature was compared. Fewer instances were found than might be expected. It was concluded that a lack of susceptibility in a certain proportion of people could explain the discrepancy.

Macklin,[17] a Canadian author on hereditary influence, has been interested in the different incidence of tumors in the male as compared to the female. When considering the appearance of neoplasm only in a system common to both sexes (gastrointestinal tract), she has seen that there are twice as many tumors in males as in females. As concerns endocrine relationships her conclusion is that "the explanation of this increased incidence in the male appears to rest upon factors inherent in the male constitution; factors which are genetic [sex-linked] in their basis, and not merely dependent upon hormonal influences arising from male gonadal tissue."[17]

The importance of inherited factors is shown by investigative procedures. Last year a genetic explanation was advanced for the rhythms of growth noted in malignant tumors. Instead of a variation in the 'virulence' of the cancer cell, the mendelian characters of the host are perhaps responsible.[18] It is apparent that "animals of controlled genetic constitution are necessary for tumor transplantation investigations," since "hereditary factors determine the characteristics of both the host and the tumor cell."

Conclusions

1. In the light of present information the glands of internal secretion must be considered secondarily causative in the development of malignant tumors in tissues under their regulatory control.

2. The mode of this influence is apparently not direct, but in the nature of antecedent hyperplastic activity.

3. Actual introduction of autonymous cell growth takes place upon innovation in cellular constitution, primarily in chromosomal conversions which (through the resultant system of genic determinants) instigate for the cell a "cancerous equilibrium."

4. Always the value of the inherited susceptibility factor should be estimated, since this index of the inclination of cells to assume a parasitic nature prognosticates the danger of endocrine dysfunction.

REFERENCES

1. Babcock, W. W.: Organic Control of Growth and New Growth, Amer. J. Surg., 28: 67-70, April 1935.
2. Bischoff, F., Maxwell, L. C., & Ullman, H. J.: Hormones in Cancer; Effect of Glandular Extirpation, J. Biol. Chem., 92: lxxx-lxxxi, June 1931.
3. Samuels, L. T. & Ball, H. A.: Hypophysectomy and Tumor Growth, Am. J. Cancer, 23: 801-803, April 1935.
4. Paik, T. S.: Relationship Between Parathyroid Hormone and Growth of Rat Carcinoma, Am. J. Cancer, 15: 2756-2764, October 1931.
5. Zondek, H., Zondek, B., & Hartock, W.: Inhibiting Influence of Prolan (pituitary preparation) on Growth of Cancer in White Mice, Klin.Wchnschr., 11: 1785-1786, Oct. 22, 1932.
6. Cockayne, E. A.: Heredity in Relation to Cancer, Cancer Rev., 2: 344, 1927.
7. Loeb, Leo: Estrogenic Hormones and Carcinogenesis, J. A. M. A., 104: 1597-1601, May 4, 1935.
8. Cook, J. W., Dodds, E. C., & Greenwood, A. W.: Sex Change in the Plumage of Brown Leghorn Capons Following the Injection of Certain Synthetic Estrus-Producing Compounds, Proc. Roy. Soc., ser. B, 114: 286, January 1934.
Cook, J. W., Dodds, E. E., Hewett, C. L., & Lawson, W.: The Estrogenic Activity of Some Condensed Ring Compounds in Relation to Their Other Biological Activities. Proc. Roy. Ser. B, 114: 272, January 1934.
Cook, J. W., & Dodds, E. C.: Sex Hormones and Cancer Producing Compounds, Nature, 131: 205, February 11, 1933.
9. Dodds, E. C.: (Goulstonian Lecture) Hormones and Their Chemical Relations, Lancet, 1: 987-992, May 12, 1934.
10. Jaisohn, P.: Do Normal Cells Change to Cancer Cells Under Hormonal Influence? W. Va. M. J., 30: 414-415, September 1934.
11. Yates, J. L.: Therapeutic Portent of Biology of Cancer, Ann. Surg., 100: 852-882, October 1934.
12. Berman, Louis: Clinical Experiences Indicating Relation of Tissues to Endocrine Growth Inhibitors, M. J. & Rec., 131: 7-10, Jan. 7, 1931.
13. Gricouroff, G.: Can Cancer be Considered a Cellular Mutation? Paris Med., 1: 237-244, March 19, 1932.
14. Mottram, J. C.: Effects of Cancer-Producing Agents on Chromosomes, Brit. J. Exp. Path., 15: 71-73, April 1934.
15. Rodman, J. S.: Chronic Cystic Mastitis, Amer. J. Surg., 28: 452-459, May 1935.
16. Bugher, J. C.: Probability of the Chance Occurrence of Multiple Malignant Neoplasms, Am. J. Cancer, 21: 809-824, August 1934.
17. Macklin, M. T.: Sex Incidence of Entodermal Tumors, Amer. J. Surg., 21: 438-446, September 1933.
18. Bittner, J. J.: Genetic Studies on Transplantation of Tumors; Genetic Explanation of "Rhythms of Growth," Am. J. Cancer, 20: 834-847, April 1934.
19. Roberts, C. W. & Roberts, C. F.: Concurrent Osteogenic Sarcoma in Brother and Sisters, J. A. M. A., 105: 181-185, July 20, 1936.

BROMIDE INTOXICATION*

Report of Cases

W. G. ELLIOTT, M.D.
Cuthbert

Intoxication from bromides in therapeutic doses is more frequent than is generally thought. According to G. T. Harding, Jr. and G. T. Harding, III, 3 to 5 per cent of admissions to State hospitals are for this condition. In 500 admissions to the Colorado State Psychopathic Hospital 7 per cent were for bromide intoxication. Wuth found twenty cases in 238 admissions to the Henry Phipps Psychiatric Clinic.

Bromide action is based on the relation between chloride and bromide. Sodium chloride in the body remains at a rather constant concentration normally. It is constantly excreted, mainly in the urine and therefore must be constantly replenished. The excretion varies somewhat with the intake. The normal amount of sodium chloride in the blood is 450 to 500 mg. per 100 cc. If the supply of salt is stopped excretion falls within three days to a lower level but the body retains its normal salt content. The excretion of chloride can be hastened by giving the patient bromides or iodides; also the administration of chloride hastens the elimination of bromides and iodides. When bromides are taken into the body their excretion starts rapidly but proceeds slowly. Twenty days after medication has stopped the excretion of the drug is not complete. This shows that there is a retention of bromides due to the fact that bromides replace chlorides in the body, thus diminishing the chlorides. Bernoulli believes that a replacement of more than 40 per cent of the chlorides of the blood by bromides is fatal. Intoxication symptoms usually appear when 25 to 30 per cent of the chlorides have been replaced by bromides, although this may vary. In any condition indicating the diminution of chloride intake in which bromides are being given there is a hastening of the bromide retention.

The symptoms of bromide intoxication vary with individual personality make-up but

*Read before the Third District Medical Society, Cuthbert, June 10, 1936.

are essentially that of a toxic reaction with some neurologic signs. Drowsiness or even stupor which may deepen into coma is usually present. Confusion, disorientation, loss of memory for recent events, hallucinations, delusions and fabrication are some of the usual symptoms. There may be ideas of persecution. Some patients show evidence of mania while others are depressed. The speech is slurred, swallowing may be difficult, diplopia may be complained of and the pupils may be unequal; the reflexes are usually sluggish and some may be absent.

This syndrome must be differentiated from a number of nuerologic and toxic states. The patient may be unable to give any history and in that case the diagnosis can only be made by examination of the blood or urine. However, the clinician who considers the possibility of this intoxication should be able to make a tentative diagnosis without laboratory examination. The laboratory examinations consist of urine and blood examinations for bromides or one may make a blood chloride examination to determine if the chloride content is reduced.

The urine test is simply a test for detection of bromide in the urine as described by Belote. This is useful in doubtful cases. An estimate of the amount of bromide in the blood may be made by the gold chloride test as described by Wuth. In the cases known to have taken bromide one may get some information about how much chlorides have been replaced by bromides by doing the ordinary blood chloride test as described by J. C. Whitehorn. One must remember, however, that there are several other conditions that cause a lowering of the blood chloride, such as alkalosis fever, obstruction to the upper gastro-intestinal tract, etc.

The treatment of this condition consists of (1) omitting the drug; (2) elimination by means of saline laxatives and enemas; (3) giving sodium chloride; (4) sedatives as barbiturates (when necessary), paraldehyde, chloral and occasionally morphine; (5) fluids; (6) good nursing care. If the patient can and will take sodium chloride by mouth it may be given in the form of saline but if they can not take it in this way it should be given intravenously or subcutaneously in the form of normal saline. This promotes very

rapid elimination of bromide. Fluids should be forced in order to make the kidneys act freely as bromides are principally excreted through this route.

The following cases are given to illustrate this syndrome and its treatment:

Report of Cases

Case 1. A white female, 60 years old, had been suffering from hypertension and was treated in another town for this trouble. From the history there was a suggestion of her having taken bromides for a considerable period. She had also been on a restricted salt diet. She was drowsy, talked at random, there was partial loss of memory, loss of appetite and general weakness. Her blood pressure was below normal. Her pulse was fast and the reflexes were sluggish. She was treated at home and no laboratory work was done except routine urinalysis. She was put under the care of a trained nurse, given sodium chloride solution by mouth, barbiturates for rest, elixir of iron, quinine and strychnine to stimulate her appetite and put on a full diet. She recovered to about normal in one week and was fully recovered in two weeks. There has been no recurrence of these symptoms.

Case 2. Mrs. H. L. P., aged 42, was first admitted to the hospital October 6, 1934, with an attack of acute appendicitis. She had suffered with bronchial asthma for years and had had several attacks of gallbladder disease. She suffered from considerable indigestion and constipation. She was more or less nervous at all times and for this reason she was given a prescription of sodium bromide, aromatic cascara and tincture of belladonna, hoping to relieve nervousness, indigestion and to keep the ephedrine and adrenalin that she was having to take from making her so very nervous. This was very satisfactory and she wanted some of the medicine when she left the hospital. She was advised not to take it continuously but it was such good medicine she continued to take it for several weeks.

Finally, about one month later, she returned, accompanied by her daughter, who said her mother's mind was not good. She would keep repeating the same things over and over. Her memory was poor, there was a loss of appetite, weakness, she had peculiar ideas about the family, etc. She would not remain in the hospital. A blood chloride examination showed diminished chloride content of the blood (about 340 mg. per 100 cc. of blood). She was advised not to take any more of the medicine and to drink saline. I heard from her a few weeks later and she was fully recovered from the mental trouble but was still having bronchial asthma.

Case 3. A white female, aged 65, was admitted to the hospital for rather severe hypertension. She was put on a prescription of sodium bromide, sodium nitrite, etc., and kept in bed for several days. When she was dismissed she seemed much better but was kept on the bromide treatment. She came back three weeks later with the clinical symptoms of mild bromide intoxication. There was weakness, drowsiness, loss of appetite, loss of memory, slurring of speech, talking at random, etc. General routine examination revealed nothing of importance and her blood pressure was low. A blood chloride examination was made and found to be about 350 mg. per 100 cc. of blood. She was put on a full diet, given elixir of iron, quinine and strychnine before meals, sodium cacodylate intravenously daily, saline purge and sodium chloride by mouth. The bromide prescription was of course discontinued. She improved slowly for the first five or six days and then improved very rapidly and seemed to be normal mentally and in good condition physically upon leaving the hospital ten days after the second admission. She has remained in good health since that time.

Case 4. A white female, aged 55, was admitted to the hospital December 17, 1934. She had fallen and injured her left knee and arm. Her family physician gave her a mixture of bromide and paragoric for relief of pain. For five or six days before admission the patient had been talking foolishly and her husband thought that she was going crazy from taking the medicine. Other history was essentially negative except her father died of insanity. General physical examination was essentially negative except for bruises on arm and leg. Blood chloride was 290 mg. per 100 cc. of blood. Treatment: Elixir of iron, quinine and strychnine before meals, acetyl salicylic acid and codein for pain, full diet, saline by mouth, H. M. C. No. 2 for rest and magnesium sulphate for elimination. She showed some improvement but was discharged before she was entirely recovered. The last report on her condition was favorable.

Summary

1. Bromide intoxication is more frequent than is generally thought.
2. The syndrome can usually be diagnosed clinically if suspected.
3. Laboratory tests are available when necessary in obscure cases.
4. Bromide should be given cautiously, particularly when there is some indication for the reduction of sodium chloride in the diet.
5. Four cases are reported to illustrate the syndrome and its treatment.

REFERENCES

1. Todd & Sanford: Clinical Diagnosis by Laboratory Methods. Sixth edition.
2. C. E. and L. T. De M. Sajour: Revised by J. Warren Hutley, The Cyclopedia of Medicine, Vol. II, 1934.
3. Wuth, Otto: Rational Bromide Treatment: New Methods for Its Control, J. A. M. A. June 25, 1927, 2013:2018.
4. Harris, Titus H. and Abe Hauser: Bromide Intoxication: Its Significance in Toxic and Delirious States. J. A. M. A. July 12, 1930. 94:96.
5. Wagner, Carl F. and D. Elizabeth Bunbury: Incidence of Bromide Intoxication Among Psychotic Patients. J. A. M. A. December 6, 1930, 1725:1728.
6. Wile, Udo J.: Bromide Intoxication, J. A. M. A. 89:340, July 30, 1927.
7. Craven, E. B., Jr.: The Clinical Picture of Bromide Poisoning, The American Journal of the Medical Sciences, 186:525, October, 1933.
8. Harding, G. T., Jr. and Harding, Geo. T., III.: Bromide Intoxication, The Ohio State Medical Journal, 30:310, May 1, 1934.
9. Sippe, Clive and Bostock, John: Some Observations on Bromide Therapy and Intoxication, The Medical Journal of Australia, 1: 85-90, January 16, 1932.

ANTENATAL ADMINISTRATION OF QUININE

LINTON SMITH, M.D.

Atlanta

Antenatal administration of quinine salt was first reported by Dr. Philip Jones, of Coleford, England. He and his coworker, Bradbrook, later reported over 400 cases in which quinine was administered with excellent results. Ganner[1] stated in reviewing Mitchell's[2] reports which were in line with Bradbrook's cases that: "If Mitchell's claims can be confirmed we have at our disposal a simple method of reducing the great dangers of everyday obstetrics, namely, the abuse of forceps, hemorrhage, and sepsis." I am unable to find anything in the American literature regarding the antenatal administration of quinine.

I have used this method in sixty of my private cases of normal pregnant women and I am reporting my results, just as they are, from carefully kept records. I regret that I am unable to show a series of control cases, but I am using a like number of cases I attended before beginning the use of this method, although they are far from satisfactory because records were not made of many things necessary for ideal comparison.

The uterus contracts throughout pregnancy with more or less periodicity and in the later stages shows greater irritability in many patients. The painless contractions of the last weeks of pregnancy force the head into the pelvis and soften the structures there and the descending portion of the fetus seems to burrow its way. Labor begins very gradually; we say that labor actually begins when the contractions become sensible to the patient. Therefore, in the first stage of labor the uterus does all of the work with gradual increasing force and develops the lower uterine segment; the hydrostatic bag of water is formed, the cervix effaced and the os is dilated. In the second stage of labor the work is largely done by the voluntary abdominal muscles, not concerned in this study. The pains may be too weak or too strong, too short or too long, too seldom or too frequent, or irregular, all of which promote an abnormal labor. Weak pains or inertia uteri may become evident by infrequent contractions, or too short contractions, and often by a combination of all three. These cause an unduly prolonged first stage of labor and may prolong the second stage, because the presenting part is not forced against the perineum strong enough to cause vigorous muscle contractions. Anything that will cause consistent normal contractions of the uterus will also assist in softening and dilating the soft tissues of the pelvis and thereby shorten labor and substantially lessen the suffering of the mother as well as lessen the mortality and morbidity, all of which are of great importance[3].

Quinine administered in small doses for three weeks before the expected onset of labor will act as a true tonic and increase the basic tone of the uterine muscle fibres, and thus reinforce contractions which are excited by other endogenous means. The increased tone of the muscles will hasten the development of the lower uterine segment and more positively develop the hydrostatic bag of water which will earlier efface the cervix and dilate the os. In my opinion, the very tone which is imparted to the uterine muscles seems to act inversely on the soft structures of the pelvis and they dilate more easily and more rapidly although there can be no positive measure of such action.

The general health of the patient is definitely improved by small doses of quinine and Green-Armytage, Johnson and others state that this is the chief good effect. Patients usually express a definite feeling of being stronger, their appetite is improved and indigestion and heartburn of which many patients complain in the late stages of pregnancy are often entirely or greatly relieved, which I think is caused by the increased flow of digestive juices in the stomach and particularly of the hydrochloric acid.

Labor is definitely shortened and made easier as shown by the table below:

Number of cases:
  Primiparas 45
  Multiparas 15

placenta, but I have been unable to observe any difference in the firmness of the uterus in these cases and in those not receiving the drug and have abandoned the routine administration of pituitrin and ergot in my quininized patients.

In no sense should this method of administering small doses of quinine be considered a method of inducing labor and I believe that it is now agreed by pharmacologists and clinicians that quinine is not an oxytoxic nor is it of any value in inducing labor. There was no apparent tendency of these patients to go into labor prematurely, and the estimated dates of confinement varied both ways just as the cases did in which no quinine had been given. I did not have a case of precipitate labor although several patients were delivered in a remarkably short time, but I attribute this to a mild or a relatively painless first stage of labor and to the prompt and thorough softening and relaxation of the pelvic soft parts previously mentioned. So many patients are ready for delivery before they are expected that I have made it a rule to stay with the patient given quinine once she is in labor.

There was no case of retained placenta in this series and the number delivered by Crede's method was 37 whereas in a similar group not quininized I delivered 52 by this method. This is a matter governed largely by the obstetricians temperament and patience but I feel sure that I used expression less often because it was not needed. The improved muscle tone seems to facilitate normal or spontaneous expulsion of the placenta. Afterpains are uninfluenced by this treatment.

There was only one laceration of the perineum in this series although one bilateral and 21 unilateral episiotomies were done with 37 or 61 per cent of undamaged perineums, which is far better than my previous equal number of cases. I attribute this better result to the fact that the patient does not have to use all of her accessory muscles to the limit. In addition the assistant who is applying pressure to the fundus is not subject to ready control and with the uterus fully capable of completing the delivery, the obstetrician is free to devote himself to exerting the necessary pressure on the crowning head and, with

deeper anesthesia, "ease" the head over the perineum and through the birth canal. False pains were a negligible consideration in this series and the tone of the muscle seems so good that when pains started real progress was made and true labor followed.

Only normal cases were selected for the quinine treatment and apparently many obstetric problems were simplified. There was so little to do for the larger number of patients during the first stage of labor that only the fear of not being available when needed prevented attending to other affairs. There was so little pain during the early stages that frequently patients were not seen until fully dilated and it was necessary to question them carefully to ascertain the time labor began. Normal cases are considered to be those without disproportion between passage and passenger, the presence of albuminuria, flat pelvis, or mal-positions. One patient with a transverse presentation which resisted early correction was quinine treated with the intention of doing a correction of the presentation when pains began but when she was admitted to the hospital the shoulder had come down into the pelvis with the arm enclosed in the unruptured bag of water; the soft tissues had completely dilated and on converting the presentation into a breech, prompt delivery was made. There is probably a large field for this treatment in abnormal cases but further experience is needed.

When a long, slow labor is desired, so that the head may be molded or the passage be dilated more slowly to accommodate itself to the passenger or for some other definite reason, this treatment is contra-indicated.

I have used quinine dihydrochloride in doses of one and one-half grains three times a day beginning three weeks before the expected confinement, and I have found only one patient who could not take the drug. She had a violent reaction after being given one dose. There was a rash, intense itching, a high fever, photophobia and the treatment was discontinued. This simplified form of treatment should be adhered to; and Mitchell[a] warns that a further simplification of this method, such as five grains daily or larger or smaller doses, will mean certain failure. I have not used more than the one and one-half grain doses in my cases.

King reports infant mortalities from the mothers having ingested quinine. Gellhorn also quotes cases as do several others, but both of these authors adverse cases could have resulted from large doses of the drug administered in a short period of time. For example, one case received thirty grains in eight hours. Taylor and others mention partial or permanent deafness of infants caused by quinine given to the mothers, who, in most instances were given the drug in an attempt to induce labor. It is conceivable that if an idiosyncrasy existed serious trouble might follow, even the small doses suggested; but I have had no case of death or deafness.

I hope that this method will be tried in this country and with a larger number of cases reported we shall be in a better position to evaluate the attempts to alleviate suffering and to lower mortality and morbidity.

REFERENCES

1. D. N. Mitchell and H. N. Bradbrook, Br. Med. Journal, 1935, 1, 206.
2. P. J. Ganner, Br. Med. Journal, 1935, 1, 205.
3. J. W. Williams, Obstetrics, 1912, Appleton & Co., New York, N. Y.

CARDIOVASCULAR DISEASE PRESENTATION OF CASE*

Student Gallemore
Augusta

A negro, 27 years old, was admitted on December 22, 1935. His chief complaint was shortness of breath with fluttering of heart. He gave no history of syphilis. Two months ago he had first noticed shortness of breath while working and also upon lying down. His heart began to palpitate, later there was tenderness in epigastrium. He began coughing and expectorating blood-tinged sputum. His feet, legs and abdomen became edematous.

He was well nourished and developed, dyspneic, orthopneic and edematous. The mucous membranes and finger tips were pale, slightly cyanotic. The precordium bulged. Breath sounds were bronchovesicular at left lung base. No precordial heaving was present. The apex impulse was diffuse over the fourth and fifth interspace, the left border of cardiac dullness was in the fifth interspace about 10 cm. from the midsternal line. The rate was accelerated, the rhythm was irregular. The pulmonic second sound was greater than the aortic second. The force was irregular, some beats were louder. There was slight hardening of the vessel walls. Tenderness was elicited in the left lumbar region. The liver edge was 6 cm. below the ensiform cartilage.

The non-protein nitrogen was 22.4, the blood

*Conducted by the Department of Pathology and Clinical Departments of the University of Georgia School of Medicine, Augusta, for the Fourth Year Class.

Wasserman and Kahn tests were negative. Examination of the urine shown albumin 2+, with many white blood cells and an occasional granular cast. The sputum was positive for blood. X-ray showed widening of the aortic arch and marked general cardiac enlargement. The temperature ranged from 97 to 100°. The blood pressure was 138/104.

The case was diagnosed as syphilitic cardiovascular disease with congestive heart failure. The patient was treated symptomatically and dismissed improved, on the twenty-fifth day after his admission.

Five weeks later he again entered the hospital complaining of a vague pain across the base of the ribs which on breathing localized in the epigastric notch. About two weeks previously he had suffered gastric distress and vomited. Occasionally he had pain extending from the sternum down the left arm which would last one or two hours. He had a cough with expectoration. The finger tips and mucous membranes were pale; the feet and legs were edematous. Slight nystagmus was present. There was slight pulsation above the clavicles and fullness over the left precordium with breathing free and equal. There was a diffuse cardiac impulse and retromanubrial dullness 5 cm. to the right and 4 cm. to the left of the midsternal line in the second interspace. The left border of the heart was 9.5 cm. to the left of the midsternal line in the fifth interspace. Arrhythmia with extra systoles was noted. The abdomen bulged in the flanks, was distended but no fluid wave was demonstrable. Tenderness could be elicited in the epigastrium. The liver was not palpable. While in the hospital he suffered a sudden attack manifested by stupor, and followed by hemiplegia on the left side.

The electrocardiogram revealed pulsus bigeminus, left ventricular extra systole, right axis deviation, severe myocardial damage. Examination of the urine was essentially negative. No growth was obtained from blood culture. The temperature varied between 97 and 100.2°.

He was dismissed improved six weeks later with diagnoses of rheumatic cardiovascular disease, congestive heart failure, and cerebral embolism with hemiplegia.

He was readmitted after three months with the same complaints. He had experienced a severe pain in the chest four days previously and expectorated bright red blood.

He was extremely dyspneic, the respiration was Cheyne-Stokes in type. Arterial pulsation and venous engorgement were noted in the vessels of the neck. The precordium bulged. Percussion note was impaired, tactile fremitus increased, and a few scattered moist rales were heard over the base of the right lung.

The cardiac apex beat was diffuse in the third to sixth interspaces. Cardiac dullness extended 5 cm. to the right and 14 cm. to the left of the midsternal line. A loud blowing systolic murmur was heard at the apex over the sternum and was transmitted to the left axilla. Pulse rate was 76, pulsus alternans in type. Blood pressure was 170/120. The liver was palpable 5 cm. below the costal margin and slightly tender. Paralysis of the left arm and leg and marked pitting edema of both feet and ankles were noted.

The blood Wasserman reaction was negative and blood culture was sterile. Passive congestion of the retinae was observed. The urine at various times contained albumin 2+. Leukocyte count was 5,000 and the red cell count was 3,300,000. Blood was present in the sputum. The temperature ranged between 97 and 102°. He responded well and was dismissed with the diagnosis of hypertensive cardiovascular disease.

His fourth and final admission occurred approximately three months later. Added to his previous complaints was pain in the right lumbar region radiating forward to the region of the right nipple. At this time a history was elicited of recurrent sore throat nine years ago. At eleven years of age he had had a severe cough, the description of which would indicate pertussis. Three years earlier he had expectorated blood following an injury to the chest from being struck by a baseball. Following the attack of hemiplegia his gait has been seriously impaired. During his married life of ten years his wife had had five pregnancies, three resulted in miscarriages and two in normal births. Previous to his illness he had worked hard as a common laborer. During the past year he had lost 35 pounds.

Three days after his third dismissal from the hospital he again suffered from dyspnea and anasarca. He was at this time orthopneic and had Cheyne-Stokes respiration. His facies were apprehensive, the conjunctivae pale, a slight tremor of the tongue was present and the tonsils were reddened and slightly enlarged. Arterial pulsation and venous engorgement were again noticable in the vessels of the neck and pulsation was noted in the suprasternal notch. The thorax was asymmetrical because of the bulge of the precordium. Expansion was limited on the left side and respiration was irregular, 30 per minute. Tactile fremitus was slightly diminished and the percussion note was impaired at the left base. A few crepitant rales were heard in the left axilla and a slight respiratory wheeze over the left apex. The pulse was 78. The point of maximum intensity of the apex beat was in the fifth interspace 11 c. from the mid line. Cardiac dullness extended 4 cm. to the right and 15 cm. to the left of the midsternal line. Cardiac pulsation was palpable in the seventh interspace in the midaxillary line. A loud harsh blowing systolic murmur was heard over the mitral area. The pulmonic second sound resembled the sound produced by forcibly bending a stiff steel saw blade. It was high pitched, musical, and loud. The aortic sounds were weak so that the pulmonic second was greater than the aortic. Extra systoles were heard and the cardiac rhythm was irregular. A fluid wave and a flat percussion note were noted upon abdominal examination. The liver was tender and palpable 5 cm. below the costal margin. Reflexes were increased in the paralyzed left arm and leg.

His blood pressure on admission was 135/80 and five days later 115/70. There was no increase in the non-protein nitrogen, again the blood Wassermann and Kahn reactions were negative. His hemoglobin was 65 per cent and the red blood cell count 3,300,000. Albumin 2+ was noted in the urine.

He was treated by a low protein-salt poor diet, restricted fluid intake, morphine when necessary. Ammonium chloride grain 60 was administered three times daily, and an ampule of mercupurine was given intravenously.

His condition did not improve and on the fifth day, following a severe pain in the left lower chest, he expectorated blood and his temperature rose from normal to 100.4° and leukocyte count increased from 5,000 to 15,400. Following this he was placed in an oxygen tent. His respiratory distress and pain continued and he died on the tenth day of his admission.

Final Clinical Diagnosis

Cardiovascular disease, hypertensive. Cardiac dilation and hypertrophy. Congestive heart failure. Left pulmonary infarction. Hemiplegia, left.

Discussion by Student Hitchcock: We had here a man whose chief complaint was shortness of breath of a year's duration. Upon his first admission there were no remarkable changes in his cardiovascular system. So despite the negative Wassermann and the denial of a primary sore, a diagnosis was made of syphilitic heart disease and he was treated symptomatically. Other than the shortness of breath there was no evidence of congestive cardiac failure.

Four months later anasarca developed but the heart was not demonstrably enlarged. There were no symptoms of rheumatism but because of the congestive heart failure a diagnosis of rheumatic carditis was made.

Two months later congestive heart failure, cardiac enlargement, and hypertension were noted. While the onset of his previous attacks were gradual, this one was fulminating. Infarction of the lungs occurred either because of an embolus or as a result of passive congestion from left sided heart failure. The occurrence of cerebral and pulmonary embolism suggests degenerative changes in the heart involving both sides.

At the fourth admission he suffered from marked cardiac failure. At this time some criticism of the treatment may be made. Insufficient treatment to rid the body of fluid is evidenced by failing to use purgatives. Venesection was probably not indicated because of the low red blood cell count. I would think that more frequent ophthalmoscopic examinations should have been made to confirm the diagnosis of hypertensive cardiac disease.

I consider the diagnosis of hypertension with congestive heart failure correct. The precipitating cause of death was pulmonary infarction. Renal involvement was evident by the persistent albuminuria.

Discussion by V. P. Sydenstricker, M. D.: It is a pity that someone did not make a diagnosis of bacterial endocarditis upon one admission, because then all of the possible diagnoses would have been made.

At his first admission the low blood pressure led us to the diagnosis of syphilis. Later it became evident that hypertension was the primary cause. He persistently showed a high diastolic pressure. This then is a case of a large man who cracked up rapidly from hypertensive cardiac disease.

None of the physicians who examined this patient at his first admission had a clear idea of the diagnosis. At a second admission the loud mitral murmur and the accentuated second pulmonic sound led us to the consideration of rheumatism. The diagnosis still was unsatisfactory. The blood pressure was excessive. Later the suspicion of rheumatism was strengthened by the occurrence of pulmonary and cerebral infarction.

From subsequent events it is probable that the loud mitral murmur was due to the dilation and hypertrophy of the heart. Cerebral infarction however is unusual in hypertensive cardiac disease. Later it became increasingly evident that hypertensive cardic disease was the proper diagnosis and the infarctions were due to mural thromboses. He had the loudest type of pulmonic second sound that one ever hears. This would suggest some change in the pulmonary arteries.

This case illustrates the fulminating or malignant type of hypertension with the development of cardiac lesions. Respiratory embarrassment precipitated his death. In reference to the criticism at the last admission this man was too sick for much treatment. Venesection of course was contra-indicated because of the state of his blood. 65 per cent hemoglobin and 3,000,000 red blood cells.

Pathological Discussion by Edgar R. Pund, M.D.:

Anatomic Diagnoses. Hypertensive vascular lesions. Arteriosclerosis of small pulmonary arteries. Cardiac hypertrophy and dilation. Cardiac mural thromboses. Multiple red infarcts of lungs. Sero-fibrinous pleurisy. Subcutaneous edema. Chronic passive congestion of virceria. Adynamic distension of stomach. Fibrosis of mural endocardium. Old infarcts of kidneys. Fibrous pleural adhesions.

The autopsy confirmed the clinical diagnosis that were made at the last admission. Evidence of hypertension was indicated by the enlarged heart (635 Gm.), and arteriolar sclerosis in sections from the thymus, kidney, seminal vesicles, and pancreas. Mural thromboses were present in the apices of both ventricles. The fibrosis of the endocardium of the left ventricle was in part due to an organized thrombus, probably the site of detachment of the cerebral embolus. The healed infarcts of the kidneys probably occurred at this time also.

Dr. Sydenstricker was right about sclerosis of the pulmonary arteries. This sclerosis involved the small arteries and was therefore secondary to hypertension in the lesser circulation.

The National Medical Council on Birth Control was organized in June, 1936. It proposes to control and supervise all medical policies of the American Birth Control League.

Great work is being done in some of our schools. Holidays are given to those classes where 100 per cent of the children have had their teeth cared for. But the educational efforts of the profession should not be limited to the instruction of children. Adults should be trained in the proper care of their teeth and in the avoidance of those things which are proven irritants. An occasional smoke possibly does no harm, but the short stemmed pipe carried in the mouth is a menace.

Blackwater Fever. Fernan-Nunez (Ann. Int. Med. 9: 1203, March, 1936) has written a stimulating paper on blackwater fever based on a clinical review of 52 cases and the observation of an equal number of patients of other physicians. In his opinion, blackwater fever is practically the one remaining tropical disease whose etiology has not been definitely solved. He submits the theory that it is an allergic manifestation of estivo-autumnal (malignant subtertian) malaria. The author gives a good description of the symptoms and pathology of the condition. The differential diagnosis includes paroxysmal hemoglobinuria, yellow fever and bilious malaria. The discussion of treatment is particularly full. Great emphasis is laid on the importance of nursing care and the tremendous importance of putting the patient to bed and keeping him there lest the hemoglobinuria increase, or, if already stopped, recur. The patient should be kept absolutely quiet and fluids forced. The weakened heart muscle requires that the patient be kept in absolute relaxation for from 3 to 6 weeks after the acute attack. The writer uses neoarsphenamine in small doses and has practically abandoned quinine. Sodium thiosulphate seems to have a specific effect on hemoglobinuria. It is of course vital to prevent acidosis and to give fluids parenterally in case of severe vomiting. Occasionally blood transfusions are necessary. Fernan-Nunez is not impressed with the use of other drugs.

Prognosis in Acute Glomerular Nephritis. Arthur B. Richter. Ann. Int. Med., Feb. 1936.

Since most studies regarding the prognosis of patients with acute glomerular nephritis have been carried on with children, the author decided to study adults and determine their status after follow-up for a number of years. One hundred adolescents and adults were studied. Of this group 10 died during the acute stage—of the remaining 90 the renal status of 77 was determined and it was found 62 had been cured whereas 15 had developed chronic nephritis. The one clinical feature of most importance was the degree and duration of albuminuria—if it decreases this denotes healing, but if it persists for a year or longer, the chances of chronic nephritis developing are 6 to 1.

Abstract by Wm. R. Minnich, M.D.

Association meets, Macon, May 11-14, 1937.

THE JOURNAL
OF THE
MEDICAL ASSOCIATION OF GEORGIA
Devoted to the Welfare of the Medical Association of Georgia

478 Peachtree Street, N.E., Atlanta, Ga.

JULY, 1936

ACUTE OSTEOMYELITIS

Several years ago an accomplished surgeon described a bone-grafting operation to repair a defect in a humerus almost totally destroyed by osteomyelitis. Another surgeon equally as brilliant remarked that the operation as designed and carried out to remedy the loss of bone was all that could be desired but inquired: "why was the child allowed to get in such condition?"

Pathologists teach the destructive nature of acute pyogenic osteomyelitis and just what may be expected if the process is allowed to proceed to its ultimate termination; bacteriologists have demonstrated the causative organisms, the foci from which they originate, and that it is a blood borne infection; clinicians have tabulated a symptomatology that is as classic as that of acute appendicitis; and surgeons have devised operative procedures which when carried out in the early stages of the inflammation will prevent, in a great majority of cases, bone destruction, multiple operations for chronic osteomyelitis with its attendant invalidism and expense and the unfortunate sequels of prolonged suppuration. It remains for the profession as a whole to be alert to recognize the disease at its inception and "it should be the aim of all practicioners to make a diagnosis sufficiently early that subsequent destruction of bone might be avoided" (Starr).

Acute osteomyelitis is primarily a disease of childhood, it being encountered most frequently between the ages of two and ten years. Given a child whose history is that of a convulsion or chill, followed by high fever, a leukocyte count of from twenty to thirty thousand, with an increase in the polymorphonuclear cells, a distinct point of tenderness over the end of one of the long bones *(the most frequent site of infection)*, without joint involvement, and the history of a recent injury, boil, sore throat, sinus infection or other focus from which infection might originate, the assumption of acute osteomyelitis is justified. There are probably two reasons why a correct diagnosis is not made earlier; one is that parents treat the child for a few days before calling a physician; and secondly, the failure to distinguish the condition from "rheumatism," "arthritis," "neuritis," et cetera. One should bear in mind that the roentgen ray is powerless to furnish aid during the first week of the illness, as sufficient time has not elapsed for the inflammatory process to produce structural changes which will register on an x-ray film. Those of large experience in seeing and caring for these cases state that the diagnosis should be made on the history and clinical findings in the first twenty-four hours.

Acute osteomyelitis is a surgical disease. Having made the diagnosis the proper treatment is an incision over the bone involved and the making of a trap-door through the cortex. The curette should not under any circumstances be employed and every effort should be made to avoid entering the medullary cavity, for if this is done, it will very likely mean that the infection will extend to other parts of the bone.

If the physician will mentally catalog acute osteomyelitis as a probability when symptoms as outlined present themselves much suffering, expense and invalidism will be avoided.

GEO. A. TRAYLOR, M.D.

MEDICAL DEFENSE

While the Committee on Medical Defense reports encouraging results from their efforts to curtail malpractice suits against physicians of this State, it is regrettable to note that during the past year two physicians were sued who were not eligible for aid. These good doctors were too busy with their work to think of medical societies and meetings and they allowed their membership in the Association to lapse.

The rule is: Pay your dues by April 1 each year and have full protection.

The JOURNAL would like to record the scientific work of Georgia doctors. It earnestly requests, therefore, that each physician in the State who publishes a contribution in some other medical periodical submit an abstract of the article for these columns.

BETTER COOPERATION AMONG PHYSICIANS

In 1804, seventy-one years after Oglethorpe came, eighteen Savannah physicians petitioned the Senate and House of Representatives of Georgia to incorporate their society, the Georgia Medical Society. This was the beginning of organized medicine in the State, the Medical Association of Georgia being organized forty-five years later, in 1849.

From this small beginning organized medicine has grown in this State and, today, we point with pride to an honorable history in the affairs of our people. It is interesting to note that at the eighty-seventh annual session of the Medical Association of Georgia, held in Savannah, the Secretary reported to the House of Delegates that 70 per cent of the 159 counties in the State had medical societies or were affiliated with counties having active organizations, that 66 per cent of the 2616 white physicians eligible for membership in the Association continued their support to organized medicine and that the membership roll had increased 112 during the past year.

At the same time the Committee on Medical Economics reported that a large number of physicians in the State, to whom questionnaires had been sent requesting suggestions for the improvement of medical practice, had written on their replies "Better Cooperation Among Physicians." Ninety-three per cent of these suggestions came from members of the Association and one of every five replies made the same statement. It is apparent, therefore, that while the medical profession of this State has made great progress during the past hundred years, there are many physicians who believe that a full understanding and better cooperation among themselves would solve many of their problems.

When these reports are studied and explanations sought, it is not surprising to find that cooperation among physicians is in proportion to their activity in organized medicine. In counties having active medical societies, problems are met with frank discussion by the majority of the members and the ultimate result is: Georgia physicians do what they have always done—the right thing.

ADMISSION TO MEDICAL SCHOOL

Under the present program of medical education, plans to study medicine should be worked out well in advance of the time of actual registration in the medical school. This is important from two standpoints:

The first is that of requirements for admission. Practically all schools now require three years of premedical college work. This work must be done in a college which is approved, and it is well to find out in advance whether any particular college is acceptable to the medical school to which the student intends later to apply. Furthermore, there are certain requirements in regard to subjects which must be taken for admission. These, at the present, apply to certain subjects such as physics, chemistry, biology, English, foreign language, and others. The premedical student should, therefore, make sure that he is including the necessary hours' credit in subjects which he will need to present for admission to medical school.

The large number of men applying for admission to medical school also makes it important for the student to do such a quality of work in his premedical career that his record will stand well in comparison with the records of other applying students. It is quite natural for medical schools to compare the records of applicants, and the student with a poor premedical record will receive less consideration than the student with a good record. It must be borne in mind also that practically all medical schools have a certain established standard of work which must be met by the premedical record presented by the student.

The question is frequently asked, "What is the most important thing for the student in his premedical training?" The real answer can not be given in terms of one or more subjects, but is to be found in the cause for the failure of medical students. In many instances failure can be traced to lack of application and lack of sound methods and habits of study. We recognize the fact that we are creatures of habit. Yet, in the face of this some students feel that they can do their premedical work in an unorderly fashion without sincere application but with the idea that when they enter medical school they will settle down and get to work. Unfortunately, this is seldom possible, the student before long finding himself in a hopeless muddle. He has no organized habits of study and application and there is no time to develop them. The effect of this deficiency is felt not alone in the earlier years of the medical curriculum; there are junior and senior year students who show they can not set themselves logically to approach the problem of the patient. It is probable that the same defect may never be overcome but will handicap them as doctors throughout their entire professional life.

The second factor which the prospective medical student must keep in mind is concerned with making application for admission to the freshman class in medicine. There are many applicants for every possible place in the freshman classes of the medical schools of the United States. Thus, it is important that his application be made sufficiently early to receive consideration. The time for making application varies in different schools; in general, it is advisable to make application by the middle of January preceding the fall when the student hopes to enter medical school. This can be determined by communicating with the individual school in which the student is interested.

RUSSELL H. OPPENHEIMER, M.D.

PSYCHIATRY

As the clocks tick off the seconds and the world spins 'round and round,' phychiatry continues to unfold dramas more colorful and fascinating than those on any stage. They are the dramas produced by the peculiarities of human behavior. Their effect upon the lives of every one of us is of vital importance. Mythologies, legends and histories abound with them. They create the current news of the day. Health and happiness are destroyed, business and professional careers are ruined, kaliedoscopic changes made in governments, world-wide conflagrations started and opinions in every land are influenced by these dramas.

The denouement of smallpox, yellow fever and diphtheria have been written by the immortals of medicine. Surgical difficulties are being rendered hors de combat by antisepsis.

WOMAN'S AUXILIARY

OFFICERS, 1936-1937

President—Mrs. Wm. R. Dancy, Savannah.
President-Elect—Mrs. Ralph H. Chaney, Augusta.
First Vice-President—Mrs. B. H. Minchew, Waycross.
Second Vice-President—Mrs. Clarence L. Ayers, Toccoa.
Third Vice-President—Mrs. J. A. Redfearn, Albany.

Recording Secretary—Mrs. Warren A. Coleman, Eastman.
Corresponding Secretary—Mrs. Lee Howard, Savannah.
Treasurer—Mrs. W. A. Selman, Atlanta.
Historian—Mrs. Grady N. Coker, Canton.
Parliamentarian—Mrs. John E. Penland, Waycross.

COMMITTEE CHAIRMEN

Student oLan Fund
Mrs. Robert C. Pendergrass, Americus.

Health Films
Mrs. A. J. Mooney, Statesboro.

Legislation
Mrs. Dan Y. Sage, 47 Inman Circle, Atlanta.

Press and Publicity
Mrs. J. Harry Rogers, 134 Huntington Rd., Atlanta.

Research in Romance of Medicine
Mrs. D. N. Thompson, Elberton.

Jane Todd Crawford Memorial
Mrs. Eustace A. Allen, 18 Collier Rd., Atlanta.

Doctors' Day
Mrs. Ernest R. Harris, Winder.

EXECUTIVE BOARD MEETING

The Executive Board met with the Advisory Committee of the Association at the Academy of Medicine, Atlanta, June 4th. Dr. James N. Brawner, Atlanta, Chairman, presided.

Dr. Brawner spoke briefly of the importance of the Auxiliary, then introduced Mrs. Wm. R. Dancy, Savannah, President. She outlined her aims and plans for the year. Dr. B. H. Minchew, Waycross, President of the Association, urged the members to continue to work for the Student Loan Fund; study the provisions of the Social Security and Child Welfare Acts,. and to think in terms of public health and talk in terms of the people.

Mrs. Ralph H. Chaney, Augusta, President-Elect, gave a sketch of her plans to organize an Auxiliary in each county of the State and to assist the weak Auxiliaries, also the importance of stressing the privilege and value of being a member.

Dr. Wm. R. Dancy, Savannah, the original advocate of the Student Loan Fund, and Dr. Benjamin Bashinski, Macon, stressed the importance of the Student Loan Fund and the necessity to continue the work.

Others present, each of whom made a short talk, were: Mrs. Ernest R. Harris, Winder, Past-President; Mrs. C. W. Roberts, Atlanta, Past-President; Mrs. Warren A. Coleman, Eastman, Recording Secretary; Mrs. Grady N. Coker, Canton, Historian; Mrs. Cleveland Thompson, Millen, First District Manager; Mrs. E. B. Davis, Byromville, Third District Manager; Mrs. Eustace A. Allen, Atlanta, Chairman, Jane Todd Crawford Memorial; Mrs. J. Harry Rogers, Atlanta, Chairman, Press and Publicity; Mrs. Robert B. Crichton, Augusta, President, Richmond County

Auxiliary; Mrs. Charles E. Boynton, Atlanta, President, Fulton County Auxiliary; Mrs. C. B. Almand, Winder, originator of "Doctors' Day;" Dr. Edgar D. Shanks, Atlanta, Secretary-Treasurer of the Association.

Third District

The Woman's Auxiliary to the Third District Medical Society met at Cuthbert, June 10th. Mrs. E. B. Davis, Byromville, presided.

The Auxiliary to the Randolph County Medical Society was reorganized. Officers elected were: Mrs. Loren Gary, Shellman, President; Mrs. W. G. Elliott, Cuthbert, Vice-President; Mrs. T. F. Harper, Coleman, Secretary-Treasurer.

Mrs. Ralph H. Chaney, Augusta, related the requisites and objectives of the Auxiliary in an interesting manner. Mrs. B. H. Minchew, Waycross, reported the proceedings of the Savannah convention, held April 21-24.

Mrs. E. B. Davis, Byromville, quoted excerpts from a talk by Dr. J. L. Campbell, Atlanta, Chairman of the Cancer Commission, made at the Savannah convention on "Cancer Control."

Mrs. J. C. Patterson, Cuthbert entertained at tea following the business session.

Burke-Jenkins-Screven Counties

The members of the three counties met at Millen on June 11th. The President, Mrs. L. F. Lanier, Sylvania, presided.

Mrs. Lee Howard, Savannah, State Corresponding Secretary, and Mrs. Cleveland Thompson, Millen, First District Manager, were guests. Mrs. Howard made a report on the recent Savannah convention.

The members and visitors of the Auxiliary and Society were entertained at dinner, served at the Community House.

GEORGIA DEPARTMENT OF PUBLIC HEALTH

T. F. ABERCROMBIE, M.D., *Director*

TYPHOID VACCINE

A period of three years has elapsed since the "Mitchell Strain" typhoid vaccine was put into circulation in Georgia. This was in January, 1933. Prior to that time typhoid vaccine was prepared from the Rawlings strain of B. typhosus, a descendent of the old Rawlings strain brought to this country in 1908 by Colonel F. F. Russell of the U. S. Army Medical School. It was the vaccine prepared from this famous culture that established beyond controversy the efficiency of prophylactic immunization in the ranks of the Army and Navy in 1912 and subsequently among the civilian population. Indeed the Rawlings vaccine proved so effective that it soon began to rank with smallpox vaccine. The exceedingly low incidence of typhoid among the soldiers and sailors during the World War bears eloquent testimony of this high regard.

About 1928 there began to drift into the headquarters of the Georgia State Health Department reports of unexplainable instances of the failure of typhoid vaccine to protect. The strength of the vaccine suspension was increased, but this brought complaints of more severe reaction. The method of preparation was subjected to careful study, but, in spite of certain improvements, reports of vaccine failure continued to mount during the period of 1929-1932.

Then came the announcement of certain investigations, notably, Larkum, Grinnel and Arkwright, that the Rawlings strain was lacking in immunizing power and that more recently isolated strains were more efficient. The sequence of events which led to the final abandonment of the Rawlings culture and the adoption of the Mitchell strain isolated from a Georgia case of typhoid fever from Mitchell County have already been recounted in a previous issue of the JOURNAL (December, 1934, p. 463). Experimental use of the Mitchell strain began late in 1932, but the new vaccine was not officially begun until January, 1933.

Since no method has yet been devised for determining the presence or absence of specific immunity produced by typhoid vaccine in man, there is, therefore, no laboratory measuring stick whereby the relative protective power of one brand of vaccine can be compared in terms of another. Such a method has been devised for diphtheria vaccines and we have the Schick skin test. Smallpox vaccine can be titrated very accurately by its ability to produce "takes" both in man and certain animals. But there is no such method applicable for typhoid. Hence the desired information must be gained slowly and awkwardly by studying the incidence of vaccine failures among relatively large groups of vaccinated people over a long period of time.

As stated above, during the three year period 1929-1931, inclusive, increasing numbers of vaccine failure reports were received. These came from private practitioners and health officers throughout the State. An investigation of these reports by the writer revealed the following information summarized in Table 1.

TYPHOID AMONG VACCINATED
TABLE I.

RAWLINGS VACCINE

Summary of cases among vaccinated reported voluntarily by physicians and health officers.
1929-1931

ALL HAD RECEIVED RAWLINGS VACCINE

Year	Total cases reported	ONSET AFTER VACCINATION			
		Within 30 days	30 days to 12 mos.	1 to 2 years	Longer than 2 years
1929	21	2	9	5	7
1930	21	10	17	3	1
1931	23	4	11	6	5
Total	65	16	37	14	13

There is good reason to believe that the peak of immunity is not reached for several weeks after the last injection of vaccine and that this peak may begin to subside after several months. Hence it is logical to assume that the period of greatest immunity must be within the interval of one month to twelve months after vaccination. It should be noted in Table 1 that 37 of the total of 65 cases previously vaccinated developed within this optimum period.

Then in 1932, a series of 216 cases of typhoid were studied in the course of investigating several small and widely distributed outbreaks. Of the number 21 or 9.7 per cent had been inoculated with the old Rawlings type vaccine within a period of 12 months. Among these 21 there were five deaths (23.8%).

Soon after the Mitchell strain vaccine was put into use in 1933, the writer undertook to obtain vaccination histories of all cases of typhoid fever reported. This study was continued for a three year period ending in December, 1935, and the results are summarized in Table 2.

TYPHOID AMONG VACCINATED
MITCHELL STRAIN
TABLE 2

Year	Number cases studied	Total cases among vaccinated	Within 30 days	ONSET AFTER VACCINATION			
				30 days to 12 mos.	1 - 2 years	2 - 3 years	Longer than 3 years
				5 R)			
1933	626	55	6	4 M) 9*	19†	9†	13†
1934	670	53	9	5	7	11†	21†
1935	628	58	2	7	10	14	25†
Total	1,924	166	17	21	36	34	59

*Of these only 4 received the new vaccine (M) while 5 received the old vaccine (R).
†These received the old Rawlings vaccine.

Data given in Table 1 was obtained from unsolicited reports prior to the change in the antigen, while that in Table 2 resulted from a systematic survey of all typhoid cases on record. Hence the two tables are not correlative. But if this same kind of systematic survey had been made prior to the change in antigen, it is reasonable to expect that a great many more instances of vaccine failure would have been discovered. Keeping in mind that the period of greatest protection should be during the first year, after vaccination, discounting the first thirty days, note that there were 37 failures during this period with the vaccine, as compared with 16 with the new. See Table 3.

TABLE 3
VACCINE FAILURES BEFORE AND
AFTER CHANGE OF ANTIGEN

PRIOR TO CHANGE OF ANTIGEN CASES REPORTED WITHOUT SOLICITATION		AFTER CHANGE OF ANTIGEN CASES DISCOVERED BY SYSTEMATIC SOLICITATION	
Year	Cases	Year	Cases
1929	9	1933	4
1930	17	1934	5
1931	11	1935	7
Total	37	Total	16

It is apparent, therefore, that the incidence of typhoid fever among persons vaccinated within one year has greatly decreased since the adoption of the new antigen in 1933. On the other hand, it should be borne in mind that for the past three years the estimated number of persons immunized each year per 1,000 population has been 75, compared with 50 per year per 1,000 population during the period 1929-30 and 31. Also the total incidence of typhoid fever as based on the death rates for the last three years has decreased to 9.1 deaths per year, as compared with 15.5 for the period of 1929-30-31. These factors may account to some extent for the decline in vaccine failure incidence. Nevertheless, there appears to be sufficient evidence of improvement to justify the change of antigen.

In all fairness to the Rawlings strain of B. typhosus, it has been recently shown that descendents of this famous culture greatly vary among each other in virulence and antigenic power. Certain Rawlings sub-strains are exceedingly high in these two essentials, while others are lacking. Since it is now possible to determine the presence or absence of these antigenic virtue in any strain, be it called Rawlings or Mitchell or by any other name, there should be no further controversy.

T. F. SELLERS, M.D.,
Chief, Division of Laboratories.

BOOK REVIEWS

Medical Papers Dedicated to Henry A. Christian, M.D., From His Present and Past Associates and House Officers: Waverly Press, Inc., Baltimore.

There are many physicians who are truly great, but few live to see their many students compile a volume of 1,000 pages in their honor. Doctor Christian must feel fully rewarded for his labors when he notes the fine work done by his past and present associates, much of which is recorded in this book. The text is handled well, the illustrations are excellent and every reader takes pride in the development of American medicine.

The Surgical Clinics of North America, Chicago Number (February) 1936. W. B. Saunders Company, Philadelphia, Pa. The Chicago number of the Clinics of North America contains 27 papers by well known physicians. The most interesting article is a symposium on cancer of the uterine cervix. There are seven separate phases of uterine cervical cancer discussed: Symptomotology, diagnosis, treatment, complications, control of pain in inoperable cases, treatment of preoperative complications and carcinoma complicated by pregnancy. Several drawings are shown illustrating different stages of cervical carcinoma.

CHARLES E. RUSHIN, M.D.

Gynecological and Obstetrical Tuberculosis by Edwin M. Jameson, M.D., Fellow of Trudeau Foundation, Attending Surgeon Saranac Lake General Hospital and Reception Hospital. Lea & Febiger, Philadelphia, Pa. Price $3.50.

The author presents a critical study of tuberculosis

of the female genital tract from his own experience and from the accumulated evidence at the great tuberculosis sanatorium at Saranac Lake. In addition he presents a very extensive bibliography.

He divides the work into three parts:

Part 1.—The effect of pulmonary tuberculosis on the physiology of the female genitalia.

Part 2.—The infection of the genital organs and peritoneum.

Part 3.—The problem of pregnancy in a tuberculous woman.

Part three should be of special interest to all doing obstetrics, to internists and to phthisiologist. The author's discussion is from his own experience and wide study of the literature both American and foreign.

The conclusion one draws from this discussion is that there is no fixed rule as to whether or not every pregnant tuberculous woman should be aborted, but a decision should be made in each individual case, consideration being given to the location, the extent of the disease and the desires of the patient. Many cases are quoted where pregnancy has caused little or no advance of the disease.

The small space given in most textbooks on Gynecology to tuberculosis of the genital organs justifies such a monograph as the author presents.

JOHN F. DENTON, M.D.

NEWS ITEMS

Commentator of the Owensby Clinic, "published by-monthly for the information of the affiliated examiners of the Owensby Clinic and for the extension of neurpsychiatric education and research," Atlanta, Vol. 1, No. 1, was published June 15th. "Address all communications to Newdigate M. Owensby, M.D., Medical Arts Building, Atlanta." The articles and abstracts published in the bulletin show some excellent editorial work and deserve attention.

Dr. Eugene E. Murphey, Augusta, spoke before a meeting of the Kiwanis Club at Hotel Richmond on "The Unfinished Problems of Public Health Work," June 12th.

The Colquitt County Medical Society met at Hotel Colquitt, Moultrie, June 9th. Dr. Henry M. McGehee and Dr. A. G. Funderburk, both of Moultrie, read scientific papers.

Dr. J. R. McCord, Atlanta, spoke at a meeting of the Tennessee Valley Medical Association at Knoxville on June 12th.

The Thomas County Medical Society met in the Methodist church at Meigs on June 17th. Dr. Harry Ainsworth, Thomasville, President, presided. Minutes of the previous meeting were read and adopted. Dr. Ernest F. Wahl, Thomasville, read a paper entitled "The Effect of Nervous Influences on Digestion;" discussed by Dr. Roy A. Hill, Dr. W. W. Jarrell and Dr. H. M. Moore, all of Thomasville. Dr. Jarrell spoke on "The Treatment of Rural Syphilis;" discussed by Dr. E. F. Wahl, Dr. H. M. Moore, Dr.

Georgia," Dr. W. W. Young, Atlanta; *"Localized Myxedema,"* Dr. J. K. Fancher, Atlanta; *"Secondary Anemia,"* Dr. Francis P. Parker, Emory University; *"A Clinical and Epidemiological Study of One Hundred Cases of Undulant Fever in Georgia,"* Dr. T. F. Sellers, Atlanta; *"Hemorrhagic Nephritis in Negro Children—Lantern Slides,"* Dr. Joseph Yampolsky, Atlanta; *"Surgical Treatment of Pulmonary Tuberculosis,"* Dr. Cleveland D. Whelchel, Gainesville. Address by Dr. B. H. Minchew, Waycross, President of the Medical Association of Georgia. Physicians who led discussions on the various papers were: Dr. A. H. Hilsman, Albany; Dr. E. B. Davis, Byromville; Dr. J. M. Barnett, Albany; Dr. F. K. Boland, Jr., Atlanta; Dr. Frank P. Norman, Columbus; Dr. Jno. D. Blackburn, Thomaston; Dr. J. A. Redfearn, Albany; Dr. Guy J. Dillard, Columbus; Dr. T. E. Rogers, Macon; Dr. Jno. W. Oden and Dr. H. D. Allen, Jr., both of Milledgeville; Dr. Geo. F. Klugh, Jr. and Dr. T. L. Byrd, both of Atlanta; Dr. H. M. McKemie, Albany; Dr. Thos. M. Adams, Montezuma; Dr. John E. Walker, Columbus; Dr. Wm. R. Minnich, Atlanta; Dr. E. B. Saye, Macon; Dr. E. H. Greene and Dr. S. T. Barnett, Jr., both of Atlanta; Dr. Enoch Callaway, LaGrange; Dr. Olin S. Cofer, Atlanta; Dr. Chas. H. Watt, Thomasville; Dr. Geo. F. Eubanks, Atlanta; Dr. Chas. C. Harrold, Macon; Dr. J. C. Keaton, Albany; Dr. Steve P. Kenyon, Dawson; Dr. Benj. Bashinsky, Macon; Dr. Wm. W. Anderson, Atlanta; Dr. E. F. Fincher, Dr. R. B. Wilson, Dr. J. Calvin Weaver, Dr. Ben H. Clifton and Dr. Dan Elkin, all of Atlanta; Dr. E. F. Wahl, Thomasville; Dr. T. C. Davison, Atlanta. Dr. J. C. Keaton, Albany, was First Vice-President, and Dr. Frank K. Boland, Atlanta, Secretary-Treasurer.

Dr. Everett L. Bishop, Atlanta, returned recently from a tour of each of the congressional districts of Georgia for the United States Department of Public Health. He spoke on Cancer and delivered twenty lectures to lay and medical audiences. *"Cancer and Its Control"* was the subject of his address at the University of Georgia Institute of Public Affairs in Athens on July 1st.

OBITUARY

Dr. George Byron Hack, Hinesville; member; Atlanta College of Physicians and Surgeons, Atlanta, 1910; aged 49; died of heart disease at his home on June 14, 1936. He practiced at Ludowici after he received his degree in medicine until sixteen years ago then removed to Hinesville. Dr. Hack was a successful practitioner and had numerous friends who held him in high esteem. He was a member of the Tri-County Medical Society, President and member of the Third District Medical Society, Hinesville Lodge, F. & A. M. and the Walthourville Methodist church. Surviving him are his widow, two sons, Fred and Orion Hack; one daughter, Jane Hack, all of Hinesville. Rev. J. F. Merrin conducted the funeral services from the Walthourville Presbyterian church. Interment was in the churchyard.

Dr. James Leslie Cheshire, Damascus; member; Atlanta College of Physicians and Surgeons, 1908, age 53, died after several weeks illness of cardiac and respiratory complications at his home on June 17, 1936. He was a descendant of one of the prominent families of Miller County, Georgia. At the time of his death he was a member of the Tri-County Medical Society, the Masonic fraternity and the Free Will Baptist church. Dr. Cheshire had been engaged in the practice of medicine at Damascus for 28 years and was deeply beloved by the entire community. He is survived by his wife and one daughter, Mrs. Peyton Keaton, his father, one sister and three brothers. Funeral services were conducted at Macedonia Church by Rev. S. T. Shutes assisted by Rev. David Cripps. Interment was in Macedonia cemetery. The following physicians, members of the Tri-County Medical Society, were active pall bearers: Doctors Sharp, Arlington; Barksdale, Gunter and Standifer, Blakely; Shepard, Bluffton; Baughn, Hays and Houston, Colquitt; Beard, Edison; and Bridges, Leary.

Dr. Benjamin Lynn Bridges, Ellaville; member; Emory University School of Medicine, Emory University, 1895; aged 63; died at his home on June 24, 1936. He was a native of Schley county. Dr. Bridges practiced medicine in Ellaville and Schley county for more than forty years. The people of his home community paid a glowing tribute to his memory and will remember his work as a friend and physician. He was a member of the Sumter County Medical Society, Third District Medical Society and the Ellaville Methodist church. Surviving him are his widow, two sons, Burton and Russell Bridges, both of Atlanta. Funeral services were conducted from the Ellaville Methodist church. Interment was in the city cemetery.

Dr. William M. Cawhern, Atlanta; Atlanta College of Physicians and Surgeons, Atlanta, 1899; aged 69; died at a private sanitarium in Atlanta after a brief illness on June 24, 1936. He was a native of Atlanta and resided here almost all his life. Dr. Cawhern on several occasions was active in politics. He was charitable and held in high esteem by many acquaintances. He was a member of the St. James Methodist Episcopal church. Surviving him are his widow, three daughters, Mrs. Edith McCormack, Mrs. P. A. Hussey and Miss Nell Cawhern, all of Atlanta; one son, Roy Cawhern, Atlanta. Funeral services were conducted by Rev. W. H. Boring from the St. James Methodist Episcopal church. Burial was in Casey's cemetery.

Dr. Daniel L. Moore, Nahunta; member; Emory University School of Medicine, 1894; aged 62; died at his home on June 24, 1936. He practiced for more than forty years in Nahunta and Brantley county. Dr. Moore was the most devoted friend to the poor and rich alike. His life was truly that of a Christian and his efforts were directed to the aid of his people with an earnest desire to add something for their relief in the practice of his profession and for the improvement of their community. He was a member of the Ware County Medical Society and First Baptist church of Nahunta. Surviving him are his widow, three daugh-

CAL ASSOCIATION OF GEORGIA, and a copy sent to the family.

W. B. EMERY, M.D.
CECIL STOCKARD, M.D.
W. L. THOMASON, M.D.
THEO TOEPEL, M.D., *Chairman*
Resolution Committee.

Resolutions on the Death of Dr. Francis Gilchrist Jones

After a long illness Dr. Francis Gilchrist Jones, a well known and active member of the Society and a beloved and honored friend, died at a private hospital in Atlanta, March 2, 1936.

Dr. Jones was born May 17, 1886, and was the son of R. H. Jones, a resident of Atlanta, formerly of Liberty County, Georgia. His mother, Susan Baker, was the daughter of Judge James M. Baker of Jacksonville, Fla. His paternal grandfather was Major Andrew Maybank Jones of the Confederate Army and formerly of Liberty County Georgia. His maternal grandfather was Judge Baker who served as a senator in the Confederate Senate during the Civil War.

Dr. Jones' family, moved to Atlanta in 1892. He entered the Calhoun Street School and later graduated from the Boys High School where he won recognition for his scholastic work and as a public debater. He later attended Washington and Lee University where he received his A.B. degree. His medical education was obtained at the Atlanta College of Physicians and Surgeons, now Emory University, from which he was graduated in 1910. He served his internship at Grady Hospital. He practiced his profession in Atlanta for several years as a general practitioner, later specializing in dermatology.

He was President of the Phi Chi Sigma fraternity and later National President of the Chi Zeta Chi which was changed to Phi Rho Sigma.

He was a member of the Piedmont Lodge No. 447 F. and A. M., the First Presbyterian Church, the Fulton County Medical Society, the Medical Association of Georgia, and the American Medical Association.

Due to his health Dr. Jones, for the past few years, had not been able to take an active interest in medical affairs. Prior to his failure of health he was associated with many of the hospital staffs and other medical organizations.

He was married to Miss Lucia Jeter, October 31, 1911. To them were born two children, a daughter, Susan Baker, who is now the wife of C. E. Medlock, and Francis G., who is a senior at Boys High School. He is survived by his widow and two children.

Dr. Jones' elegance of manner showed a cultural background of long standing. He was a sterling personality with great ability for fellowship and helpfulness toward his associates. His life and work stand as a solid memorial to the best in medicine and as a tribute to his family and friends.

Whereas, the Fulton County Medical Society and organized medicine suffered a grievous loss in the death of Dr. Jones, and

Whereas, his family lost a devoted husband and father and many of us lost a friend, therefore

Be it Resolved: That we extend to them our heartfelt sympathy and that a copy of these resolutions be spread upon the minutes of this Society, printed in the Bulletin of the Society, the JOURNAL OF THE MEDICAL ASSOCIATION OF GEORGIA, and a copy sent to his family.

J. C. McDOUGALL, M.D.
BEN H. CLIFTON, M.D.
C. C. AVEN, M.D., *Chairman.*
Resolution Committee.

Resolution on the death of
Dr. Willis F. Westmoreland

Dr. Willis Foreman Westmoreland was born in a farmhouse near the village of Milner, Ga., fifty-four miles south of Atlanta, on the evening of July 22, 1864. He died December 4, 1935, at his home in this city. But for the exigencies of war his birth would have occurred in Atlanta.

Dr. Willis Westmoreland, senior, a fearless soldier and the ranking surgical officer of the Confederate forces, evacuated the sick and wounded on July 18, proceeding toward Macon. His little family and servants were transported by private conveyance in advance of the hospital corps.

Mrs. Westmoreland was in daily expectation of confinement. The expedition reached Milner on the morning of July 22, and at sundown on that historic day the soldier husband officiated at the birth of his only son.

Distraught, but unafraid, in those long hours of anxiety, he knew that the Battle of Atlanta was raging and that in a few hours his every earthly possession and this beautiful city would be reduced to ashes.

Young Westmoreland was educated in the schools of Atlanta, the Kirkwood Military Academy and Georgetown University. He graduated in medicine at the Atlanta Medical College in 1885. The breadth of medical education in that era was exemplified by this father's insistence that two years should be spent as a graduate student in the offices of the leading medical and surgical men of the nation.

His first six months were with Dr. J. Solis Cohen of Philadelphia, the leading throat specialist of his day. Then to New York with Janeway and Loomis in medicine. His second year was in the marvelous general surgical environment of Dr. Henry B. Sands and Dr. Wm. T. Bull, accompanying them daily at the Roosevelt and New York Hospitals. Finally he was a house guest and assistant to Dr. Lewis A. Sayre and his distinguished son, the late Dr. Reginald H. Sayre.

The Sayres were the leading orthopedic surgeons of that period. This branch of surgery had a special appeal to Dr. Westmoreland and for many years he stood alone in this section in the practice of orthopedics in connection with his general surgical work.

It is felt that this detailed narration of Dr. Westmoreland's thorough and unusual medical education is appropriate, as only a small circle of his intimate friends, at this time, are acquainted with this phase of his career.

Following the death of his father in 1890, he was elected to succeed him as the Professor of the Principles and Practice of Surgery in the Atlanta Medical College.

At the age of twenty-six years he assumed the responsibility of this honorable promotion and for twenty-five years maintained with dignity and brilliancy all the traditions of a great family of physicians and surgeons. In 1915 he retired from active teaching and was appointed Emeritus Professor of Surgery in his Alma Mater.

In chronicling the achievements of an outstanding surgeon and teacher his success is measured by the ability to impress and inspire his students in the ideals of the art and science of surgery and of the observance of the high principles of conduct obtaining amongst his confreres.

There was no need of his subscribing to the oath of Hippocrates, nor the necessity of following written rules governing and guiding his sense of professional fairness and honesty. His scrupulous respect for the opinion of all medical men and his unswerving defense of them, whether prominent or obscure, endeared him to them in a manner impossible for the written word to describe.

His enthusiasm for everything pertaining to medicine was an inspiration to all of us and in the development of medical education and medical organization his talents were unexcelled. In medical politics he was a fair but relentless opponent and in defeat was as generous and magnanimous as in the full enjoyment of victory.

Dr. Westmoreland was an idealist in the practice of his profession. Never a moment in his life was given to the thought of making money. To him money was a fleeting thing to be used only as a means of giving happiness to his friends, and to hold the ever open hand to the sick and afflicted poor.

It may safely be said for him that surgery was indeed the Queen of the Arts.

Therefore, be it resolved that the sympathy of the Fulton County Medical Society is extended to his family, and that a copy of this resolution be forwarded them and a copy be spread upon the minutes of this Society.

E. D. HIGHSMITH, M.D.
J. CALVIN WEAVER, M.D.
W. S. GOLDSMITH, M.D., *Chairman.*
Resolution Committee.

"STONE WALLS DO NOT A PRISON MAKE NOR IRON BARS A CAGE"

Winter is a jailer who shuts us all in from the fullest vitamin D value of sunlight. The baby becomes virtually a prisoner, in several senses: First of all, meterologic observations prove that winter sunshine in most sections of the country averages 10 to 50 per cent less than summer sunshine. Secondly, the quality of the available sunshine is inferior due to the shorter distance of the sun from the earth altering the angle of the sun's rays. Again, the hour of the day has an important bearing: At 8:30 A.M. there is an average loss of over 31 per cent, and at 3:30 P.M., over 21 per cent.

bordered with flowering oleanders. and for many miles running through pine forests and broad expanses of the beautiful marshes of the Coastal regions.

Everything combines to make this beach the most prominent and unrivalled seashore resort on the South Atlantic. Five miles of splendid beach swept at all times by cool refreshing and health retaining breezes, entices thousands of bathers daily. Nowhere on the Atlantic Coast has nature bestowed more favors than Savannah Beach. affording an almost ceaseless enjoyment of the ocean. From early spring until late fall the water is of an even temperature, and bathing is excellent. Health and happiness abound here.

The beach is only thirty minutes drive from Savannah and to the pleasure loving visitor or permanent homeseeker offers every advantage. The health of Savannah Beach is not surpassed by that of any resort. The resort abounds with an abundant supply of artesian water, tested monthly by the State Board of Health, and its drainage and general conditions are under the direct supervision of the health officer of Savannah.

Pleasures of every type are enjoyed at Savannah Beach. In addition to the surf bathing there is still-water bathing for those who prefer it. Boating and fishing is excellent. One of the largest pavilions on the Atlantic Coast affords dancing day and night with music furnished by orchestras of national reputation. There are many other pavilions of every type with most modern and excellently kept bath houses. A magnificent board walk and amusements of all types greet the visitor. The hotels and boarding houses furnish good accommodations, at reasonable cost. The entire island is well lighted by electricity, and ample police protection is furnished throughout the year.

Two of the South's most attractive golf courses, with a length of 6,135 yards, are only fifteen minutes ride from the beach. These courses, with their wonderful fairways and grass putting greens, have won the praises of famous golfers from all parts of the country, The green fee is $1.00 per day on one course and 50 cents on the other.

Savannah Beach is adjacent to one of the South's most beautiful, historic and charming cities, which has become known as one of the country's greatest and most popular all year round resorts.

For rail fares to Savannah inquire of any Central of Georgia Railway Agent.

CALCIFICATION OF AORTIC VALVE

In a Negro, aged 37, with a long history of cardiac pain and a relatively short history of congestive heart failure, L. Minor Blackford, William W. Bryan and Emory D. Hollar, Atlanta, Ga. (*Journal A. M. A.,* July 4, 1936), made the diagnosis of calcification of the aortic valve during life. They state that Osler first divided calcification of the aortic valve into "those with and without arteriosclerosis." In their case arteriosclerosis as singularly lacking in the retinal and coronary arteries, and in the aorta. From the history and microscopic studies they feel justified in saying that it belongs to the group Osler described as of rheumatic origin. They have diagnosed but one other case of calcification of the aortic valve, and this was in a man of 59 who is still living: it was typical of the more common type. A calcified aortic valve is a matter of importance in differential diagnosis because in the South as soon as an aortic diastolic murmur is detected, particularly in a Negro, a diagnosis of syphilitic aortic insufficiency is apt to be made. One of the authors has studied more than 140 cases of the syphilitic type of valvular involvement but has not heard such a harsh murmur in any of them. nor has the occasional aortic thrill (noted by Corrigan) even been so intense. The electrocardiograms gave evidence of severe myocardial damage and a serious prognosis: the "T-1 and S-2 combination" remarked on by Proger and Minnich, the bundle branch block and the increase in the PR interval. It has often been said that the Negro is not subject to angina pectoris. Aside from the frequency of retrosternal pain in syphilitic cases, the authors have noted cardiac pain in a number of cases of hypertension and arteriosclerosis, and in one case of biventricular aorta with pulmonic stenosis. They have also seen several cases of angina in rheumatic heart disease, although rheumatic heart disease is not common in Atlanta. This patient suffered from classic angina pectoris.

Stewart-Webster Counties Medical Society

The Stewart-Webster Counties Medical Society announces the following officers for 1936:

President—C. E. Pickett, Richland.
Secretary-Treasurer—A. R. Sims. Richland.
Delegate—C. S. Lynch, Lumpkin.
Alternate Delegate—J. M. Kenyon, Richland.

The American Medical Association will hold its eighty-eighth annual session in Atlantic City in 1937.

DIARRHEA

"the commonest ailment of infants in the summer months"

(HOLT AND McINTOSH: HOLT'S DISEASES OF INFANCY AND CHILDHOOD, 1933)

One of the outstanding features of DEXTRI-MALTOSE is that it is almost unanimously preferred as the carbohydrate in the management of infantile diarrhea.

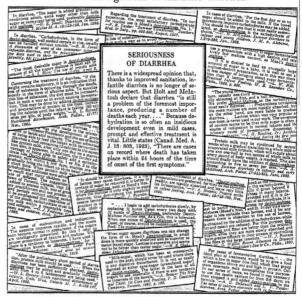

SERIOUSNESS OF DIARRHEA

There is a widespread opinion that, thanks to improved sanitation, infantile diarrhea is no longer of serious aspect. But Holt and McIntosh declare that diarrhea "is still a problem of the foremost importance, producing a number of deaths each year. . . ." Because dehydration is so often an insidious development even in mild cases, prompt and effective treatment is vital. Little states (Canad. Med. A. J. 13: 803, 1923), "There are cases on record where death has taken place within 24 hours of the time of onset of the first symptoms."

THE JOURNAL
OF THE
MEDICAL ASSOCIATION OF GEORGIA
DEVOTED TO THE WELFARE OF THE MEDICAL ASSOCIATION OF GEORGIA
PUBLISHED MONTHLY under direction of the Council

| Volume XXV | Atlanta, Ga., August, 1936 | Number 8 |

A YARDSTICK TO MEASURE ARTIFICIAL FEEDINGS FOR INFANTS†*

WM. A. MULHERIN, M.D.

Augusta

I shall endeavor to simplify in a practical manner our present knowledge of the artificial feeding of infants. In this age of intensive propaganda and exploitation of half-baked medical truths by some of the unethical pharmaceutical houses, it is well to establish a yardstick by which we can evaluate the merits and demerits of the various methods of infant feeding. With such a procedure faulty feedings can be detected and corrected.

Yardstick

There are four fundamental requisites that every correct infant feeding should possess. They are:

1. Sufficient Calories—enough of food units in the formula on which the baby can thrive.
2. Sufficient Proteins—carbohydrates, fats, mineral salts, water and vitamins A, B, C, D and G to permit normal growth and development of the baby.
3. The formula shall not contain a sufficient amount of pathogenic bacteria to make the baby ill (the best safeguard against this occurrence is to boil clean fresh cow's milk 3 to 5 minutes).
4. The food must be digestible, in amounts sufficient for normal growth and development.

Requisite No. 1

Calories—The usual number of calories needed during the first year of life for the

†From the Department of Pediatrics, University of Georgia School of Medicine, Augusta.
*Read before the Medical Association of Georgia, Savannah, April 22, 1936.

normal infant are: 50 to 55 calories per pound of body weight per day (110 to 115 calories per kilogram). During the first three months the caloric requirement is a little greater than this, and after six months is somewhat less. Calculations of calories for the undernourished, or overnourished, infant should be based on the expected weight for the age. *The caloric requirements of the breast fed baby is met when approximately 2.5 to 3 ounces of breast milk per pound of weight per day are given the baby. In the artificially fed infant it is advisable that about two-thirds of the total caloric requirements be met by milk and one-third by added carbohydrates.*

To calculate the number of calories in a formula is quite simple. In the average milk formula for babies three ingredients are usually used—milk, sugar and water. The milk and sugar have food values; the water none. The caloric value of average strength cow's milk is 20 calories for each ounce. The caloric value of evaporated unsweetened, unskimmed cow's milk is 44 calories for each ounce. One level tablespoon of Karo syrup (corn sugar) contains approximately 60 calories. Granulated sugar (cane sugar) has the same caloric value as Karo syrup, 60 calories for each level tablespoonful. Dextri Maltose, or sugar of milk (lactose) has 40 calories for each level tablespoonful.

Now if a formula contains 21 ounces of whole cow's milk, 9 ounces of boiled water and cane sugar 4 level tablespoonfuls, its caloric contents would be:

21 ounces of cow's milk x 20 calories per ounce	= 420 calories
4 level tablespoonfuls cane sugar x 60 calories per tablespoonful	= 240 calories
Total calories in mixture	660 calories

If this formula were given to a 3 months' old baby weighing 12 pounds, giving six feedings of 5 ounces in each bottle, the number of calories per pound weight, in 24 hours, may be easily obtained by dividing the total number of calories in food, which is 660, by the weight of the baby (12 pounds) which would be 55 calories per pound weight of the baby for each 24 hours.

Requisite No. 2

Protein—The most important ingredient in the formula is the protein. It causes cell proliferation, such as tissue and muscle growth; also multiplication and generation of blood cells. *When 2.5 ounces of breast milk per pound of baby weight are given to the baby in 24 hours, the protein requirement of the baby is adequate.* This corresponds to approximately 2 grams of protein per kilogram in the breast fed, and 3.5 grams per kilogram in the artificially fed infant. *As far as we know a moderate excess of protein does no harm. In the undernourished infant the amount of protein given should be proportionate to the expected rather than the actual baby weight.*

Carbohydrates—The physiologic purpose of carbohydrates in nutrition is to furnish heat and energy to the baby. There are two kinds of carbohydrates: soluble (sugars) and insoluble (starches). *An infant should receive not less than 1 per cent of his body weight in carbohydrates per day* (0.15 ounces per pound or 10 grams per kilogram). *This amount is received by the breast fed baby in breast milk. In the artificially fed baby it is well to have one-third of the carbohydrates furnished by cow's milk and the remainder from sugar or starch.* Roughly calculated, the proportion of carbohydrates added to the formula of cow's milk should be approximately one part of carbohydrates for each 10 to 15 parts of milk.

Sugars of the dextrin and maltose type, also cane sugar and milk sugar, are to be preferred in early infancy. After the fifth or sixth month a part of the carbohydrate given should be in the form of starch.

Fats—Fats are somewhat interchangeable with carbohydrates and are a valuable source of energy. *Unless a reasonable amount of fats is included in the formula, excessive amounts*

or Karo syrup. As we apply our yardstick to this formula we find it measures up to No. 1 requirement: it contains enough calories. It contains in sufficient amounts all the necessary ingredients required for normal growth and development, except vitamin C, which is killed by boiling the milk, and which is usually supplied by giving the baby sufficient amounts of orange or tomato juices, therefore it measures up to requisite No. 2 when orange juice is given the baby. The milk has been boiled, for 3 minutes, thereby preventing trouble from pathogenic organisms, and therefore meets requisite No. 3. The formula is well-balanced and will likely be digested by the baby and will make the baby gain in weight the expected weekly amount, therefore requisite No. 4 would be satisfied. Of course, No. 4 can not be definitely calculated, like requisites Nos. 1, 2 and 3, but has to be determined by observing the results of weekly gains in weight and noting if the physical development of the baby is normal. Formulas made from unsweetened evaporated cow's milk, with a ratio of one part of the milk to 2 parts of boiled water, or equal parts of the milk and water with 2 to 4 level tablespoonfuls of cane sugar, or Karo, to the pint or quart, would meet the yardstick requirements. The same might be said of whole lactic acid milk, made with milk boiled 3 to 5 minutes and then cooled, with the same ratio of sugar added as in the two preceding formulas.

Now, when we apply the yardstick to a formula made with sweetened, condensed milk, it is found that No. 2 requisite is not complied with, for the reason that when the heavily sweetened, condensed milk is diluted with boiled water, sufficiently to cover caloric requirements and to make the milk digestible and palatable, the protein and fat in the formula are reduced to the point where they are deficient for normal growth and development. Therefore the formula is a poor baby food, even though it measures up to requirements Nos. 1 and 3, and frequently to No. 4.

Normal Expectations in Physical Development

To properly evaluate the merits or demerits of an artificial infant feeding it is necessary that elementary knowledge be possessed

of the normal physical and mental development of infants; for if the normal is not
known the abnormal can not be recognized.
It is necessary to know that a baby usually
doubles his weight at 5 months and triples
his birth weight at 1 year of age. After the
initial loss of about 10 ounces in the first
two or three days of life, the baby should
regain his lost weight when 10 days to 2
weeks of age. From 2 weeks of age to 5
months, the baby should gain 4 to 8 ounces
a week and from 5 months to 9 months, 3
to 6 ounces a week is a natural expectation.
From 9 months to 1 year, 2 to 4 ounces a
week is a normal gain in weight.

During the second year of life a baby's
total gain in weight should be 6 pounds,
which means a half pound a month or, approximately 2 ounces per week. During the
third year 5 pounds is a normal gain. From
the end of the third year to 8 years of age
a child is expected to gain only 4 pounds a
year.

Other normal physical developments are:
the baby should hold up its head at 3 months;
sit alone at 7 or 8 months; stand holding to
a chair at 10 months; walk, holding to
mother's hand, at 12 months; and step out
by itself at 14 to 15 months. It will awkwardly reach for a toy at about 4 months,
and recognize its mother at about 5 months.
A baby will say "mama" and "papa" and use
other monosyllables at about 1 year. At 2
years of age short sentences can usually be
spoken.

With knowledge of these fundamental
facts regarding the normal physical and mental development of babies, and the practical
application of the proposed yardstick to our
present and future methods of infant feeding,
I feel that the profession will be able to feed
babies and children in a more intelligent and
successful manner, thereby contributing materially to the production of a stronger,
healthier, happier and more representative
race.

Discussion on Paper of Dr. Wm. A. Mulherin

DR. BENJAMIN BASHINSKI (Macon): There is
one thing Dr. Mulherin did not mention. That is
the concentration. I remember several years ago we
had an idea that we must feed all babies with percentage feeding. As you know at the present time,
babies two months of age or one month or three

milk. At the same time we will unquestionably be aiding the allergic infant who oftentimes has trouble with the proteins of cow's milk.

I also feel that the fats in evaporated milk are more readily tolerated and enable us to feed a formula with a more uniform fat content.

The type of added carbohydrates and the amount used, I think, depend largely upon the individual infant.

I would further emphasize the addition of Vitamins A, B, and C to every infant's diet.

DR. M. A. EHRLICH (Bainbridge): In Dr. Mulherin's paper he gave you a yardstick for infant feeding. There are two points in my feeding that I add to his yardstick. First, is the child good or is the child bad? A well-fed child is ordinarily a good child, and if you have a bad child, you know that you are not feeding your child properly.

The second thing that I add is: Later, during the second, third, fourth and fifth years of life, is that child healthy? If you feed your children in the first year and get big, fat, fine babies that all the mothers want, so much for the mothers. But in the second, third and fourth years if your children are sickly, do not respond to ordinary external stimuli as they should, do not learn properly, and do not control their emotions and their activity properly, look back upon your infant feeding and you will realize that you have fed that child incorrectly.

One of the discussors mentioned evaporated milk in infant feeding, and that digestion, as I understood him to say or mean, was the keynote of allergy. Digestion is not and never will be and never has been the keynote of an allergic child. They may be allergic at times from digestion, only when they are over-fed and cannot take care of the amounts that are given to them, but if you have a child in which the most minute quantities of a food cause an allergic reaction, as one that I have tested allergically, in which the egg-white on zwieback toast gives and has given an eczema, you know that the digestion is not the whole sheet anchor to an allergic child.

DR. JOSEPH YAMPOLSKY (Atlanta): I believe that in order to develop successful feeding we must call attention to the fact that the doctor must be as well educated as the public in the problem of feeding.

We must again re-educate the mothers that breast feeding is an old time custom and is not as bad as is thought to be by some of them. There is enough breast milk left in Georgia to raise every baby born in this State. So much time has been spent on having the doctor learn formulas on how to use different forms of raw milk, dry milk and evaporated milk, that as a result of this the practitioner has become somewhat befuddled.

We must teach them again the chemistry of breast milk and cow's milk in order that they may know the effects of it on the child's digestion. Most of the doctors still feed babies although many of them do not claim to be child specialists. It is to those doctors that we must bring a message which is simple in its form,—first, let us advise them to use breast milk

whenever possible and when that can not be done
then they can follow the simple yardstick outlined.

DR. WARREN QUILLIAN (Miami, Florida): The
experience in Florida and South Florida is certainly
similar to that in North Georgia, in respect to infant
feeding. We find confusion generally in respect to
modification of milk, elaboration of formulas of various kinds, and we find that the average mother comes
to her bed of confinement with a preconceived idea
that she must employ someone to prepare a formula
for her baby. On two occasions already this week
there have been mothers who have informed me when
I first was taken into the room that they wanted the
baby fed in other ways rather than breast-fed.

This formula that has been stressed this afternoon,
(evaporated milk in infant feeding) is certainly a
practical one: it is simple; it combines all the advantages of simplicity, safety, freedom from bacteria,
and for that reason it is valuable for general usage.

There is one other phase that I should like to
stress about evaporated milk feeding that we have found
in clinical cases in staff hospitals. The average staff
patient is unable to afford refrigeration after going
home. They are also unable to purchase these elaborate
formulas that are prepared. As a result of that, a
certain stock formula is frequently supplied to those
mothers upon their leaving the hospital, and this is
carried out during the early months of the infant's
life. We have prepared some figures on that and have
a few slides to show tomorrow that may be of general
interest concerning the results obtained in the feeding
of evaporated milk formulas to normal infants born
on the general staff service.

DR. WILLIAM A. MULHERIN (Augusta): I appreciate the generous discussion given my paper, and
wish to thank the physicians who were kind enough
to enter the discussion. I am sorry the title of my
paper was not perfectly understood, for the paper deals
with artificial infant feeding, and not infant feeding.
However, I am glad that Drs. Yampolsky and Quillian
stressed the importance of breast feeding. We all know
that it is the best form of infant feeding, and as
shown by Grulee of Chicago, in his analysis of some
20,000 cases of infants, some artificially fed and some
breast fed, there was a very decided increase in infant
mortality in the artificially fed baby, when compared
to the breast fed ones. Also, I would like to keep the
record straight by mentioning the fact that the yardstick referred to in my paper is intended for the average normal baby, not the allergic, fat, intolerant, difficult feeding cases. These are special cases and differ
from the average normal baby. My paper was not intended to deal with these types of different babies.

The same remarks might be applied to the children
mentioned by one of the physicians discussing my
paper, namely, the negative calcium balance child. This
type of child, as you know, will eliminate as much
calcium salts as you put in its body, therefore this
type of child requires special study, and differs from a
normal average child. In these cases, sun baths,
furnishing plenty ultraviolet rays, and cod liver oil.

condition. Because one blows some secretion from his nose, or has some dripping into the nasopharynx, by no means signifies that this individual is a sufferer from the unfortunate word catarrh. Various pathologic lesions in the nasal cavities will produce these symptoms, but when the word catarrh is used it signifies, in the minds of most people, a foul smelling discharge which only occurs in a very limited number of cases. Let us avoid this word and speak of nasal conditions more from the symptomatic and clinical significance than with the euphonious word *catarrh*.

In my forty-two years of practice, the management of nasal diseases has made but few changes and these mostly from a conservative standpoint and in the refinement of surgical technic.

The Septum

In the beginning of my rhinolaryngologic practice, there was a great furor as to the best method of straightening the nasal septum. That this septum played a prominent part in the ventilation of the sinuses and middle ear is well recognized. Just when a nasal septum needs to be operated upon is by no means a settled question, especially in the attempt to make this organ conform to anatomic perfection.

For many years septum deviations were corrected by cutting through the cartilaginous portion of this organ, straightening the then movable parts of the septum with forceps and the insertion of nasal splints to hold the parts in position. Later, Morris Asch devised a cutting forcep to accomplish the same purpose and for many years, after 1892, this was a well recognized procedure. All of these operations were only applicable to the anterior cartilaginous portion of the septum and had no effect upon the posterior bony part of the same structure. For this latter reason, there was developed the so-called submucous resection operation and which was brought to an almost perfect surgical technic by my old friend, Otto Freer of Chicago. This now constitutes the recognized operation for this condition with modification in its technic.

Some twenty-five years ago, the submucous resection operation was frequently performed for the most trivial deviation. When necessary, the results of this operation have proven most beneficial to patients. But the cases must be carefully selected. Time and experience have taught us that slight deviations should not be subjected to this operation, as the final results are sometimes more annoying to patients than the original deviation. I know of no operation in rhinolaryngology which requires more dexterity in its performance.

The Turbinate Bodies

As we all know, the turbinates play an important role in the comfort of the patient by warming and moistening the atmosphere we breathe and by giving us a freedom of air ventilation when they are not enlarged or congested. In the early years of my practice, there was a great enthusiasm for removing the inferior turbinate whenever there was marked stenosis of the nasal cavity. This was especially the case before the introduction of the submucous operation on the septum. An instrument known as the spoke-shave was used, which was nothing more than a ring curet with the cutting edge on the inside, by which the posterior end of the turbinate could be engaged, and with a forward pull the turbinate could be entirely removed. Scissors and biting forceps were later substituted for the spoke-shave so that the amount removed could be limited. Later, however, it was discovered that while the patient would have decidedly more air space, there was a marked feeling of discomfort due to the scabby condition at the seat of operation and also due to the fact that the inspired air lacked the warmth and moisture engendered by the erectile tissue of the turbinates. Hence partial removal in selected cases superseded these radical procedures. The removal, however, of the middle turbinate is a well recognized procedure when there is a blocking of the ethmoidal cells and frontal sinus.

Allergy

In the early years of my practice, nothing was known of that systemic condition denominated as allergy. In following these cases of nasal stenosis, I was convinced in my own mind that there was some obscure systemic condition which existed at the bottom of these nasal symptoms. Toxic condition was a term frequently used, but even then, this term did not signify the importance which exists today. We know now that these turbinates, in fact the whole lining membrane of the nasal cavities, may be greatly swollen through this mysterious allergic reaction peculiar to the individual. Hence it is entirely unsurgical in many of these cases to remove or operate upon the turbinates when this condition can be remedied by more conservative measures. In fact, much of our nasal pathology has been found to be closely related to allergic reactions, and for this reason, surgical operations are much less frequent today than they were twenty years ago.

Nasal Sinus Disease

The word sinus disease has almost reached the stage of obsession. The public has become so imbued with the prevalence and importance of nasal sinus disease, that a sensation of fear passes through these individuals whenever there is a pain about the head. The importance of this condition must not be underestimated, but the fact must be borne in mind that a diagnosis of nasal sinusitis is not always easy to make. Too many rhinolaryngologists depend upon the x-ray as a final criterion. That this diagnostic procedure is a distinct aid in some cases, must be admitted by every rhinolaryngologist, but that such is absolute in its findings, would lead many of us into error.

Dr. Shambaugh, of Chicago, in a recent comment, has expressed very forcibly the ideas of the majority of men who have had a large clinical experience. I shall take the liberty of quoting him, verbatim. "Roentgenograms properly made are a valuable adjunct in the diagnosis of sinus disease. It does not occupy the all-important position in making a diagnosis, however. In the first place, using any technic does not assure satisfactory results. Most of the skiagraphs brought in by patients are unsatisfactory and are not an aid in making diagnosis. Certain of the sinuses lend themselves more readily to skiagraphy than do others. The rhinologists gets important assistance in skiagraphs of the frontal sinuses. They give one the size and the depth, important facts to have in mind if one is contemplating operative interference; also skiagraphs of the frontal sinuses give one very definite data regarding the contents of the sinuses. The same holds true to the maxillaries. Skiagraphy of the ethmoids and of the sphenoid sinuses is much less definite than of the frontal and maxillary sinuses and in the case of the ethmoid and sphenoid sinuses, a much more accurate conclusion can be obtained by other methods. The surgeon who relies for his diagnosis entirely upon skiagraphy is going to meet with a great deal of grief if he undertakes surgical relief."

In other words, experience and clinical observation are much more reliable than x-ray plates. The frequency of sending patients to the roentgenologist for a final diagnosis of sinus involvement, is certainly not always necessary in the light of the uncertainty of these skiagraphs.

What has been said above in reference to nasal sinuses, is equally applicable to skiagraphs of the mastoid. I consider that skiagraphs of the mastoid are usually unnecessary in making a diagnosis of mastoid involvement. Any middle ear which has had a purulent discharge for over two weeks, with severe pain and some rise in temperature and with practically no diminution in the discharge in acute cases, or for years in chronic cases, will always show an involvement of the mastoid. Consequently, x-ray plates only show us what our clinical knowledge has already demonstrated. The question of operation in such cases must depend upon other clinical symptoms and not upon the x-ray. If all mastoids were operated upon because the skiagraphs showed them to be involved, the otologist would be operating upon nearly every case of middle ear involvement. The younger men in our profession should not be taught to put too much confidence in x-ray plates. Just at this point, I wish to call attention to the prevalence in the consultation room of patients who frequently imagine that they are suffering from some mastoid disease. Most frequently pain around the ear is referable either to some acute tonsillar infection or more often as a reflex from bad teeth. If people could be taught that mastoid disease never occurs unless there has been a previous discharge from the middle ear, there would be less fear about these occasional pains.

The question of sinus disease as the focal point of infection for many systemic diseases will always need careful consideration. As a causative factor, sinus involvement can not be placed in the same category as the tonsils, teeth, gallbladder and prostate gland. The absorption of infected material through the lymphatic drainage depends upon its close relationship to the parts involved. The fact that the submaxillary glands enlarge when the tonsils and teeth are infected, shows how easy it is for the infection to travel along the lymphatics. In sinus involvement, there is no close relationship and my experience does not justify me in regarding these parts as a causative factor in so-called focal infection in but a limited number of cases.

Lymphoid Tissue in the Pharynx and Nasopharynx

This subject resolves itself into a discussion of adenoids, faucial and lingual tonsils. It is a subject for unlimited discussion and I shall only give some of my clinical observations on certain points which have been rarely considered. The final word has not yet been spoken in reference to the medical and surgical treatment of these lymphoid structures. I have been firmly convinced for many years of the importance of this tissue in its relationship to the human economy. I am also convinced that a more thorough preliminary and after treatment of these cases should be made before the operative removal of this tissue. My experience shows me that there is a close relationship between this lymphoid tissue and the functional activity of the endocrines.

Whether or not the tonsil is an endocrine organ is a question which has not as yet been answered with certainty. Peller of Vienna, in the Monatschr. f. Ohrenh. 1934, is firmly convinced after a thorough study of 3,200 cases, that the question can be absolutely answered in the affirmative. Physicians and patients often wonder why, after a supposedly thorough removal of tonsils and adenoids, in a few years there is a return of this same tissue in the back part of the pharynx and even frequently extending into the nasopharynx. This occurs in the practice of the most skilled operators. Years ago, I had a patient whose tonsils had been removed three times. This of course is an exceptional case, but such actually occurred. All laryngologists are familiar with the experience of having patients develop a large amount of lymphoid tissue in the pharynx after the removal of tonsils. Compensation in the human body is a well recognized fact. If one is completely blind, there is a compensatory development in his hearing and tactile sense. If he is deaf, there is a compensatory development in his eyes, as for instance, in lip reading, and so it is true in other portions of the body. For instance, Dr. Abel, of John Hopkins University, has shown that when one adrenal gland is removed, there is a compensatory enlargement of the other gland. The inter-relationship of the hormones of the various endocrine bodies is now a well recognized fact. So that when the tonsils have been removed, there is a compensatory development in the form of islands of lymphoid tissue in the pharynx and especially along its lateral walls. Consequently, many patients have almost as much trouble after the removal of tonsils as they did before, but with a different kind of inflammatory process.

Such individuals are apt to suffer with a nasopharyngitis or a laryngitis, having been deprived of the protection afforded by the tonsils. I believe that much of this complication could be avoided if the patients are thoroughly iodinized before and after the operation. The treatment of this condition, when it does occur besides the administration of iodine, often finds its relief in x-ray therapy. Some years ago, this treatment was advised for the reduction of large tonsils, but this latter method has been largely abandoned. In compensatory outgrowths of lymphoid tissue in the pharynx and nasopharynx, after tonsillectomy and adenoidectomy, this treatment by x-ray has been reported by many rhinologists as giving most excellent results. In addition to this, I think it very advisable for some endocrine test to be made before the removal of tonsils in children, as it has been repeatedly shown that there is a close relationship between the thyroid glands and this lymphoid tissue in the throat. The removal of tonsils have too often been considered a simple operation, but the after results have not been duly considered. There are many other conditions in the field of rhinolaryngology which the writer would like to consider and in this way call your attention to the fallacy of routine treatment.

that way. After thirty days had gone by and I had not heard from him, I asked, "Where are those deaf women you were going to bring here?" He said, "I declare to de Lawd, Doctor, I can't find a deaf negro woman in this town."

DR. DUNBAR ROY (Atlanta) : The points which I have tried to bring before you have been the things which have accumulated in my experience for the last forty-four years. And I have long ago determined that it is experience in medicine in the long run that enables one to discern and to tell the difference between various conditions of the human body. You can not find them in textbooks; you can not find them in writings, but it is a practical intuitive knowledge which you get by long and continued experience.

So that the whole intent of this paper was to give you the conclusions of my own experience along this line and to try, if possible, to make the internist and the specialist come closer together so that one can be benefited by the other.

HONOR ROLL FOR 1936

1. Randolph County, Dr. W. G. Elliott, Cuthbert, October 30, 1935.
2. Dougherty County, Dr. I. M. Lucas, Albany, December 27, 1935.
3. Monroe County, Dr. G. H. Alexander, Forsyth, February 14, 1936.
4. Hancock County, Dr. H. L. Earl, Sparta, February 25, 1936.
5. Elbert County, Dr. A. S. Johnson, Elberton, March 6, 1936.
6. Worth County, Dr. G. S. Sumner, Sylvester, March 12, 1936.
7. Rockdale County, Dr. H. E. Griggs, Conyers, March 21, 1936.
8. Morgan County, Dr. W. C. McGeary, Madison. March 30, 1936.
9. Turner County, Dr. J. H. Baxter, Ashburn, March 30, 1936.
10. Ware County, Dr. Kenneth McCullough, Waycross, March 30, 1936.
11. Georgia Medical Society· (Chatham County), Dr. Otto W. Schwalb, Savannah, April 17, 1936.

R. H. Jaffe, Chicago (*Journal A. M. A.*, July 11, 1936), asserts that the improvement in the technic of biopsies of the bone marrow has added a valuable method to the diagnostic laboratory procedures to which the clinician can resort in the cases in which the examination of the peripheral blood fails to give definite information. The importance of the examination of the bone marrow in vivo becomes evident if one considers the fact that the circulating blood does not always reflect the condition of the bone marrow. Great differences exist sometimes between the cellular content of the blood and that of the bone marrow which may be the source of diagnostic errors. Since the biopsy of the bone marrow is expected to become widely used in clinical medicine, he presents a brief discussion of the normal bone marrow and of the changes that are observed in some of the important disturbances of blood formation.

PRIMARY BRONCHIAL CANCER AND THE DIFFICULTY IN EARLY DIAGNOSIS*

Case Report

STEWART R. ROBERTS, M.D.
Atlanta

J. DEWEY GRAY, M.D.
Augusta

This case is worthy of attention because of the difficulty in making a diagnosis. Only a few of the usual clinical features of primary bronchiogenic carcinoma were present in this case and the unusual symptoms deserve emphasis. The differential diagnosis between pulmonary tuberculosis with pleurisy and effusion and primary bronchiogenic carcinoma may at times be very difficult.

Report of Case

A white woman was admitted to the Emory University Hospital Jan. 12, 1935. Her illness definitely began in September, 1934. At this time she had an attack of pain beginning in the back and extending around the seventh rib on each side almost to the anterior axillary line. The pain was more severe on the right side. On Oct. 8, 1934, the patient experienced severe muscular pains in muscles parallel to the vertebral column and low in lumbar region. Again the pain was severe and bilateral. This lasted several days and disappeared, and was followed by some residual muscular soreness. There were no shooting pains and no paresthesia or anesthesia of the skin. Most of pain was at the level of floating ribs. On Oct. 18, the patient had another attack of pain in back in same region and as high as the right shoulder; and some pain around as far as abdominal wall. The pain was bilateral. Again there was residual soreness. On Nov. 12, she had the most severe of all attacks. Pain was severe and there was spasm of muscles all along the vertebral column on both sides, with radiation to the hips. She was in bed eleven days, during which time morphine was required. This would relieve the pain but would not relax the muscle spasm. On Nov. 7, she had an attack of pain in right upper chest, anteriorly and posteriorly. At this time the pain began as a burning sensation, increasing in intensity in the right side of chest anteriorly, and finally passing to back in dorsal area, and down in lumbar region, and then into hips. The attacks persisted but with less frequency. She was usually comfortable between attacks.

Examination showed a well developed and fairly well nourished woman of 45 in semi-recumbent position in no respiratory distress. Eyes, ears, nose and throat were normal. Thorax: There was a definite

*Read before the Medical Association of Georgia, Savannah, April 22, 1936.

point of tenderness in the paravertebral muscles to the right of midline about 4 cm. at level of axillary fold. Also another point of tenderness over the first and second lumbar vertebrae. Kronig's isthmus on the right equal 7.3 cm.; on the left 9.5 cm. P. N.: Hyper-resonant over entire left chest. Excursion left base, 4.2 cm., right 4 cm. There is a slight increase in the cardiac dulness to the left. The left axilla is normal. Posteriorly from the spine to a line from the lower 1/3 clavicular line, resonance is present; then rather abruptly the note changes to extreme dulness to flatness. This extends around the axilla anteriorly from the base to axilla and upward to the second rib anteriorly. The dulness here is continuous with the cardiac dulness. Breath sounds over the resonant area are distant but audible. Over the dull and flat area breath sounds are practically absent.

No rales are heard except on very deep inspiration. No bronchial breathing except over the anterior thorax and rather close to the mid-line. No amphoric breathing anywhere. Whispered voice on right 2 plus. over apex. and barely heard over flat area. Spoken voice: left base increased, right greatly diminished.

Heart: Sounds good. Rate 80. No murmurs. Rhythm regular.

Pelvis: Normal except old transverse tear of cervix. Rectum normal.

Blood Count

White Blood Count	6,950
Red Blood Count	4,820,000
Hemoglobin	73 per cent
Myelocytes	2 per cent
Juveniles	3 per cent
Bands	21 per cent
Segmenters	57 per cent
Lymphocytes	13 per cent
Monocytes	1 per cent
Basophiles	2 per cent
Eosinophiles	1 per cent

Kahn on blood negative.

Tuberculin test (intracutaneous) strongly positive.

X-ray films taken at this time show fluid on right side almost to apex; also an infiltrative mass that seems to arise from the hilus region. Films made at a previous examination suggest a malignant lesion more than tuberculosis.

Bronchoscopic examination: There was no growth in the tracheobronchial tree as far as could be seen. There was evidence of pressure on the carina from without. The bifurcation was rounded instead of sharp.

On Jan. 21, 1935, thoracentesis was done. About 500 cc. of fluid was removed. The fluid clotted very quickly and there was some pellicle formation. Specific gravity, 1,017. A guinea pig was injected and, after six weeks, an autopsy showed no evidence of tuberculosis. There were no mitotic figures found.

She was in the hospital about one month during which time there was never any fever. It was not possible to be absolutely sure of the diagnosis but it was felt that the diagnosis was either tuberculosis or pulmonary neoplasm. It was thought wise to replace the fluid with air. Thorascentesis was done several times followed by pneumothorax. Never was the fluid bloody

and each time it clotted very quickly. It was decided that she should continue the same treatment in Augusta.

There was no improvement in her condition after withdrawing the fluid and replacing it with air. On March 21, 1935, it was decided to take more pictures and it was now possible to make a positive diagnosis of a neoplasm of lung. Fluid removed about this time was examined by Dr. Greenblatt at the Medical School in Augusta and mitotic figures were found. There was not any fever from the time she was dismissed from the hospital. The attacks of pain persisted but were less severe. On April 29, 1935, the red blood cells had dropped to 3,240,000, hemoglobin, 70 per cent.

On May 28, 1935, she was seized by a rather sudden severe dyspnea. There was marked cyanosis. Oxygen was administered but she died May 29th, 1935.

It was felt that x-ray treatments for this patient would be of no permanent value. Certainly it was out of the question to consider pneumonectomy.

In review, then, it is seen that cough, a very common symptom in tuberculosis and bronchiogenic carcinoma. was not found to any extent in this case. There was never any blood streaked sputum.

Dyspnea was never distressing until twenty-four hours before death.

Autopsy was limited to the thorax.

The body was that of a fairly well developed and nourished female of about 45 years of age.

Pleural cavities: The left contained a slight excess of clear yellow fluid; the surfaces were smooth and glistening. The right contained about 200 cc. of fluid and semi-solid yellowish material anteriorly. Posteriorly and inferiorly the cavity is obliterated and the parietal and visceral surfaces are fused in a dense white sheet.

Lungs: The left crepitated throughout and was heavy and soggy. On section it was uniform, dark reddish purple in color and wet; much blood stained frothy fluid flowed from the cut surface. The right lung consisted apparently of only two lobes. It was solid and hard except in the posterior portion of the inferior lobe where the lung was solid but much less firm than in the remaining portions. On section the firmer portions were whitish in color, very firm in consistency, and the normal lung markings were obliterated. The less firm portions on section were solid but moist and reddish-brown in color and a few of the lung markings remain.

Pericardial cavity: It contained about 350 cc. of clear straw fluid. The surfaces are smooth except on the right side where there are numerous small, firm, white nodules projecting into the cavity.

Heart: The myocardium was flabby and brownish-red in color; the endocardium was smooth; the aorta was smooth and elastic; the coronary arteries showed nothing unusual.

Esophagus: Nothing unusual. Trachea and bronchi: the trachea and left bronchial tree showed only congestion. The right bronchial tree could be followed only a short distance into the solid mass of lung tissue but no new-growths were demonstrable arising therefrom.

Tracheobronchial lymph nodes: Slightly enlarged, all of them were firm and on section were replaced by firm white new-growth.

Liver: On palpation the capsule was smooth except for a few small whitish nodules on the upper surface; on section one of these was firm, white and circumscribed.

The gallbladder on inspection was normal.

The remaining abdominal viscera on partial inspection and palpation appears to show no noteworthy changes.

Anatomic diagnosis: Carcinoma of the right lung; extension of the carcinoma to the tracheobronchial lymph nodes, pleura, pericardium, diaphragm and liver; pericardial effusion; hydrothorax; edema of left lung.

Microscopical Examination: Right Lung: Adenocarcinoma, widespread invasion, in the older parts stimulating much new-growth of connective tissue. The cells were cuboidal, not only from new tubular structure but also line the alveolar walls. The tumor resembled bronchial epithelium.

Left Lung: Lymphogenous spread of the new-growth. Congestion and edema.

Diaphragm: Metastatic adenorcarcinoma of the pleural surface spreading by way of the lymphatics through the muscular coat and into the peritoneal surface.

Pericardium: Metastatic adenocarcinoma spreading by way of the lymphatics. Simple pericarditis, lymphocytic infiltration. Heart: Nothing unusual. Aorta: Medial degeneration. Tracheobronchial Lymph Node: Metastatic adenocarcinoma, destroying the entire lymph node, much production of connective tissue.

Liver: Metastatic adenocarcinoma. Fatty degeneration of the liver cells.

Microscopic Diagnosis (additional): Metastatic carcinoma of left lung; fatty degeneration of liver.

Discussion on Paper of Doctors Gray and Roberts

DR. MURDOCK EQUEN (Atlanta): Those of us who are interested in the pathology of the lung have found the case reported by Dr. Gray of great interest.

Malignant tumors of the lung may be either primary or secondary. We were inclined to think of them more as being secondary, until the bronchoscope came along; now we can look down in the bronchus and frequently find a lump of malignant cells which we are able to remove. We may implant radon seeds, and with intense radiation, using the Coutard technic, literally burn up the malignant cells, thereby adding many years of life to these individuals.

Carcinoma of the lung is essentially of bronchiogenic origin. It may arise from the mucous glands in the wall of the bronchus or from the respiratory epithelium lining the bronchus. If it arises from a large bronchus, the primary mass will be at the hilus, and if from a small bronchus it may be situated in any part of the lung. Those arising at the hilus will shortly disseminate through the lung substance, giving the appearance of multiple seats of origin. When the patient first complains of symptoms, this has probably already taken place in most instances. Therefore the physician should remember that the average case of lung tumor is a late case at the time of his first observation.

The tumor may produce early obstruction of a large bronchus, resulting in collapse, lung abscess or bronchiectasis. It may project as a papillary mass into the lumen, but more often it grows outward instead of into the lumen, so that the only clue to its existence may be only roughening of the bronchial mucosa at the point of its origin. This is early in the case. Later on, of course, as the tumor grows, one is bound to get some obstruction of the bronchus, which can be easily picked up by the bronchoscope.

Boyd states that he has found the anaplastic group is most common, there being three groups, the anaplastic, the glandular and the epidermoid. The metastases are more anaplastic than the primary tumors. It may spread through the lung by direct extension to the draining lymph nodes or to distant organs. It metastasizes in order of frequency to the following organs: the liver, brain, bone, kidney, adrenal and, more rarely, to the pancreas and thyroid.

When you have a patient who is in the cancer age and you cannot find any symptoms of cardiac, renal or arterial disease, and he has a cough and is short of breath, you should think of a possible growth in the bronchus.

The symptoms of this condition are, first of all, a cough, due to bronchial irritation; bloody sputum, due to actual hemorrhage, because of bronchial ulceration; atelectasis, due to bronchial occlusion; dyspnea, due to interference with cardiac action and replacement of lung tissue; pain, due to pleurisy, pressure on the nerves, or metastases in the vertebral column; pleural effusion, due to pleural involvement; loss of weight; fever and leukocytosis.

If these cases are gotten early enough, the best thing, of course, is to do radical surgery. I noticed in the paper last night that in New Orleans a lung had been completely removed. This is the second time an entire lung has been removed in the South. Several years ago at the meeting of the American Bronchoscopic Society in Boston, a physician was shown who had been operated on by Dr. Graham for carcinoma of the lung. The lung had been completely removed and he had been able to resume his practice, doing work that was not very strenuous. The interesting part about this was that he drove over 150 miles to attend this meeting and said afterwards he was going to drive back. So I think the future of the treatment of carcinoma of the lung is more radical surgery, because it is like cancer anywhere else, if not completely removed there is nothing of value accomplished. As practitioners become more suspicious of lung cancer and refer their patients for early bronchoscopic examination and as the thoracic surgeons advance with their technic I think more and more of these cases can be cured.

DR. ALLEN H. BUNCE (Atlanta): This case report of Dr. Gray's stresses a very important point. That is the necessity of early diagnosis in certain conditions. In those conditions where the history, physical examination, x-ray examination, examination of the sputum if there be any, fail to make a diagnosis, although the patient has evidences of pathology, some pathological indication in the chest, I think we will use more and more the services of those who can examine the bronchi with the bronchoscope. We have recently had an experience of this kind, where a very early bronchial carcinoma was diagnosed, where a positive diagnosis was found. If first the examination be negative, do not be afraid to repeat it again and again, in the presence of symptoms. That refers not only to a physical examination, but an x-ray examination and a bronchoscopic examination.

Of course, only a few of these patients will be cured. Most of us will never see more than one or two. But if the life of one person is saved in a hundred examinations, I think we are well repaid.

DR. EDGAR PUND (Augusta): I wish to further emphasize what Dr. Bunce has said about the diagnosis. I may illustrate how often a diagnosis is missed in bronchial carcinoma by citing four cases in which the diagnosis was made or confirmed at autopsy; in only one of these was the correct diagnosis made before death. This was the case Dr. Gray reported. Dr. Gray deserves more credit for the diagnosis in this case than he gives himself. He made it quite early when he first saw the case although this is not evident in his paper.

The other cases illustrate the rapidity with which carcinomas of the lung may spread to other portions of the body and the difficulty of diagnosis. When one considers the lymph and blood supply of the lungs, we can see the only hope for such cases rests in a very early diagnosis. In most of these cases this is practically impossible. Yet one should always consider, of course, the possibility of a carcinoma of the lung in individuals of the cancer age. Most commonly it is confused with tuberculosis. In one of our cases a diagnosis was made of pulmonary tuberculosis with tuberculous meningitis. Here again we see the relation of the symptoms to pathology, because so frequently these tumors metastasize to the brain. This case was a primary carcinoma of the lung with metastasis to the cerebellum and symptoms referable to the intracranial trouble; hence the diagnosis of tuberculous meningitis.

Frequently a metastatic tumor will outgrow the primary tumor. In another case the primary tumor was 3 cm. in diameter, while the secondary tumor formed a large mass in the liver, and a diagnosis of intraabdominal malignancy was made. In the third case the mediastinal metastases overshadowed the picture of the primary tumor of the lung so that a diagnosis of primary mediastinal tumor was made.

DR. R. B. GREENBLATT (Augusta): The difficulties in arriving at a diagnosis of malignancy within the chest cavity are evident because of the varied and bizarre syndrome each case affords. This, which is important in itself, is particularly borne out by the interesting and quite baffling case just reported by Dr. Gray.

It is to be deplored that one important vehicle of great aid in the diagnosis is not more frequently employed in such cases where pleurisy is an important and complicating feature and that is examination of the aspirated fluid. The procedure is quite simple.

in any condition necessitating this procedure,
Fowler in 1898 and Martin in 1899 suggested methods of valve formation at the site
of anastomosis. Neither of these technics
proved entirely satisfactory, nor did their
authors accomplish their purpose. In 1911
Robert C. Coffey, of Portland, Oregon, described his method of construction of a physiologic valve mechanism at the site of implantation of the severed ureter or common
bile duct into the intestine. Coffey alone has
been accorded full credit for the development
of the present day solution of the problem.
Two additional technics, but retaining his
original principle of valve construction, were
later advanced by the same author. Various
modifications and adaptations of these three
technics have been advocated and successfully
employed, but the original principle has been
retained in all. The original technic, as well
as its modifications, is essentially as follows:
a linear incision is made in the wall of the
intestine through the serous and muscular
layers, down to but not through the mucosa.
The uterer is fixed in the interlamellar space
(between the mucosa and muscular layers)
for a distance of 4 cm. and empties into the
lumen of the intestine through a small opening in the mucosa at the caudal end of the
incision.

Coffey's outstanding accomplishment widened the field of applicability of uretero-intestinal implantation to include not only exstrophy of the bladder, but the following
lesions as well: as a palliative measure or as
an essential step preliminary to cystectomy
for malignancy of the bladder; advanced
tuberculous cystitis; extensive ulceration and
contracture of the bladder; incurable vesico-
vaginal fistula; certain types of traumatic injuries of the bladder or ureter; or in any affection in which it is necessary to dispense
with the bladder as a reservoir for urine.

Several hundred cases in which ureteral
transplantation has been done clearly demonstrate that the mortality and morbidity of
the procedure have been so markedly lowered
that the risk of subsequent renal infection
need no longer be considered as a contraindi-
cation. Walters and Braasch reported the occurrence of mild, transitory symptoms of
renal infection in only a small percentage of

a large series of cases several years after operation. It has also been reported that the operation would not seem to contraindicate pregnancy with a reasonable degree of safety. Eberbach and Pierce; Randall and Hardwick reported cases proceeding to full term without clinical evidence of renal disturbance.

Re-absorption of urine and fluid feces, lesions of the bowel wall and changes in the bacterial flora of the colon have been advanced as arguments against ureteral transplantation. Evidence has been repeatedly demonstrated, by many different surgeons, that these fears are largely unfounded and that colitis of a truly serious nature occurs but rarely. Most reports have shown that urine is passed from the rectum three to four times during the day and once or twice at night, that in the presence of a competent anal sphincter there is no leakage of urine and fluid feces through the anus, and that the presence of urine in the rectosigmoid does not of itself give rise to discomfort.

Uretero-intestinal anastomosis has been shown to be a procedure offering relief, added years of life and the ability to carry on with their duties to those suffering from any one or more of the several afflictions stated herein. More than one author has stated that experimental surgery upon animals should be done prior to the performance of the operation upon the human subject, not so much with the idea of gaining skill in technic but to familiarize one's self with the many phases of the procedure.

Report of Case

A white boy, aged 16 years, was admitted to the surgical division of the University Hospital, Dec. 3, 1932. Three hours prior to admission the patient had received an accidental shotgun wound of the lower abdomen and upper right thigh. At operation, by Dr. G. A. Traylor, the symphisis pubis and both rami of the left pubic bone were found to be considerably damaged. There was a rent, 2 cm. long, in the dome of the bladder. The greater portion of the wound extended to the left of the bladder into the left ischio-rectal fossa. The peritoneal cavity was apparently not entered. Debridement was done and hemorrhage was controlled by gauze packs. A Pezzar catheter was fixed in the bladder wound for drainage. Convalescence was long and stormy. Nine months after operation a suprapubic fistula was draining pus and urine. A large calculus and a primary sequestrum were removed from the bladder by the resident on surgery, Dr. W. J. Williams. Roentgenograms revealed considerable destruction and osteomyelitis of the left pubic

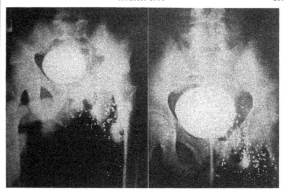

FIG. 1.
The radio-opaque fluid instilled into the bladder has filled the lower left ureter and the large fistulous tracts. Note numerous lead shot.

FIG. 2.
Results of cystography fifteen days after operation. Note filling of stump of left ureter and absence of fistulous tracts.

any other reasonable procedure. Urine was recovered from the rectum 36 hours after operation.

Post-operative excretory urograms showed only moderate left hydronephrosis, comparing favorably with the size of the opposite kidney. Phenolsulphonphthalein excretion from the left kidney (the side upon which the ureter had been transplanted) in 2 hours was 20 per cent. From the right kidney, 30 per cent. The opening on the left posterior thigh closed spontaneously. Non-protein nitrogen and uric acid determinations of the blood at regular intervals were within normal limits. Three months after operation, the patient had gained 20 pounds in weight, excretory urograms and renal function tests were essentially the same as on previous occasions. Control of urine in the rectum was perfect.

REFERENCES

1. Brenizer, A. G.: Ureteral Transplantations: Modifications of Methods, Am. J. Surg. 28: 210, 1935.
2. Coffey, R. C.: Physiologic Implantation of the Severed Ureter or Bile Duct into the Intestine, J. A. M. A. 56: 397, 1911.
   A Technic for Simultaneous Implantation of the Right and Left Ureter into the Pelvic Colon which does not Obstruct the Ureter or Disturb Kidney Function, Northwest Med. 24: 211, 1925.
   Transplantation of Ureters into Large Intestine, Surg. Gynec. & Obst. 47: 593-621, 1928.
   Production of Aseptic-Ureteroenterostomy, J. A. M. A. 94: 1748, 1930.
3. Eberbach, C. W., and Pierce, J. M.: Pregnancy Terminated by Caesarean Section After Ureteral Transplantation into the Sigmoid, Surg. Gynec. & Obst. 47: 540-542 (Oct.) 1928.
4. Furniss, H. C.: Uretero-Intestinal Anastomosis; A Simplification of the Coffey Technic, Am. J. Surg. 13: 12-14, 1932.
5. Kirwin, T. J.: A Study of Ureteral Implantation with a Description of a New Procedure, Am. J. Surg. 8: 1-27, 1930.
   Clinical Value of Experimental Ureteral Implantation, Am. J. Surg. n.s. 23: No. 1: 14-25, 1934.
6. Lower, W. E.: Disposition of the Ureters in Certain Abnormal Conditions of the Urinary Bladder, J. A. M. A. 80: 1200, 1928.
7. Mayo, C. H.: Exstrophy of the Bladder. Contributions to Medical and Biological Research: Dedicated to Sir William Osler: II: 1095-1110, New York: Paul B. Hoeber, 1919.
8. Randall, L. M., and Hardwick, R. S.: Pregnancy and Parturition Following Bilateral Ureteral Transplantation for Congenital Exstrophy of the Bladder, Surg. Gynec. & Obst. 58: 1018-1020, 1934.
9. Walters, W.: Transplantation of Ureters to Recto-sigmoid and Cystectomy for Exstrophy of the Bladder: Report of 76 Cases, Am. J. Surg. 15: 15-22, 1932.
10. Walters, W., and Braasch, W. F.: Ureteral Transplantation to the Recto-sigmoid, Am. J. Surg. 23: 255-270 (Feb.) 1934.

Discussion on Paper of Dr. George W. Wright

DR. JULIAN QUATTLEBAUM (Savannah): Dr. Wright is to be commended for bringing this subject to the attention of the Association and I congratulate him upon the excellent result obtained in the case reported.

It is gratifying to see the older views on ureteral injury changing. Previously it was considered that any serious injury to the ureter demanded the immediate removal of the ureter with its kidney, which more often than not was entirely normal. The procedure of uretero-intestinal anastomosis which now makes possible the conservation of the kidney and the restoration of normal health in such cases as Dr. Wright's, is directly attributable to the principle of a valve action developed by that great surgeon of whom we in the South should be especially proud and of whom Lord Moynihan spoke as "a surgeon of great sagacity," the late Dr. Robert C. Coffey of Portland; a native of North Carolina. By encouraging a careful selection of patients, emphasizing the indications and contraindications for the operation, and by perfecting the technical procedure, they have greatly reduced the risk even in less experienced hands.

While the principle of uretero-colostomy is well established, there is still some debate as to the best method of performing the anastomosis, particularly as to the need of using catheters as in the Coffey No. 2 technic, or doing the operation without them as performed by the Mayo group. There is also a difference of opinion as to whether the operation should be done in one or several stages. This is a matter of individual judgment and for those who have only an occasional opportunity to do the operation, necessitates the most thorough preoperative study with attention to all details that might make for success in that particular case. The risk of the operation will be less in the hands of experienced surgeons of course, but other factors also play a prominent part. Probably the most favorable cases for uretero-intestinal anastomosis are those individuals who have some congenital anomaly of the urinary tract with normal ureters and kidneys. This is most often found in children with exstrophy of the bladder. However, one must be certain that an associated defect of the nervous mechanism controlling the rectal sphincters is not present since it goes without saying that a competent anal sphincter is most necessary for the success of the operation.

The operation should not be performed on children until they are old enough to have voluntary control of the bowel. Another very favorable group of cases for this operation are those with injuries to the bladder or ureter. If only one ureter is injured the outlook is especially good since the uninjured ureter and kidney are sufficient to take care of normal function for the time necessary for operative recovery. Extensive injuries to the bladder require bilateral transplantation of course. The operation has a field of usefulness in non-tuberculous chronic cystitis as well as in the tuberculous variety. Perhaps the greatest mortality and poorest result will be found in those cases of cancer of the bladder, obviously because the patients are older and their general physical condition considerably weakened by their disease. It is well known that the presence of cancer seems in some mysterious way to lower the vitality of the patient and the mortality of this operation will always remain high among those patients on whom the operation is done for cancer. The mortality rate also will be high in those cases in which the ureters are abnormal. Given gross abnormality with dilatation and hypertrophy of the ureter, uretero-intestinal anastomosis takes on a risk which is rarely justified even in the most expert hands and some other type of operation for the diversion of urine, such as cutaneous ureterostomy, must be done.

From a review of the literature it would appear that the lowest mortality can be obtained by doing the operation in two stages and by making the operation substantially extra-peritoneal. It is certainly desirable to use the catheter technic of Coffey in transplanting the sole ureter in those cases where one kidney and ureter have been previously removed, the catheter preventing the postoperative edema from blocking the urinary flow even temporarily.

It is well to point out here that there are female patients on whom this operation has been done who have gone through repeated pregnancies without difficulty and as time goes by they will increase in number. The advisability of performing a cesarean section on such patients is influenced by the absolute necessity of preserving the integrity of the anal sphincters and should such patients be permitted to go through a normal labor, every attention should be given towards preventing a perineal laceration that would involve the sphincters.

DR. L. G. BAGGETT (Atlanta): The field of operation for this type of condition has been greatly enlarged in the last two years, since the dangers attending that operation have been greatly eliminated, and especially by our good friend the late Dr. Coffey, who I think is due a great deal of credit.

(Slide) This shows a case which I operated on two years ago.

(Slide) This was done in the single stage, and the bilateral transplantation was done in one sitting. Three of these cases are living and well today.

(Slide) You notice here that the transplantation on the one side is a little lower than the one on the other side, the inch and a half incision referred to by the essayist being made through the two coats of the intestine, and later making a second drainage transplantation.

(Slide) Here you see the two openings made before the ureter had been put into the mucosa. The catheters had been put into the ureter, as you see there, and there the little fine-pointed knife is put in, in order that the intestine may cover the ureter to that area, so that there is a valve-like action and it develops into a very fine incision.

(Slide) Here is where the ureter was transplanted into the last little dip, where it goes into the bowel.

(Slide) Here is the completed operation, done with a peritoneal flow on the one side. The entire operation now is retroperitoneal.

(Slide) This shows a diagram in which the rectum is packed with gauze.

(Slide) This is just a diagram showing where the ureters have been transplanted, out through the rectum.

(Slide) This shows the result in this boy.

DR. GEORGE W. WRIGHT (Augusta): As Dr. Quattlebaum has stated, the existence of a competent anal sphincter is necessary for a successful outcome. Disease of the large intestine should be ruled out. The operation should never be performed upon greatly debilitated individuals nor upon those who are obviously poor risks. The condition of the kidneys should be determined as accurately as possible prior to operation. Intravenous urography is a most useful procedure. Comparison of preoperative and postoperative roentgenograms is of importance.

Because the mucosa of the large intestine is thought by some to be relatively immune to tuberculosis, uretero-intestinal anastomosis has been done because of the intractable pain of tuberculous cystitis.

Experimental transplantation of the ureter into the upper portion of the small intestine has invariably resulted in death.

It would seem that the rectosigmoid is the portion of the intestinal tract best suited for this operation.

PUBLIC HEALTH PROBLEMS
IN GEORGIA*

T. F. ABERCROMBIE†, M. D.

Atlanta

To get a perspective of Georgia's public health problems, it will be necessary for us to take a retrospective view of health work in our State. Georgia has had state health work continuously since 1903 and has spent $2,155,351 from the State Treasury for this purpose. To some, this may appear to be a large expenditure, but by comparison let's see how it looks. Georgia has spent seventy-one cents per person for health work in thirty-three years, less than 2½ cents per person per year. The total amount expended by Georgia for health work in thirty-three years would build just one hundred and fifteen miles of hard surface roads. How far out of the mud would we be now if we had only one hundred and fifteen miles of good roads? None of us would have driven to this beautiful city in our seventy-five, ninety, or one hundred horsepower automobile.

However, let us see what this $2,155,351 expenditure has helped to purchase for Georgia. On September 10, 1903, the State Board of Health began operation under the able direction of Dr. H. F. Harris with the magnificent sum of $3,000 and a microscope owned by Doctor Harris. If the same death rate had prevailed in Georgia in 1935 as in 1903, there would have been 14,658 more deaths than actually occurred. There was a saving of 4,002 lives from tuberculosis in 1935, 779 from typhoid fever, and 805 from diphtheria over the 1903 rates. In 1917, the laboratory examined 7,034 specimens; in 1935, 187,725.

Within the past year, we have obtained in Georgia an insight into the benefits to be derived from a broad program of public health activities, through resources of the Federal government and contributions from the Rockefeller Foundation. The result has been an awakening of vision of the full possibilities of health service to all the people. These emergency aids can not be expected to continue permanently, however, and with their withdrawal there will necessarily follow a lessening of safeguards and benefits. It is to establish a permanent program that we are seeking. It is our desire to enlarge our organization to carry health service to all of the people all of the time. Most of the counties in Georgia are unable to pay for local health protection, and the State must assume the cost of this service if it is to be adequately provided.

During 1935, every county in Georgia was given public health nursing service, tuberculosis x-ray clinics, and sanitary engineering service for the prevention of malaria, typhoid fever, dysentery, and hookworm disease. In addition, county health work has been supervised and promoted, outbreaks of communicable disease have been suppressed, the laboratory has aided in the detection and control of communicable disease, and dental health education and venereal disease programs have been carried on.

The nurses made 132,537 visits in promoting maternity and child hygiene, gave 212,729 inoculations against preventable disease under supervision of the local medical profession, supervised and instructed the midwives who attended thirty-two per cent of the births last year, and carried on a general health education program. Although the infant and maternal mortality rates are declining, much remains to be accomplished. There was one maternal death for every 145 live births in Georgia last year.

There were 1,717 deaths from tuberculosis in Georgia in 1935. It is conservatively estimated that there are 10,000 cases, with only 700 hospital beds available for the treatment of this disease. The inadequacy of a system of tuberculosis control which does not give the fullest consideration to home treatment is apparent. The Department's x-ray unit made 13,503 x-ray examinations last year. The splendid cooperation of the medical profession made possible this immense amount of work. The tuberculosis death rate has declined thirty-two per cent since 1903, but there still remains much to be done as this disease takes sixth place in the deaths from all causes.

The drainage of malarial areas, construc-

*Read before the Medical Association of Georgia, Savannah, April 23, 1936.
†Director, Department of Public Health, State of Georgia.

tion of sanitary privies, and the extension of water mains and sewer lines are the primary functions of the sanitary engineering program; 2,639 ponds were drained, 10,461 standard pit privies were installed, and 38 miles of sewers were constructed. It has been assumed by some that the amount of malarial drainage during the past several years should have reduced the malaria problem to a greater extent than it has. This assumption fails to consider that the work carried on was an emergency measure, and not under professional administration. The prevalence of malaria is governed primarily by rainfall conditions and the number of malaria deaths each year closely approaches the average expectancy of 8.62 deaths per inch of annual rainfall. Malaria is also a disease of cyclic occurrency, the cycle about seven years in length, and 1935 was a year of approximate cyclic maximum. Heavy rainfalls occurred in the summer months in South Georgia. In spite of unfavorable influences, the malaria death rate per inch of rainfall was held below the average expectancy.

A comparison of the county health officers' reports for 1935 with the previous year shows a marked increase in activities from 5.0 to 210 per cent. The Ellis Health Law provides every county with a board of health. Upon two successive recommendations of the grand jury, a full-time county health unit is established. There are thirty-two counties operating under this law, leaving 127, comprising more than fifty per cent of the State's population, without local health service.

A division of epidemiology was established in Georgia in 1931 through a grant from the Rockefeller Foundation, which division is responsible for the study of disease epidemics to determine the cause of spread and to recommend control measures, and for research work to aid the Department in combatting communicable diseases. Increasing demands for this type of work make expansion of this program necessary.

The laboratory functions to aid physicians and health officers in the detection and control of communicable diseases. With the present appropriation the laboratory is able to distribute free only a few products for safeguarding the public health. No free diph-

In our county two successive grand juries have recommended that we have a county health commissioner and establish the Ellis Health Law, but when we go to the county commissioners we fail to get the appropriation necessary to finance this. In my county the tax necessary for carrying out this law would be about fifty cents per capita.

I should like to ask Dr. Abercrombie in closing what he would recommend and what plea to carry before a set of county commissioners by which we could get this law established. In my county it is a law but we cannot get it financed, so therefore we cannot carry it out. We pay about $1,800 to $2,000 a year for an agricultural agent, while to my mind a health commissioner would be more valuable to the county.

I wish to mention another thing. Recently a lady referred her nurse for her child to me for examination. She had a primary sore, with a florid eruption, all over her body. The Wassermann test was strongly positive, and there she was, having her baby under the care of this nurse. I mentioned the fact to her after I got a report of the Wassermann and she has done nothing about it. I informed her of the danger to this child, and of course they put the woman under treatment.

I think we ought to carry on an educational campaign through the women's clubs and Parent-Teachers Association. We doctors going before these women should inform them of the dangers of venereal diseases among their servants, to get them to demand before they employ them that they have a health certificate from a reputable, competent authority as to whether or not they are fit for service. I think that ought to be carried out and should be emphasized.

In my little town of Arlington, I have roughly estimated that there are 75 per cent of the negro population who are syphilitic.

I should like to ask Dr. Abercrombie, in closing, what is the danger of syphilitics in employment? If there is any danger in closed cases, that is cases where there is no open lesion, or anything like that, whether or not there is danger to the people from cooks like that.

DR. GEORGE L. ECHOLS (Milledgeville): I do not know what Dr. Abercrombie will say in regard to the question my good friend Dr. Sharp asked in closing, but I heard Dr. Solomon discuss that point in one of his lectures in Boston. He says where there are open lesions, primary lesions, there is very great danger. After the primary lesion has healed, the danger is less. After the syphilis has gone on for a year, there is still less danger, and the second year there is still less, and the third still less, and so on, and after a number of years the possibility for contracting syphilis in an innocent manner of that sort is very, very limited. While there is an open lesion, you had better look after it.

DR. GUY G. LUNSFORD (Atlanta): There is one problem in public health that probably Dr. Abercrombie forgot to mention or did not have time for.

I am sure all of you are familiar with the provisions of the Social Security Act, the fact that we have some money available, as he mentioned, for rural health work. One of our real problems is the finding of qualified men to carry on this work. At present, we could place from eight to a dozen health officers, physicians who are trained in public health and preventive medicine. Possibly most of you remember reading in the State JOURNAL some time last year, I think about March or April, the qualifications that are set out by the Conference of State and Provincial Health Officers and the United States Public Health Service, for these officers. We are very anxious to secure capable and qualified county health officers. They must have special training, and in order to get that special training they must be 35 years old or younger when they start in public health work. So that if you refer to us young men who want to make this a life work, interested in this particular specialty of medicine, we would be appreciative. As an incentive to this work we will be in a position to at least pay them enough to live on while they are taking some special training. I just want to mention this as a problem that possibly you might help us to solve.

DR. T. F. ABERCROMBIE (Atlanta): Just one point in reference to what Dr. Lunsford said. We will give preference to Georgia doctors every time if we can get them.

In answer to Dr. Sharp's question about the ditches and malaria, you may remember that I said a great deal of that work was done without professional supervision. You will recall at that time we had lots of relief work that was done to give people work, and this was one method of giving it to them, and we realized, at the time, we were digging a lot of ditches that did not have any relation to malaria, and in the case of a lot of them there was no provision made for keeping them open, but from now on there is to be. It will be under professional supervision and engineering, and we will determine whether malaria exists or whether it is economically feasible to drain.

Another question is as to how to get small counties to finance it. I wish somebody would answer that for me. I can not answer it. It is a question of education, getting your people to want it. I will refer to another statement in my address, that the two million and some odd dollars would have built only 115 miles of good roads. Why do we have good roads all over this state? It is because we wanted them, we wanted them a long time, we wanted them bad enough to pay for them. If we want public health we have to want it, want it bad enough to pay for it. And when we get to that state we will get it.

Dr. Echols answered the other question as to the communicability of venereal diseases.

The Southern Medical Association, Birmingham, Ala., will hold its thirtieth annual meeting at Baltimore, Md., Tuesday, Wednesday, Thursday, Friday, November 17-20, 1936. The Lord Baltimore Hotel, corner of Hanover and Baltimore Streets, will be general hotel headquarters.

his visit as a guest of the Association,
May 8-10, 1935 . . . .   84.65

2374—Alliance Printing Company
Printing and mailing 1900 copies of
the May, 1935, issue of the JOURNAL 339.00

2375—Alliance Printing Company
250 Programs for Woman's Auxiliary;
50 cards with names of Honorary
Advisory Board 39.50

2376—Miller's Book Store
1 Copy of Roberts Rules of Order for
and in possession of Parliamentarian .   1.50

2377—Ivan Allen-Marshall Company
Wrapping paper, T. W. paper, T. W.
ribbon and twine 4.85

2378—Southern Bell Telephone & Telegraph
Company
Telephone account to May 11, 1935   34.25

2379—Southern Press Clipping Bureau
News clippings for April and May,
1935 . . . .   10.00

2380—Allen H. Bunce, M.D.
Salary as Secretary-Treasurer, May 1-
15, 1935 . . . .   75.00

2381—Edgar D. Shanks, M.D.
Salary as Secretary-Treasurer, May 15-
31, 1935 . . . .   75.00

2382—H. L. Rowe
Salary as Executive Secretary for May,
1935 . . . . 175.00

2383—Wm. H. Myers, M.D.
Payment on expenses as delegate to
the Atlantic City session of the American Medical Association, June, 10-14,
1935 . . . . 100.00

2384—C. W. Roberts, M.D.
Payment on expenses as delegate to
the Atlantic City session of the American Medical Association, June 10-14,
1935 . . . . 100.00

2385—Olin H. Weaver, M.D.
Payment on expenses as delegate to
the Atlantic City session of the American Medical Association, June 10-14,
1935 . . . . 100.00

2386—Walter Wilson
Gold leaf sign for the door at the
Academy of Medicine 4.50

2387—Cathcart Allied Storage Company
Moving office furniture and all equip-
ment and supplies from 139 Forrest
Avenue, N. E., to 38 Prescott Street,
N. E., Atlanta 17.50

2388—Logan Clarke Insurance Agency, Inc.
Premium on surety bond, No. FB-
1021, for Secretary-Treasurer, for one
year to May 25, 1936 . . . .   10.00

2389—J. N. Reisman
Rent at 139 Forrest Avenue, N. E.,
Atlanta, May 1, to June 6, 1935 . . .   17.10

2390—Master Reporting Company
Reporting the Atlanta session, May 7-
10, 1935, original and carbon copies

of minutes of Council, general meetings and House of Delegates....... 276.15

2391—L. F. Livingston, Postmaster
Postage 30.00

2392—Fulton County Medical Society
Balance due on the Scientific Exhibit,
Atlanta session, May 7-10, 1935... 150.00

2393—Fulton County Medical Society
Rent for June and July, 1935.... 20.00

2394—Alliance Printing Company
Printing and mailing 1925 copies of
the June, 1935, issue of the JOURNAL 323.25

2395—W. H. Evans
Lumber and carpenter work building
shelves in supply room........... 1.20

2396—L. F. Livingston, Postmaster
Deposit for mailing the JOURNAL... 25.00

2397—Dixie Seal & Stamp Company
Rubber Stamp for endorsing checks.. 1.40

2398—Western Union Telegraph Company
Telegraph account for May, 1935... 2.05

2399—J. F. Thompson Engraving Company
2,000 Letterheads and 2,000 envelopes
for President, James E. Paullin..... 40.80

2400—Service Engraving Company
4 Copper halftones for illustrations
and repairs on electros for advertisers 20.18

2401—Edgar D. Shanks, M.D.
Salary as Secretary-Treasurer for June,
1935 .... 150.00

2402—H. L. Rowe
Salary as Executive Secretary for June,
1935 .... 175.00

2403—Southern Bell Telephone & Telegraph
Company
Telephone account, May 11- June 21
and moving charges.............. 10.20

2404—Atlanta Envelope Company
24,985 Envelopes for mailing the
JOURNAL 85.46

2405—Alliance Printing Company
10,500 Letterheads 25.75

2406—J. L. Campbell, Chairman, Cancer
Commission
Commissions on insurance appropriated
for expenses of the Cancer Commission 156.70

2407—C. L. Smith
One 9' x 12' Colonial rug......... 23.12

2408—H. F. Linder
One Sterling cup with engraving,
"Health Trophy Medical Association
of Georgia to Georgia Congress of
Parents and Teachers for Best Work
in Health," Cost of cup.......... 100.00
Less donations as follows:
W. L. Champion.......$ 5.00
Grady E. Clay.......... 10.00
F. P. Calhoun.......... 10.00
T. C. Davison......... 5.00
Hugh Lokey 2.50
E. G. Ballenger 5.00
Calhoun McDougall 5.00
Jas. E. Paullin.......... 7.50

Less total contributions 50.00
Balance paid by the Medical Association of Georgia................. 50.00

2409—L. F. Livingston, Postmaster
Postage 30.00

2410—Miss Annie Jacks
Commission on advertising orders... 48.58

2411—Alliance Printing Company
Printing and mailing 1760 copies of
the July, 1935, issue of the JOURNAL 308.40

2412—Service Engraving Company
Copper halftones and repairs on electros
for advertisers 23.27

2413—Southern Bell Telephone & Telegraph
Company
Telephone account to July 21, 1935 6.15

2414—Edgar D. Shanks, M.D.
Salary as Secretary-Treasurer for July,
1935 .... 150.00

2415—H. L. Rowe
Salary as Executive Secretary for July,
1935 .... 175.00

2416—Ivan Allen-Marshall Company
Cards for addressograph plates, writing
pens, rubber bands, twine, wrapping
paper, T. W. ribbon............. 5.35

2417—Southern Press Clipping Bureau
News clippings for June and July,
1935 .... 10.00

2418—Fulton County Medical Society
Rent for August and September, 1935 20.00

2419—The Geographical Publishing Co.
25 Maps of Georgia showing new
Congressional districts 4.11

2420—Empire Letter Shop
8,000 Letterheads and 5,000 envelopes
for officers and committees......... 43.50

2421—R. L. Goodman
Fire proof safe to prevent loss of
valuable records 55.00

2422—L. F. Livingston, Postmaster
Postage 30.00

2423—J. E. Penland, M.D.
Expenses incurred as Councilor for the
Eighth District 17.00

2424—Alliance Printing Company
Printing and mailing 1775 copies of
the August, 1935, issue of the
JOURNAL 318.50

2425—Southern Bell Telephone & Telegraph
Company
Telephone account to Augusta 21,
1935 .... 6.15

2426—Bryan, Middlebrooks & Carter, Attys.
Suit of J. J. Mashburn vs. Dr. J. C.
Rollins, Dalton, fee for attorney Mitchell employed by Dr. Rollins...... 75.00

2427—Associated Mutuals, Inc.
Premium on $1000.00 fire insurance 7.60

2428—American Surety Company
Premium on surety bond for H. L.
Rowe, September 6, 1935, to September 6, 1936................ 5.00

2429—Edgar D. Shanks, M.D.
Salary as Secretary-Treasurer for August, 1935 .... 150.00

2430—H. L. Rowe
Salary as Executive Secretary for August, 1935. .... 175.00

2431—L. F. Livingston, Postmaster
Postage 30.00

2432—Empire Letter Shop
Multigraphing 150 letters to county secretaries: 600 copies of letter from American Medical Association in reference to Directory and dues also stationery $8.40; stationery and multigraphing 400—3 page questionnaires (1200) for the Committee for the Study of Maternal Mortality—$9.45   17.85

2433—S. J. Lewis, M.D.
Expenses incurred as Councilor for the Tenth District 15.00

2434—J. W. Simmons, Clerk, Fulton Superior Court
Certified copy of the original charter of the Medical Association of Georgia   2.05

2435—E. B. Paille
Commission on advertising order....   3.60

2436—Alliance Printing Company
Printing and mailing 1775 copies of the September, 1935, issue of the JOURNAL 318.50

2437—Miss Annie Jacks
Commission on advertising orders and collections 21.75

2438—L. F. Livingston, Postmaster
Deposit for mailing the JOURNAL... 25.00

2439—Southern Press Clipping Bureau
News clippings for August and September, 1935 .... 10.00

2440—Alliance Printing Company
2,500 Reprints of editorial by Dr. Jas. E. Paullin published in the July, 1935, issue of the JOURNAL....... 14.75

2441—Service Engraving Company
Repairs on electros for advertisers...   3.85

2442—L. F. Livingston, Postmaster
Postage 30.00

2443—Edgar D. Shanks, M.D.
Salary as Secretary-Treasurer for September, 1935 .... 150.00

2444—H. L. Rowe
Salary as Executive Secretary for September, 1935 .... 175.00

2445—Southern Bell Telephone & Telegraph Company
Telephone account to September, 21, 1935 .... 6.15

2446—J. F. Thompson Engraving Company
Copper halftone for illustration, printing 500 postal cards, mortising and mounting electros for advertisers.....   8.26

2447—Empire Letter Shop
450 Letters multigraphed for delinquent members; signature plate for Dr.

Shanks to run on multigraph machine and signature on stamp..........   7.25

2448—Addressograph Company
Addressograph ribbon and 500 B Alloy plates 2.79

2449—L. F. Livingston, Postmaster
Postage 30.00

2450—Alliance Printing Company
Printing and mailing 1825 copies of the October, 1935, issue of the JOURNAL 285.19

2451—Miss Annie Jacks
Commission on advertising orders.... 10.08

2452—Miss Annie Jacks
Commission on advertising orders.... 11.00

2453—J. F. Thompson Engraving Company
Chart and copper halftones for illustrations 19.89

2454—Alliance Printing Company
500 Reprints for Dr. L.
Minor Blackford ....$ 5.75
Balance on October, 1935,
JOURNAL 9.10   14.85

2455—Empire Letter Shop
Stationery and multigraphing letters in reference to Medical Economic Survey —$3.25: multigraphing letters mailed to delinquent and former members— $3.00 ....   6.25

2456—Southern Bell Telephone & Telegraph Company
Telephone account to October 21, 1935 ....   6.15

2457—Ivan Allen-Marshall Company
Gem clips, erasers, wrapping paper and stamp pad 2.15

2458—L. F. Livingston, Postmaster
Postage 30.00

2459—Edgar D. Shanks, M.D.
Salary as Secretary-Treasurer for October, 1935 .... 150.00

2460—H. L. Rowe
Salary as Executive Secretary for October, 1935 .... 175.00

2461—L. F. Livingston, Postmaster
Postage (Medical Economic Survey). 30.00

2462—L. F. Livingston, Postmaster
Deposit to pay postage on business reply envelopes. (Medical Economic Survey) Permit No. 1387, Section 510, P. L. & R................ 30.00

2463—Alliance Printing Company
Printing and mailing 1875 copies of the November, 1935, issue of the JOURNAL 297.30

2464—L. F. Livingston, Postmaster
Postage (Part for Medical Economic Survey) 30.00

2465—M. M. McCord, M.D.
Expenses incurred as Councilor for the Seventh District 17.40

2466—Miss Annie Jacks
Commission on advertising........   6.00

2467—Bryan, Middlebrooks & Carter, Attys.
One-half the court reporters cost for
reporting trial of suit W. A. Welchel
vs. Dr. J. W. Ellis, Kennesaw 31.39

2468—Ivan Allen-Marshall Company
Journal for registering names of members, index tabs, pencils, T. W. ribbon, folders for files, letter and stamp
moistener 7.70

2469—Empire Letter Shop
Stationery and multigraphing 5,000
letters with two signatures to physicians in Georgia; 5,000 business reply
envelopes (Medical Economic Survey)   43.00

2470—Southern Bell Telephone & Telegraph
Company
Telephone account to November 21,
1935 . . . .   6.15

2471—Journal Engraving Company
Mounting and mortising electros for
advertiser 1.92

2472—Wrigley Electrotyping & Sterotyping
Company
Repairs on electros for advertisers . . .   2.00

2473—Edgar D. Shanks, M.D.
Salary as Secretary-Treasurer for No-
vember, 1935 . . . .   150.00

2474—H. L. Rowe
Salary as Executive Secretary for No-
vember, 1935 . . . .   175.00

2475—Photo Process Engraving Company
Cuts for illustrations. 8.35

2476—Alliance Printing Company
5,000 Questionnaires for Medical Eco-
nomic Survey 15.00

2477—Fulton County Medical Society
Rent for October, November, Decem-
ber, 1935 . . . .   30.00

2478—Southern Press Clipping Bureau
News clippings for October and No-
vember, 1935 . . . .   10.00

2479—James E. Paullin, M.D.
Honorarium for President, 1935-1936 150.00

2480—Empire Letter Shop
10,000 No. 10 Maxwell
bond envelopes $32.50
400 Letters multigraphed to
be sent to delinquent and
former members 3.20
100 Letters multigraphed to
county secretaries in reference
to Directory 1.65   37.35

2481—Alliance Printing Company
Printing and mailing 1900 copies of
the December, 1935, issue of the
JOURNAL, pasting in one insert, fold-
ing and inserting questionnaire in reference to Medical Economic Survey . .   306.45

2482—L. F. Livingston, Postmaster
Economic Survey — $18.50; regular
postage $11.50 . . . .   30.00

2483—William McKinley, Janitor
Painting and repairing office furniture
and cabinets 3.00

2484—Ivan Allen-Marshall Company
Filing cabinet with lock, two sets of
guides, 5,000 yellow second sheets,
stamp pad and T. W. ribbon 35.65

2485—Empire Letter Shop
Multigraphing letters to county secretaries in reference to reporting officers
and members, program for the Savannah session, scientific exhibit, and Medical Defense 3.00

2486—Southern Bell Telephone & Telegraph
Company
Telephone account to December 21,
1935 . . . .   6.70

2487—Edgar D. Shanks, M.D.
Salary as Secretary-Treasurer for De-
cember, 1935 . . . .   150.00

2488—H. L. Rowe
Salary as Executive Secretary for De-
cember, 1935 . . . .   175.00

2489—Alliance Printing Company
Taking questionnaires for Medical Economic Survey out of JOURNALS and
re-inserting JOURNALS in envelopes for
mailing 8.36

2490—L. F. Livingston, Postmaster
Deposit for postage to mail the JOUR-
NAL 25.00

2491—L. F. Livingston, Postmaster
Postage 30.00

2492—Miss Annie Jacks
Commission on advertising orders . . .   14.79

2493—Alliance Printing Company
Printing and mailing 1900 copies of
the January, 1936, issue of the JOUR-
NAL 320.67

2494—Alliance Printing Company
Printing 2000 membership c a r d s;
2000 reprints of editorial, "Malpractice Suits;" 2000 blue slips mailed
with JOURNAL in reference to dues . .   33.50

2495—L. F. Livingston, Postmaster (Dr.
Paullin's letter)
Postage 30.00

2496—S. H. Benedict
Reducing drawing and making 100
blue prints of floor space to be used
in Hotel DeSoto, Savannah, during
the Savannah session for commercial
exhibits 12.00

2497—L. F. Livingston, Postmaster
Postage 30.00

2498—Miss Annie Jacks
Commission on advertising order 9.75

2499—Fulton County Medical Society
Rent for January, February, March,
1936 . . . .   30.00

2500—Southern Press Clipping Bureau
News clippings for December and Jan-
uary, 1935-6 . . . .   10.00

2501—Bryan, Middlebrooks & Carter, Attys.
Retainer as attorneys for the Medical
Association of Georgia from January
1 to December 31, 1936 . . . . .1000.00

2502—Southern Bell Telephone & Telegraph
Company
Telephone account to January 21,
1936 . . . . 6.15

2503—Wrigley Engraving Company
Mats of three ads for the Georgia
Power Company — ads run in the
JOURNAL 2.25

2504—Service Engraving Company
Cuts for illustrations and repairs on
electros for advertisers 6.66

2505—Edgar D. Shanks, M.D.
Salary as Secretary-Treasurer for Jan-
uary, 1936 . . . . 150.00

2506—H. L. Rowe
Salary as Executive Secretary for Jan-
uary, 1936 . . . . 175.00

2507—Empire Letter Shop
Multigraphing 1900 letters in reference
to Savannah session and dues in name
of Dr. J. E. Paullin, President; 150
letters in reference to commercial exhibit space at Savannah session 14.50

2508—L. F. Livingston, Postmaster
Postage—Dr. C. F. Holton's invita-
tion 30.00

2509—Alliance Printing Company
Printing and mailing 1925 copies of
the February, 1936, issue of the
JOURNAL 320.16

2510—L. F. Livingston, Postmaster
Postage 30.00

2511—Southern Bell Telephone & Telegraph
Company
Telephone account to February 21,
1936 . . . . 6.15

2512—J. F. Thompson Engraving Company
1000 Envelopes, 1000 letterheads in
name of Dr. J. E. Paullin, President,
used in mailing letters to delinquent
and former members in reference to
Savannah session and dues; steel die
signature of Dr. Edgar D. Shanks for
printing membership cards and repairs
on electros for advertisers 21.50

2513—Ivan Allen-Marshall Company
Carbon paper, paste, T. W. paper,
filing cards, blue prints of floor space
in Hotel DeSoto, index for filing cab-
inet and folders 10.90

2514—Service Engraving Company
Copper halftones for illustrations and
repairs on electros for advertisers 10.95

2515—Empire Letter Shop
2000 Letters multigraphed in name of
Dr. C. F. Holton, Savannah, President, Georgia Medical Society, inviting members and former members to
attend the Savannah session; signature

plate for Dr. Holton and stationery;
100 letters to county secretaries in reference to delegates; 150 letters in reference to program 15.40

2516—Edgar D. Shanks, M.D.
Salary as Secretary-Treasurer for Feb-
ruary, 1936 . . . . 150.00

2517—H. L. Rowe
Salary as Executive Secretary for Feb-
ruary, 1936 . . . . 175.00

2518—James E. Paullin, M.D.
Telegraph and telephone account of
the President in the interest of the
Association 11.80

2519—J. L. Campbell, M.D., Chairman,
Cancer Commission
For use of Cancer Commission in pro-
moting its work 50.00
(From insurance Commissions)

2520—Herff-Jones Company
"Badge of Service" for President, Jas.
E. Paullin 3.82

2521—L. F. Livingston, Postmaster
Postage 30.00

2522—Alliance Printing Company
Printing and mailing 1975 copies of
the March, 1936, issue of the JOUR-
NAL 323.40

2523—Mrs. G. R. Sims
Compiling data in questionnaires for
Medical Economic Survey 50.00

2524—L. F. Livingston, Postmaster
Postage (Mailing JOURNAL $9.50—
notices to delinquent and former mem-
bers, $15.00) 30.00

2525—J. A. Redfearn, M.D.
Expenses incurred as Councilor for the
Second District 25.00

2526—Empire Letter Shop
Three sets of letters multigraphed with
signature of Dr. Jas. E. Paullin,
President; one to doctors in counties
where there were no organizations; one
to secretaries of county societies and
Councilors; one to county societies in
reference to Medical Defense and collection of dues: 750 letters to all
delinquent and former members with
names of Dr. J. W. Daniel and Dr.
Wm. R. Dancy, Past Presidents, inviting them to Savannah, with note
from Secretary-Treasurer in reference
to dues; letters for county secretaries
enclosing Delegate's Credentials 16.50

2527—Southern Bell Telephone & Telegraph
Company
Telephone account to March, 21, 1936   6.15

2528—Bryan, Middlebrooks & Carter, Attys.
Attorneys' fee for B. P. Gaillard, Jr.,
and W. P. Whelchel in suit of Irvin
vs. Dr. W. A. Palmour, Gainesville . 100.00

2529—Southern Press Clipping Bureau
News clippings for February a n d
March, 1936 .... 10.00
2530—Southern Typewriter Company
Repairs on typewriter............ 6.00
2531—Service Engraving Company
Cuts for the JOURNAL and repairs on
electros for advertisers........... 9.29
2532—Alliance Printing Company
500 Extra copies of the March, 1936,
issue of the JOURNAL $40.00—less
error on Merck and Company's ad.. 22.00
2533—Edgar D. Shanks, M.D.
Salary for March, 1936, as Secretary-
Treasurer 150.00
2534—H. L. Rowe
Salary for March, 1936, as Executive
Secretary 175.00
2535—L. F. Livingston, Postmaster
Postage 30.00
2536—Miss Annie Jacks
Commission on advertising orders... 25.75
May 20, 1935: Check on Dr. Laetus
Sanders, Commerce, returned unpaid
and paid later............... 6.00
May 20, 1936: Check J. Weyman
Davis, Athens, returned unpaid and
charged to balance to credit of his
account as Secretary-Treasurer of the
Clarke County Medical Society... 15.00
April 2, 1936: Check Ware County
Medical Society post-dated and re-
turned unpaid and paid later..... 6.00
Exchange deducted by the Fulton
National Bank on non-par checks. 9.36

Total disbursements $13,051.89

CASE FINDING METHODS FOR DIAGNOSIS OF
TUBERCULOSIS

According to J. Burns Amberson, Jr., New York
(Journal A. M. A., July 25, 1936), pulmonary tuberculosis remains the first cause of death in young adults.
From 60 to 70 per cent of tuberculosis people, even
intelligent ones, are unaware of symptoms of serious
disease until the pulmonary lesions are moderately or
far advanced. Most cases will not be diagnosed early
except by case finding methods based on a familiarity
with the characteristics of tuberculosis as a community
disease as well as an individaul lesion. The simplest
and most effective method of case finding consists of
x-ray surveys of the chests of selected susceptible groups,
in some instances with preliminary tuberculin testing.
In the yield of cases from such surveys, the proportion
found in the earliest stage is 70 per cent or more. If
the cases found are skilfully studied and promptly and
properly treated, when necessary, the accomplishment
of actual care of the disease and prevention of spread
of the infection to others exceeds that of any other
known methods.

PRESENTATION OF THE "BADGE OF
SERVICE" TO THE PRESIDENT,
JAMES E. PAULLIN*

F. PHINIZY CALHOUN, M.D.
Atlanta

I am proud and deeply honored that the
opportunity has been given me tonight to
say publicly what has been in my heart for
a long time, to a man who has been a true
friend to my family and to me, ever since
we both began the practice of medicine in
Atlanta.

It has been said that a sound student is
of more value to a state than a half dozen
grain elevators or a new transcontinental railroad.

This statement, still true, can be para-
phrased by saying that a doctor who keeps
abreast of the time by hard study and application, who unselfishly devotes himself to
the promotion of his profession and of humanity, who considers the profession of medicine as a consecrated calling, and who in civil
life feels that it is his duty to take some part
and to vote regularly and conscientiously, is
an asset to his state. Such is the man about
whom I speak. Were there more like him,
the honor and dignity of our profession
would reach its height, its influence would be
greater, and there would be reflected into the
minds of most citizens a higher regard for
good government, good office holders and
good leadership. How badly are they needed!

But first listen to the accomplishments of
this man:

He was born in Fort Gaines, Georgia, in
1881, and if the records are straight, he attended school five days in the week from eight
o'clock in the morning until four o'clock in
the afternoon, and on Saturdays his chief
duty was to weed the garden.

He graduated from Mercer University in
1900 with the degree of Bachelor of Arts,
and in medicine from The Johns Hopkins
Medical School in 1905. He received his hospital training and was pathologist at the

*Presentation of the "Badge of Service" to the President
before the Medical Association of Georgia, Savannah, April 22,
1936.

oratory methods is well known. He did the
first Wassermann test for syphilis in the
State. He was the first to recognize and report typhus fever in the South. His early
work on diabetes attracted attention, and he
gave the first dose of insulin in Georgia. From
the beginning of his teaching, he stressed the
importance of accurate histories, the correlation of one's own laboratory work with
clinical findings and the follow up of autop-
sies. His original investigations on the subjects of coronary disease, arterial hypertension
and diabetes are monumental achievements,
and his papers on these subjects are still
quoted in the literature.

Carlyle said, "Science is as deep as etern-
ity; speech is as shallow as time." My words
will soon be forgotten but his influence in
this Association will be felt beyond this generation.

His success as a practitioner of medicine has
not altogether been due to his erudition and
fine personality, but to his gentleness and
tenderness, and to his honesty and fair dealing
with his patients. Of a kindly disposition and
considerate of his fellow man; affable and
with a born ability to make and keep friends;
calm on the surface but with a courageous
display of Irish blood and loving a good
fight when it is necessary; helpful and never
shirking duty; a dutiful son, a firstclass husband and a devoted father, are some of the
many fine qualities of the man who is your
leader.

He must have known of the epitaph on the
tomb of Kiser Willhelm der Grosser, and accepted it as his motto—"I have no time to be
tired." Only his family and immediate
friends appreciate the tremendous kinetic
drive under which he daily works. Indeed,
I become fatigued when I learn of his weekly
program.

A great physician and philosopher, in his
farewell address to the physicians of Canada
and America, once said that he had three personal ideals; one, to do the day's work and
not bother about tomorrow; the second, to
act the Golden Rule towards his professional
brother and to his patients committed to his
care; and third, to cultivate such a measure
of equanimity as would enable him to bear
success with humility, the affection of his

friends without pride, and to be ready when the day of sorrow and grief came to meet it with courage befitting a man. These were the ideals of William Osler, and the man about whom I speak was one of his last students. I have often listened to him talk about that great physician with admiration and affection, for he was his model.

Early he hitched his wagon to this brilliant star, and by precept and example he has tried his level best to follow.

Still young and ambitious, I prophesy that other nation-wide honors will justly come to him.

With this background of achievement and the personal qualities which I have inadequately described, is there any wonder that his friends drafted him and this Association sought out this man to elect him President?

James Edgar Paullin, I am happy to present to you the President's "Badge of Service" of the Medical Association of Georgia.

ACCEPTANCE OF THE "BADGE OF SERVICE" BY THE PRESIDENT*

JAMES E. PAULLIN, M.D.
Atlanta

Friends and Distinguished Guests:

I am embarrassed beyond words. There is this to be said, that I can still eat three meals a day, sleep eight hours at night, and accept bountifully of Savannah's hospitality.

The things which Dr. Calhoun, in the magnanimity of his spirit, has said concerning my feeble efforts toward the advancement of medicine, are due to the inspiration which has come to me in years past from the wonderful ideals, the wonderful example of those who have gone on before us in the practice of medicine. I simply carry on the traditions of that wonderful galaxy of individuals who have participated in the advancement of medicine and the individuals who stand for those things which are for the public good.

Dr. Calhoun, I thank you for your kind remarks, for your prejudiced remarks, and I assure you I only wish that I were worthy of what you have said.

*Acceptance of the "Badge of Service" before the Medical Association of Georgia, Savannah, April 22, 1936.

The Anatomic Diagnosis Was, Syphilitic Aortitis
Aneurysm of Abdominal Aorta with Rupture

DR. V. P. SYDENSTRICKER: The necropsy findings came as a surprise to the clinical group; we failed to give syphilis its due consideration in the presence of what seemed acute inflammatory disease. It is enlightening to see the extent to which bone erosion can go without pain: the posterior wall of this man's aneurysm was formed by the deeply eroded lumbar vertebrae, this was an old process certainly of many months' duration. Actual rupture took place three weeks ago with the production of the large false aneurysm which proved so puzzling to us. It is remarkable that the extensive infiltration of the left abdominal wall gave no more signs. The secondary rupture into the peritoneum caused death from shock more than from actual loss of blood.

AMERICAN MEDICAL DIRECTORY

The new Fourteenth Edition of the American Medical Directory has just been published by the Biographical Department of the American Medical Association and contains accurate information in regard to 183,312 physicians and 7,200 hospitals. It separates the legally qualified practitioners from many other varieties of "doctors."

The facts given about each physician are abbreviated and condensed in an accessible plan and contains more data than would ordinarily be given in many times the space.

The Directory is geographically arranged with all states, cities, and names of physicians listed alphabetically.

More than 7,200 hospitals and sanatoriums are listed. The capacity and official rating of each institution is shown.

The Directory contains: National and Interstate Information, Directory of Physicians and Hospitals, Index of Physicians; list of American Physicians in Foreign Countries, State and County Health Officers, Medical Journals, and a Complete Alphabetical Index of All Physicians.

It would be difficult to estimate the value of the Directory. With a copy in your office, you have authentic information in reference to any physician or hospital in the United States, its possessions, and Canada. To own a copy of the new Fourteenth Edition of the American Medical Directory, may increase your pride in the profession to which you belong and enhance your own self esteem.

THE JOURNAL
OF THE
MEDICAL ASSOCIATION OF GEORGIA
Devoted to the Welfare of the Medical Association of Georgia

478 Peachtree Street, N.E., Atlanta, Ga.

AUGUST, 1936

PROTAMINE INSULINATE*

The announcement some six months ago of H. C. Hagedorn and N. B. Krarup from The Steno Memorial Hospital, Copenhagen, of the discovery of a compound of insulin hydrochloride with protein which is more slowly absorbed and consequently slower in its action than regular insulin, has stimulated further interest in the treatment of diabetes mellitus. The new insulin was soon made available for clinical investigation in this country to a group of workers interested in diabetes.

The ideal treatment hoped for and sought after for patients suffering with diabetes mellitus is a procedure which will not only keep the urine sugar free but at the same time will prevent wide fluctuations in the blood sugar. It has been known for many years that even in patients with mild diabetes there is, within a twenty-four hour period, marked variations in the blood sugar; consequently with the average diabetic, even though the urine remains sugar free during a twenty-four hour period, the blood sugar level is far from normal. Should this diabetic's condition be of sufficient severity to require insulin for control of the glycosuria, then the blood sugar fluctuations would vary even more. In an attempt to control the severe forms of diabetes it frequently is necessary to administer three, four or more doses of insulin within twenty-four hours to keep the urine sugar free. Such a procedure is made necessary because of the fact that when insulin is injected subcutaneously it is rapidly absorbed and is rapid in its action. Soon after the administration of insulin the blood sugar declines and the "peak effect" of the dose is reached within five or six hours. Should a continuous insulin effect be desired it becomes necessary to give frequent doses of insulin to accomplish complete control of the glycosuria and hyperglycemia.

*Investigations which have been carried on by me with this product have been made possible by the Eli Lilly Company, Indianapolis, and by E. R. Squibb Company of New York.

The study of an hourly blood sugar curve from a moderately severe diabetic receiving insulin will show striking variations, or "peak effect" due to the rapid action of insulin.

With protamine insulin the story is quite different: this product when injected subcutaneously is more slowly absorbed and its action is greatly prolonged. In other words, it more nearly approaches the normal physiologic action of the pancreas in furnishing a constant supply of insulin to the body thereby avoiding "peak effects." So far the observations of quite a few physicians interested in diabetes have confirmed these expectations. It has been demonstrated in patients with mild diabetes that it is possible to keep them sugar free and with practically a normal blood sugar on one dose of protamine insulinate. It is necessary to supplement this with a small dose of regular insulin which, in some patients, may be given at the same time as the protamine insulinate but injected into a different location. With severe cases it has been found possible to keep the patient sugar free by giving two doses of protamine insulinate each day, one in the early morning and one in the late evening.

The original protamine insulinate was made by precipitating insulin hydrochloride with a buffered protein derived from the rainbow trout. At the present time a protamine compound containing calcium and another containing zinc are seemingly more efficacious than the product originally used. When the buffered solution is added to the insulin a whitish precipitate is formed which, when injected into the subcutaneous tissue, is more slowly absorbed.

This wonderful remedy is most useful in controlling the glycosuria and in preventing hypoglycemic reactions, particularly in children and young adults. In times past it has been most difficult to keep children sugar free and with a normal blood sugar, and avoid frequent hypoglycemic reactions. With the new insulin, although our experience still is not sufficient to warrant dogmatic conclusions, it would seem that this difficulty is greatly minimized.

It is needless to point out the advantages which will occur to the metabolism of a diabetic patient when the blood sugar is kept within the limits of normal; suffice it to say,

graduate courses. It is not presumed that such courses could be made sufficiently comprehensive to qualify one for the management of conditions arising in this field. It would seem feasable, however, that such instruction might include the more common diseases and the practical phases of diagnostic interest.

For example, otitis media in its several forms constitutes a malady of the utmost frequency and gravest importance. As a consequence of it, hearing is often impaired or lost, and life itself may be sacrificed by reason of its complications. Indeed, acute inflammatory aural disease so commonly presents infection of the mastoid bone that every occurrence of this affection should be regarded as potential mastoiditis. Certainly, a disability of this magnitude should be accorded instant recognition and prompt effort toward its alleviation. With improved armamentarium and better understanding, the sufferer is entitled to this type of effective service.

It is universally conceded that abnormal tonsils and adenoids are not conducive to good health. By many it is thought that adenoids are capable of more mischief during the early years of life than are the tonsils. At any rate, only those who have stirred themselves to special inquiry in this respect does full appreciation of the pathologic significance of these lymphoid infections and hypertrophies seem evident. All too frequently parents are advised by their physicians to postpone surgical interference with these structures until the patient attains more age. Such counsel may be justified as regards tonsils, but is manifestly pernicious in the proper disposition of adenoids. Through their effectiveness in occluding the pharyngeal orifices of the eustachian tubes, adenoids are a most prolific source in the causation of deafness, and should be removed at any time when it is suspected that auditory aeration is restricted by their presence. It is estimated that 10 per cent of all school children are affected with more or less impairment of hearing. Moreover, evidence undoubtedly demonstrates that a very large percentage of auditory difficulties experienced in adolescence began in childhood because of nasopharyngeal abnormalities. While this is appalling, there is reason for optimism in future generations because of present-day methods of caring for pharyngeal and otologic disturbances. In deafness, as in many other situations, prevention is better than cure.

From an ophthalmologic viewpoint, much injury has been inflicted because of a lack of understanding concerning certain ocular manifestations, particularly iritis and glaucoma, and of the remedial agents employed. The principles in the treatment of iritis being directly opposed to that of glaucoma, the misapplication of drugs unhappily terminates in blindness. The same, of course, applies to glaucoma as regards iritic involvement. It is obvious, therefore, that in conditions of such momentous issue extreme caution must be practiced. While it is urgently necessary that the treatment of these maladies be reserved for ophthalmologists, it is very desirable that the general consultant be informed concerning them. In this and other respects, he can be of much help.

S. J. LEWIS, M.D.

MENTAL HYGIENE IN GEORGIA

The present-day mental hygiene movement started when Mr. Clifford Beers recovered after being confined in mental hospitals. His disclosures of many abuses prevalent led to the founding of the National Committee for Mental Hygiene. This instituted nationwide reforms and a shift from custodial care in "asylums" to treatment in "hospitals." Stress on treatment led to intensive study of cause. Causes so frequently start in childhood, therefore, clinics were set up and Child Guidance and Parent-Education have taken a leading role in prevention. From these experiences evolved a mental hygiene philosophy: to handle situations and individuals on the basis of motives and causes back of behavior rather than behavior itself.

Georgia has no mental hygiene program. A strong department is sorely needed to administer such a program. Our commitment laws are archaic, placing commitment of the mentally sick in the same category as trial and sentencing of criminals. No mental hygiene program can succeed until these laws are changed. Our well-staffed State Hospital is overcrowded and dozens of sick are confined in jails. Hospitals and wards should be maintained in large centers to relieve the load of acute cases. The institution for feebleminded in Gracewood is cluttered with untrainables.

cancer. Likewise that cancer never develops
from a healthy area but always from some
diseased spot and particularly if this diseased
area is irritated. Of all organs of the body
the skin receives the greatest amount of accident and injury. It is the intermediary between the body proper and the outside world.
Throughout life it is continuously the object
of blows, cuts, bruises and abrasions and is
exposed to all the extremes of cold and heat.
It is here that cancer should and does find a
most fertile soil. The weather-beaten skin
tends to become senile at the age of forty
or under. It dries out, becomes hard and
wrinkled and begins to develop keratoses.
Ten per cent of these keratotic spots will
become cancerous. Seborrhoeic warts, moles,
scars either from trauma or from the healing of burns or previous ulcers, discharging
sinuses, pigmentations,—any or all of these
lesions are definitely pre-cancerous. Pigmented
moles and naevi may give rise to melanoma,
the most malignant of all neoplasms. Each
and every one of these conditions can be cured
or removed. Surely our methods of prevention will find their greatest scope in lesions
of the skin.

The diagnosis of skin cancer is, as a rule,
easy. Occurring mostly in middle aged or
older people, developing always on some pre-
cancerous base and presenting the two cardinal
symptoms of *induration* and *ulceration*, it is
recognized most readily. In case of doubt
biopsy is easily performed.

The prognosis in cancer of the skin depends on the type of growth, its size and
duration and the efficiency of the treatment
applied.

Of all cancers of the body, is it not a remarkable thing that skin cancer should be
so prevalent and that it should continue to
kill so many people? In plain view where
it can be seen daily, its steady advance under
constant observation, always developing from
some unhealthy place that was not cancer in
the beginning, it is a sad commentary on the
intelligence of our people that the cancer
problem, as applied to the skin, should be
a problem at all. *Early cancer should be
curable in a high percentage of cases. The
neglected cancer pushes the patient inevitably
towards his grave.*

G. T. BERNARD, M.D.

WOMAN'S AUXILIARY

OFFICERS, 1936-1937

President—Mrs. Wm. R. Dancy, Savannah.
President-Elect—Mrs. Ralph H. Chaney, Augusta.
First Vice-President—Mrs. B. H. Minchew, Waycross.
Second Vice-President—Mrs. Clarence L. Ayers, Toccoa.
Third Vice-President—Mrs. J. A. Redfearn, Albany.

Recording Secretary—Mrs. Warren A. Coleman, Eastman.
Corresponding Secretary—Mrs. Lee Howard, Savannah.
Treasurer—Mrs. W. A. Selman, Atlanta.
Historian—Mrs. Grady N. Coker, Canton.
Parliamentarian—Mrs. John E. Penland, Waycross.

COMMITTEE CHAIRMEN

Student Loan Fund
Mrs. Robert C. Pendergrass, Americus.
Health Films
Mrs. A. J. Mooney, Statesboro.
Public Relations
Mrs. Wallace Bazemore, Macon
Doctors' Day
Mrs. Ernest R. Harris, Winder.

Legislation
Mrs. Dan Y. Sage, 47 Inman Circle, Atlanta.
Press and Publicity
Mrs. J. Harry Rogers, 134 Huntington Rd., Atlanta.
Research in Romance of Medicine
Mrs. D. N. Thompson, Elberton.
Jane Todd Crawford Memorial.
Mrs. Eustace A. Allen, 18 Collier Rd., Atlanta.

PROGRAM FOR YEAR'S WORK

Mrs. William R. Dancy, President of the Auxiliary, has compiled the following aims for the year's work, which were approved by the Advisory Committee:

1. To secure an Advisory Committee or a Councilor for each county and district Auxiliary and to be guided in all State activities by the Advisory Committee of the Medical Association of Georgia. Without their sanction, no changes are to be made in the educational program.

2. For county and district Auxiliaries that have not done so, to file copies of their Constitutions and By-Laws with the State Auxiliary.

3. In each County Auxiliary to have, if feasible, Chairmen corresponding to the State, Southern, and National Auxiliaries.

Organization, Health Education, Public Relations, Hygeia, Press and Publicity, Historian, Student Loan Fund, Health Films, Legislation, Doctor's Day, Research in Romance of Medicine, Jane Todd Crawford Memorial.

4. To contribute generously to the Student Loan Fund, in order that a sufficient capital sum may be promptly raised, the interest from which is to be used to educate Georgia students in Georgia medical schools. These students are limited to the families of Georgia physicians. This objective has been the great incentive, which has moulded the State Auxiliary into a functioning unit; and it should be kept as our principal objective. It is planned to instruct the Student Loan Committee to carry out plans for building up this principal sum.

5. To contribute to the Health Library and provide this form of education for Auxiliaries and for the public.

6. To assist in the entertainment at county, district, and State meetings, and promote unity and friendliness through social contact. This is conceded to be one of our most important functions. It is our duty to encourage and preserve fellowship.

7. To present the health education program outlined for us by the Medical Association of Georgia, to all lay organizations; the Medical Association and local societies to appoint the speakers, the Auxiliary to supply approved educational material. The educational scope of the Auxiliary includes programs on heart disease, cancer, tuberculosis, and maternal care, with certain brief three minute talks on other phases of health. These three minute talks are available through local health education chairmen. These may be used as monthly topics or radio talks. To read them carefully until familiar with them.

8. To increase our subscriptions to Hygeia, the Health Magazine published by the American Medical Association.

9. To accept chairmanships of health and public welfare in other organizations, or any office that will advance the work of the Auxiliary.

10. To read the news letters and the Auxiliary pages of the Journal of the Medical Association of Georgia, and the same in the Southern Medical Association and American Medical Association Journals. To contribute to them and send items of interest to district and State Scrapbook Chairmen.

11. To re-enlist former members and secure the membership of every eligible wife by an active membership campaign.

12. To cooperate with the recommendations of the Southern and American Medical Auxiliaries.

13. To observe March 30th, as Doctor's Day. On this day to have programs or suitable exercises honoring the men who have dedicated their services to the welfare of hu-

Martin, Mrs. Luther A. DeLoach, Mrs. S.
Elliott Wilson, Mrs. A. A. Morrison, Jr.,
Mrs. Herman Hesse, Mrs. R. E. Graham,
Mrs. H. H. McGee, Mrs. Walter E. Brown,
Mrs. J. S. Bolten, Mrs. C. Y. Bailey, Mrs.
Charles Usher, Mrs. G. T. Olmstead, Mrs.
E. S. Osborne, Mrs. W. H. Myers, Mrs. L.
W. Williams, Mrs. V. H. Bassett, Mrs. H.
J. Morrison, Sr., Mrs. Harry M. Kandel,
Mrs. C. G. Redmond, and Mrs. Julian K.
Quattlebaum.

Committee Chairmen

The following chairmen for the First District have been appointed by Mrs. William
R. Dancy, State President:

Health Education, Mrs. J. C. Metts, Savannah; Public Relations, Mrs. W. E. Simmons, Metter; Hygeia, Mrs. Luther A. DeLoach, Savannah; Press and Publicity, Mrs.
G. Hugo Johnson, Savannah; Legislation,
Mrs. J. Wallace Daniel, Claxton; Student
Loan Fund, Mrs. Lee Howard, Savannah;
Health Film, Mrs. A. J. Mooney, Statesboro;
Doctors' Day, Mrs. William H. Myers, Savannah; Research in Romance of Medicine,
Mrs. J. E. Mercer, Vidalia; and Jane Todd
Crawford Memorial, Mrs. Q. A. Mulkey,
Millen.

BENZEDRINE SULFATE AND ITS VALUE IN SPASM OF GASTRO-INTESTINAL TRACT

Abraham Myerson and Max Ritvo, Boston (*Journal
A. M. A.*, July 4, 1936), have found benzedrine sulfate, a sympathicomimetic drug, to be of great value
in diminishing or abolishing spasm of the gastro-intestinal tract. This effect is observed when the spasm
is due to whatever cause, such as unpleasant emotion,
organic disease of the gastro-intestinal tract, and reflex
spasm due to disease elsewhere in the body. This effect
greatly facilitates the roentgen study of the gastro-intestinal tract, makes differential diagnosis between
functional and organic spasm more certain and gives
better visualization of organic lesions. The effect is
almost immediate and is, on the whole, unattended
with any side effects of importance. Clinically it has
been found useful in relaxing spasm, such as is found
in spastic colitis and pyloric spasm, and this has been
of therapeutic benefit to the patient. The dosage for
the average patient is 30 mg. of benzedrine sulfate
orally; very stout patients may require 40 mg., while
thin and very young individuals are given from 10 to
20 mg. Unpleasant effects may occur in a very small
number of cases and consist of chilly sensations, flushing, diarrhea and general malaise. The authors have
administered the drug to more than 200 patients and
in only one instance was there a severe reaction. There
may be sleeplessness or restlessness during the following
night if the drug is administered late in the afternoon.
The drug causes moderate rise in blood pressure (about
20 to 50 mg. of mercury) and therefore it should be
used with caution in the presence of severe cardiac
disease.

GEORGIA DEPARTMENT OF PUBLIC HEALTH

T. F. ABERCROMBIE, M.D., *Director*

"A COOPERATIVE HEALTH PROGRAM

There has always been close cooperation between the Georgia Department of Public Health and the medical profession of this State. Any public health benefits that have come to the people of Georgia are, to a very large extent, due to the pleasant relationship existing between those specializing in public health and those engaged in the practice of medicine.

One result of this spirit of cooperation was the appointment by the Medical Association of Georgia of an Advisory Committee to the State Board of Health. This Committee formulated certain policies for the operation of county health departments, which were submitted to the Association and adopted by it. So far as has been ascertained, no other state medical association has done this. Georgia is leading the way to greater accomplishments in the field of public health.

The policies adopted follow:

(1) *Control of Preventable Diseases*—It is the proper function of a public health department to use every known scientific means for the prevention of disease, especially the communicable or infectious diseases. This is to be done by educational campaigns, isolation and quarantine, sanitation, immunization, and sterilization of carriers by drugs and other measures.

The department should see that all laws, ordinances and regulations governing communicable diseases are duly carried out.

While the diagnosis of a regularly licensed physician is usually accepted without question, the health officer has the right to confirm or change it, as the facts justify. Diagnoses of others than physicians will not be accepted without investigation.

Visits may be made for the purpose of supervision, isolation, disinfection or release, in the judgment of the health officer. Visits for any other purpose, such as giving bedside care and instructing other members of the family on this subject, will be made only with the consent of the attending physician.

It shall be the duty of the health officer to promote immunization of all persons who have been or might become exposed to smallpox, diphtheria, typhoid fever and other infectious or communicable diseases for which an immunizing agent may be of definite value in their prevention. It is desirable that these agencies be administered by the family phy-

sician. However, the prevention of such diseases is the duty of the health officer, under the direction of the board of health. The health officer is required to enforce the laws and regulations set up by statute acts.

(2) *Child Hygiene* — One-fifth of all deaths of all ages occur in persons under one year of age, and one-third under five years of age. The average age at death has been raised largely by saving the lives of children. Therefore, it is an important function of the public health department to promote child hygiene, beginning with prenatal care. The per cent of births attended by midwives ranges from 10 to 70 per cent in different localities. It is, therefore, an important function of the health department to instruct and supervise midwives, and to limit their practice in accordance with recognized standards.

(a) *Prenatal*—It is a proper function of the health department to contact and instruct expectant mothers, to teach them the importance of early and regular medical supervision by a physician, and to assist the physician in giving the expectant mother proper instruction in the hygiene of pregnancy; also, to stress the necessity for regular physical examination by the physician, including urinalysis, blood pressure readings, etc., and to give instruction concerning the danger signs occurring during pregnancy.

In those cases that will use a midwife, a closer supervision by the health department may be allowed, to include regular check-up by the health officer with regard to blood pressure, kidneys, weight and danger signs. In no case shall the health officer or nurse prescribe any treatment, but if abnormal conditions are found or suspected, the patient is to be referred to her physician; she and the midwife are to be notified that such case should have attention by a physician. A postnatal examination by the physician should be advised in all cases.

(b) *Infant and Preschool*—It is the function of the health department to assist the attending physician in giving instructions as to the general care of infants, to demonstrate baths, and see that his directions as to these and the diet are properly carried out. The health department shall promote regular physical examination of infants and preschool children by a physician, and when defects are found, do such follow-up work as will secure the needed correction.

(c) *Schools and School Children*—The health officer shall make an annual examina-

NEWS ITEMS

The First District Medical Society met at Hotel Savannah, Savannah, July 15th. Titles of papers on the scientific program were: *First Aid Treatment of Fractures*, Dr. Laurence B. Dunn, Savannah; *The Use of Protamine Insulin in the Treatment of Diabetes*, Dr. Harold Bowcock, Atlanta; *Back Injuries Other Than Fractures*, Dr. Geo. A. Traylor, Augusta, President-Elect of the Association; *Some Practical Points About X-Ray Therapy*, Dr. Wm. A. Cole, Savannah; *Address*, Dr. B. H. Minchew, Waycross, President of the Association; *The Autonomic Nervous System in Its Relation to Clinical Medicine*, Dr. Cleveland Thompson, Millen; *Plasma Proteins in Various Forms of Kidney Lesions*, Dr. John W. Daniel, Savannah. Program Committee: Dr. Lee Howard, Dr. A. A. Morrison, and Dr. H. L. Levington. Entertainment Committee: Dr. Lee Howard, Dr. J. C. Metts, and Dr. Julian K. Quattlebaum.

Dr. H. B. Jenkins, formerly of Thomasville and recently of Fort Barrancas, Florida, has moved to Donalsonville and opened offices for the practice of medicine.

Dr. W. K. Stewart, formerly of Donalsonville, has moved to Damascus. Dr. Stewart is quoted in the Donalsonville, Ga., News, as follows: "The cordial reception extended by the people of Donalsonville is appreciated, and the friendships developed while here are treasured."

Dr. Guy G. Lunsford, Atlanta, Director of County Health Work for the State Board of Health, spoke at a luncheon of the Kiwanis Club at the Ansley Hotel, Atlanta, on *Activities of the State Board of Health*, July 7th.

Members of the Cherokee County Medical Society entertained Dr. F. B. Murphy, Canton, at a fish fry at Pettit's Lake, on June 29th. Dr. Murphy has been associated with Dr. N. J. Coker and Dr. Grady N. Coker, Canton, for seven years in the practice of medicine. He has removed to his former home in West Virginia.

The Secretary-Treasurer has just had inquiries for two physicians for different locations, also one drug clerk. If interested write the office of the Association.

The Coffee County Medical Society met at Douglas June 30th. Titles of papers on the program were: *Anatomy of the Face*, L. Davis, D.D.S.; *Treatment of Facial Injuries*, Dr. W. A. Sibbett, Douglas. Dr. Alton M. Johnson, Valdosta, will speak at the meeting to be held on August 25th on *Pylorospasm in Infancy*. At the September 29th meeting, Dr. Sage Harper, Wray, will speak on *The Management of Fractures*. At the December 29th meeting. Dr. J. G. Crovatt, Douglas, will discuss *Dietary Treatment of Diabetes*; Dr. B. O. Quillian, Douglas, *Other Measures in the Treatment of Diabetes*.

Dr. M. K. Bailey announces the association of Dr. Charles A. Eberhart with him in the practice of urology. Offices located at 1106 Medical Arts Building, Atlanta.

The Fulton County Medical Society met at the Academy of Medicine, Atlanta, July 16th. Dr. E. D. Highsmith reported cases, *The Necessity of Follow-Up Work on Plastic Surgery of the Face;* Dr. Jack C. Norris, clinical talk, *Demonstration of New Test (Lewis Test) for Quick Diagnosis of Syphilis;* Dr. Shelley C. Davis read a paper, *The Chronically Diseased Cervix as a Focal Point of Infection.* The discussion was led by Dr. Edgar H. Greene, Dr. Mark S. Dougherty, and Dr. Lewis M. Smith.

New officers of the Chattahoochee Valley Medical Association elected at the close of its meeting at Radium Springs, Albany, July 15th were: Dr. Marion T. Davidson, Birmingham, Ala., President; Dr. Edgar H. Greene, Atlanta, First Vice-President; Dr. Clayton E. Royce, Jacksonville, Fla., Second Vice-President; Dr. Frank K. Boland, Atlanta, Secretary-Treasurer. Dr. C. W. Roberts, Atlanta, is member of the Council from Georgia.

Dr. C. W. Roberts, Atlanta, spoke before a meeting of the Lions Club at the Henry Grady Hotel, Atlanta, July 13th on *Doctors and Hospitals—an Atlanta asset.*

Dr. and Mrs. W. W. Turner, Nashville, entertained the members of the South Georgia Medical Society at a barbecue at their home on July 14th. The Society is composed of the counties of Berrien, Clinch, Cook, Echols, Lanier and Lowndes. The scientific meeting of the Society was held at the Nashville Woman's Club House. Dr. J. R. Paulk, Moultrie, read a paper on the *Use of the Bronchoscope with Report of Cases.* The discussion was led by Dr. A. M. Johnson and Dr. T. H. Smith, both of Valdosta.

Awards to scientific exhibitors for the best displays in the scientific exhibit at Savannah during the annual session, April 21-24, 1936, were: first, Grady Hospital, Atlanta, *Thyroids;* second, Dr. Wm. G. Hamm, Atlanta, *Plastic Surgery;* third, Dr. Walter A. Stultz, Augusta, *Transplantation of Organs.* Exhibitors to receive honorable mention were: Dr. V. P. Sydenstricker, Augusta, *Blood Pictures,* and Cancer Commission of the Association, *Cancer.*

The Southern Medical Association (home office Empire Building, Birmingham, Ala.) will hold its thirtieth annual meeting in Baltimore, Maryland, November 17-20, 1936. Georgia physicians who are members of the Council and various sections of the Association are: Council—Dr. Edgar G. Ballenger, Atlanta. Section on Pediatrics—Dr. M. Hines Roberts, Atlanta, Chairman. Section on Pathology—Dr. Roy R. Kracke, Emory University, Secretary. Section on Dermatology and Syphilology—Dr. Jack W. Jones, Atlanta, Chairman. Section on Railway Surgery—Dr. J. W. Palmer, Ailey, Vice-Chairman. Section on Ophthalmology and Otolaryngology—Dr. Grady E. Clay, Atlanta, Vice-Chairman. Section on Medical Education—Dr. Russell H. Oppenheimer, Emory University, Vice-Chairman. Allergy Clinic and Round Table—Dr. Hal M. Davison, Atlanta, Chairman.

Dr. Bernard McH. Cline announces the association of Dr. James Laurence Jennings with him in the treatment of diseases of the eye, ear, nose and throat. Offices are located at 400-01-02 Grand Theater Building, Atlanta.

If interested in what is claimed to be an excellent location for a practicing physician, write the Secretary-Treasurer.

Dr. Chevalier Jackson, of Philadelphia, has accepted an invitation to deliver an initial lecture in the Jonte Equen Memorial Lectureship in ear, nose and throat, the date and subject to be announced at a subsequent time. Dr. Jackson is an outstanding authority in the field of bronchoscopy and is internationally known. This lecture is given under the auspices of the Fulton County Medical Society and a general invitation to attend is extended to the medical profession.

Dr. G. A. Holloway announces the opening of his offices at 512 Grand Theater Building, Atlanta. His practice will be general medicine and surgery.

The Fulton County Medical Society met at the Academy of Medicine, Atlanta, August 6th. Dr. Everett A. Bancker, Jr., reported a case, *Treatment of Hypertension with Alloton;* Dr. Hugh Cochran made a clinical talk, *Brain Injuries;* Dr. J. Gaston Gay read a paper entitled *Present Status of Surgery of Thyroid in Children.* The Discussion was led by Dr. L. Minor Blackford, Dr. Floyd W. McRae and Dr. Ben H. Clifton.

Dr. Joseph Yampolsky, Atlanta, recently addressed the Griffin Exchange Club on the subject of *Romance of Syphilis,* which was well received by a large audience composed of laymen, dentists and physicians.

The Fourth District Medical Society met at Warm Springs, August 10th. Titles of papers on the scientific program were: *Handling of Accidents Occurring During the Administration of Anesthesia,* Dr. Wilmer Baker, New Orleans, La.; *The Principles of Plastic Surgery,* Dr. Neal Owens, New Orleans, La.; *Cardiac Pain,* Dr. L. Minor Blackford, Atlanta; *The Immediate Care of Fractures,* Dr. Frank K. Boland, Atlanta; *Presentation of Cases* by members of the Society.

OBITUARY

Dr. James Madison Baird, Columbus; member; Kentucky School of Medicine, Louisville, Ky., 1892; aged 67; died at a private hospital in Atlanta on July 10, 1936. He was born in Daviess County, Kentucky. After he graduated in medicine and practiced for a few years, he went to Europe and studied pediatrics, and again later studied in Europe and limited his practice to diseases of the eye, ear, nose and throat. Dr. Baird was a member of the State Board of Medical Examiners

The author has approached a big job and one that was greatly needed in the field of mycology. He has made a splendid attempt to classify various fungi so that investigators in the future will be better able to recognize the parasites they may encounter. In the past *utter confusion reigned supreme* in this regard.

Therefore, the book is one of monumental importance and will be received with great appreciation by the mycologist and research workers in the field of botany and medicine.

JACK C. NORRIS, M.D.

Exophthalmic Goiter and Its Medical Treatment. By Israel Bram, M.D., Medical Director, Bram Institute, Upland, Pa. With a foreword by R. G. Hoskins, Ph.D., M.D. Second Edition. Cloth. Price, $6.00. Pp. 456, with 79 illustrations. St. Louis: The C. V. Mosby Co., 1936.

In spite of the strong partisan viewpoint expressed by the author of this splendid monograph, it immediately commands the attention of internist and surgeon alike. The internist will welcome such a clear, forceful presentation of "his side" of the controversy, while the surgeon must consider carefully the methods and results of one who admittedly finds no place for their services. A personal experience with over 5000 cases certainly enables him to speak with authority, and it behooves all of us to listen well to what he has to say.

He has revived the ancient argument as to whether the "toxicity" that accompanies the so-called toxic adenoma is one and the same with Graves' Disease, and presents many strong points in favor of the two being separate and distinct disease conditions. These are based upon clinical impressions almost entirely without much consideration of the pathological picture presented by each, and no mention is made of some rather exhaustive studies that have been made upon a comparison on this basis.

The text is well written, and the large type is easy to read. The illustrations are rather small, somewhat crowded in places and are none too numerous.

D. HENRY POER, M.D.

Passive Vascular Exercises and the Conservative Management of Obliterative Arterial Disease of the Extremities. Louis G. Herrmann, A.B., M.D. Assistant Professor of Surgery, College of Medicine of the University of Cincinnati; Director of Vascular Disease Clinic of the Cincinnati General Hospital. With a foreword by Mont R. Reid, M.D. Cloth. Price $4.00. Pp. 288, illustrated with 80 engravings and 4 colored plates. Philadelphia: J. B. Lippincott Company, 1936.

This splendid monograph of Herrmann's has been long waited for by workers in vascular diseases, and is sure to create increased interest in the proper treatment of these conditions by all practitioners. It represents an impressive contribution to the meagre literature upon this subject, and the unfortunate sufferer of many types of arterial disease of the extremity is quite sure to benefit by this addition to our armamentarium of therapy.

The author reviews the history of the development of the method that he adapted to clinical use in a most thorough manner, and has carefully given credit to every contribution. Perhaps the mechanical details will not be of great interest to many, but it is well that it is set down for historical reference. The physiology of the circulation is included, with special emphasis upon the development of the collateral circulation in the extremeties.

A brief but concise classification of the obliterative arterial diseases of the extremities is given, but there is nothing to help the general practitioner, who sees only an occasional vascular conditions, in the differential diagnosis of these conditions. While all the general and medicinal measures of any therapeutic value are discussed briefly, the author has scientifically limited his experiences to the use of alternate pressure and suction, and his results are therefore all the more valuable. Perhaps for economic or other reasons it may be necessary for physicians to use one or more measures in combination with the passive exercises in order to secure more permanent relief of symptoms.

The subject matter is well arranged, and the references are very complete. The illustrations are clear, well arranged, and add much to the understanding of the text. The colored plates are particularly good.

D. HENRY POER, M.D.

Allergy of the Nose and Paranasal Sinuses. By French K. Hansel, M.D. C. V. Mosby Company, St. Louis, Missouri. 820 pages, 58 illustrations, 7 charts and color plates. $10.00.

The title is misleading since the book includes an excellent discussion of immunology and full discussion of practically all phases of allergy.

Special attention is given to allergic manifestations of the nose, paranasal sinuses, ears, and eyes. The relation of these conditions to the allergic manifestations in other parts of the body is made clear.

There is a full and detailed report on experimental work, showing how to differentiate between allergic conditions of the nose and paranasal sinuses, and other conditions affecting the same, both in infant children and in adults.

Indications and contraindications for operative procedures on the nose and paranasal sinuses are given.

The author has analyzed from both theoretical and practical viewpoints the work that has been done with iontophoresis of the nasal mucosa, and gives the results of experimental work done by himself and by others. The limitations and possible usefulness of this therapeutic procedure are fully outlined. No one unfamiliar with this work should attempt it without first reading this book.

This book is invaluable for the allergists and rhinologists and is desirable for the library of the pediatricians, dermatologists, and internists.

HAL M. DAVISON, M.D.

Wish Hunting in the Unconscious. By Milton Harrington, M.D. The MacMillan Co., N. Y. This is an interesting indictment of Freudian psychology which is apt on occasion to degenerate into cultism. On the

of pregnancy there is only about a 25 per cent chance of the patient giving birth to a living baby, even if pregnancy is continued to the stage of viability, and there is almost 100 per cent chance of permanent vascular-renal injury developing. If toxemia precedes the twenty-eighth week of pregnancy and is not accompanied by retinitis, the prognosis is slightly better.

7. A previous hypertensive toxemia of pregnancy contraindicates a future pregnancy; the chance of the patient developing eclampsia is less, but the prospect of a live baby is not as good, and the chance of developing permanent vascular-renal injury is greater.

8. Retinal detachment occurs in about 2 per cent of hypertensive toxemias of pregnancy. The detachments usually become reattached within ten days after termination of the pregnancy.

THE KNOWLEDGE OF A LIFE TIME

A surgeon was forced to resort to the courts in order to collect his fee from a recalcitrant client.

The counsel for the defense brought out the fact that the operation was performed in fifteen minutes.

"The labor of fifteen minutes, then, is that for which you ask one hundred and fifty dollars?"

"No," the surgeon replied, "I ask it for the knowledge of a lifetime."

In the medical profession there is something more than the examining of a patient, prescribing medicines or performing an operation. The Physicians and Surgeons put *themselves* into their work.

The true worth of any product is neither greater nor less than the measure of the men creating it. The men creating the medical profession of the South are physicians and surgeons who have brought to their work "the knowledge of a lifetime"—a rare combination of outstanding ability and practical experience. To them we dedicate this publication.—Commentator of the Owensby Clinic, Atlanta, June, 1936.

ANTIVENIN

Concurrent with the reports of more than 600 persons being bitten by the "Black Widow Spider" with a mortality record of 40, comes the announcement that E. R. Squibb & Sons are now supplying Antivenin (Anti-Black Widow Spider Serum.) Widespread professional interest has been shown in methods of treating these bites, especially with the steady increase in the number of cases reported from southern, southwestern and western sections of the United States.

Antivenin is prepared by the hyperimmunization of sheep with repeated doses of venom from the black widow spider. The serum is standardized by determining its neutralizing effect when mixtures of it with venom are injected into young rats. Clinical reports upon this important product as well as information as to dosage and administration are contained in literature supplied by E. R. Squibb & Sons upon request.

Antivenin is available in ampuls of sufficient content to permit the withdrawal and administration of 10 cc. of the serum.

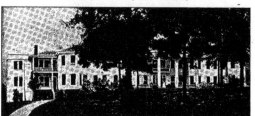

THE JOURNAL
OF THE
MEDICAL ASSOCIATION OF GEORGIA

DEVOTED TO THE WELFARE OF THE MEDICAL ASSOCIATION OF GEORGIA
PUBLISHED MONTHLY under direction of the Council

| Volume XXV | Atlanta, Ga., September, 1936 | Number 9 |

FUNDAMENTAL ASPECTS OF THE DIAGNOSIS AND TREATMENT OF ANEMIA*†

WM. BOSWORTH CASTLE, M.D.
Boston, Mass.

The patient suffering from anemia usually has either a condition for which appropriate treatment is brilliantly successful or one for which there is no specific remedy and for which the best available measures merely forestall temporarily the fatal issue. These diametrically opposed possibilities render precision in diagnosis in this field of internal medicine of especial significance. Recognition of those conditions for which specific therapy is available is obviously of primary importance. The possibility of obtaining from adequate treatment complete relief for patients suffering from such types of anemia offers an opportunity which will appeal to any physician who has the good of his patients at heart. For this reason I believe it is worth while to present briefly to you some of the salient facts concerning the fundamental aspects of the diagnosis and treatment especially of those anemias which can be successfully treated.

Anemia may be divided on an etiologic basis into two main groups. In the first group, acute blood loss or increased blood destruction is the cause of such inordinate demands that the blood-forming organs are unable to supply the requisite number of red blood cells. The peripheral blood and the bone marrow present evidence of an intensive regenerative effort. The anemia of acute blood loss needs no treatment unless as a result of sudden decrease in the blood volume there is

circulatory failure. For this condition, copious fluids or blood transfusions are urgent necessities. The successful treatment of the anemia of increased blood destruction obviously depends on the elimination of the blood-destroying agent whether organic (e. g., malaria, streptococcus) or chemical (e. g., lead). For congenital hemolytic jaundice splenectomy is almost a specific. In other types of hemolytic anemia in which the cause of the blood destruction is obscure, treatment is largely by the judicious use of transfusions.

In anemias of the second group failure of the supply of cells or of hemoglobin is the dominant cause for anemia. The bone marrow, whatever its morphologic appearance, is functionally inadequate to keep up with the natural rate of blood destruction. The inactivity of the blood-forming organs is usually emphasized by the lack of signs of active blood production in the peripheral blood. The success of the treatment depends on whether or not the cause of the bone marrow failure is remediable. If failure is due to toxic inhibition by poisons of external origin (e. g., benzol) or of internal metabolism (e. g., chronic infection or nitrogen retention) transfusions may keep the patient alive until the underlying cause has been removed. If due to destruction of the bone marrow by invading neoplasms (e. g., carcinomatosis, leukemia) the life of the patient may be prolonged by irradiation provided the tumor cells are sensitive to such a measure. If due to aplasia of the bone marrow (e. g., idiopathic aplastic anemia) in a physiologic sense and sometimes morphologically as well, no specific treatment is available, though frequent transfusions may be a means of lengthening the period of the patient's useful existence.

In striking contrast to the unsatisfactory methods of treatment of many varieties of

*Abner Wellborn Calhoun Lecture read before the Medical Association of Georgia, Savannah, April 22, 1936.
†From the Thorndike Memorial Laboratory, Second and Fourth Medical Services (Harvard), Boston City Hospital, and the Department of Medicine, Harvard Medical School, Boston, Massachusetts.

anemia are the therapeutic successes attainable in conditions of the second group in which the failure of cell or hemoglobin production is due to defective nutrition of the blood-forming organs. Thus, in certain types of macrocytic anemia what the marrow needs for a return to normal function is a substance contained in preparations of liver or stomach tissue. In all types of hypochromic anemia the diminished production of hemoglobin will be corrected by providing an adequate supply of iron. In certain instances of scurvy with macrocytic anemia vitamin C deficiency appears to be the basis of the bone marrow starvation. In thyroid deficiency a general lowering of the metabolism is in some way responsible for inadequate activity of the blood-forming organs. Patients with anemias of these types are, then, those most important to recognize early and to treat thoroughly.

It is well to suspect anemia as a possible cause or contributing factor of disability in every patient. The appearance of the patient is not necessarily an indication of the existence of anemia. Pale individuals may have normal blood counts and patients with "good color" may have well-advanced anemia. Therefore if nothing more is done, at least a determination of the hemoglobin of every patient should be made by some reliable method. A hemoglobin determination is more useful than a red blood cell count because in every type of anemia the hemoglobin is decreased, although in the common hypochromic anemia the red blood cell count may be little below normal. Digestive symptoms are usually present in anemia of nutritional deficiency. Sore mouth, dysphagia or "hyper-acidity" may, upon analysis, turn out to be associated with gastric anacidity and anemia. A "nervous breakdown," mental depression or neural symptoms, including "neuritis" and "locomotor ataxia," may be the manifestations of degenerative processes associated with pernicious anemia. The symptoms of congestive heart failure or of angina pectoris are sometimes due to an underlying anemia. Swelling of the ankles, albuminuria and some nitrogen retention may seem to indicate a diagnosis of nephritis but in reality may be the manifestations of anemia. Enlargement of the liver and spleen may suggest cirrhosis

marrow. The failure of this mechanism may obviously be brought about by (1) defective nutrition, (2) defective gastric secretion, (3) defective absorption from the intestinal tract and (4) in theory, defective utilization of material after absorption. In any case of macrocytic anemia one or more of these mechanisms may participate in variable proportions. For purposes of illustration it may be said that disturbance of the intake of food is an important factor in the macrocytic anemia of pellagra, sprue and pregnancy. Disturbance of the gastric secretion is predominantly of importance in pernicious anemia but is also involved to some degree in certain cases of sprue and of the pernicious anemia of pregnancy. Disturbance of intestinal absorption is to some extent probably involved in all such conditions, but is a significant feature of certain cases of anemia in sprue, idiopathic steatorrhea and unusual instances of macrocytic anemia in which intestinal anastomoses or stenoses of the gut are present. All these mechanisms may be involved to variable degrees in states of chronic malnutrition associated with gastro-intestinal disease, whether in extensive cancer of the stomach or of the large bowel, or in intestinal tuberculosis, ulcerative colitis or chronic dysenteries. With these facts in mind it is not difficult to understand the occasional instance of the development of macrocytic anemia or of sore tongue or diarrhea, or of neuritis in pathologic conditions of the alimentary tract. Such conditions sometimes develop after operations, preceding which the patient has been in a prolonged state of chronic malnutrition.

The factors involved in the production of hypochromic anemia are somewhat similar, with the outstanding difference that blood loss, whether by actual bleeding, by transfer of hemoglobin-building materials to the fetus, or by a relative reduction of the amount of hemoglobin in circulation through rapid growth, is the dominant factor. Blood loss due to these mechanisms would not alone be effective in producing hypochromic anemia were the supply of iron in the food or its absorption from the intestinal tract adequate. It is for this reason that poor diets and gastric anacidity are so frequently associated with many instances of hypochromic anemia in which loss of blood does not seem to have been an outstanding phenomenon. However, since the male adult does not ordinarily need more than 1 mg. of iron a day, it is necessary to have blood loss by one of the methods mentioned above in order to deplete the available iron significantly. The menstrual loss of women is probably the feature causing the higher incidence in this sex.

Hypochromic anemia, unlike most other types of anemia, can usually be diagnosed from the blood examination alone, for in the absence of chronic infection the finding of a low color index usually indicates a failure of hemoglobin production, which can be relieved by the administration of iron. In contrast to this is the fact that pernicious anemia and related macrocytic anemias are by no means the only conditions in which macrocytosis of the red blood cells is observed. Following acute hemorrhage the red blood cells are temporarily increased in size, and in most conditions in which a depression of bone marrow function takes place the red cells are normal or somewhat increased in size and contain a normal concentration of hemoglobin unless blood loss has occurred. Thus, in aplastic anemia, aleukemic leukemia, benzol poisoning, chronic nitrogen retention and cirrhosis of the liver the blood picture may distinctly resemble that of pernicious anemia, but the anemia will not respond to the administration of liver or stomach preparations. In the differential diagnosis of pernicious and related anemias, the final proof is a therapeutic test with effective liver or stomach preparations. Because orally administered material may not be adequately absorbed, the original therapy should perhaps always be given parenterally in the form of liver extract.

In the treatment of pernicious and related macrocytic anemias, the administration of liver or stomach preparations in adequate amounts is essential. The effectiveness of the treatment may be quickly confirmed by discovering whether or not significant increase of reticulocytes occurs at about one week after the treatment was begun. Since liver and stomach preparations are expensive compared with iron compounds, it is worth knowing at once whether the former are going to be effective in treatment. Whereas it may be justifiable to give iron empirically to

blood loss is responsible for the hypochromic anemia, marked temporary improvement in the patient can often be brought about by abolition of the anemia. It is of practical interest that the disability in hookworm disease is largely due to the associated hypochromic anemia. This can be successfully abolished, with or without removal of the hookworms, by the administration of efficient doses of iron. When patients are severely anemic, the anemia should be treated before removal of the hookworms is attempted because of the increased danger from vermifuges when the patient's general condition is poor. Elimination of the hookworms is, of course, desirable, but this alone in many cases does not lead to rapid recovery and should therefore always be combined with therapy with iron. Because following the administration of liver or allied products in certain macrocytic anemias, especially in sprue, a change to hypochromic anemia may develop, the administration of iron is probably indicated as a routine procedure until the blood has returned to normal. In patients with pellagra or sprue and hypochromic anemia, therapy with iron does not relieve the intestinal symptoms, though the blood may be improved.

In conclusion, I should like again to emphasize the importance of recognizing those types of anemia for which there are specific remedies. In no type of condition is treatment so regularly effective as in the so-called nutritional deficiency diseases. Certain types of anemia clearly fall into this category and benefit in such conditions is no less certain than in other types of deficiency disorder.

WALTER D. ABBOTT, Des Moines, Iowa (*Journal A. M. A.*, June 20, 1936), cites a case of compression of the cauda equina by the ligamentum flavum in which there was persistence of root pain with a paucity of demonstrable objective changes. In the event of progression of symptoms, spinal manometric readings and injections of lipoiodine are justified to determine the existence of an underlying pathologic process which may be removed before severe damage to the nerve roots has taken place. The case illustrates the role of antecedent trauma in which the ligamentum flavum was torn and, in the reparative process, scar tissue had caused a compression of the cord. One month after laminectomy was performed the patient stated that she was driving a car, walking one or two miles daily, had attended a dance without recurrence of pain, and to all appearances had recovered completely.

EXAMINATION OF PROSTATE*

RUDOLPH BELL, M.D.
Thomasville

In placing the proper emphasis upon the desirability of making rectal examinations, one can do no better than to repeat Osler's well known dictum that "The difference between a good doctor and a poor doctor is that a good doctor knows how to make a rectal examination." The extent of the examination to be made on the prostate depends on the leading symptoms and the findings noted on rectal examination.

The resection era has focused a great deal of attention to the prostate with particular reference to the type of gland suitable for resection. However, it has fallen short of calling sufficient attention to the endless chain of symptoms and disabilities produced by the various types of pathologic prostates. To do this, it is imperative that the structures of the posterior urethra, vesical neck, trigone, seminal vesicles and prostatic secretion be included in the examination of the prostate.

Digital Examination

The insertion of the gloved finger into the rectum is for the purpose of recording the sense of touch in its proper place of the structure felt on examination, and not to hastily reach the prostate and apply hard pressure with the tip of the finger to see if secretion can be punched from that area. For the benefit of the patient the anus, anal sphincter, and rectum should be carefully examined and if hemorrhoids, fissures, ulcers, etc., are noted the patient should be advised of such and sent through his selective channel for treatment. On further inserting the finger one encounters the perineum, Cowper's glands and triangular ligament, lateral and medium portions of the prostate, seminal vesicles and the spaces around the seminal vesicles and prostate.

Any change in the consistency of the prostate from that of its normal elasticity implies that one is dealing with an abnormal gland. The enlarged, hot, boggy prostate indicates that the gland is acutely inflamed. An en-

largement with definite areas of fluctuation is indicative of prostatic abscess. Adhesions on either side of the prostate are suggestive of inflammation of the prostate and seminal vesicles of long standing. When the distended vesicles can not be stripped easily they show severe infection. The nodular prostate is often a "bugaboo" because the physician wants to convince himself as to its nature before proceeding with treatment. The diagnosis should be made much easier by considering separately the four conditions that will produce a nodular prostate, namely, (1) inflammation, (2) stone, (3) cancer and, (4) tuberculosis. I prefer to consider the tuberculous nodule separately from the nodule produced by all other types of inflammation.

The inflammatory nodule has a consistency somewhat similar to that of a thick piece of wet leather, which yields a little to pressure, and is usually located on the lateral aspects of the gland. One usually finds adhesions about the prostate on the corresponding side with the nodule. The early malignant nodule has a third degree, or board-like resistance, and according to Moore[1] is predominantly a lesion of the posterior lobe, but may arise in any other portion of the gland. The consistency of the tuberculous nodule and the stony nodule is similar to that of carcinoma, but is more likely to be in a different locality from that in which carcinoma is found. An x-ray examination is of value in noting the metastases of malignancies and also in demonstrating stones. In cases of suspected malignancies, the biopsy needle is of inestimable value in securing tissue for examination. According to Lowsley and Duff[2] there has been but one case of primary tuberculosis of the prostate gland reported; therefore, one may conclude that the condition is tuberculous only after the acid-fast bacilli have been demonstrated in other portions of the urogenital tract. According to Bell[3] stones should be considered much more often than is commonly thought.

The aforementioned structures may impart nothing on digital examination from that of normal, yet the prostatic secretion may show pathologic changes. The prostatic secretion is best obtained by passing the finger well over the lateral portion on one side of the pros-

*Read before the Medical Association of Georgia, Savannah, April 22, 1936.

Urinary Obstruction

In considering the obstruction to the urinary outflow produced by the prostate one should learn not to rely too much on the size of the gland as felt per rectum. A very large prostate may not produce any urinary symptoms; on the other hand, a prostate that feels no larger than that of the usual size to digital examination may produce acute urinary retention. One case was referred to me while the patient was in an acute urinary retention. On examining the prostate per rectum it felt very small. On further examination the gland proved to be an extremely large one. One peculiar fact noted on rectal examination was that the lateral lobes of the gland could not be felt, and the area of the sulcus, or prostatic urethra, was distended with a portion of the prostate giving it a round appearance. The prostate was found to lie almost entirely in the bladder cavity.

A simple procedure to give one an idea of the amount of prostatic obstruction present is to instruct the patient to void and then pass a catheter and withdraw the residual urine. Immediately after the amount of residual urine is determined, several syringes full of a clear solution should be injected through the catheter and then withdrawn so as to determine the amount of pus that has collected on the floor of the bladder in front of the prostatic obstruction. It should be remembered that digestive disturbances, headaches, weakness and cardio-respiratory symptoms often over shadow the urinary symptoms, as a result of which the outstanding symptoms are treated symptomatically, and no attention paid to the underlying factor. To illustrate that all patients with residual urine do not have urinary symptoms, I should like to cite a case reported by Young*: "In one of my patients with over 2,000 cc. of residual urine, micturition occurred at normal intervals and he did not have to get up at night. The residual urine was 2,100 cc. the bladder capacity 2,600 cc. He had, therefore, a functioning bladder of 500 cc. which was normal."

A cysto-urethrogram is at times of great aid in locating the obstruction and in differential diagnosis, but to determine accurately the condition of the posterior urethra and the degree of obstruction one has to resort to urethroscopy.

Urethroscopy

Although urethroscopy and cystoscopy have justly acquired a renown reputation for being a painful procedure, they can and should be done with very little discomfort to the patient.

After introducing the urethroscope, the bladder should be inspected. A trabeculated bladder wall and hypertrophied trigone are indicative of an obstruction to the lower urinary outflow. An inflamed trigone without any evidence of upper urinary tract infection is conclusive proof of an infected posterior urethra. As the instrument is slowly withdrawn and rotated, the vesical portion of the prostate and the neck of the bladder can be inspected. Any intrusion into the bladder or inflammation of the prostate can be readily determined. The classification of prostatic hypertrophies has been so thoroughly covered that one only has to review the literature of recent years to acquire a knowledge of their grouping. However, the unilateral intrusion and the protrusion that is not uniform should receive some consideration at this time. It is true that the markedly enlarged prostate may not protrude uniformly, but this protrusion can be readily determined as being composed of prostatic tissue. A case that I was called in to see had a protrusion from the space between the middle lobe and the right lateral lobe which fluctuated as the instrument was pressed over it. From rectal examination there were no signs of prostatic abscess, but while I was trying to determine the nature of the intrusion it ruptured; about two drachms of pus drained from it. Such abscesses about the vesical portion of the prostate are not uncommon. Cysts are found more often than is commonly thought; they can be transilluminated as the urethroscope is slowly withdrawn and the light pressed against them.

On urethroscopic examination, the areas of the prostatic urethra about the verumontanum should receive very close attention, for it is in this area that numerous pathologic conditions of obscure origin arise and produce untold anguish. The verumontanum may be enlarged or contain a polyp. Its base

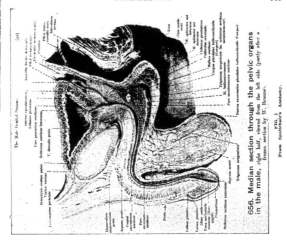

656. Median section through the pelvic organs in the male, right half, viewed from the left side (partly after a frozen section by W. Braune).

FIG. 1
From Spalteholz's Anatomy.

introducing a finger into the rectum, it is a simple procedure, and one that any physician is capable of doing. Why not prevent untold suffering and save countless lives with the information that can be obtained by examining the prostate of all adult males?

Summary

1. No examination of an adult male is complete without a digital rectal examination of the prostate.
2. One can not determine the degree of prostatic obstruction to the urinary outflow from rectal examination alone.
3. An obliteration of the sulcus, or prostatic urethra, is indicative of a very large prostate.
4. It is just as essential to examine the prostatic secretion of an adult male as it is to examine the urine.
5. Pus in the prostatic secretion is accompanied by pathologic changes in the posterior urethra which can be determined only with the aid of the urethroscope.
6. An inflamed trigone with no evidence of upper urinary tract infection is conclusive proof of infection in the posterior urethra.

REFERENCES
1. Moore, R. A.: J. Urol. *33:* 224-233 (March) 1935.
2. Lowsley, O. S., and Duff, John: Ann. Surg. (Jan.) 1930, 106-114.
3. Bell, Rudolph: J. M. A. Georgia, *24:* July, 1935.
4. Young, H. H.: Nelson Loose Leaf Living Surgery—Urol. Vol. 6, P. 215.
5. Lowsley, O. S., and Kirwin, T. J.: Text Book of Urology, Philadelphia: Lea & Febiger, 1926.

Discussion on Paper by Dr. Rudolph Bell

DR. MONTAGUE L. BOYD (Atlanta) : It is difficult to compose a paper for presentation to the general practitioner upon the subject about which Dr. Bell has addressed you since its discussion necessitates the inclusion of so many details. On that account and because of the limited time at his disposal, he does not have a chance to give due emphasis to the many essential points. I saw Dr. Bell's paper before I came here and I did not see how he could leave out anything but it was evident that many of the points which he presented needed much more discussion. I shall attempt to elaborate upon only one of these, namely the anatomy of the prostate in relation to disease, diagnosis and treatment.

This illustration (No. 1) shows the prostate and the adjacent urogenital organs. You can see that at rectal examination the part of the prostate immediately accessible to the palpating finger is the part lying back of the ejaculatory ducts. The part of the prostate

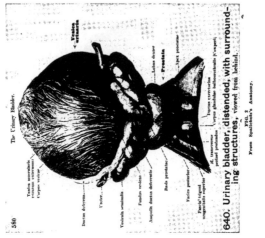

lying behind and on each side of the neck of the bladder is beneath this layer and it is in this portion of the prostate that benign hypertrophy occurs, and occasionally cancer. Fortunately, cancer begins in most cases in this most accessible, posterior layer.

This illustration shows also why it is often difficult to discover by rectal palpation those changes which occur in the prespermatic portions of the prostate unless they are extensive enough to be palpated at the side of the posterior layer or through it.

A skilled urologist is able to palpate many of these conditions, but many of them can be found only at cystoscopic examination.

You are also able to observe in these illustrations why massage of the prostate is ineffective when the prespermatic portions are solely or principally involved *unless* the massage is given so as to express the secretion from these portions and the effect of the massage is augmented by adequate urethral dilatations.

Abscesses which arise in the prespermatic portions are difficult to feel, produce urinary obstruction early, and rupture into the urethra or bladder.

DR. WALLACE L. BAZEMORE (Macon): It will be only repetition for me to comment on the points that the essayist has so clearly made in his comprehensive paper on examination of the prostate gland.

I shall confine my remarks to examination of the prostatic patient confronting operation. Assuming that physical and laboratory tests suggest an uneventful sur-

gical recovery, there is that personal individual equation in the preoperative summary of these cases that I am convinced plays no small part in our prognosis. From time to time I continue to lose that patient following prostatectomy (the so-called second operation), who presents a near normal dye excretion with no nitrogen retention. Invariably my foresight has made me apprehensive, and my hindsight has convinced me that with all our urologic armamentarium there is one unmeasurable and indescribable test that is far more important than our measurable ones. I refer to: Does our patient look and act like his neighbor who successfully submitted to this same surgical procedure?

The active, alert old gentlemen with markedly impaired kidneys, is certainly surer of Ponce de Leon's dream than his neighbor presenting normal laboratory tests but lacking in that something we gather from observation, but cannot describe.

The surest way that I know to improve that personal test is prolonged bladder drainage. Should irreparable renal damage take place, we still operate with the feeling that our patient looks and acts like a good surgical risk.

I contend that the prostatic patient who can successfully undergo suprapubic drainage, can with sufficient drainage time undergo successful prostatectomy. Should we depend entirely on our laboratory test, our operative judgment will frequently prove disastrous. Until our patient "looks good" regardless of normal urologic test, he is not ready for operation.

APPENDICITIS*

CHARLES USHER, M.D.
Savannah

It has been fifty years since the first case of appendicitis was diagnosed and operated on as such. It is still an unsettled question from the fact that in the last four years there have been about 800 articles on appendicitis that have been published in the journals[1]. Recently, such men as Charles W. Mayo[2], Haggard[3], Arthur Dean Bevan[4] and many others have written on this subject.

When you begin to review the books and journals on appendicitis it is readily seen that the mortality is entirely too high, as some of the authors report, approximately 25,000 annually for the United States and Canada. In the Year-Book of Surgery and numerous articles the mortality is said to be about the same as it was several years ago, some even say that it has increased in the past few years. For pus cases a mortality of 10 per cent was given.

In reviewing my own cases I began to realize that in the beginning my records were very poor, and I am not able to report them all, but I would like to report my observations from 1,546 cases.

	Number of Cases	Mortality	Per Cent
Uncomplicated	501	2	.039
Ruptured	242	19	7.85
Appendix and other operation	803	28	3.4

At the same time I would like to report 2,757 cases of general abdominal operations with a mortality of 80 or 2.9 per cent.

Deaths from 1917 to 1925	none
1925	3
1926	1
1927	0
1928	1
1929	0
1930	1
1931	1
1932	3
1933	3
1934	4
1935	1
Deaths from embolus	2
from peritonitis	11
from pneumania	6

(2 plain cases and 4 ruptured cases.)

1. Aged 47, 6-5-26, sick one day, ruptured gan-

---

*Read before the Medical Association of Georgia, Savannah, April 22, 1936.

grenous appendix, peritonitis. Local anesthesia; died 3 days postoperative from embolus.

2. Aged 30, 3-25-30, sick 5 days, ruptured appendix, general peritonitis, local anesthesia, died from peritonitis.

3. Aged 12, 12-5-33, acute appendicitis, died 6 days postoperative from bronchopneumonia. Ether anesthetic. This case had epilepsy and probably died from aspiration pneumonia.

4. Aged 14, 6-24-34, ruptured appendix and peritonitis, abdomen full of pus, ether anesthetic, died from peritonitis.

5. Aged 22, 6-26-34, acute appendicitis, ether anesthetic, died 7 days postoperative from pneumonia, had hookworms.

6. Aged 15, 5-17-31, ruptured appendix and peritonitis, no protective barriers, ether anesthetic, on 5-29-31 intestinal obstruction, perfringens antitoxin given 5-29-31, relieved for a time, spinal novocaine 120 mg. at 11:30 P. M., 5-30-31 relieved, 600 cc. blood transfusion 5-31-31. Patient developed double bronchopneumonia, 2 weeks later died 6-28-31.

7. Aged 80, 4-15-32, ruptured appendix and peritonitis, local anesthesia, died 4 days postoperative from peritonitis.

8. Aged 25, 7-1-32, ruptured appendix and peritonitis, 6 days standing, ether anesthetic, died next day from peritonitis.

9. Aged 10, 12-25-17, sick one week, ruptured appendix and peritonitis, ether anesthetic, died 5 days postoperative from lobar pneumonia.

10. Aged 10, 5-18-28, ruptured appendix and peritonitis, ether anesthetic, died 2 days postoperative from peritonitis.

11. Aged 30, 12-12-32, ruptured appendix and peritonitis, 400 cc. blood transfusion on 12-13-32, died 2 days postoperative from peritonitis.

12. Aged 42, 6-2-33, ruptured appendix and peritonitis, ether anesthetic, died 23 days postoperative from bronchopneumonia.

13. Aged 18, 5-14-33, sick two weeks, ruptured appendix and peritonitis, abscess drained, died the next day from peritonitis.

14. Aged 40, 11-16-33, sick about two weeks, ruptured appendix and peritonitis, localized abscess, appendix removed, general condition of patient poor, wound scarcely drained any at all, patient absorbed the toxic material, died 4 days postoperative from peritonitis.

15. Aged 30, 7-10-25, ruptured appendix and peritonitis, drainage only, local anesthesia, died the next day from peritonitis.

16. Aged 25, 7-19-25, ruptured appendix and peritonitis, local anesthesia, died the same day from peritonitis.

17. Aged 30, 9-28-25, large pus appendix and peritonitis, died 8 days postoperative from general peritonitis.

18. Aged 60, 1-9-35, ruptured appendix and peritonitis, died 7 days postoperative from embolus.

19. Aged 5, 1-7-32, acute appendix gangrenous, retrocecal abscess to kidney pouch, 1-30-32; 250 cc.

blood transfusion, 200 cc. later, bronchopneumonia right, empyema, bronchopneumonia left, died 2-18-32 from pneumonia.

In making a diagnosis of appendicitis, it is not as easy as it first appears on the surface; one may be very easy, the next very hard. A very careful history is most important and I think one should consider; in making a differential diagnosis some of the other diseases which are non-surgical cases of an acute abdomen. These are:

1. Metabolic [5]
   a. Diabetic acidosis.
   b. Tetany.
2. Cardiovascular.
   a. Referred from the heart (angina pectoris, coronary occlusion, pericarditis).
   b. Embolism and thrombosis (mesenteric occlusion, subacute bacterial endocarditis, polycythemia).
   c. Intraabdominal arterial disease (periarteritis nodosa, dissecting aneurysm, abdominal angina).
3. Hematologic
   a. Hemolytic icterus.
   b. Purpura (Henoch, Osler).
   c. Sickle-cell anemia.
   d. Splenic enlargements with perisplenitis or infarction (leukemia, Banti's disease, Hodgkin's disease, etc.)
4. Infectious
   a. Occasionally, at onset of acute infections (influenza, typhoid and paratyphoid fevers, poliomyelitis, malaria, acute tonsillitis).
   b. Dysentery (amebic, bacillary).
   c. Rheumatic peritonitis.
   d. Tabetic crises.
   e. Arachnoidism.
5. Gastro-Intestinal
   a. Cholangitis.
   b. Acute gastro-enteritis (foods, heavy metals, acids, alkalies, etc.)
   c. Pylorospasm.
   d. Intestinal parasites.
6. Genito-Urinary
   a. Dietl's crises.
   b. Pyelitis.
   c. Distended urinary bladder.
7. Pulmonary
   a. Pleurisy.
   b. Pneumonia in children.
8. Abdominal-Wall disorders
   a. Early herpes zoster.
   b. Intercostal neuralgia.
   c. Trichinosis.
   d. Trauma.
9. Hysteria and malingering.
   The symptoms of appendicitis, acute and chronic as given by Kitchens[6] are as follows:
1. Pain, abdominal, general.
2. Pain, epigastric.

oratory will aid considerably. I have found
that the Schilling count will help very much
in doubtful cases. The white blood count is
not so reliable, you may have a normal white
count and still have a gangrenous or ruptured appendix.

In making a differential diagnosis between
appendicitis and ruptured duodenal ulcer, as
a rule in duodenal ulcer the liver dullness is
absent. In making a differential diagnosis
between appendicitis and kidney stones, a
urinalysis, an x-ray and a cystoscopic examination will be of great value. The mere presence of pus and blood, especially blood in
urine does not mean that there is a stone in
the kidney or ureter, and that the appendix
is normal.

Bastianelli[1] wrote: "When physicians are
discussing whether a case is appendicitis or
not, it is; when they are inclined to admit
the possibility of appendicitis without being
sure of it, it not only is but is about to perforate; when the diagnosis is sure, there is
already perforation, with more or less circumscribed peritonitis."

In making a physical examination, a rectal and vaginal examination should not be
neglected. In some cases when the appendix
is in the pelvis, the abdomen may not be
rigid. Without a rectal and vaginal examination a diagnosis may be missed.

Whenever pregnancy occurs and the patient has appendicitis, the appendix should
be removed at the earliest moment possible.
To try to tide the patient over with appendicitis in a case like this, is a great mistake, because, if the appendix happens to rupture, you would not only have peritonitis to
deal with, but a vicious circle also. *When a
diagnosis of appendicitis is made, that is the
time when the appendix should be removed;
there should be no delay.*

The incision is a very important part of
the operation. In an acute case of appendicitis, I like to use the McBurney incision in
men, but for women I prefer to use a right
rectus incision. By right rectus incision I
mean that you may split the muscle or push
it to one side; using this incision you can
always examine the adnexa, which is a point
that should not be forgotten. In cases that
present a mass it is advisable as a rule to make
the incision over the mass, but not always.

Sometimes it is wise to make an incision over one edge of the mass, for instance when you have a ruptured appendix with a pelvis full of pus; in these cases it is better to use a McBurney incision. Sometimes it is very difficult to decide which incision to make; if you make a McBurney you may wish that you had made a right rectus and vice versa.

Drainage is also a very important item, and in cases where the pelvis contains pus, it is a good idea to put in a long drain into the pelvis. The surgeon should dress his own cases and pull out the tube a little each day, sometimes cut a piece off and sometimes not, but it should be moved each day. The tube should not be left in one place too long because it is resting over the iliac artery and by leaving it too long in one place it might cause an erosion into the artery. The advantages of a McBurney incision are; you are not so liable to have a hernia, even where there is drainage, and if the wound breaks down, viscera are not so apt to escape.

In doing an operation for chronic appendicitis and gallbladder, or appendicitis and stomach operation I prefer to use two small incisions rather than a long right rectus incision. In doing general abdominal work, especially pelvic work in women, when the operation is confined to the pelvis, I believe it advisable to remove the appendix when it is easy accessible and does not add to the mortality.

In doing an operation for ruptured appendix, I think the appendix should be removed, whenever you can do it without breaking down the protecting barriers, whenever there is pus in the abdominal cavity, whether a ruptured appendix or where the appendix is mixed up in pelvic sepsis and adherent I do not think the stump of the appendix in cases of this kind should be inverted, because where there is sepsis, each time that you put in a stitch to invert the appendix, that point becomes the site that might become infected. However, in all other cases after tying the appendix with cat gut, I think the stump should be inverted and if practical a little piece of omentum should be tacked over the site of the appendix stump, because I have seen a few cases where some little diverticulum became attached to the appendix stump and caused intestinal obstruction; or the ap-

When after an operation a patient's abdomen becomes ballooned up and he is not doing so well, they generally have a dilated stomach and I think a stomach tube should be used. When I say a stomach tube, I really mean Levine's small duodenal tube, and it should be passed not through the mouth, but through the nose. These patients should have enough morphine to keep them quiet, and should have some atropine to dry up secretions when indicated. You can not lay down hard and fast rules that will cover all cases; every one should be considered as an individual case and should be treated accordingly.

I have found morphine superior to all other narcotics; however, there is an occasional case where pantopon, codeine, or dilaudid may be used with an advantage. Wangensteen[8] states that these drugs are only efficient in proportion to the amount of morphine that they contain.

Another important point to remember is, the patient should not be given enemas before or after an operation, early before or early after. If you are going to give an enema, give it the night before or the day before, because it has been proven that too much washing of the colon before an operation is not advisable because it is better to have solid rather than liquid feces.

Purgatives should be avoided in appendicitis cases because they may blow off the ligature around the appendix stump. A little mineral oil is about all that should be given. In acute cases nothing except morphine and atropine. Some recommend only atropine until the diagnosis is made. It has been proven that when cathartics are used before an operation more appendices perforate than when they are not used.

After an operation it is better not to use enemas too early because there have been reported cases where the enema would blow off the ligature around the appendix stump. It is better to let them have the Murphy drip rather freely and if they expel a little fluid it is better because they generally expel some gas. A rectal tube may be used with great advantage. There are no vaccines or serums that will prevent appendicitis; however, after the appendix has ruptured and the surgeon has operated, the use of the serum of Weinburg of the Pasteur Institute has been reported on favorably.

REFERENCES

1. Hobler, L. L.: Appendicitis: Analysis of 4,833 Cases, Ann. Surg. 103: 86-96 (Jan.) 1936.
2. Mayo, C. W.: Mayo Clinic, 1934.
3. Haggard, W. D.: Am. J. Surg. 28 (April) 1935.
4. Bevan, A. D.: The Present Status of the Problem of Appendicitis, Surgical Clinics, N. America 16; 63-79 (Feb.) 1936.
5. Comroe, B. L.: Ann. Surg. 101: (Jan.) 1935.
6. Kitchens, W. L.: Definite Diagnosis in General Practice.
7. Babcock, W. W.: Text Book of Surgery, ed. 2. Philadelphia.
8. Wangensteen, O. H.: The Postoperative Control of Distention, Nausea and Vomiting, J. A. M. A., 100: 1910-1917 (June 17, 1933).

Discussion on Paper of Dr. Charles Usher

DR. GRADY N. COKER (Canton): During the past nine years I have removed a total of 827 appendices. Four hundred sixty of these were uncomplicated acute cases, without mortality. One hundred thirty-four of them were ruptured, with a mortality of eight. Two hundred thirty-three of them were a combination with other operations.

We do not make a definite routine of always removing the appendix while doing other surgery in the abdomen. If it is easily accessible, we remove it; if not, we leave it alone. In that way you are lowering the mortality rate on the rest of your abdominal surgery.

In regard to the diagnosis, I think there are four things to remember. The first is that the patient has pain, as a rule acute pain, and as a rule it does not start in the right lower quadrant. If it does, you had better look for another diagnosis. The next thing is nausea and vomiting, abdominal tenderness, localized to the right lower quadrant, and elevation of temperature. The patient may have an elevation of temperature, and he may not. I have seen several cases without any elevation of temperature. I have seen it without any elevation of the white cell count. I think it is very important to do a differential count.

In regard to the incision in an operation for appendicitis, I think that possibly is a matter of personal choice, but I prefer the right rectus incision. I think if all would adopt that routine it would save a lot of grief, when you get a retrocecal appendix six or eight inches long. Statistics show that you have more incisional hernias following other incisions than you do following a right rectus or paramedian incision.

In regard to postoperative care, you have heard the proverb: When in doubt, to drain or not to drain. When in doubt about this drainage business, we just don't drain. We have more tendency not to drain than ever before.

In the December issue of the A. M. A. Journal there is an important piece about appendicits that I think it would be well worth our while to study several times. We do not use anything in our cases but the Mikulicz's drain. We have not used the soft rubber drain in many years. I think our low mortality justifies that procedure.

The postoperative care of the perforated cases is very important. I do not think the Fowler position is

twenty-seven more cases. We think this has materially reduced the mortality, has reduced the length of stay in the hospital and the patients have been very much helped. You can get fluids in them easily, get drainage: the abdomens stay flat and we have not had a fistula that refused to heal.

I noticed in *The Southern Surgeon* for February, an independent paper by Dr. G. A. Hendon, of Louisville, who uses the same technic.

The technic is simple. All you have to do is take about a 15 umbrella catheter, and after the appendix has been removed slip it in the appendix stump and put a purse-string suture of plain catgut around it and then connect it up to a bottle. We have made a rule to put anywhere from 4 to 6 ounces of fluid in the catheter every four to six hours if it is necessary for fluids, sometimes clamping it off and sometimes letting it drain. We feel it has helped us out a great deal, and, as you know, some of these cases are desperate when you get hold of them. We feel like recommending it more each year.

DR. CLEVELAND THOMPSON (Millen): With regard to the symptomatology of appendicitis, Dr. Usher's paper is so thorough and so inclusive that it is a little confusing to some of us who have to decide for ourselves when and where we meet these cases. The only fault with the symptoms that he gives us is that there are too many. I know of no better description of appendicitis than that of Murphy's original description of it: First, bellyache, not pain in the side, but pain over the abdomen—it may be in the epigastrium, is usually around the umbilicus—but pain over the abdomen. Dr. Murphy particularly emphasized the *sequence of symptoms in appendicitis.* The next symptom that comes on is nausea—always nausea in acute appendicitis, and usually vomiting, but not always. Then, after a long or shorter time, depending on the rapidity of the spread of the infection, the pain shifts to the right flank, and soreness, tenderness and fever come on. First, pain over the abdomen, then nausea and usually vomiting, then the pain shifts, and soreness, tenderness and fever come on. And along with it, there is a leukocytosis, as a rule.

If you have this *sequence* of symptoms, you do not need a blood count to make a diagnosis of appendicitis. You do not need a urinalysis, although you ought always to have these.

When a patient comes in, suspected of having appendicitis, I ask: "When did you get sick?" "How did you get sick?" Then, "What happened?" Then, "What happened?" And "Then, what happened?" Asking these questions, your diagnosis in 80 per cent of the cases is absolutely certain from the beginning.

A lot of these patients could be saved and complications prevented if every doctor realized that *any acute abdominal pain not promptly relieved without narcotics demands at least a surgical consultation.*

There is one symptom that I have not seen described in the literature that invariably indicates a rupture of the appendix. When a patient comes in with a history of appendicitis, and the nurse says, "The patient cannot void; we will have to catheterize him to get a

specimen of urine"—or if he says he was not able to void, invariably that indicates that the appendix has ruptured. There is pus in the culdesac, in contact with the bladder, causing the inability to void.

DR. EDGAR H. GREENE (Atlanta): The classic history, symptoms and findings, that have been so ably described today, tend to make the diagnosis relatively simple, but one occasionally encounters the patient with suspected appendicitis presenting an extremely difficult problem for diagnosis.

Hence further regard may be taken here concerning the diagnosis of appendicitis by mentioning two conditions that are of importance:

1. The appendix is often displaced. At times it is found in the neighborhood of the gallbladder; sometimes it is in the region of the right ovary and rarely it is found in the left side of the abdomen. In concurring pelvic inflammatory disease I have often found the appendix adhered to the uterus, ovary and tube on the right.

2. A girl or young woman may have an attack which is presumably appendicitis, but at operation an acute salpingitis is found on the right. The appendix may or may not be involved.

It seems very important, therefore, in cases of suspected appendicitis, to make a thorough vaginal examination in every female past the age of puberty. A careful examination of the right adnexa will frequently reveal an acutely inflamed fallopian tube and no definite appendiceal involvement.

It should be borne in mind, however, that the two pathologic conditions may co-exist.

WOUNDS OF THE THORACIC VISCERA

Daniel C. Elkin, Atlanta, Ga. (*Journal A. M. A.*, July 18, 1936), discusses the 553 patients that have been treated in the last five years (1931 to 1935 inclusive) at the Emory University Division (Negro) of the Grady Hospital (municipal) for penetrating chest wounds. In the nine years previous to 1931, 511 similar cases were treated in the same hospital. Treatment was attempted by conservative methods. Except in wounds of the heart, operative procedures have been rarely carried out. Aspiration of blood or air has been practiced only in those patients having pain and dyspnea. With these methods the mortality was 6 per cent. Of 148 patients who were in shock most of them had hemothorax or pneumothorax on entrance to the hospital. Treatment of this class of patient presented the most difficult problem and eighteen of them died, usually within the first twenty-four hours after admission, without reacting from shock. Some of that number might have been saved by operation. This would have necessitated open thoracotomy and lung suture. Had this method been carried out on a large number of patients, it is doubtful whether the mortality would have been as low as 6 per cent. Thoracotomy with exteriorization and extrapleuralization of the lacerated lung has been advocated and practiced by Connors and Stenbuck. By this procedure they have unquestionably saved a number of lives, but their mortality in a small series of thirty-two cases was 12.5 per cent. Thoracic injuries in civil life are different from those seen in war injuries and are less severe. In the former a knife, ice pick or pistol bullet are the usual weapons, and large sucking wounds, such as are made by shrapnel, are less frequently seen. The lodgment of clothes, ribs and shell, giving rise to serious infection, is therefore more rarely a complicating factor.

ANTERIOR POLIOMYELITIS

A Review of Recent Studies

WILLIAM A. SMITH, M.D.
Atlanta

Anterior poliomyelitis is a disease of great public interest, especially when an epidemic occurs. The problems involved have been the subject of extensive investigations. It is my purpose to present a brief review of some of these experimental studies which have added much to our knowledge. It is now considered to be a disease primarily and exclusively of the central nervous system. In spite of intensive studies, preventive control remains an unsolved problem.

Etiology

The etiology is a filterable virus which has been found in the nasopharynx in both paralyzed and non-paralyzed types of cases. It can also be isolated from the nervous system of those infected, but Brodie[1] did not find it anywhere else in the body, neither in the blood, cerebrospinal fluid, salivary glands, liver, spleen, mesenteric lymph nodes nor kidneys. In the nasopharynx, the virus usually disappears in a short time, but may persist for as long as seven months; in such cases, there may be a recurrence of acute symptoms, which usually occurs within a period of three months[2]. Second attacks after many years occur in rare instances.

Epidemiology

The epidemiology of this disease has always been confusing, as it is seldom possible to trace the infection in one case to contact with other cases. Most cases occur between July and October. The incubation period is seven to ten days. The greatest susceptibility occurs in the first six years of life. Paul and Trask[3] found that from 70 to 95 per cent of urban adults possess specific antibodies against the virus in their blood serum. This may be due to previous contacts with subinfective doses of the virus. Protection may depend upon the presence of such antibodies in the mucus overlying the olfactory mucosa. The transmission of the disease apparently is through contact with healthy carriers or with abortive cases by so-called droplet infection.

the virus was injected into the brain, the lower cord was not involved, as judged by the absence of lesions and the inability to recover the virus. Thus proof seems complete that this disease is one exclusively of the nervous system, its invasion and spread occurring along the axones of nerve fibres.

Symptoms

In accordance with these facts, Faber[9] and others proposed a new interpretation of the symptoms, on an entirely neurologic basis. The early symptoms are due to cerebral involvement; they include fever, disturbance in sleep, such as drowsiness during the day and restlessness at night, headache, generalized hyperesthesia, vomiting, constipation or diarrhea, tremor, prostration, pallor, tachycardia and marked sweating. There is often a characteristic mental state of apprehension, fear and irritability when disturbed. All these symptoms are referable to a disturbance of the sensory and vegetative centers of the diencephalon.

In the next stage, some hours or several days later, occur symptoms from involvement of the posterior horns of the spinal cord. These include localized pains and tenderness, stiffness of the neck, Kernig's sign, pain on flexion of the spine and exaggerated tendon reflexes. This is followed in a few hours or days by involvement of the anterior horn cells and the production of flaccid paralysis, with loss of tendon reflexes. The extent of the paralysis usually reaches a maximum within 24-48 hours; less commonly, paralysis may progress for several days to two weeks. Following this there is a tendency for steady improvement, which may continue for as long as two years. In the so-called abortive cases, the virus apparently dies out and the disease does not progress beyond the first or second stage.

In the first stage, the fever may reach 101 to 103° F. In some cases the fever disappears several days after the onset, reappearing with the paralysis. Rarely there is no fever, the paralysis being the first symptom. There is a leukocytosis varying from 10,000 to 30,000. The nasopharynx may appear congested. The spinal fluid is under increased pressure but is clear and contains from ten to several hundred cells per cubic millimeter. The cell count averages about 50; in the early stages as many as 50 per cent may be leukocytes; later they are all lymphocytes. The spinal fluid also shows an increased globulin and a normal sugar content. Within two or three weeks the spinal fluid becomes normal.

The paralysis is always segmental, involving groups of muscles, and usually asymmetrical. Seldom is an entire limb paralyzed. Many varieties may occur involving groups of muscles in the extremities, back and abdomen as well as those of facial and bulbar muscles. If recovery does not occur, atrophy may begin in two or three weeks. The sphincters are seldom involved; urinary retention may occur. The majority of patients paralyzed are left with some permanent residual defect. In adults the paralysis tends to be more extensive and with less tendency for improvement.

A diagnosis before paralysis may be difficult when the disease is not prevalent, but in an epidemic the characteristic early symptoms should suggest examination of the spinal fluid to confirm the diagnosis. Differential diagnosis is not within the scope of this review.

Treatment

In regard to treatment, much hope was placed in the use of serum of normal adults or of those who had the disease, since the serum of such individuals contains antibodies to the virus. The serum of horses and goats immunized to this disease has also been studied. Clinically, serum was given in various ways with results difficult to interpret. As pointed out by Harmon[11] 71 per cent of cases do not develop paralysis even when untreated. In careful studies Kramer and Aycock[12], Park[13] and Fischer[14] have shown no difference in the course of the disease in a large series of cases treated before paralysis and in a control group untreated. Furthermore, Schultze and Gebhardt[15] and also Brodie[16] have shown that even large amounts of serum given after the nasal instillation of virus has no effect in the monkey. The newer conception of the disease is that the virus is fixed in the nerve cells beyond reach of antibodies in the serum and that serum can be of no value after infection occurs. The intraspinal treatment with serum produced a marked meningeal inflammation, an undesirable complication. Serum therapy has therefore been abandoned: only a few still advo-

resistance of the central nervous system. Hudson, Lennette and Gordon[34] also emphasized that antibodies in the blood serum were formed outside of the nervous system by virus escaping from the nerve cells, and that these antibodies do not protect the nervous system from infection. An effective immunity must be developed in the nervous tissue itself, and probably occurs only through infection.

The danger involved in vaccination, especially in view of the low attack-rate of the disease, and the doubtful protection conferred by antibodies in the blood serum, has shifted interest to measures aimed at the portal of entry in the nasal mucosa. Armstrong and Harrison[35] found that a nasal spray of 4 per cent sodium aluminum sulphate and also 0.32 per cent picric acid (1.5 cc.) would protect the monkey for four to seven days. Such a spray has been used extensively in the present epidemic in nearby states. The results of its use are not yet known. Directions for this spray are as follows[36]:

"Solution A: Dissolve one gram (1 Gm.) of picric acid in 100 cc. of physiologic salt solution (0.85 per cent). (Warming facilitates solution of the picric acid.)

Solution B: Dissolve 1 gram (1 Gm.) of sodium aluminum sulphate (sodium alum) in 100 cc. of physiologic salt solution (0.85 per cent). Any turbidity in this solution should be removed by filtering one or more times through the same filter paper.

Mix solutions A and B in equal amounts. The resulting mixture, which contains 0.5 per cent piric acid and 0.5 per cent alum, is sufficiently antiseptic to prevent the growth of organisms and is ready for use as a spray. Home-made concoctions are not favored. The solution should be sprayed into the nostrils three or four times on alternate days and thereafter weekly during the presence of poliomyelits. The spray tip should be pointed upward and backward at an angle of about 45 degrees, and the spraying should be thorough enough to reach the pharynx as well, when a bitter taste will be noted."

Summary

Anterior poliomyelitis is a primary infection of the central nervous system by a specific virus, which enters directly by way of the olfactory nerves, spreading through the nervous system along the axones of nerve fibers. The nerve cells are directly attacked by the virus, and inflammatory changes are secondary to the injury to the nerve cells. After infection occurs, there is no specific virucidal therapy which can affect the disease. Preventive vaccination is both dangerous and of doubtful benefit, since the mere presence of antibodies in the blood serum is no evidence of resistance on the part of the nervous system. Methods of prevention aimed at the portal of entry in the olfactory mucosa by use of a nasal spray are of interest at this time.

BIBLIOGRAPHY

1. Brodie, M. and Elvidge, A. R.: Portal of Entry and Transmission of Virus of Poliomyelitis. Science 79:235 (Mar. 9) 1934.
2. Quigley, T. B.: Second Attacks of Poliomyelitis. J. A. M. A. 102:752 (Mar. 10) 1934.
3. Paul, J. R. and Trask, J. D.: Neutralization Test in Poliomyelitis. Comparative Results with Four Strains of Virus. J. Exp. Med. 61:447 (Apr.) 1935.
4. Draper, G.: Anterior Poliomyelitis, Blakiston's Son & Co., Phila., Pa. 1917.
5. Flexner, S. and Amoss, H. L.: Localization of the Virus and Pathogenesis of Experimental Poliomyelitis. J. Exp. Med. 20:249, 1914.
6. Fairbrother, R. W. and Hurst, E. W.: The Pathogenesis of and Propagation of the Virus in Experimental Poliomyelitis. J. Path. and Bact. 33:17, 1930.
7. Jungeblut, C. W. and Spring, W. J.: A Note on the Propagation of the Virus in Experimental Poliomyelitis. Proc. Soc. Exp. Biol. and Med. 27:107 (June) 1930.
8. Faber, H. K. and Gebhardt, L. P.: Localization of Virus in Poliomyelitis in Central Nervous System During Preparalytic Period after Intranasal Instillation. J. Exp. Med. 57:933 (June) 1933.
9. Faber, H. K.: Acute Poliomyelitis as a Primary Disease of the Central Nervous System. Medicine 12:83 (May) 1933.
10. Schultze, E. W. and Gebhardt, L. P.: Olfactory Tract and Poliomyelitis. Proc. Soc. Exp. Biol. and Med. 31:728 (Mar.) 1934.
11. Harmon, P. H.: Poliomyelitis—Results of Treatment in Acute Disease; Analysis of Reports on 4,400 Patients Treated with Serum; Observation on 2,660 Untreated Patients. Am. J. Dis. Child. 47:1216 (June) 1934.
12. Kramer, S. D., Aycock, W. L., Solomon, C. I. and Thenebe, C. L.: Convalescent Serum Therapy in Preparalytic Poliomyelitis. New Eng. J. Med. 206:432 (Mar. 3) 1932.
13. Park, W. H.: Therapeutic Use of Antipoliomyelitis Serum in Preparalytic Cases of Poliomyelitis. N. York State J. Med. 33:91 (Jan. 15) 1935.
14. Fischer, A. E.: Human Convalescent Serum in the Treatment of Preparalytic Poliomyelitis. Am. J. Dis. Child. 48:481 (Sept.) 1934.
15. Schultze, E. W. and Gebhardt, L. P.: On the Prophylactic and Theraupetic Value of Specific Immune Serum in Experimental Poliomyelitis. Proc. Soc. Exp. Biol. and Med. 31:260 (Nov.) 1933.
16. Brodie, M.: The Role of Convalescent Serum in Preparalytic Poliomyelitis. J. Immun. 28:353 (May) 1935.
17. Harper, P. and Tennant, R.: Treatment of Respiratory Failure in Poliomyelitis. Yale J. Biol. and Med. 6.31 (Oct.) 1933.
18. Landon, J. F.: An Analysis of 88 Cases of Poliomyelitis Treated in the Drinker Respirator with a Control of 68 Cases. J. Ped. 5:1 (July 1) 1934.
19. Retan, G. M.: Some Applications of Forced Drainage to Various Infections in Inflammatory Conditions in the Central Nervous System. Arch. Neurol. and Psych. 29:404 (Feb.) 1933.
20. Henry, J. M. and Johnson, G. E.: Acute Anterior Poliomyelitis in Philadelphia. A Comparative Study of the 1916 and 1932 Epidemics. J. A. M. A. 103:94 (July 14) 1934.
21. Brodie, M.: Rate of Antibody Formation in Monkeys Actively Immunized with Poliomyelitis Virus. J. Immun. 27:395 (Oct.) 1934.
24. Brodie, M.: Active Immunization of Children Against Poliomyelitis with formalin Inactivated Virus Suspension. Proc. Soc. Exp. Biol. & Med. 32:300 (Nov.) 1934.
26. Brodie, M.: Active Immunization Against Poliomyelitis. Am. J. Pub. Health 25:54 (Jan.) 1935.
27. Kolmer, J. A., Klugh, G. F. and Rule, A. M.: A Successful Method for Vaccination Against Acute Anterior Poliomyelitis. J. A. M. A. 104:456 (Feb. 9) 1935.
28. Brodie, M. and Park, W. H.: Active Immunization Against Poliomyelitis. J. A. M. A. 105:1089 (Oct. 5) 1935.
29. Kolmer, J. A.: Susceptibility and Immunity. Its Relation to Vaccination in Acute Anterior Poliomyelitis, With

spread use of ovarian remedies and the lack of uniformity in nomenclature and method of extraction of the active principles. This confusion has resulted in unnecessary and unwise use of ovarian products. Since the isolation of the three or more active principles from the urine of pregnant women, treatment of ovarian disorders has become more rationalized. These substances from pregnant urine are called anterior-pituitary-like substances because it is unknown whether or not they derive from the pituitary. According to Collip, they are formed in the placenta. Although all are derived from the urine of pregnant women, they are isolated through different chemical routes and possess different chemical formulas. It has been suggested by Collip that perhaps all of these are but variations of the original unknown hormone in the urine, but changed by reason of the various processes employed for isolation and purification. It is a clinical fact that the administration of whole ovary extract will in some cases accomplish what single purified hormones can not do. According to Frank[4] in the normal female the following hormones require consideration: (1) —a—the bisexual trophic hormone of the anterior pituitary, b—the bisexual a-p-l hormone found in the blood, urine and placenta, (2)—the estrogenic factor, (3)—the corpus luteum hormone (progestin), (4)—the testis hormone (found in both ovaries and testes).

In the normal menstruating female the estrogenic factor increases to 25 mouse units per liter of blood before menses and disappears within 2 to 6 hours of onset of flow. Estrogenic substances injected into the blood disappear rapidly but concentrate in menstrual blood 5 to 6 times the concentration in circulating blood. When the physiologic menopause is fully developed, no estrogenic substance is found in the blood or urine, but in half of the cases the gonadotrophic factor is greatly increased in the blood. This factor differs from the a-p-l factor of pregnant urine and resembles the pituitary. In artificial menopause estrogenic substance is absent from blood and urine. The gonadotrophic factor is increased as early as the 10th day after operation and always after 8 weeks.

By ovarian insufficiency is meant either the absence of the ovaries, or their functioning at such a low level activity that clinical symptoms appear. The physiologic ovarian failure of the menopause is not considered here because it may be anticipated, and in many cases therapy is unnecessary. The age at which the menopause may occur varies greatly, but rarely occurs as early as does ovarian failure of the types to be considered in this discussion. Here we shall deal with early ovarian failure.

In amenorrhea, oligomenorrhea, purely functional sterility and often in dysmenorrhea, ovarian inactivity is easily recognizable. Werner[5] and others, however, have called attention to the benefits of female sex hormonal therapy in many cases of nervous women with various symptoms in whom ovarian insufficiency had not been suspected.

As to the age incidence, in the experience of a series of several hundred patients with early ovarian insufficiency, it is evident that the average age ranges from 25 to 35 years, although it may be found at puberty.

The predisposing factors are: influenza, measles, pneumonia, pelvic infections, underdeveloped sex organs, frigidity due to mechanical or psychologic causes, surgical interference with the ovaries, secondary anemia, excessive social activity with insufficient rest, too frequent childbirth and ovarian cysts.

The symptoms are variable. Extreme nervousness, fatigue, despondency and weakness are usually prominent. The variableness of the symptoms at menopause is reflected in the other forms of ovarian failure. The types are numerous, yet the symptoms are recognizable. Severe suboccipital headache is often a characteristic symptom. Riley Bricker and Kurzok[6] found prolan in the urine of 20 of 29 cases of migraine. The two cases presenting statusmigrainicus the excretion of prolan was uninterrupted. There was, therefore, a continuous relationship between the appearance of prolan and the occurrence of the headache.

The following protocols will serve to illustrate some of the most common types classified according to symptomatology, since the findings are all of insufficient ovarian secretion.

Report of Cases

Case 1.—(Gastro-intestinal type). A female, aged 23 years. She complained of stomach trouble. Her family considered her hysterical. She had been suffering with indigestion for two months and had been in bed 8 days. Her birth weight was 6½ pounds at term. She had had measles, pertussis, mumps, chickenpox, influenza, and sore throat until her tonsils were removed at 12 years. An embedded wisdom tooth had been extracted. She ate chiefly fruits and vegetables. She never used tobacco, alcohol or drugs. She had a good appetite and was not constipated. She slept fairly well for eight hours but usually dreamed and sometimes had nightmares. However, she felt rested in the morning. Her menses began at 13 years, occurring every 28 days. There was seldom any pain. The duration of the flow was six days, but the last three days were always very scant. The patient was more nervous before and during her menses. She had choking and tightness in right side of the neck occasionally. She felt very weak. The diet had been liquid for four weeks. She could not eat much. The bowels were slightly loose after going on a full diet three days previously. The patient at times dieted and then went on a sugar spree. She gained weight easily. Her greatest weight was 135 pounds and the lowest was 113 pounds. The examination revealed slight obesity, weakened heart action, marked tenderness over both ovaries, and cold feet and hands. The hymen was intact. The patient had never experienced sexual gratification during three years of married life! Response to ovarian hormonal therapy was satisfactory. The patient became strong enough to leave her bed and come to the office after three weeks. She reached normal in about six months. Marital relations are now quite pleasurable and she is planning for a new member of the family. A year after treatment, she is still well in every respect. This case is an example for a rather large group of women suffering with symptoms referable to the G. I. tract, but who on careful examination are found to have no other disorder but a disturbed ovarian activity.

Case 2.—(Goitre). A female of 18 years, complaining of convulsions since puberty at the age of 12. The menses were regular, with a flow of 5 to 7 days. It was formerly profuse, but later quite scanty. The convulsions were always associated with the menses, either three days prior to or one week after menses. At each attack, there was experienced severe choking, cyanosis, and unconsciousness for about fifteen minutes. The examination showed the patient to be 50 pounds overweight. The tonsils were infected. The thyroid gland was enlarged symmetrically to two and one-half its normal size. There was a rapid pulse (120). Pronounced exophthalmos was present. The patient was extremely nervous. There was a marked tremor of the outstretched fingers and the protruded tongue. All of the findings of exophthalmic goitre were present except loss of weight. The basal metabolic rate four days prior to menses was plus 60. After treatment and her menstruation had become established the rate was plus 18. The following month before menses the basal was plus 24, and one week later it was plus 8. The convulsions, which were but choking attacks due to the greatly enlarged thyroid gland, were controlled by ovarian hormonal therapy. Operation was contraindicated in this case as it would have produced myxedema.

THE TREATMENT OF ACNE VULGARIS*

Cosby Swanson, M.D.
Atlanta

The condition known as acne vulgaris is a chronic, inflammatory disorder of the pilosebaceous follicles, characterized by comedones, papules, pustules and cystic nodules. The most common locations are the cheeks and forehead. In many cases all parts of the face, chest, upper arms, shoulders and back are involved. In the severe types the lesions often extend to the back and buttocks. In a few cases the face is not involved, the lesions are found only on the chest, shoulders and back. It is one of the commonest and most polymorphous of skin diseases, usually manifesting itself at the age of puberty, most frequently in those who have coarse, oily, seborrheic skin of the face and seborrhea of the scalp.

The lesions usually present are comedones, papules and pustules; they vary greatly in shape, size and number. In severe cases the pustules especially vary in size, shape and depth. In a few cases, inflamed nodules, deep granulomatous infiltrations, pustular cystic lesions, atrophic and hypertrophic scars are also encountered.

Acne is thought by the majority of physicians to be due to changes in the consistency of sebaceous secretions. It is often spoken of as the disease of the adolescent, the majority beginning at puberty when all the glands of the body, including the skin are hypersensitive. The increased activity of the endocrine system, gonads, thyroid and other glands affect the secretions of the sebaceous glands. This relation is also manifested during menstruation, preceding and following which time the eruption is likely to be aggravated.

This hyperactivity and enlargement of the glands of the skin cause the formation of comedones and their subsequent infection. In those with lowered resistance from this infection there follows the development of the different types of inflamed lesions found in acne. The inflammation from the infection

*Read before the Ninth District Medical Society, Gainesville, September 18, 1935.

often causes destruction of the tissues of the skin which heals with the formation of scars.

Acne is considered by most dermatologists to be a syndrome and not a disease. In the majority of cases there are a number of contributing factors. The advocates of primary local bacteria (acne bacillus) as a cause has not been proven after many years of careful research by the leading men of this and other countries. Opinions differ as to the primary cause of the pustules and abscesses found in acne. All agree as to the type of organisms found, staphylococcus and acne bacillus. These organisms are present at all times in persons with normal healthy skin and it is only when certain conditions are present that they form the inflamed lesions found in acne.

Why some have and others do not have the disease we do not know, so we use the terms, lack of resistance and predisposition; therefore some unknown cause or causes are present other than the abnormal conditions found. When more is known of the action of the hormones, we may then have more knowledge of the cause of acne.

Clinical observation has led the majority of observers to contend that while there is a certain inherited predisposition to acne (large pored oily skin) along with certain internal factors such as the physiologic and pathologic activities of the internal secretions taking place at this time, there are in the majority of patients other disorders present, such as constipation, so-called intestinal toxemia, foci of infection, error of diet, over-eating, especially excess of carbohydrates derived from sweets and cold drinks; lack of outdoor life, exercise and sunshine; diseases such as the anemias, tuberculosis, malaria, diseases of the liver, kidneys, spleen and toxic states in which no particular disease can be located.

In the majority of cases of acne the symptoms vary and they are usually classified accordingly. In acne sexualis the eruption is limited to the face, especially the cheeks and chin; seborrhea is slight or absent; menstrual disturbances are usually present and new lesions of acne nearly always occur at the menstrual period. In acne intestinalis the lesions are found mostly on the trunk; constipation, intestinal toxemia, colitis and diseases of the digestive organs are the most out-standing symptoms. In seborrheic acne, as a rule, all locations on which acne occurs are involved, face, chest, shoulders and back; we find oily skin, a very large number of small lesions and often hyperactivity of the thyroid glands. Neurotic acne occurs in persons who have unstable nervous systems; the majority of cases seen are in young girls and an acne phobia usually is present. Nervousness and undernourishment are the outstanding symptoms. Patients with this type of acne continue to traumatize the lesions by picking and scratching with their finger nails, causing more infection, ulceration and scarring. Acne artificialis usually develops in persons as a result of external irritants connected with their occupations or the taking of drugs especially bromides, iodides and many of the hypnotic and sedative drugs; there is a difference in the appearance of the eruption from other types seen. Pustular acne develops after adult age, twenty-three or more years. In this type of acne no comedones and very few papules are found. The majority are due to foci of infection or so-called intestinal toxemia, or both. In acne cacheticorum the lesions are indolent, deep seated, purplish, nodular, pustular, healing with scars; they are found on various parts of the body especially shoulders and back. As a rule marked symptoms of cachexia, error of diet and foci of infection are present. The majority have, or have had infection of the lungs or pleura or both.

Of the different types of acne there are all stages of the disease from the mild to the very severe types; the different types often merge making it difficult to classify.

Acne is a chronic and obstinate disorder, prone to relapse and recurrence. In a few cases it disappears without treatment after adult age is reached; this is true only in healthy individuals. Others improve, but a large number of neglected cases persist well into middle life. To get the best results it is necessary to continue the treatment for several months and the general hygiene and diatetic treatment for years. When we consider the many conditions that enter into the causes, and complications that are associated with acne, it is obvious that the treatment of acne cannot be accomplished by any one formula if the best results are to be obtained. To prevent disfigurement and often an inferiority

TOXIC AMBLYOPIA*

*Tobacco-Alcohol-Focal
Infections-Diabetes*

HENRY M. MOORE, M.D.
Thomasville

It is with an interest of bringing out discussion that I present this paper to you. I have had in my limited experience what to me seems an unusually large number of toxic amblyopias, compared to reports by physicians in larger centers and with correspondingly larger practices. It is generally agreed that most symptoms are subjective; in fact, the patient comes to the doctor and complains of dimness of vision or loss of vision in either one or both eyes. A fundus examination will show practically a normal looking fundus; external eye clear, pupils often slightly dilated.

History is very important, the age of patient, habits as to eating, smoking and drinking. Males predominate; they smoke, drink, eat and are excessive in all habits more than women and have more focal infections: throat, sinus, teeth, prostate, and are more subject to diabetes. A careful history should be taken back for several months. The patient may truthfully tell you he doesn't smoke or drink, or very little; but on questioning he may tell you he has done both to excess up to a few days prior to your seeing him. Refraction will show little error compared to impairment of vision. Lenses will aid very little, if any, and it is not advisable to attempt at first to give any corrective lens.

The diagnosis is suspected and to a great extent made on the history of the patient and by elimination of other causes, a practically normal looking fundus with refractive error not in keeping with the degree of amblyopia, in what had been a seeing eye.

I am indebted to The Chemical Journal of London, The British Journal of Ophthalmology, Archives of Ophthalmology, U. S. A., The Transactions of the Ophthalmological Society of the United Kingdom, and an article in Northwest Medicine, 1932, by Richard W. Perry, of Seattle, for some of my

*Read before the Second District Medical Society, Quitman, April 10, 1936.

data. This material was loaned me by the A. W. Calhoun Library of Emory University.

The clinical part of this condition is the one of greatest interest to me; the theoretical and laboratory part is an attempt to explain the etiology and pathology of the parts affected.

Observation of Cases: The first case was a railroad man, aged 45, a moderate drinker and heavy user of tobacco. On eliminating tobacco and alcohol the vision cleared up to 20/20 in about six weeks. He resumed moderate smoking and had an immediate relapse. On discontinuing tobacco he again cleared up. He was warned that if tobacco was continued he would eventually go permanently and totally blind.

A recent case: A man, aged 41, could only see gross objects. His vision improved so on discontinuing tobacco that with the aid of plus .50 sph. he had 20/20 vision. On moderate use of tobacco he had beginning diminution of vision. Needless to say, he decided to divorce Lady Nicotine permanently. The patients all improved in their general health; some were very much underweight and gained as much as 20 pounds in six weeks.

Dr. Perry says that the use of pilocarpine in nephritis and hobnailed livers is well known, and reasoning along this line, after seeing cases of alcoholic amblyopia improve with the administration of 1/4 grain of pilocarpine daily for two days, then 1/3 grain for five days, this was repeated for an additional two weeks in amblyopic cases with good results.

Pilocarpine stimulates sweat glands, removes toxins, and liquefies deposits of infiltration on interstitial connective tissue of the optic nerve. Removal of the cause is most important. I have never used pilocarpine, but in the event I have a stubborn case, I think I shall do so. Dr. M. B. Ray, of London, notes that toxic amblyopias have very small refractive errors, and correction with lens helps very little or none. Of course, it is possible to have refractive error prior to the amblyopia, and that should be corrected.

I have had twelve cases of this trouble, most of them men over 40 years old. All used tea, coffee, Coca-Cola, all were tobacco users except one woman, all had hypertension, all had some dental foci of infection and hypertrophied tonsils, and three had diabetes. Of these cases there were ten recoveries. Two diabetic patients who were also hypertensive, discontinued alcohol, tobacco and other stimulants, were put on a suitable diet, referred to their family physicians, and did not have to take insulin. Their general condition improved, blood pressure was lowered to safety, but the glycosuria was unchanged. One woman's general condition improved but her vision was not improved. The diabetic patient would improve if given insulin and made sugar free. These diabetics happened to be the oldest patients under observation and under treatment the shortest time.

The etiology in the case of one woman was unde-

unilaterally. Central vision may be normal in one eye and peripheral vision affected. There is a great discrepancy in distance and near vision, the distance vision being relatively better. The optic disc is normal or shows a slight temporal pallor.

According to H. M. Faruair, toxic amblyopia is a partial blindness due to absorption of external poisons. He divides toxic amblyopia from diabetic amblyopia and toxic retrobulbar neuritis of pregnancy, though he admits the line is more artificial than real, as the pathologic lesions that have been found are much the same. He states that in toxic amblyopia both eyes are always affected and that in his country when toxic amblyopia is mentioned it nearly always means tobacco and alcohol emblyopia as 1 per cent of all eye diseases come under this head. (This looks to me like a pretty high per cent). The patients, generally men over 50 years of age, give a history of vision failing for weeks or months.

When the patient ceases to use tobacco the defect improves in about six weeks in mild cases; two to three months may elapse in more severe cases of longer standing, and the condition may become worse before improvement shows up. Years may be necessary for complete restoration of vision. Large amounts of tobacco is the general cause, though some people may have an idiosyncrasy and have an amblyopia though moderate users of tobacco. Chronic alcoholics who are non-tobacco users do not seem to be affected.

The true cause of the disease is tobacco, but the disease is determined in nearly every instance by a depression in the patient's health. The age incident shows disease appears when health begins to fail. Tobacco amblyopia may complicate other diseases. Prognosis: good.

Conclusion

Toxic amblyopia is more common in men, in chronic tobacco users of long years. Age is an important factor. Tobacco plays a more important part in health than is generally realized. I think it may cause its trouble by affecting the central nervous system, not only in amblyopia but many other conditions. No negroes with toxic amblyopia have been observed by me.

THE JOURNAL

OF THE
MEDICAL ASSOCIATION OF GEORGIA
Devoted to the Welfare of the Medical Association of Georgia

478 Peachtree Street, N.E., Atlanta, Ga.

SEPTEMBER, 1936

CORONARY INSUFFICIENCY

Attention has been called on many occasions to the increasing prevalence of coronary arterial disease. Leading pathologists throughout the world, and particularly in this country, are emphasizing the increasing number of myocardial infarcts found at necropsy. Most of the conditions described are unquestionably the end results of preexisting coronary disease and in the many thorough and comprehensive articles written on this subject, the very earliest stages of this disease have been neglected. Since 1912, and the splendid observations of Herrick, the general attitude toward this condition has undergone change. No longer does one hear a physician use the term "acute indigestion" for that sudden dramatic clinical picture, which we now know to be due to coronary occlusion. No longer do we believe that the coronary arteries are strictly end-arteries and no longer do we believe that the diagnosis of occlusion of one of these arteries is dependent upon a particular group of signs and symptoms. We know now that many occlusions are gradual in onset; that many occur without ever causing substernal pain and that the vast majority of them occur without ever producing that time-honored sign, a pericardial friction rub. The electrocardiogram has done much to verify the diagnosis and to enrich our knowledge of the late stage of coronary disease.

Coronary insufficiency, sometimes called stenocardia, may be *functional* or *organic*. It means that a given system of coronary vessels in a patient is not able to deliver the required amount of blood to his myocardium when it is needed. A certain amount of physiologic insufficiency of the coronaries may be present in every individual; for example, the sharp substernal pain that one experiences after some extreme effort, such as running a quarter-mile race at top speed. This

hydrochloride on heart muscle precludes its routine use.

The results obtained by a rational persistence in the use of a series of amebicides justifies the conclusion that under the present diagnostic standards any chronic diarrhea of unproven cause deserves prolonged and varied antiamebic therapy.

CRAWFORD F. BARNETT, M.D.

THE STUDY OF DISEASE

Too often the so-called modern physician travels the beaten path to the laboratory to prove or disprove something without first taking a good look at his patient. While he is willing to acknowledge the greatness of such clinicians as Hippocrates, Galen, Paracelsus, Sydenham, Laennec, Richard Bright, Graves and James MacKenzie, he forgets the picture of Sir William Osler sitting at the bedside of a patient, surrounded by young doctors and nurses, all of whom are observing and meditating. He forgets Theodore Janeway, Sr., who staked his reputation on his knowledge of aneurysms, simply stating that the patient under discussion was aged 55 and, therefore, she was not in the age group in which this condition commonly occurred.

Witness for example, the erroneous diagnoses made of common skin diseases. Scabies has been mistaken for some allergic phenomenon and numerous skin tests were applied to determine the patient's sensitivity to foods, face powder, dust and bacteria. A patient with exophthalmus, enlargement of the thyroid gland, tremors, tachycardia and who gives a definite history of losing weight and being too nervous to sleep, is treated for "nervousness" because the basal metabolic reading was near normal.

"Unfortunately the popular idea that the severity of symptoms will in some degree be proportional to the seriousness of the disease is quite incorrect." The patient with coronary occlusion may be comfortable and willing to get out of bed and go to work at the very time the infarction in his heart muscle is softening. To permit such activity for this patient is inviting certain disaster. Contrariwise, the psychoneurotic patient may insist that she is unable to feed herself.

Laboratory tests should be performed and should not be discredited, but more careful study of the signs and symptoms of disease is required if one keeps faith with the old masters in medicine.

URINARY BACK PRESSURE AS A CAUSE OF TOXEMIA OF PREGNANCY

Due to lack of knowledge as to the cause of the toxemias of pregnancy, such as pernicious vomiting, chronic nephritis, and eclampsia, little headway has been made in the treatment of these symptoms except in a symptomatic way. Numerous theories have been advanced, discussed and dropped as they have been considered inadequate by those who were in position to judge their merits.

In the Urologic and Cutaneous Review of August, 1936, Hayes presents a study of seventy patients to determine: first, whether or not there was sufficient evidence of kidney damage to account for the symptoms; second, whether or not such damage was of the type usually caused by back pressure; and third, whether or not it could be remedied by proper treatment. The results of his investigations were surprisingly conclusive and point to an entirely new conception of the toxic symptoms of pregnancy. He assembled collateral evidence to support this concept. For example, Baird examined forty-three pregnant women and found indigo-carmine excretion to be delayed in all and when obstruction was found this delay was greater. Numerous investigators have observed that the ureters are dilated and tortuous during pregnancy and Rush has reported one hundred fifty cases of pernicious vomiting cured by ureteral dilation.

Hayes' studies included sixty-two living patients and eight autopsy findings. He summarizes the results of the treatment of thirty-nine cases of pernicious vomiting, preeclamptic toxemia or eclampsia as follows: "All the mothers showed an immediate improvement after the kidneys were drained and all ultimately recovered, with some of them showing more or less permanent kidney damage. Among nineteen pernicious vomiting cases, only one miscarriage was observed and that was in a syphilitic mother. Among fourteen preeclamptic cases, five miscarriages occurred or a percentage of 35.7. Among the eclamptic cases, one miscarriage occurred, or

type known as pyelitis and pyelonephritis. Hydronephrosis and residual urine may seriously damage the kidney function before albumen, casts, blood, pus, or bacteria direct attention sharply to the primary cause. Anemia, edema and high blood pressure may reach a serious stage before the primary cause is suspected or attacked.

To regard the presence of pus as a proper line of demarcation between the so-called medical and surgical nephritis often brings disaster. Premature aging, anemia, advanced cardiac, circulatory, infectious and toxic symptoms often arise from congenital as well as acquired obstruction before adequate urologic studies are made.

No organism has been found to have a selective action for the kidney, the kidney pelvis, or the bladder unless there is a congenital or acquired obstruction or pockets which do not drain properly and which render the organ vulnerable to infection. It is not only desirable, therefore, but necessary in the treatment of nephritis to know the type of genitourinary disability present as well as to know the source which feeds the infection. Intelligent treatment requires knowledge of predisposing as well as exciting causes. Kidney disease is rarely a disease involving the kidney primarily. The kidney is like an innocent bystander hurt in a fight he did not start.

All physicians admit that inadequate drainage plays a definite part in causing diverticulitis of the intestines, in the production of chronic gallbladder disease, in sinus infections, etc. It is equally true that nonspecific urethritis, cystitis, nephritis, pyelitis and pyelonephritis are most often caused by obstructive lesions. More rational measures would be employed in the management of these disorders if they were regarded merely as symptoms and not as diseases. Properly interpreted their rational treatment necessitates an attack on the primary causes.

EDGAR G. BALLENGER, M.D.

The JOURNAL would like to record the scientific work of Georgia doctors. It earnestly requests, therefore, that each physician in the State who publishes a contribution in some other medical periodical submit an abstract of the article for these columns.

GEORGIA DEPARTMENT OF PUBLIC HEALTH

T. F. ABERCROMBIE, M.D., *Director*

MALARIA CONTROL

That malaria is on the decrease in Georgia should be of interest to everyone. There is an annual fluctuation of malaria mortality and morbidity, but this is of minor consideration when we consider that over a period of years there is a decided reduction trend in malaria mortality. Although malaria control work by the State Board of Health has been intensive, it is realized that the practicing physician plays an important part in our program. Prevention and cure must proceed together in order that malaria may be reduced to a minimum.

Drainage for the reduction of malaria in Georgia precedes scientific knowledge of the cause and transmission of this disease. Some areas in the State possess a history of drainage for malaria control more than a century old. The State Department of Health has been concentrating on the promotion of this program for fifteen years, and in 1930 was able to stimulate considerable activity in the protection of urban areas. A widespread program originated the following year and numerous counties having a high malaria rate were aroused to the fact that the economic loss from malaria was a more serious threat to their people than was inadequate maintenance and construction of county roads. County convict crews were furnished for drainage construction. This drainage program proved so popular that with the start of the 1933 RFC relief program practically every county in malarial areas assigned most of their work-relief forces to malaria drainage operations.

Malaria drainage work in 1935 dealt with the end of the FERA program and with the beginning of the WPA, and operations have been principally confined to work-relief programs. However, considerable activities of a maintenance character have been carried on by local governments and an expansion of this work is contemplated as soon as work-relief is eliminated. Throughout the year State funds were not available for field service on the malaria drainage or community sanitation programs. During the first half of 1935 funds were not available from any source for field service in 145 of the 159 counties. Limited funds made available by the United States Public Health Service in fourteen full-time county health departments permitted the use of sanitary engineers in these counties for direction of sanitation and malaria drainage. On July 1, 1935, the budget

for these engineers expired and all field service was suspended with the exception of that provided by two assistant state directors, acting in the capacity of division engineers.

On September 1, 1935, provision was made for the establishment of three divisions and twelve district supervisors, to exercise technical supervision over WPA community sanitation and malaria drainage local projects. These positions were filled with funds provided by the United States Public Health Service, but difficulty was experienced in the resumption of the field service. The salaries offered on the new budget were markedly inferior to those offered on comparable positions in the new work-relief program. The trained engineers who had served in previous years had secured better positions. The background of experience and training in the specialties of epidemiology, botany, entomology, drainage engineering and public relations, required of a public health officer in the projection of county-wide malaria drainage programs is so extensive that it has been possible to extend limited service on the malaria drainage program, although it is anticipated that with further training and experience the department will again be able to offer effective service in this field.

This problem has been further complicated by the fact that more than 9,000 ponds have already been drained in the State. Because there has been no opportunity to record the location of these ponds and attendant drainage construction, new engineers assigned to districts are faced with the necessity of carrying on several months intensive field activity in each county before they are in a position to intelligently advise local authorities in matters of malaria control practice. Because of time limitations prohibiting the development of this background, certain field personnel have been concentrated on the supervision of the community sanitation program, and for all practical purposes the amount of service available on malaria drainage during the latter part of 1935 has been reduced to the equivalent of two or three full-time supervisors.

It is apparent that the people of Georgia are receiving benefits of great value and it is evident the volume of genuine malaria control protection received by them greatly exceeds what they would have accomplished during the same period through dependence upon local resources.

NEWS ITEMS

A practicing physician with an excellent established practice wants an associate. Numbers of other locations where physicians are wanted are available. If interested write the Secretary-Treasurer.

Dr. Samuel Y. Brown, Atlanta, returned recently from New York City where he took post-graduate study in surgery, and announces the opening of offices at Suite 501 Doctors' Building, Atlanta.

Dr. T. H. Chesnutt, Moultrie, Colquit County, Commissioner of Health, reported that health conditions in that county had been better for the past twelve months than for many years, not a single case of typhoid fever had been reported and only one case of diphtheria.

The Ware County Medical Society met at the Ware Hotel, Waycross, on August 5th. Dr. K. C. Walden, Chief of the A. C. L. Hospital, spoke on *Gallbladder Diseases.*

Dr. C. L. Ayers, Toccoa, Past President of the Association, has been elected Chairman of the Stephens County Hospital Committee. It has been planned to build and equip the hospital during the fall season and have it ready for occupancy by early winter.

Dr. S. L. Waites announces the opening of his new offices in the City Pharmacy Building, Covington.

The Fulton County Medical Society met at the Academy of Medicine, Atlanta, August 20th. The program consisted of address, *Observations of European Clinic,* by Dr. Wm. Perrin Nicolson; clinical talk, *Headaches of Nasal Origin,* Dr. T. S. Burgess; paper, *Treatment of Cholecystitis,* Dr. Olin S. Cofer. The discussion was led by Dr. C. W. Roberts, Dr. Edwin S. Byrd and Dr. Lon W. Grove.

Dr. Geo. F. Klugh, Jr., has removed his office from the Healey Building to 139 Forrest Avenue, N.E., Atlanta.

The visiting staff of the Crawford W. Long Memorial Hospital, Atlanta, entertained Dr. L. C. Fischer as an honor guest at the Druid Hills Golf Club at a barbecue on August 18th.

The Colquitt County Medical Society at a recent meeting made plans to entertain the Second District Medical Society at its fall meeting to be held on October 13th at Moultrie.

Dr. A. G. DeLoach was elected President of the Atlanta Chapter of the Sons of the American Revolution; Dr. W. A. Selman was elected to the Board of Managers.

The Entertainment Committee of the Crawford W. Long Memorial Hospital, Atlanta, entertained the nurses of the Hospital to a watermelon cutting and swimming party at Cooley's lake on August 27th.

Dr. Thos. R. Aycock, Monroe, has resumed his practice after taking several weeks post-graduate study in some of the foremost clinics of New York City.

Dr. Rance O'Neal, Dr. J. L. Weldon and Dr. C. O. Williams have been appointed on the Rules Committee to draft rules and by-laws for the management of the Valley Hospital at West Point.

Dr. Michael Hoke has completed his undertaking with the Georgia Warm Springs Foundation and announces his association with Dr. Lawson Thornton and Dr. Calvin Sandison in the practice of orthopedic surgery in Atlanta, offices at 551 Capitol Ave., S.W.

The Coffee County Medical Society met at Douglas on August 25th. Dr. A. M. Johnson, Valdosta, read a paper entitled, *Pylorospasm in Infancy.*

The Fourth District Medical Society met at Warm Springs on August 10th. Titles of papers on the scientific program were: *Handling of Accidents Occurring During the Administration of Anesthesia,* by Dr. Wilmer Baker, New Orleans; *The Principles of Plastic Surgery as Applied to the Immediate Handling of Accidents,* Dr. Neal Owens, New Orleans; *Cardiac Pain,* Dr. L. Minor Blackford, Atlanta; *The Immediate Care of Fractures,* Dr. Frank K, Boland, Atlanta. Dr. Enoch Callaway, LaGrange, President of the Society, offered a silver cup to the winner in a golf tournament which was played at the Foundation's Golf Course after the scientific meeting. Dr. Hugh McCulloh, West Point, won the trophy.

Dr. Jack C. Norris, former Associate Professor of Pathology at Emory University School of Medicine— Grady Hospital, announces the opening of offices in Suite 810 Doctors' Building, 478 Peachtree Street, N.E., Atlanta. His practice will be limited to diagnostic procedures in pathology and clinical pathology.

Dr. Leo Smith, Homerville, entertained the members of the Ware County Hospital at the Musgrove Hotel, Homerville, on September 2nd. Dr. T. J. Ferrell, Waycross, read a paper entitled *The Significance of Auscultation in the Diagnosis of Abdominal Conditions.*

The Crawford W. Long Memorial Hospital, Atlanta, will open its nurses' training school at an early date. Applications will be accepted from competent young women.

The Fulton County Medical Society met at the Academy of Medicine, Atlanta, September 3rd. Dr. George A. Williams reported a case, *Contusion of the Heart with Aortic Regurgitation and Complete Recovery;* Dr. T. F. Sellers made a clinical talk, *Analysis of One Hundred Cases of Undulant Fever in Georgia;* Dr. J. H. Kite, Atlanta, read a paper, *Tuberculosis of*

BOOK REVIEWS

The Art of Treatment. By W. R. Houston, A.M., M.D., F.A.C.P. Formerly Professor of Clinical Medicine, University of Georgia. Formerly Visiting Professor of Medicine, Yale-in-China. The Macmillan Company, New York. Price $5.00. Houston's book should be a delight to the practitioner of medicine. Instead of the dull statistical treatise made so familiar to us in America by Teutonic influence, he approaches the treatment of disease with a broad philosophy and with a charmingly lucid style.

The treatment of the sick patient rather than the label of disease is the main thesis of the book; and this thought is elucidated with a clarity seldom encountered since the time of Osler. Each chapter shows profound learning and an intimate care for the details of treatment, but the scholarly ideas are brought out with such ease and grace of manner that the reader absorbs a great deal of knowledge almost painlessly. The chapter on psychotherapy forms a short treatise of itself and shows by its many angles of approach the wide culture of the author.

This is a book that should be in the hands of everyone interested in the treatment of disease.

H. M. MICHEL, M.D.

Clinical Heart Disease. By Samueal A. Levine, M.D. 443 pages, price $5.50. W. B. Saunders Company, Philadelphia. Concepts as regards heart disorders have changed markedly in the past decade. As a result much has been written, a great deal of which has been highly misleading. This has left the general practitioner and surgeon in a state of mental confusion when attempting to secure information regarding such subjects as systolic murmurs, functional heart disorders, etc. Dr. Levine, an outstanding authority, has written a book which is purely clinical and which covers the entire subject of cardiology, including etiology, pathology, diagnosis, prognosis and treatment. The chapters on the development of rheumatic heart disease, acute cardiac emergencies, factors concerning prognosis and treatment of congestive heart failure are especially interesting. The section on electrocardiography is adequate. The book contains enough ideas of a controversial nature to stimulate the reader to further work and thought. In writing this book Dr. Levine has rendered a genuine service to the general practitioner and specialist alike.

C. M. WEST, M.D.

Parenteral Therapy; Walten F. Dutton, Director, Medical Research Laboratory, Amarillo, Texas, and George B. Lake, Editor Clinical Medicine and Surgery. Published by Charles C. Thomas, Baltimore, Maryland. Price $7.50.

Parenteral Therapy deals with all methods of extra-oral medication and gives details of technic and discusses freely indications, complications and formulas. It is one of the most valuable books of the year and should be on the desk of every practicing physician, whether general practitioner or specialist; it will also prove valuable to dentists and nurses. This volume deals with anesthesia administered intravenously, subcutaneously, spinally or nerve-block and gives details as to methods, doses, dangers and complications. It describes in detail the injection method for obliteration of varicosed veins, varicocele, hydrocele, hemorrhoids and hernia. This book also contains a valuable therapeutic index and pharmacologic notes which will be very helpful to the busy practitioner for a quick reference.

Parenteral therapy is rapidly becoming the modern method of treatment in the hospital, in the office and in the home. Drs. Dutton's and Lake's treatise will familiarize you with its indications and methods.

T. C. DAVISON, M.D.

Synopsis of Diseases of the Heart and Arteries. By George R. Hermann, M.D., Ph.D., Professor of Clinical Medicine, University of Texas, Member Association of American Physicians, etc. 344 pages with 88 illustrations and 3 color plates. Price $4.00. St. Louis: The C. V. Mosby Company, 1936.

Dr. Hermann set out to write a book for the student and general practitioner. He has aimed to put into concise form every fundamental about the heart. He carefully selected the illustrations, selecting some "not so much for their novelty as for their value." The publisher moreover, has collaborated in the manufacture of the book, so that it can be easily slipped into one's coat pocket.

Although the book will be of no particular assistance to one who wishes to delve deeply into cardiology in the preparation of an ambitious paper, it is recommended without reservation to all those who wish to increase or to refresh their knowledge of the heart.

L. M. B.

This Sixth Edition of the National Formulary is of particular interest. As it marks the completion of about 50 years of National Formular history as a published authority, a comparison with former editions is instructive as indicating the development of pharmacy during this period.

This edition contains 689 monographs on drugs, chemicals and preparations; 232 of these items are new to National Formulary VI and 321 monographs included in National Formulary V have been dropped from this new edition. The greatest increase has been in ampule and tablet preparations. Glandular products make their initial appearance in this edition. The deletions have been mostly in the fluidextracts, mixtures and miscellaneous preparations.

The outstanding features of the Sixth Edition may be summarzied as follows:

1—The admission of monographs for drugs and chemicals which are not included in the U. S. Pharmacopoeia XI or in the formulas of National Formulary VI.

2—By the establishment of nation-wide surveys, a basis of definite extent of use has been determined which governs admissions and omissions.

3—The simplification of formulas of simple preparations. This was done to eliminate restrictions on their manufacture.

4—The extensive development of ampule and tablet monographs and of the section on Diagnostic Materials and Preparations.

5—The admission of glandular powders and the development of histologic descriptions of them.

6—The development and use of many additional assays of the chemical proximate and biologic types.

The arrangement of the subject matter has been excellently handled. It is an important and very necessary work, in that it authoritatively covers a wide field of well known and frequently used preparations for which standards are not provided in the U. S. Pharmacopoeia.

J. D. KITCHENS, PH.G.

Medical Dictionary. Gould's Pronouncing Medical Dictionary, Fourth Edition. Thoroughly revised with many new words and definitions. It has the quality and quantity of medical words and terms with definitions generally used in medicine and allied sciences and a valuable asset for quick and accurate references. *New Definitions* are carefully checked. *Gould's Dictionary* holds steadfastly to accuracy, real scientific content and service. *Pronunciation* is represented by simple English phonetics. *Revisions* are always to keep the dictionary up-to-date. *Contents* include all words that belong in a modern medical dictionary. *Illustrations* are ample. *Tables* include arteries, bones, measures, muscles, weights, also breath sounds in health and disease, diet lists, dose-lists which have been revised according to the latest pharmacological and medical research. The dictionary contains 1538 pages, 273 illustrations and 175 tables. Publishers: P. Blakiston's Son & Company, 1012 Walnut Street, Philadelphia, Pa. Price $7.00, or with thumb index $7.50.

ABSTRACT

"Variations in glycogen content of vaginal mucosa as a relative index to the quantitative amount of Ovarian Hormone available in the organism."—John F. Krumm, Chicago—American Journal Obstetrics and Gynecology, June, 1936.

The principle of the Schiller-Gram test in diagnosis of cervical and vaginal malignancies is used to determine ovarian function. This test is based upon the reaction of iodine to the glycogen stored in the vaginal mucosa. Positive tests are graded as number 1, number 2, normal, and exaggerated, depending upon the density of the staining reaction. This test was made in a large series of women and the presence or absence of ovaries were definitely known to be absent either alone or as a part of a panhysterectomy the strain was invariably negative. It was also found to be negative in girls before puberty and in women past the menopause—both physiologic and artificial. Variable results were obtained when the test was made upon patients in whom a hysterectomy had been done and the ovaries left intact. Many patients as late as 5 to 11 years after operation showed positive reaction while others as recent as 3 to 18 months after operation reacted negatively to the test and were annoyed with hot flashes and an increase in the waist line. The impression is

hat in the former the ovaries continued to function
while in the latter they had generated or were degen-
rating. It is hoped by further study to be able to
etermine the effect of subtotal or total hysterectomy
pon the length of viability of the remaining ovary or
varies.

In a number of post-menopausal patients with a
egative test it was possible after a number of injec-
ions of concentrated follicular hormone to obtain a
ositive Gram test. This would indicate that the pres-
nce of glycogen in the vaginal mucosa is dependent
pon the presence of ovarian hormone in the organism.
'he test was found positive in pregnancy, varying in
ntensity at different stages in the same individual. In
he presence of uterine fibroids the test was highly
ositive. Further study is to be made in constitutional
iseases such as tuberculosis, diabetes and malignancies.

In a large number of cases with trichomonas vaginalis
: was noted that the Gram test was negative or only
ildly positive. In one patient with severe and per-
istent trichomonas the vaginitis cleared up spontane-
usly during pregnancy. It is well known that tri-
homonas proliferate rapidly after menstruation at a
ime when ovarian hormone is low in the body. Mas-
ive doses of ovarian follicular hormone in oil were
iven to a number of patients 3 to 6 days before
enstruation with very excellent results in checking the
richomonas infestation. It appears that increased ova-
ian function is a factor in checking trichomonas vagin-
lis. Abstract by C. B. Upshaw, M.D.

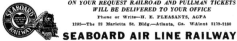

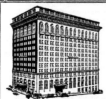

THE JOURNAL

OF THE

MEDICAL ASSOCIATION OF GEORGIA

DEVOTED TO THE WELFARE OF THE MEDICAL ASSOCIATION OF GEORGIA
PUBLISHED MONTHLY under direction of the Council

| Volume XXV | Atlanta, Ga., October, 1936 | Number 10 |

THE PROBLEM OF THE DIAPHRAGM*†

ARTHUR M. SHIPLEY, M.D.
Baltimore, Md.

The surgical problem of the diaphragm has a number of phases that should be considered. There is the question of disease of the diaphragm itself, but the more important factor is the relation of the diaphragm to disease in either the abdomen or chest. The position of the diaphragm is often an important diagnostic problem and at times it is difficult to locate clinically or in a roentgenogram in its relationship to a lesion in its immediate vicinity. The pathologic changes may be evident enough, but it may be most difficult to say whether the diaphragm is above, below, or is a part of them.

The diaphragm may be found high or low without any serious inconvenience and at times such unusual positions are without real significance. It is apt to be relatively high in short, broad-chested individuals and the converse of this is true, so that in reading an x-ray plate these facts should not be overlooked. The diaphragm is high in fat individuals and in patients with ascites and in the late months of pregnancy. On the other hand, the diaphragm is high in many conditions within the chest independent of abdominal disease; in pulmonary tuberculosis with fibrosis the diaphragm is not only apt to be elevated, but it is also apt to be thickened, adherent and irregular. In massive collapse of the lung it is elevated. In shock, because of superficial breathing, the diaphragm may be found elevated and much of the postoperative discomfort following operations in

the upper abdomen is due to a combination of paralytic ileus plus a high diaphragm caused, in part, by increased pressure from below, as well as partial collapse of the lung because of shallow and painful breathing, together with increased areas of atelectasis created by plugging of small bronchi by mucus. Such a patient is unwilling to breathe deeply or to cough and the areas of poorly areated lung may become infected. It was common practice in past years to speak of such a condition as ether pneumonia.

The diaphragm may be found high without any explanation as to the cause and if this elevation is marked the condition is spoken of as eventration. It may be paralyzed. Rarely birth palsy will involve the phrenic nerve or toxic paralysis may be seen in diphtheria or lead poisoning. Tumors of the cervical cord involving the cord itself, where the symptoms are due more to localized destruction than to pressure, may involve the phrenic nerve.

In approaching this subject one has to consider whether the diaphragm itself is at fault and if that is so, whether it is the muscle and tendinous part or its pleural or peritoneal covering, or whether there may be some dysfunction due to paralysis spasm or irregular action, or whether there is some form of herniation through it. Generally none of these things is present, but the diaphragm is playing a relatively passive part and enters into the problem because of pathologic changes in the abdomen or chest, or both.

The diaphragm performs a three-fold service to the body. It separates the abdomen from the chest and in so doing accomplishes two important things: it prevents the contents of the abdomen from entering the chest, and its most important function is to make possible a differential pressure mechanism within the celom. The diaphragm as a com-

*Read before the Medical Association of Georgia. Savannah, April 22, 1936. Invited guest.
†From the Surgical Clinics of the University Hospital and the Baltimore City Hospital. Baltimore, Md.

plete septum between the abdomen and chest came into existence because of changed conditions within the torso brought about by the mammalian solution of the continuity of species at the time when animals began to give birth to live offspring. The simple cloaca was no longer an efficient apparatus and the necessity of bringing live offspring into the world able to look out for themselves, in part at least, made it necessary for the mother to carry her young in utero for relatively long periods in order to perfect their development. Some mechanism was necessary to protect the respiratory and circulatory organs from pressure during the later periods of intra-uterine gestation and especially to make safe the very great increase in intra-abdominal pressure during delivery, so that the diaphragm as a complete differential pressure mechanism between the abdomen and chest is not found until one encounters the mammals.

The most used function of the diaphragm is the least essential. It is a very important muscle of respiration, but is not necessary to life as both sides of the diaphragm may be paralyzed and an individual still get along without much handicap. On the other hand, if all other muscles of respiration are paralyzed the diaphragm alone is able to maintain sufficient respiration to support life. The muscle of the diaphragm ranks next to heart muscle in the high quality of its ability to perform its work. By all laboratory tests the properties of diaphragm muscle stand at the top of the skeletal muscles. Lee, Guenther and Meleney have shown this conclusively and list a long series of tests in which this extraordinary muscle outranks all the rest.

Joannides believes that eructation of gas is a function of the diaphragm. Air is swallowed along with food and liquids, especially if ingestion is rapid, or gas may be formed in the stomach, if there is interference with proper emptying at the pylorus and also in ileus, either paralytic or mechanical, as there may be reverse peristalsis allowing intestinal gases to enter the stomach.

After phrenic neurectomy eructation may be difficult or altered and observation with the fluoroscope supports the belief of Joannides. He has observed that during eructation there is contraction of the left diaphragm and he believes that at the same time there

is relaxation of the right side. This is an interesting observation of contralateral behavior of the two sides. Cardiospasm is very likely a diaphragmatic dysfunction as the esophageal opening is entirely surrounded by the decussating crurae. The prevention of regurgitation of food is a function of the diaphragm and vomiting is a phenomenon in which the diaphragm plays a role. Habliston, Aycock and Shaw in a paper published in the University of Maryland Bulletin do not agree with Joannides. Their report is based on a careful postoperative study from the Departments of Surgery and Tuberculosis at the Baltimore City Hospital, of 48 cases of phrenic avulsion with hemidiaphragmatic paralysis.

The embryologic development of the diaphragm seems to be a confused and intricate matter and congenital defects are better understood when this fact is borne in mind. The anterior portion of the diaphragm is formed from the septum transversum, a mass of mesoblastic tissue which begins its growth high up toward the head and gradually descends. The septum transversum contains also the anlage of the veins of the heart and of the liver. There is a second mass of primitive cells, the pleuroperitoneal membrane which forms the dorsolateral portions of the diaphragm. In between these two masses there grows forward a portion of the dorsal mesentery and a small portion of the periphery of the diaphragm is formed by infolding of the lateral walls of the torso. That part of the diaphragm formed by the body wall has given rise to very considerable controversy as to whether or not the diaphragm receives any motor nerve supply from the lower intercostal nerves.

The stomach begins its development as an enlargement of the foregut within the thorax and gradually descends below the diaphragm. Its rate of descent is controlled by the growth of the esophagus. If the esophagus fails to lengthen before the diaphragm is formed the stomach remains a thoracic organ and the intestinal tract opening in the diaphragm is for the duodenum instead of the esophagus.

The motor supply to the diaphragm is believed by most anatomists and surgeons to come entirely from the phrenic nerve. The sensory supply is from the phrenic nerve which supplies the central portion of the diaphragm and from the lower sixth intercostal nerves which chiefly supply the periphery. The lymphatics of the diaphragm play a very important part in its pathologic changes and in the relationship between abdominal disease and chest complications. Both infection and metastasis spread very easily from abdomen to chest, but the reverse is not common. There is abundant clinical and experimental proof of the rapidity and ease with which infection reaches the chest from the abdomen. If particulate matter, dyes or organisms are injected into the peritoneal cavity they may be recovered very soon afterwards in the lymphatic spaces of the diaphragm and in the mediastinum.

The lower ribs slant sharply forward and downward, while the tilt of the diaphragm is backward and downward. This brings the lower ribs obliquely across the plane of the diaphragm. This makes it necessary to clearly define the cephaladcaudate axis of the body in locating the diaphragm in relation to the ribs that cross it. The shape of the diaphragm is due to three factors: the diameter of the leaflets is greater than the diameter of the body at that level and the minus pressure in the chest, together with the increased intraabdominal pressure, give the diaphragm its characteristic dome-shaped form:

"On the right side, the convexity extends upward to the level of the fourth interspace anteriorly and to the level of the eighth rib posteriorly. On the left side, the convexity reaches to the level of the fifth interspace anteriorly and to that of the eighth interspace posteriorly."

The attachment of the diaphragm to the body wall is fixed and does not change with its varying positions. It is the central portion of the two halves of the diaphragm that is elevated or depressed under varied conditions of physiologic action and pathologic change. When the diaphragm is depressed the costophrenic angles broaden out and when the diaphragm is elevated the costophrenic angles become sharp and narrow. Any attempt to locate the attachment of the diaphragm and the level of the costophrenic angle along a rib line is confusing, unless the vertical axis of the body is borne in mind. One gets a very good idea of this fact when it is remembered that the approach to the splanchnic

nerves in the Peet operation for their resection above the diaphragm in the treatment of hypertension, is along the eleventh rib, which is resected for about 7.5 cm., from its attachment to the spine. This approach holds good for both the right and left sides. In the midline in front, the level of the diaphragm is the junction of the second portion of the sternum with the ensiform. This is an important landmark as it forms the lower boundary of the triangle of safety through which the usual approach is made to the pericardium in operating for suppurative pericarditis.

The diaphragm is in relation above with the lower lobes of both lungs covered by pleura and with the contents of the anterior, middle and posterior divisions of the lower mediastinum and their contents. A wide variety of pathologic changes may be found, therefore, just above the diaphragm and in more or less intimate contact with it. Below, the liver is on the right and while the right subphrenic space does not exist as such in health, a number of collections may be found there, the chief of which are subphrenic abscess, localized pyopneumoperitoneum, adhesions between the liver and diaphragm, or some lesion of the liver pushing the diaphragm upward. Rarely there will be seen a hernia through the right side of the diaphragm in which either the stomach or a portion of the liver may be found.

On the left side the stomach, spleen and left lobe of the liver are in intimate contact with the diaphragm, while the colon, omentum and coils of small intestine may enter into the picture. The pancreas being behind the peritoneum and fixed, is usually not displaced upward but infections beginning in this organ may reach the diaphragm, so that there is a very wide possibility of mishap when all of the diseases of any of these structures are considered.

In many instances when pathologic changes are present, it is not difficult to say by clinical findings and x-ray examination that the trouble is either on the right or left and is either above or below the diaphragm, but it is sometimes difficult to know whether the diaphragm is an active or passive agent in the lesion found.

There are times, however, when it is difficult to determine what the relationship of the diaphragm is to the disease found, so that, often enough to make the problem a real one, clinicians and roentgenologists have to answer the question: where is the diaphragm?— Is it above or below, or is it a part of the mass or collection of fluid, or is there a hernia through the diaphragm, or is one side or other of the diaphragm entirely missing? Under the fluoroscope the diaphragm may be seen moving with respiration and in most instances the outline of the diaphragm is clear enough in the film, but if there is any uncertainty there are a number of procedures which may help to locate the diaphragm in relation to puzzling lesions in this region. Pneumothorax, or pneumoperitoneum, or stimulation of the phrenics, or bronchography may aid in locating it. Roentgenograms taken in different directions and the visualization of the stomach with some shadow throwing substance, or by the aid of air or fluid, may also help.

Tumors of the diaphragm are not common and by far the greater portion are secondary and metastatic. There are less than twenty reports of primary tumors of the diaphragm in the literature. Tuberculosis is common and rarely there will be weakening of the diaphragm caused by extension of infection from the lung and hernia may be a slow development.

Phrenic neurectomy has called especial attention to the position and function of the diaphragm. Suggested by Stuertz in 1911, it was first undertaken in the treatment of bronchiectasis. At the present time it is associated in the minds of most physicians with pulmonary tuberculosis, but there is a considerable list of conditions for which some form of phrenic nerve interruption is practiced with more or less success. This procedure has been undertaken for hiccough, spasm of diaphragm, persistent eructation, tic of the diaphragm, adhesions between pericardium and diaphragm, diaphragmatic pleurisy, tetanus, persistent cough, hemorrhage from the lung and in preparation for operations on the diaphragm, lung or esophagus. The approach to the nerve depends upon the condition for which interruption is undertaken. Consequently an accurate knowledge of the location and relations of the phrenic nerves is essential.

One of the reasons for failure to get the desired elevation of the diaphragm after phrenic neurectomy by the common approach above the clavicle is because in from 25 to 40 per cent of all individuals the phrenic nerve has an accessory branch that joins it below the clavicle from the nerve that supplies the subclavius muscle. Thomas B. Aycock, working in the anatomical laboratory at the University of Maryland, reports 130 dissections of phrenics and found the percentage was nearer 40 than 25. He also demonstrated by careful dissection that some communication could be found in almost every subject between the phrenic and the stellate or cervicothoracic ganglion.

The diaphragm itself is more often the site of pathologic changes than is commonly supposed. Acute infectious diaphragmitis may occur and while infections of the diaphragm usually reach it by extension from the chest or abdomen, there are almost surely a certain number of primary infections of this structure. Joannides has reported three cases and suggests that this condition be called Hedblom's syndrome. At autopsy when there is an acute infectious process in contact with the diaphragm there will be found edema and infiltration of the muscle and tendon with thickening of the peritoneum or pleura which cover its lower and upper surfaces. Our attention has been fixed on the serous coverings and we have been overlooking the diaphragm itself. There are many lymphatics that pass through this structure and it is easy to understand how infection may reach it. In the x-ray examination of such a diaphragm its appearance is quite striking. If it is pushed upward by some abdominal condition or sucked upward by collapse of the lung or elevated by eventration or paralysis without any involvement of the diaphragm itself, its outline is apt to be smooth and clear cut and the costophrenic angle sharp and visible. If, on the other hand, the diaphragm is inflamed it will have a "fuzzy" appearance with a cloudy, indistinct outline, is often thicker than normal and, if it is adherent, it is apt to be distorted.

Several years ago I was interested in a patient who was in the University Hospital, Baltimore, and under the care of Dr. M. C. Pincoffs and the late Dr. Gordon Wilson. This patient was taken acutely ill with fever and a moderate elevation of the pulse rate, but his outstanding symptom was a continuous pain on the left side of his body, chiefly in the position of the left diaphragm, and with a great deal of pain also under the left scapula with some radiation to the neck, felt chiefly along the medial margin of the trapezius muscle. This pain was not markedly worse on ordinary respiration, but very much aggravated by deep breathing. Fortunately, there was no cough, but the patient was very apprehensive lest he cough, sneeze or hiccough. The x-ray showed thickening of the pleura along the diaphragm and loss of clear diaphragm outline, but repeated auscultation failed to discover any rales or other evidence of lung disease. This patient had had attacks of gout, involving the metatarsophalangeal joint of his left great toe and he insisted that the trouble in his chest was gout of his diaphragm. This diagnosis was not certain until the fourth day of his illness at which time the left great toe became red, painful and swollen. He had been in the habit of controlling his attacks of gout with colchisat and when this drug was given for the gout in his foot, the pain in his chest promptly disappeared. About one year later this same patient had a similar attack in his right side, with the same symptoms except that the x-ray showed less involvement of the pleura, but the appearance of the diaphragm was the same. The attack was shorter, owing to the fact that treatment directed at gout was begun immediately after the beginning of the symptoms.

The only reference to gout of the diaphragm that either Dr. Pincoffs or I was able to find is in Trousseau's Clinique Medicale de L'Hotel-Dieu published in Paris in 1877. In this book Trousseau refers to observations made by him in another publication and says that W. Butter, an English physician, had described the same condition as diaphragmatic gout.

There is some confusion as to terminology when writing of hernia through the diaphragm. The most used classification divides these protrusions into three groups: *congenital, acquired* and *traumatic* and they are spoken of as *true* or *false*, depending on whether or not there is a sac.

A very excellent description of the surgical anatomy of the diaphragm in its relation to hernia was given by Hedblom in the Cyclopedia of Medicine. It is very clear and brief and is as follows:

"The diaphragm is a thin, fibromuscular septum between the thoracic and the abdominal cavities. It consists of a peripheral muscular and a central tendinous portion, and has three large openings: the esophageal, the aortic and the caval. The esophageal is the only one of the three through which hernias occur. It lies at the level of the tenth dorsal vertebra a little to the left of the midline, is oval in shape, and is bounded by two muscle bundles from the crurae which rise on either side of the bodies of the upper lumbar vertebrae. The inner halves of these bundles cross one another between the aorta and the esophagus, and then pass forward to the central tendon. The size of the muscular ring so formed varies somewhat. Hernias occur in the gap bridged by pleura and the peritoneum between it and the contained esophagus.

"There are two triangle parasternal areas anteriorly —known as the foramina of Morgagni—between the attachment of the muscle to the xiphoid and to the cartilage of the seventh ribs, where there is a gap in the muscle bridged over by peritoneum, through which diaphragmatic hernias occasionally occur.

"There are two other triangular lumbo-costal areas, between the attachment of the muscle to the vertebra and twelfth rib, called the foramen of Bochdalek, which are similarly lacking in muscle and through which a fetal hernia may develop. After birth these areas are protected from pressure by the upper poles of the kidneys and are, therefore, seldom the sites of an acquired hernia."

Traumatic hernias are usually false, but congenital and acquired hernias may be with or without a sac. Congenital hernias are due to some defect in the formation of the diaphragm from its component parts, or to widening in the esophageal opening.

There are a number of reasons why hernia occurs through the esophageal hiatus. This opening is guarded by the medial margins of the two crurae which cross between it and the aortic opening, which is really not a foramen in the diaphragm, but is behind it lying immediately in front of the body of the upper lumbar vertebrae with the crurae on either side. The thoracic duct and vena azygos major also pass through this opening. The opening through which the esophagus passes from thorax to abdomen is much larger than the empty esophagus. This larger size is to accommodate a bolus of food. The opening is to the left of the center and is poorly supported by the posterior mediastinum and is behind the heart which is in the middle mediastinum. There is also a peritoneal pouch that extends for a short distance along the esophagus. All of these factors together with the difference in pressure between the abdomen and chest favor the development of hernia at this site. When coughing, vomiting, hiccoughing and straining at stool are considered, it is surprising that hernia is not more common than it is.

It is only rarely that structures behind the peritoneum are found in the chest. Recently there was reported a large rent in the diaphragm extending from the esophageal opening backward and laterally on the left side with both the kidney and spleen lacerated and partially displaced into the thorax.

Several years ago there came into the accident room at the City Hospital, Baltimore, a man who had been injured by falling earth. He was badly shocked and x-ray examination showed the left side of the chest almost filled with abdominal contents. He had eaten his lunch just before the accident and had drunk a bottle of orange juice. A small needle was thrust between the ribs and the orange juice was aspirated. He began to recover somewhat from shock and there was no evidence of peritonitis. It was thought that the crushing injury had torn his diaphragm and that the stomach was partially in the thorax and was ruptured. He was operated on by opening the thorax through a long intercostal incision with the intention of closing the rent in the stomach, reducing the hernia and suturing the diaphragm. Very much to my surprise I opened into what seemed a normal peritoneal cavity containing stomach, spleen, colon and small intestine, except that these structures occupied the left thorax. There was no evidence of any injury whatsoever and examination showed a complete absence of the left diaphragm. The intercostal incision was closed and the patient recovered without any further mishap. He was seen recently and came into the hospital for x-ray examination which showed exactly the same findings as were seen immediately following his injury. He is not conscious of any disability, his heart is very little displaced and all that remains of the left lung is crowded into the apex of the left chest.

About the same time there came into Dr. Pincoffs service in the University Hospital a

young college student, who, since he could remember had been troubled by intermittent attacks of discomfort after eating with vomiting. At times he would be quite well, but the spells of pain and vomiting were becoming more frequent. X-ray showed the pyloric end of the stomach above the diaphragm with the hernia in front of the esophageal opening. There was considerable elongation of the duodenum. At operation, through a high left-sided abdominal approach, about one-half of the pyloric end of the stomach was found in a hernia through the ventral portion of the diaphragm near the anterior body wall and just to the left of the midline. The stomach was the only content. It was not adherent and not very much constricted and was easily reduced. There was a true sac, which was adherent medially to the pericardium and laterally to the pleura covering the lung and very adherent to the defect ring in the diaphragm. No attempt was made to free the sac, but the neck of the sac, together with the edges of the defect in the diphragm, were closed by three layers of silk sutures. This patient made a good operative recovery and has remained symptom free. The hernia was probably due to enlargement at the site of the foramen of Morgagni.

The larger congenital hernias are usually due to defects caused by failure to fuse between the septum transversum and the pleuroperitoneal folds and the opening is usually seen on the left side between the esophageal opening and the posterolateral chest wall. Such a hernia may be true or false and if there is no sac there are apt to be many adhesions between the herniated structures and the contents of the lower thorax. If the defect is large, closure may be difficult. Paralysis of that half of the diaphragm may make closure less difficult and in inoperable hernia phrenic neurectomy may be followed by marked improvement in symptoms. Rarely hernia will occur through the foramen of Bochdalek.

The most common acquired hernia is through the esophageal opening with the stomach usually the only structure in the sac. Recently we have observed the development of a small hernia of the stomach through the diaphragm following avulsion of the phrenic nerve.

A few days ago I saw a patient who is a physician and who has been partially disabled by pulmonary and intestinal tuberculosis since 1918. His chest condition has been carefully watched at Saranac and he has been seen repeatedly by Dr. Edward Archibald of McGill University. He has a large defect in the midportion of both the left and right diaphragm and the greater part of his stomach is in his thorax, lying transversely behind the heart.

Most diaphragmatic hernias in children are congenital. Truesdale has collected 303 cases from the literature; 165 were found at autopsy; 90 with the x-ray; 35 clinically and 13 at operation. Of this number 44 were operated on for cure of the hernia, with 24 recoveries. Truesdale added 13 cases of his own, 10 of whom were operated on with only one death. Most of these congenital hernias in children are due to a defect at the junction of the pleuroperitoneal fold with the septum transversum. In several reports there is evidence of a combination of congenital weakness and tearing due to trauma.

BIBLIOGRAPHY

Arey, L. B.: Developmental Anatomy. 3rd edition. Saunders, Phila., 1931.
Aycock, T. B., and Hablston, C. C.: Radical Phrenicotomy. The American Rev. of Tuberculosis, 22:757-768 (Dec.) 1930.
Hablston, D. C., Aycock, T. B., and Shaw, C. C.: Hemidiaphragmatic Paralysis as an Adjunct in the Treatment of Pulmonary Tuberculosis: Report of 48 Cases. Univ. of Md. Bulletin, 22:1-21 (July) 1936.
Harrington, S. W.: Diaphragmatic Hernia. Arch. Surg. 16:386 (Jan. pt. 2), 1928.
Harrington, S. W.: Phrenicotomy in the Treatment of Diaphragmatic Hernia and of Tumors of the Wall of the Chest. Arch. Surg. 18:561 (Jan. pt. 2), 1929.
Harrington, S. W.: Diaphragmatic Hernia Associated With Traumatic Gastric Erosion and Ulcer. S. G. & O. 51:504 (Oct.) 1930.
Hedbiom, Carl A.: Diaphragmatic Hernia. Cyclopedia of Medicine. Vol. IV, 553-565, F. A. Davis Co., Phila.
Higgins, G. M., and Graham, A. S.: Lymphatic Drainage from the Peritoneal Cavity in the Dog. Arch. Surg. 19:453 (Sept.) 1929.
Joannides, Minas.: An Extraperitoneal Transdiaphragmatic Route for Lower Intrathoracic Surgery. Ann. Surg. 84:337 (Sept.) 1926.
Joannides, Minas.: An Extraperitoneal Route of Approach for Intrathoracic Surgery. Ann. Surg. 80:908 (Dec.) 1924.
Joannides, Minas.: Acute Primary Diaphragmitis (Hedblom's Syndrome). Am. J. M. Sc. 189:566-570 (April) 1935.
Joannides, Minas.: The Mechanics of Eructation. J. Thor. Surg. 2:380-383 (April) 1933.
Lee, F. S., Guenther, A. E., and Meleney, H. E.: Cited by Lemon, W. S., Chapter on the Diaphragm. Cyclopedia of Medicine. Vol. IV:538-550, F. A. Davis Co., Phila.
Lemon, W. S.: The Function of the Diaphragm. Arch. Surg. 17:840 (Nov.) 1928.
Lemon, W. S.: The Physiologic Effect of Phrenic Neurectomy. Arch. Surg. 14:345 (Jan. pt. 2) 1927.
Lemon, W. S.: Chapter on Diaphragm. Cyclopedia of Medicine. Vol. IV:538-550, F. A. Davis Co., Phila.
Magee, Russell.: Rupture of the Diaphragm With Report of 2 Cases. Canad. Med. Jour. 32:506-509.
Stewart, Wm. H., and Illick, Earl.: Where is the Diaphragm? Radiology 22:668-673, (June) 1934.
Stuertn: Cited by Lemon, W. S., Chapter on the Diaphragm. Cyclopedia of Medicine. Vol. IV:538-550, F. A. Davis Co., Phila.
Tattersall, K. R., and Harvey, E. B.: Rupture Following Slight Trauma. Brit. M. J. 1:879, (April 27), 1935.
Trousseau, A.: Goutte. Clinique Medicale de L'Hotel-Dieu, 342-391.
Truesdale, P. E.: Anatomy of the Diaphragm. The Jour. of Thoracic Surg., 4:429-434 (April) 1935.
Truesdale, P. E.: Traumatic Rupture as a Sequence to Congenital Hernia of the Diaphragm, with an Experimental Study of Its Mechanism and the Effects of Phrenicotomy. Ann. Surg. 90:601 (Oct.) 1929.

THE EFFECT OF EMOTIONAL DISTURBANCES ON SLEEP*

GLENVILLE GIDDINGS, M.D.
Atlanta

The role of the emotions, both as causative and contributing factors in disease, is generally recognized in clinical medicine. A cursory review of medical literature suffices to impress one with the emphasis placed on emotional factors by physicians in such clinical phenomena as cardiospasm, pylorospasm, spastic colitis, angina pectoris, hypertension and other manifestations of the spasmogenic aptitude. Alvarez, in his interesting monograph on Nervous Indigestion, recites a number of cases of severe gastrointestinal disorders that evidently had no organic origin; they were due solely to worry, anxiety, fear or some other emotional state. In the physiologic laboratories, Cannon, Pavlov and others have shown that secretory activity, peristaltic movements and other physiologic processes are affected by the emotions.

These physiologic effects produced by the emotions suggest that emotional disturbances might also interfere with sleep. If such is the case, the emotions might in this way affect adversely one's health or, interfere with recovery from illness. The importance of sound sleep in maintaining good health is generally admitted. In ministering to the sick, physicians recognize that nothing favors recovery from illness more than restful sleep; it is a common clinical observation that a restless, sleepless patient makes little progress toward recovery.

Alvarez[1] says that "it is strange that so many physicians forget to ask about sleep. Especially in the case of nervous patients insomnia may be the secret of all the troubles complained of." Elsewhere he states that "in innumerable cases all the patient needs to bring back his health is relief from insomnia; but unfortunately physicians often fail even to ask about sleep, and thus miss the chance to work a cure . . . " The nervous person, he continues, "needs to get away from his tumultuous and bothersome thoughts; he needs rest, and it should be obvious that little can

*Read before the Medical Association of Georgia. Savannah, April 23, 1936.

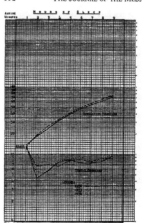

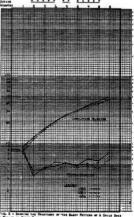

be done for him until he learns again to sleep."

> Sleep that knits up the ravelled sleeve of care
> The death of each day's life, sore labor's bath
> Balm of hurt minds, great nature's second course,
> Chief nourisher in life's feast.

Since the emotions which play such an important part in everyone's life may perhaps interfere with Nature's restorer, sound sleep, I shall attempt in the present paper to give an experimental answer to the question, "How is sleep affected by the emotions?"

In a problem of this nature the first task is to find some reliable means of gauging the depth of sleep. It may be stated at this point that no accurate method has as yet been devised for determining the exact moment when a person goes to sleep or is awakened; however, Johnson and Weigand[2], Renshaw[3], Müllin, Kleitman and Cooperman[4], and others have shown that the time spent in bodily movements after retiring serves as an accurate index of the character of one's sleep. With Renshaw and others we may assume that the depth of sleep is inversely proportional to the amount of bodily activity during sleep. In my studies I have taken the time spent in changing one's position in bed while asleep, as a comparative basis for estimating the depth of sleep. Since sleep is affected by a number of factors such as noise and quiet, light and darkness, heat and cold, I endeavored to control all extraneous factors by maintaining conditions as uniform as possible. The subjects of these experiments retired at the same hour every night and were all awakened at the same time in the morning. The dormitory in which they slept was kept dark and free of noise. In order to eliminate as much as possible any errors that might be introduced by uncontrollable variations in temperature and atmospheric conditions normal sleep records were obtained on alternate nights to serve as controls for comparison with the records obtained under experimental conditions.

The apparatus used in these experiments for recording sleep was originally described by Renshaw and Weiss[5]. A mechanism was attached to the bedspring, consisting of a perpendicular metal plate containing alternate inserts of bakelite and brass. The slightest movement of the person occupying the bed

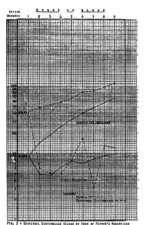

FIG. 3 - EMOTIONAL DISTURBANCE CAUSED BY NEWS OF FATHER'S REMARRIAGE

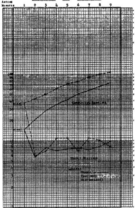

FIG. 4 - EMOTIONAL DISTURBANCE CAUSED BY BICYCLE BEING STOLEN

caused two small brush contacts to travel up and down over the plate, making or breaking an electric contact. This mechanism was connected by cables with a hypnograph in an adjoining room. The hypnograph consisted of a battery of 24 stylus pens (one for each bed) which wrote on a uniformly traveling roll of paper, 8 inches (20.32 cm.) broad. Two colors of ink were used in the pens, one for the male and another for the female subjects. As the paper moved under the pens, it was stamped electrically by a timer at one minute intervals, and each body movement accurately recorded, minute by minute, for the entire nine hours or 540 minutes that the subject was in bed. When the contacts were made or broken by the bed mechanism, electromagnets on each pen of the hypnograph made offsets from the base line on the record. Relay boxes were so arranged that if the circuit through any bed ceased functioning properly, the signal lamp flashed and remained burning until the condition was corrected. Thus when a subject left his bed for any purpose during the night, the relay lamp at once notified the operator of this fact.

The subjects used in this investigation were boys and girls in a boarding school, ranging in age from 9 to 14 years. In a study of this nature there is a distinct advantage in using children as subjects as their daily routine can be better controlled than that of adults.

At the end of each night's observations all the minutes during which there was any movement on the part of the sleeper, were counted, hour by hour, for each of the children and the total number of active minutes recorded. From this record the observations were copied daily onto the subject's chart.

All graphs have been plotted on ratio paper, as we believe that the trend can be more readily shown by using this method. The hours of sleep are listed at the top of the graph with a scale showing the number of active minutes on the left of the graph. The lower limb of the graph shows the time spent in body movements, hour by hour, of the child or children under observation. The upper limb is a summation of the active minutes throughout the night. The resultant curve may be referred to as the child's sleep pattern.

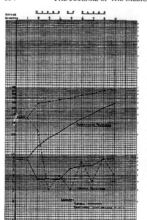
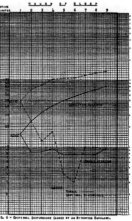

In order to obtain a normal sleep pattern we used 15 consecutive nights in which 24 children had followed their normal daily routine. The sleep pattern thus obtained was derived from 3,240 hours of normal sleep. Considering the children from an individual standpoint, we can say that no two children have the same sleep curve except in a very general way. The first hour in bed is the most active hour and the next most active period is the last regular hour of sleep. In a vast majority of children the quietest sleep is reached the second 30 or 60 minutes after going to bed. As a concrete example: if a child retires at 8:30 p.m. and arises at 5:30 a.m., it will be more restless, that is, show more active minutes between 8:30 and 9:30 p.m. and 4:30 and 5:30 a.m., than in any other two hours of the night. Aside from this, generalities cease, and what may be quite normal for one child, may be distinctly abnormal for another, assuming both to be normal children. These observations apply equally to boys and girls.

In the course of this investigation I have been struck by the constancy of the sleep pattern of the individual children. If a child is physically well, living his usual routine life in his regular environment, his sleep behavior changes only with atmospheric temperature. I wish especially to stress the statement that this is true only if the individual is in good health. When illness is impending, marked deviations from the child's normal type of sleep can be observed three or four days before the disease becomes clinically apparent. We believe that the nature of one's sleep is probably the most constant of all the factors that enter into his physiologic and psychologic behavior and that no single factor serves as a more accurate index of well being than the character of an individual's sleep.

This remarkable constancy of sleep is shown in Fig. 1 which gives the sleep pattern of a subject whom we have followed over a period of three years. It will be noted that the general character of the sleep patterns is practically identical, in fact there was a variation of only four active minutes from year to year. Each graph represents an average of 15 nights' observations which were made

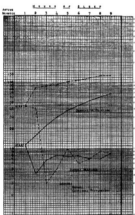

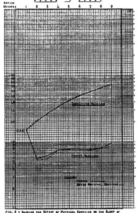

FIG. 7 - EMOTIONAL DISTURBANCE - SHOWING THE SLEEP THE NIGHT BEFORE COMMENCEMENT.

FIG. 8 - SHOWING THE EFFECT OF PHYSICAL EXERCISE ON THE SLEEP OF A GROUP OF TWELVE CHILDREN.

during the autumn of 1932, 1933 and 1934. A similar finding is noted in Fig. 2. These are two examples of 22 sets of observations, all of which confirm this statement. Because of this constancy of sleep it is easy to detect any deviations from the normal that might be induced by the emotions. Figs. 3 to 11 illustrate the effect of the emotions on sleep. Fig. 3 shows the sleep motility of a girl who was told one day that her widowed father had remarried; previous to this time she had no intimation of his intentions. As seen in the graph, her sleep that night was greatly disturbed. Fig. 4 shows the restlessness throughout the night of a boy who received a letter from home stating that his bicycle had been stolen. As the straightened circumstances of the parents made it impossible for them to replace the stolen bicycle, this was quite a calamity in the child's life. Fig. 5 is another illustration of the restless character of sleep following emotional excitement. This boy was called upon one evening to sing at a school banquet, which was for him a novel and exciting experience. Fig. 6 is the sleep record of a child following an at-

tempted burglary late in the afternoon in the dormitory where the subjects of these experiments slept. The children hearing of this occurrence were naturally apprehensive. The other children also manifested similar restlessness that night. In Fig. 7 we have a representation of the disturbed sleep of a child the night before commencement. The closing of school, as one recalls from his childhood days, arouses in a child many happy anticipations and is a time of jubilation.

From the illustrations we may conclude that the emotions, whether of a pleasurable or painful nature, interfere with normal sleep. It matters not what emotion is aroused—fear, worry, disappointment or pleasant anticipations of the future. The examples given are but a few of many observations which lead us to believe that probably no single factor affects sleep more constantly and more adversely than the emotions.

Frequently one hears it said that exercise is conducive to sound sleep; sometimes, on the other hand, it is maintained that one sleeps better if he relaxes and rests an hour or so before retiring. In a previous paper[6] I

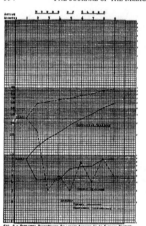
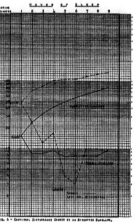

In order to obtain a normal sleep pattern we used 15 consecutive nights in which 24 children had followed their normal daily routine. The sleep pattern thus obtained was derived from 3,240 hours of normal sleep. Considering the children from an individual standpoint, we can say that no two children have the same sleep curve except in a very general way. The first hour in bed is the most active hour and the next most active period is the last regular hour of sleep. In a vast majority of children the quietest sleep is reached the second 30 or 60 minutes after going to bed. As a concrete example: if a child retires at 8:30 p.m. and arises at 5:30 a.m., it will be more restless, that is, show more active minutes between 8:30 p.m. and 9:30 p.m. and 4:30 and 5:30 a.m., than in any other two hours of the night. Aside from this, generalities cease, and what may be quite normal for one child, may be distinctly abnormal for another, assuming both to be normal children. These observations apply equally to boys and girls.

In the course of this investigation I have been struck by the constancy of the sleep pattern of the individual children. If a child is physically well, living his usual routine life in his regular environment, his sleep behavior changes only with atmospheric temperature. I wish especially to stress the statement that this is true only if the individual is in good health. When illness is impending, marked deviations from the child's normal type of sleep can be observed three or four days before the disease becomes clinically apparent. We believe that the nature of one's sleep is probably the most constant of all the factors that enter into his physiologic and psychologic behavior and that no single factor serves as a more accurate index of well being than the character of an individual's sleep.

This remarkable constancy of sleep is shown in Fig. 1 which gives the sleep pattern of a subject whom we have followed over a period of three years. It will be noted that the general character of the sleep patterns is practically identical, in fact there was a variation of only four active minutes from year to year. Each graph represents an average of 15 nights' observations which were made

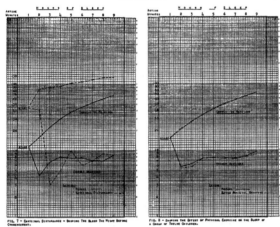

FIG. 7 – EMOTIONAL DISTURBANCE – SHOWING THE SLEEP THE NIGHT BEFORE COMMENCEMENT.

FIG. 8 – SHOWING THE EFFECT OF PHYSICAL EXERCISE ON THE SLEEP OF A GROUP OF TWELVE CHILDREN.

during the autumn of 1932, 1933 and 1934. A similar finding is noted in Fig. 2. These are two examples of 22 sets of observations, all of which confirm this statement. Because of this constancy of sleep it is easy to detect any deviations from the normal that might be induced by the emotions. Figs. 3 to 11 illustrate the effect of the emotions on sleep. Fig. 3 shows the sleep motility of a girl who was told one day that her widowed father had remarried; previous to this time she had no intimation of his intentions. As seen in the graph, her sleep that night was greatly disturbed. Fig. 4 shows the restlessness throughout the night of a boy who received a letter from home stating that his bicycle had been stolen. As the straightened circumstances of the parents made it impossible for them to replace the stolen bicycle, this was quite a calamity in the child's life. Fig. 5 is another illustration of the restless character of sleep following emotional excitement. This boy was called upon one evening to sing at a school banquet, which was for him a novel and exciting experience. Fig. 6 is the sleep record of a child following an at-

tempted burglary late in the afternoon in the dormitory where the subjects of these experiments slept. The children hearing of this occurrence were naturally apprehensive. The other children also manifested similar restlessness that night. In Fig. 7 we have a representation of the disturbed sleep of a child the night before commencement. The closing of school, as one recalls from his childhood days, arouses in a child many happy anticipations and is a time of jubilation.

From the illustrations we may conclude that the emotions, whether of a pleasurable or painful nature, interfere with normal sleep. It matters not what emotion is aroused—fear, worry, disappointment or pleasant anticipations of the future. The examples given are but a few of many observations which lead us to believe that probably no single factor affects sleep more constantly and more adversely than the emotions.

Frequently one hears it said that exercise is conducive to sound sleep; sometimes, on the other hand, it is maintained that one sleeps better if he relaxes and rests an hour or so before retiring. In a previous paper[6] I

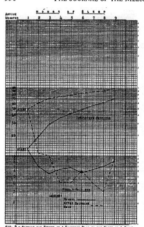

FIG. 9 - Showing the Effect of a Swimming Race on the Sleep of a Child.

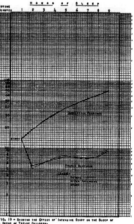

FIG. 10 - Showing the Effect of Intensive Study on the Sleep of a Group of Twelve Children.

have shown that a normal individual, accustomed to moderate muscular activity, can take intensive physical exercise in the late afternoon and even immediately before retiring without having his sleep appreciably affected one way or the other. These conclusions were deduced from a series of observations made on a group of twelve subjects. Beginning one hour before the time for retiring, or one hour and fifteen minutes after the evening meal, the group was taken out of doors on an illuminated basketball court and given hard, vigorous exercises, consisting of skipping the rope, setting-up exercises, skipping and running. The procedure was to have the group exercise three minutes and to rest two minutes. Each exercise was done in rotation, the cycles being repeated until 8:15 p.m. If a member of the group became obviously fatigued he was asked to drop out and proceed to the dormitory. At the conclusion of the hour the exercises were completed and the group was sent to the dormitory to undress and retire for the night, lights were extinguished and the recording instrument was started promptly at 8:30 p.m. These exer-

cises were done every other night in order to avoid the possibility of a carry-over effect from the exercise.

At the conclusion of the exercise period of 15 nights the sleep activities for these nights was determined and plotted against the normal nights on which no exercise was taken. We have reproduced the average of 15 nights' sleep for the entire group of 12, compared with the average of 15 nights' sleep of the same group on which no exercise was taken in Fig. 8, as we wish to show how one may be misled into attributing restless sleep to physical exercise, when the real culprit is not the exercise, but the emotions associated with it. In Fig. 9 we have the record of the sleep of a boy who had engaged in a swimming race at 4 o'clock in the afternoon. On first thought one might be inclined to the conclusion that the restless sleep was due to the physical exercise. This conclusion would go unchallenged if our other studies represented in Fig. 8 had not shown that exercise as strenuous, if not more so than the swimming, did not result in disturbed sleep. Another

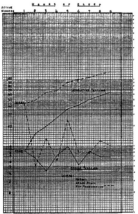

Fig. 11 • Showing the Effect of Study for An Examination on the Sleep of A Child.

promptly at 8:30 p.m. The mental work was carried on every second night during the test period. This plan made it certain that there was no carry-over effect from the previous test night. At the conclusion of the study period of 15 nights the sleep activity on these study nights was determined and plotted against 15 non-study nights.

Again. as in the foregoing discussion on physical exercise. we reproduce a graph which has been published previously (Fig. 10). It is necessary to keep this figure in mind, in interpreting the observation recorded in Fig. 11. This latter figure represents a child's sleep one night after hard study. Here again one could easily arrive at an erroneous conclusion. The child's study this night was in: preparation for an examination and no one's school days are so far removed that he does not remember how an impending examination upset his emotional equilibrium. In view of the other observations that an · equal amount of study did not affect the children's sleep, it is proper to attribute the night's restlessness to an emotional disturbance and not to mental activity.

These observations, I believe, afford unmistakable. evidence of the untoward effects of the emotions on sleep. It is hoped that they may offer some practical and· helpful suggestions to the practicing physician.

BIBLIOGRAPHY

1. Alvarez. W. C.: Nervous Indigestion. Paul B. Hoeber, New York. 1931.
2. Johnson. H. M.. and Weigand. G. E.: The Measurement of "Sleep." Proc. Pennsylvania Acad. Sci. Sc. 2:43, 1927.
3. Renshaw. S.: Children's Sleep. Macmillan Co.. New York. 1933.
4. Mullin, F. J.; Kleitman, N., and Cooperman. N. R.: Studies on the Physiology of Sleep: X. Effect of Alcohol and Caffeine on Motility and Body Temperature During Sleep. Am. J. Physiol. 106:478, (Nov.) 1933.
5. Renshaw. S., and Weiss: Journal of Psychology, 1926.
6. Giddings, Glenville: The Effect of Study and Physical Exercise on Your Child's Sleep. Hygeia 12. 1934.

Discussion of Paper by Dr. Glenville Giddings

DR. JAMES N. BRAWNER (Atlanta) : Dr. Giddings' statement about environmental influences producing sleep reminds me of a statement made by one of my teachers in neurophysiology, who said that one of the greatest factors in producing sleep was monotony. So he lectured for a half hour in a monotonous tone, and then he looked over the audience and said, "Now I notice that about half the students are asleep, proving my statement.'

The experiments made by Dr. Giddings for the purpose of demonstrating accurately, by means of graphs the effects of emotional reactions on sleep, are very instructive. and I wish to compliment him on his ingenuity and his painstaking study. His work is valuable in the fact that it shows experimentally what we have surmised for many years from clinical experience,

explanation should therefore be sought. Our records show that the race in which this boy engaged was a highly competitive one. It is reasonable then to attribute the ensuing restless sleep to an emotional disturbance resulting from that intangible something which we may call the "spirit of competition" rather than to exercise or consequent fatigue.

In like manner sleeplessness may erroneously be laid at the door of mental activity or mental fatigue. I have previously reported observations showing that intensive mental activity immediately before retiring has no appreciable effect on sleep. Beginning. one hour before the regular time for retiring, a group of children under the supervision of three instructors were given simple mathematical problems to solve. Each child worked at maximum speed and excellent cooperation was exhibited by the group throughout the experiment. These mathematical sessions were concluded at 8:15 p.m. and by 8:30 p.m. the children were in bed, lights extinguished, and instructions given to remain quiet and go to sleep. Observations with the recording instrument were begun

One very interesting observation made by Dr. Giddings is that any of the emotions, whether pleasant or unpleasant, will cause sleep disturbances. This, when correlated with experiments made by Dr. Cannon of Harvard, who demonstrated the effects of the emotions on the glands of internal secretion, explains the profound effects of strong emotions on the endocrines and other tissues of the body. It explains also the damaging effects of grief, abnormal fears and intense hatred on the functions of the heart, blood vessels and digestive organs. The experiments indicate that insomnia, which is often seen in various types of nervous and mental disorders, may be caused by disagreeable psychic experiences which stimulate strong emotional reactions. As a corollary to the above assumption, it is reasonable to believe that mental experiences which promote an attitude of composure and serenity will also promote sleep, health and happiness. This explains why suggestive therapeutics is often of value in quieting a patient which may in turn promote sleep, and why the consoling remarks of a minister may be of value in relieving certain functional disorders.

Dr. Giddings has shown, by unerring mechanical means, that "when an illness is impending marked deviations from the child's normal type of sleep can be observed three or four days before the disease becomes apparent." While it is recognized that such disturbances in sleep are, in the majority of cases, not due to emotional factors, yet the experiment shows that any illness, however slight, may affect the sleep mechanism.

In studying patients suffering from insomnia, I often try to evaluate the possible causative factors. I have noticed that nervous conditions due to toxic states, such as the infectious-toxic psychoses, delirium tremens and drug psychoses, result in very marked insomnia, the patient sleeping very little, if any, for several days. One of the first symptoms of improvement in such patients is sound, natural sleep. This fact, I think, indicates that in toxic states the sleeplessness is due to some chemical disturbance in the body fluids. When the toxin is removed or perhaps neutralized by antibodies, sound sleep and rapid recovery from the psychosis occur simultaneously. Sleep disturbances in those mental disorders due to unbearable situations, emotional shocks and other psychic factors are often marked but are not so persistent as those seen in the toxic psychoses.

I wish to state that Dr. Giddings has made a valuable contribution to scientific medicine, and he is to be complimented on his accurate and painstaking experiments.

DR. GEORGE L. ECHOLS (Milledgeville): I wish to thank Dr. Giddings very much for this study that he has made on this subject. In the first place it reminds me of the story of the party that visited his aunt. The next morning the aunt asked him how he slept, and he said, "I didn't stay awake to see."

It reminds me also of an experience I had in attending one of these medical association meetings in Athens. I got in, tired, and had a room across from the City Hall, and as I was going to bed the clock across the street was banging out ten. I had the feeling, "I am very tired, and I have eaten a big supper, and I am not going to sleep at all." I waked up with the same feeling in the morning, that I had not had fifteen minutes of sound sleep. I heard the old clock across the street banging out seven, and the thought came to my mind, "The whole night, with that clock striking every thirty minutes, I did not hear it a single time."

For that reason I realize fully how necessary it is for us to make more accurate studies, just as Dr. Giddings has been attempting to do.

For twenty-seven years it has been one of my jobs to get up in the morning and go through wards and read over the reports of how patients have slept and gotten through the night, and also to hear the story from the nurse or attendant that had observed these patients, and to see what a difference there is between the actual records as observed and what the patient tells you about sleep, and I have found their variation about as marked as my variation in my experience in Athens when I did not hear the clock all night long.

I would certainly like to see these experiments carried out on the real neurotics, with the emotions that you get in psychoses. As I gather, these observations are more or less in their infancy. Dr. Giddings' work has been, as I understand, on rather an average group of youngsters, who would be expected to sleep pretty well.

DR. GIDDINGS: Yes.

DR. ECHOLS: I should like to see this carried out further.

Back in the old days, when I first started this business of studying night reports on my wards in the state hospital and studying how the patient slept and listening to their stories, I had a notebook with just a bunch of prescriptions that would make anybody sleep, and I used those pretty freely. As time went on, the book wore out and I forgot some of the prescriptions and now I have forgotten them all. I am not looking so much to the sleep. Now I am looking more toward what the patient is eating, what sort of a diet the patient is getting, what sort of exercise he is getting, building up the general health, and I find with this type that I am talking about, the neurotic type and emotional, depressive type, there is not so much complaint about the sleep, but the thing that gives greatest pleasure, in looking over these reports, is to see that our recovery rates are much higher and death rates lower.

DR. ALLEN H. BUNCE (Atlanta): Some time ago I had an opportunity to visit this dormitory and see the way this work was carried on by Dr. Giddings. The building was erected especially for this purpose, equipped for it, and every possible outside factor was taken into consideration.

These boys and girls lead ordinary, normal, healthy lives, going to school, getting on well, and intelligent. This work of Dr. Giddings is really epoch-making, because it has never been done before. We have known very little about sleep. Dr. Giddings has been working here for a number of years, and his work has been presented before the American Medical Association, both in scientific session and scientific exhibit, and we owe him a debt of gratitude for his work along this line.

I think this is a beautiful demonstration this morning of differentiating between the emotions and exercise. In other words, where you have exercise and emotion, is it the exercise or the emotion which interferes with sleep?

I am very glad to have had the opportunity of hearing Dr. Giddings this morning. It represents a new phase of his work which has not been presented heretofore, and for us to know more about sleep, and how to control it, we should know the fundamental physiological facts which have been so clearly demonstrated by Dr. Giddings.

FIVE UNUSUAL FRACTURES*

J. H. MULL, M.D.
Rome

I wish to report five difficult and unusual cases of fractures selected from 821 cases treated at the McCall Hospital Clinic during the past five years.

Case Reports

Case 1. A young woman, Miss A. W., was brought to the hospital February 24, 1930, with a history of having passed through a cotton mill beamer. She caught her hand between the rollers and was dragged through the machine. Her fractures as shown by roentgenograms were: Fracture of the right zygomatic process, the upper six ribs in the right axillary line, middle third of both femurs and a compound comminuted fracture in the middle third of the right tibia, with laceration of soft tissues.

Due to multiple fractures, I decided it would be best to immobilize them as quickly as possible, although she was unconscious and in shock. She was put on the traction table, the compound fracture cleaned and repaired, a double spica splint was applied from the axillary spaces, including both legs, and the compound fracture was closed. The treatment of compound fractures as closed fractures has been routine for the last ten years unless excessive maceration of soft tissue prohibit. This patient was transferred to bed and the foot of the bed was elevated. Thirty pounds of weight were attached to the cross bar between her femurs. Roentgenograms on March 3, 1930, showed a satisfactory position and good alignment with about one inch overlapping in each femur. I could find no way in which to use countertraction other than her body weight, so we had to be satisfied with some shortening, as we had equal overlapping in both femurs and good alignment. She made a gradual recovery, and at the first change of plaster on April 15, 1930, I found good union in the left femur, and the right tibial fracture was healing by first intention. There was delayed union in the right femur. This was then immobilized in a Thomas splint

*Read before the Medical Association of Georgia, Savannah, April 22, 1936.

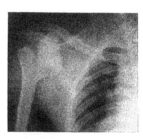

FIG. 1.
Fracture as shown when admitted to the hospital.

without traction. This patient remained in the hospital until August 11.

On leaving the hospital she had some muscular and joint stiffness in her right knee due to the long period of immobilization. This gradually improved, and she recovered with little permanent disability.

Case 2. L. S., a negro man, aged 35, during an epileptic fit fractured and dislocated the head of the left humerus on October 18, 1935. Following admission I tried to reduce his fracture and dislocation by closed methods usually used. This being impossible, I attempted an open reduction but was unable to reduce the fracture or dislocation. I then used Boehler's method of reduction, using screw traction, with an assistant placing a towel across the shoulder with the heel in the arm pit after screw traction had been applied. I then followed his technic of inserting a Kirschner wire through the olecranon process and using a screw traction appliance with a Thomas arm splint and reduced the fracture and dislocation. It was then put up in the usual position for fracture of the humerus. This patient made an uneventful recovery and was back in his laboring position about February 1. However, he still had some atrophy of his arm from disuse, but all movements were 90 per cent normal.

Case 3. S. H. was referred to the hospital on November 6, 1935, with a fragmented fracture and dislocation of the olecranon process and fracture, displacement, and dislocation of the head of the radius. An open operation was done over the olecranon and with kangaroo tendon the olecranon was fastened in place. I felt that I had reduced the dislocation at the time of operation, but the roentgenogram failed to confirm my opinion. I then applied screw traction and was able to get a satisfactory reduction of both ulna and radius. Following this reduction a skin plaster was applied. Subsequent roentgenograms showed that this held the fragments and that the dislocation was reduced. This man returned to his job as a driver of a school bus about January 1. He has about 60

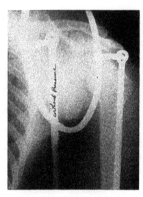

FIG. 2.
Screw traction appliance in place, pressure relieved to
allow head to slip into glenoid cavity.

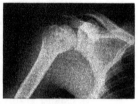

FIG. 3.
Shoulder after reduction. Check up film shows reduction
of dislocation and fracture.

per cent range of motion in his elbow with good rotation and without any noticeable deformity. The stiffness is gradually lessening in his elbow and he says he has no pain.

Case 4. E. D. S., male, aged 62, was admitted to the hospital on September 22, 1935, suffering from bruises and lacerations about the face and head as a result of an automobile accident. By roentgenogram and examination it was found that there was a fracture of the superior maxilla extending from tuberosity to tuberosity, across both maxillary sinuses and including the nasal septum. The entire maxilla was detached from its cranial attachments. Using modeling compound, an impression was taken of the upper arch. A vulcanite splint was made on the model and heavy wires were vulcanized into the splint, bending them anteriorly through the corners of the lobe of the ears. A skull cap was made of plaster and two leather straps were placed in the cast. Two straps were also placed on each splint wire. A splint was then placed in the mouth and the straps of the splint attached to those of the skull cap by use of buckles. By tightening the straps the fracture was reduced without the use of anesthesia. After a few hours the patient was able to take nourishment without any trouble. The splint and cap remained in place for three weeks at which time they were removed and the patient dismissed in a very satisfactory condition.

Case 5. J. C. M. was brought into the hospital on October 12, 1935, in a semi-conscious condition with a fracture of the middle third of the left femur, a fracture at the junction of the upper and middle third

of the right femur and a fracture of the lower and middle third of the right femur. There was an injury to the chest and abdomen and fracture of the middle third of the ulna. This man was put in Thomas splints on admission. His unconsciousness increased along with delirium. Two days after admission he was placed in a modified Russell traction with swinging cuffs around each femur and with adhesive plaster traction in the Thomas splints. Sixteen days later he cleared up sufficiently to be placed in permanent position. At this time Steinman pins were placed through the tibias just under the tibial tuberosity, and a 25 pound weight was applied to each femur with the aid of Thomas splints and the cuffs. This brought the fragments into reasonable alignment. He developed pneumonia on November 18, weathered this and apparently had firm union of all fractures on December 9. All pins and traction were removed and the right leg placed in a Thomas walking caliper to steady the leg. He was allowed to go to his home on December 16, and massage of both limbs was begun. He was out in a rolling chair by Christmas and began walking on crutches about March 1 without any noticeable disability except some weakness in his limbs and some stiffness in his knees.

Conclusion

I feel that these fractures demonstrate the extreme difficulties that we have to contend with at times. We still have to use plaster in treating femurs despite the fact that a good many men contend that it has passed its day of usefulness. The closed method of treating compound fractures is practical and screw traction, skin plaster, Steinman and Kirschner pins, and skeletal traction all have their usefulness. Good functional results can be obtained without perfect apposition of broken fragments in bone provided general alignment is good.

Discussion on Paper of Dr. J. H. Mull
DR. J. W. SIMMONS (Brunswick): Dr. Mull is

to be complimented on the ultimate results in function obtained in these rather serious multiple and comminuted fractures. That he was able to obtain and retain fair alignment with such a minimum of discomfort that is unusual in such splinting methods, is a rather obvious reason for complimenting him aside from the unusual ultimate functional result in all the cases.

In some practices I believe too much reliance is placed on plaster retention rather than mechanical ingenuity, which, with plenty of common sense are the principal personal assets in fracture work. End-results in restoration and preservation of function as near normal as possible are the sine qua non in such cases. Frequent check-ups with the x-ray, with the preservation of the "before and after" films are all important, especially in cases that might find their way into the courts.

Some twenty years ago I heard Dr. W. S. Goldsmith, I believe it was, observe: "The x-ray is both a blessing and a curse to the fracture worker, and a reliable ally sometimes of the damage suit lawyer." Certain it is that the absence of them now is inexcusable in any case brought before the court where there is the least question of disability or impaired function.

May I differ with some eminent orthopedists and fracture surgeons in the matter of stockinetting, bandaging, cotton-padding extremities under plaster casts. In my recent limited experience, I have found that reduction was more easily maintained; immobilization more secure; blebbing, excoriation, chafing and maceration of the skin a great deal less frequent; weight bearing in the lower limbs permissible earlier; and quicker recoveries the rule, in direct-to-the-skin application of a smooth fitting, wrinkleless cast in most cases of simple, easily reduced, or non-displaced fractures of the extremities. Of course, this method is only to be used where there is no marked swelling, or where it can easily be controlled under the extent of pressure and consequent skin necrosis.

We, who do any appreciable amount of industrial surgery, are always on the lookout for means and methods of reducing postfracture disabilities, as well as deformities that might be obvious. We are always grateful to anyone who presents us newer and better methods that promise such results as Dr. Mull seems to have obtained.

DR. R. C. FRANKLIN (Swainsboro): I wish to compliment Dr. Mull on his resourcefulness in handling these difficult and unusual fractures.

While handling fractures is a mechanical problem, and in a way has to be worked out from an individual standpoint, yet the end results are what we are seeking most of all.

In this day of unusual fractures, many times multiple fractures, and compound fractures, often in the same individual, it taxes our ingenuity in arriving at the best method to be used in a given case. We should consider the comfort of the patient—as nearly free of pain as possible, the length of stay in the hospital or in bed, and especially the end results.

In handling fractures of long bones, especially of the lower extremities, skeletal traction is the method of choice in most instances. This is best accomplished by inserting either the Steinman pin or Kirschner wire, and traction accomplished with some form of apparatus which suits in the case. Recently I have been using the Roger Anderson Automatic Splint. This apparatus —complete setup—may be used in the skeletal traction of any long bone of the upper or lower extremity. The advantage is that you may, more or less, accurately place the fractured ends of bones while under the fluoroscope and later apply plaster cast, incorporating the pins in the cast.

In treating compound fractures, if it becomes necessary to change the cast, you may again set the pins in the automatic splint which holds the bones in place while renewing the cast. Some such apparatus is invaluable in treating fractures of both the tibia and fibula, whether simple or compound.

In treating fractures of the upper end of the humerus, or fractures at the anatomic or surgical neck, the Hoke-Martin splint, either with adhesive skin traction, or skeletal traction, is a most successful method. Fix the cast so as to hold the humerus in line with the fractured head as shown under the fluoroscope, as you have no control of the head.

DR. J. H. MULL (Rome): I appreciate what the doctor said, that you are tempted a lot of times to do open fracture work because it appears to simplify things. I do not do more openings than necessary, and I make it a point to simplify fracture work as much as possible, due to the fact that in small hospitals and places where you haven't the nursing forces to properly take care of a lot of apparatus, you will find you get into more difficulties than you will if you do not try for such good x-ray pictures but try for functional results.

I think the point of skeletal traction is well taken, but there are times with semi-delirious patients, when you can hardly hold them on the bed, you have to resort to something that will hold those patients down. I know it is perhaps not the best thing to do at all times, but a lot of times you have to do the best you can with these fractures.

Also I think the closed method of treating fractures, which no one commented on, is a thing that we ought to do as much as possible. I think it gives us lower morbidity and better end results. If the patients do not start temperature in the first week, or excess swelling, let them alone, and when you take the cast off you find they are perfectly healed and you have shortened the time a great deal. When you have holes in your cast it will swell through and the patient will develop a secondary infection, and when there is an osteomyelitis in a fracture then it is up to the Lord. There is not much you can do.

I think we ought to recognize that the closed method of treating compound fractures is practical and that screw traction, skin plaster of paris, Steinman and Kirschner pins, skeletal traction, all have their usefulness, and good functional results can be obtained without perfect apposition of broken fragments in bone, provided general alignment is good. I think alignment is more important than any other point. Of course in double fractures of the femurs, if they overlap a little I think you get healing just about as quickly as you do if you get perfect apposition on it.

FRIEDMAN'S MODIFICATION OF THE ASCHHEIM-ZONDEK TEST FOR PREGNANCY*

GEORGE F. KLUGH, M.D.
Atlanta

The purpose of this paper is to emphasize the importance of using a proper technic for the Friedman test. Previous writers seem to have considered only the qualitative aspect of the procedure and have neglected the quantitative factor which is the basis of the test. The injection of the proper amount of urine is essential to a proper evaluation of the test and reduces to a minimum the false negative and false positive interpretations. Ten or 12 cc. in single or divided doses seems to be the optimum amount for the routine test.

The need of a reliable test for pregnancy, and especially early pregnancy, is evident when we consider the various conditions which give one or more of the signs of uterine or ectopic gestation. Most physicians and surgeons often see cases that cannot be diagnosed accurately from physical examination or from a carefully taken history. These cases may cause, and frequently have caused, the doctor concern and embarrassment. The early diagnosis of pregnancy is frequently of great value in its social and medicolegal aspects.

Numerous workers have evolved tests, but none was reliable or satisfactory until Aschheim and Zondek perfected their test. This test is based on the fact that during pregnancy the anterior-pituitary-like sex hormone is markedly increased and is excreted in large amounts in the urine. This hormone when injected in immature female mice stimulates the maturation of the graafian follicles and ovulation. The female mouse normally ovulates when about twelve weeks old and has a weight of about 12 grams. The Aschheim-Zondek test requires six female mice of about three weeks of age and each weighing about six grams. The time required for completion of this test is approximately five days.

In the Friedman modification of the Aschheim-Zondek test we have a reliable test, easy to perform and requiring only one or two

*Read before the Medical Association of Georgia, Savannah, April 23, 1936.

days for its completion. Friedman found that the female rabbit normally ovulates only after copulation with the male. Mating stimulates the anterior-pituitary body with increased production of the anterior-pituitary sex hormone. This stimulates the graafian follicles of the ovaries, ovulation occurring about eight or ten hours after copulation. In view of this normal response to the anterior-pituitary sex hormone, Friedman used the rabbit for his modification of Aschheim-Zondek pregnancy test and, with Lapham, reported a series of cases. Urines from both pregnant and non-pregnant women were used in making the tests. His results were correct in all cases. Schneider corroborated his work using 5 cc. of urine in one injection and found that the test was positive as early as twelve to twenty days after the intercourse causing pregnancy. His experiments also showed that the test rapidly becomes negative after delivery. Most of his cases were negative twenty-four hours after placental separation. An occasional case was positive as late as sixty-seven hours. This was thought to be due to fragments of retained placenta, since the anterior-pituitary-like sex hormone of pregnancy is believed to depend upon the presence of living active placental tissues. This fact adds to the value of the test in cases of missed abortion and other cases of pregnancy in which the fetus dies or placental separation occurs. Reinhart and Scott also confirmed Friedman's work using 5 to 7 cc. of urine.

The Friedman modification of the pregnancy test is also of value in diagnosing chorion epithelioma. In this condition the anterior-pituitary-like sex hormone is from ten to five hundred times as much as is usually found in the urine of pregnant individuals. The Friedman test is positive with 1 cc. of urine from patients with chorion epithelioma. False positives have been reported in disturbances of the anterior-pituitary body which may occur at the menopause, in the presence of ovarian cysts and in hyperthyroidism in which conditions an increase in the anterior-pituitary sex hormone is found the urine. This may be due to an actual stimulation of the anterior-pituitary body or possibly to a hormone imbalance. While it may not be possible to eliminate all false negatives and false positives it is highly probable that with the use of proper amounts of urine both will be reduced to a minimum. Since 5 cc. of pregnancy urine will ordinarily give a positive test even in early pregnancy, it would seem useless to use more than 10 or 12 cc. to insure against false negatives. Obviously the injection of 10 cc. of urine on each of two successive days as advocated by Mazer and Goldstein, and six doses of 4 cc. each within two days, as suggested by Friedman, would double the chances of a false positive in cases of anterior-pituitary imbalance. A single injection of 10 to 12 cc. of urine would be ideal were it not for the fact that certain specimens are toxic for the rabbit when given in large doses.

With these facts in mind and after five years of experience with the Friedman test, the following method seems advisable: Young female rabbits four or five months old and weighing about four pounds that have been kept isolated for three weeks are preferred. It is difficult to differentiate the males from females in younger animals, if the testicles have not descended. Age and development are of more importance than is weight since some breeds are very large and lack proper development at three months of age. The concentrated urine is preferable and should be carefully collected though catheterization is not necessary. While advisable to keep the specimen on ice, it may be mailed and transported a reasonable distance. Satisfactory results have been obtained on specimens twenty-four to forty-eight hours old that have been sent in by mail.

The urine is centrifuged and 5 or 6 cc. of the clear urine is diluted with an equal amount of sterile normal salt solution. Dilution with normal salt solution seems to lessen the toxicity of the urine. The diluted urine is injected slowly into the marginal ear vein of the rabbit. Another 5 or 6 cc. of the urine is prepared and injected in the same manner a few hours later. The rabbit is killed thirty to forty-eight hours after the first injection. The ovaries are inspected and, if positive, show hemorrhagic follicles macroscopically. If the follicles are not hemorrhagic the test is negative.

The urine of normal non-pregnant women frequently causes stimulation of the graafian follicles but not sufficient to cause complete ripening. The estrin or follicular ovarian hormone of normal urine causes congestion and enlargement of the rabbit uterus. The estrin content of pregnancy urine is markedly increased and in this test a marked congestion and hyperplasia of the rabbit uterus is usually found.

In a consecutive series of 75 cases in which pregnancy was considered a possibility, 40 were positive and 35 were negative to the Friedman test. These were checked by clinical findings and subsequent history and found correct in all cases. Most of the patients had missed a menstrual period after sexual exposure. The pregnancies, if present, were of five or six weeks' duration and the earliest pregnancy in this series was estimated at four weeks' duration. Several patients were going through their menopause and had missed one or two menstrual periods. None of these cases gave false positives.

The following cases illustrate the value of the test:

Case 1. An unmarried girl who loved a boy and told him she was pregnant. She wanted him to marry her. The pregnancy test was negative. They did not get married.

Case 2. Patient was seen December 13, 1935, five months after her last menstrual period. Examination revealed her uterus to be enlarged to the size expected in a three months pregnancy. Patient was sure she was pregnant and that something was going wrong. She had a similar experience several years ago, and carried a fetus seven months. She was seen again, six weeks later and examination showed the uterus had not increased in size. Still later, February 5, 1936, the uterus was much smaller and to the left side. This suggested a mass on the left side that simulated a pus tube. At a subsequent examination, February 24, the mass had decreased markedly in size and there was slight uterine bleeding. She miscarried on February 26, and was delivered of what appeared to be a dead four month fetus with membranes intact. The fetus was tough, leathery and not macerated. There was no odor of decomposition. This patient was seen by another doctor in the beginning and the Aschheim-Zondek test was positive. My test was negative on January 22.

Summary

1. The Friedman modification of the Aschheim-Zondek pregnancy test is a practical and reliable test for early pregnancy.

2. It is applicable as early as pregnancy is suspected.

3. Its use is valuable in eliminating or confirming pregnancy in conditions in which

one or more signs of early pregnancy are present.

4. It is useful in cases in which social and medico-legal aspects of pregnancy are involved.

5. In a series of 75 consecutive tests on patients showing one or more signs of pregnancy, and covering five years' experience, there were 40 positive and 35 negative reactions agreeing with subsequent history and findings.

6. The injection of 5 or 6 cc. of urine diluted with an equal amount of saline, followed in a few hours with a second injection of 5 or 6 cc. will reduce, if not entirely eliminate, false negatives and false positives.

7. The rabbit ovaries should be examined from thirty to forty-eight hours after the first injection. If saving time is a factor two or more rabbits may be used and 10 cc. given in one dose. One rabbit may be examined twelve hours after the injection and the other after twenty-four to thirty hours.

BIBLIOGRAPHY

1. Aschheim, S.: The Early Diagnosis of Pregnancy. Chorion Epithelioma and Hydatiform Mole by the Aschheim-Zondek Test. Am. J. Obst. and Gynec. 19:335-342, (March) 1930.
2. Friedman. M. H.: (1) Mechanism of Ovulation in the Rabbit. (2) Ovulation Produced by the Injection of Urine from Pregnant Women. Am. J. Physiol. 90:617-622, (Nov.) 1929.
3. Friedman. M. H., and Lapham. M. E.: A Simple Rapid Procedure for the Laboratory Diagnosis of Pregnancies. Am. J. Obst. and Gynec. 21:405, 1931.
4. Schneider. P. F.: A Hormone Test of Early Pregnancy. Surg. Gynec. and Obst. 52:56-60, (Jan.) 1931.
5. Reinhart. H. L., and Scott. Ernest: The Hormone Test for Pregnancy. Am. J. Clin. Path. 1:113-126, (March) 1931.
6. Mazer and Goldstein: Clinical Endocrinology of the Female. 383-390. W. B. Saunders Co., Philadelphia (March) 1933.

Discussion on Paper of Dr. Geo. F. Klugh

DR. G. LOMBARD KELLY (Augusta): I have quite a number of comments I should like to make in regard to this interesting paper of Dr. Klugh's. I wish to commend him for bringing this very valuable test before the society again. It seems that a test as valuable as it is is taking on entirely too slowly with the medical profession. A test with such a high accuracy for early pregnancy should be used by more physicians more frequently. I recently went over the literature to determine just how accurate most observers had found this test to be, and the percentages of accuracy varied all the way from 98 to 100 per cent. but no investigator reported an accuracy of less than 98 per cent.

In regard to one statement made by Dr. Klugh, that Friedman discovered that rabbits do not ovulate unless they copulate. I wish to say that discovery was not originally made by Dr. Friedman, but has been known for a long time. There are three animals that do not ovulate spontaneously, the ferret, the cat and the rabbit. Friedman's researches were not dealing with this particular phase of the physiology of the reproduction of the rabbit. What he discovered really was

that the same hormone that Aschheim and Zondek found would produce ovulation in a rabbit. They ovulate normally about ten hours after copulation. The pregnancy urine, however, does not ordinarily cause ovulation in less than sixteen hours.

In some cases of chorioepithelioma, much less than one cubic centimeter of urine will give a positive result. A tenth of a cubic centimeter or less, in some cases, will give a positive result.

There are, of course, variations of the Aschheim-Zondek test employing female mice. I published a paper in The Journal of the American Medical Association on the use of immature rats, the test being determined by the opening of the vaginal orifice in immature rats. A report was published later by some authors on this test and the results were reported as satisfactory, but they found, just as I did, that the Friedman test is simpler and quicker, and for that reason it still serves as the best means for the early diagnosis of pregnancy.

Recently we completed a study in our laboratory, using about 150 rabbits and employing urines from women known to be pregnant. I should like to take up some of the things we tried to determine in this investigation, which up to the present time has not been published, as we have just finished it. We tried to determine what is the lowest weight of rabbit that would react positively. Some authorities say that if you use rabbits too light you will not get a positive result. We found that rabbits weighing less than 1300 grams quite frequently would react positively just as well as rabbits of greater weight. We found that urines with specific gravity around 1.010 or less would at times give a negative reaction though the patients were known to be pregnant. We would be careful to have morning specimens. with urines of a gravity of 1.010 or higher.

Most authorities advise acidifying the urine. I do not think that is absolutely necessary. We determined this point by injecting alkaline urines in the rabbits. urines of known pregnancy origin. and getting positive results, although the urine was alkaline. We have found that it is not absolutely necessary for the urine to be acidified.

I was interested in whether you have to have ruptured graafian follicles or can determine the test simply by the hemorrhagic follicles. I have found in a large percentage of our cases actual rupture did not take place, and I think this is due to the fact that we use in about four-fifths of our cases the routine modification of the Friedman test, the ten-ten test, 10 cc. one day and 10 the next. At any rate, it is not necessary to have a rupture. I think it is advisable to examine the ovaries with a low-power binocular microscope.

DR. A. J. AYERS (Atlanta): I can not enlarge very much on Dr. Klugh's paper, which has covered the ground very thoroughly as I see it. There are one or two points I should like to bring out.

In making the test, I do the test somewhat differently than the method given by Dr. Klugh. There has been considerable improvement in the test from that used by the originators of the test. Friedman's modification of the test is practically used universally today. It is simple. and is easy to do.

I prefer using fresh morning specimens of urine, adjust the acidity, if needed and inject 10 cc. Twenty-four hours later give the second injection of 10 cc. of urine. Twenty-four hours after the second injection autopsy the rabbit. In the examination of the ovaries in doubtful cases; I find the high-powered hand lens helps me to determine whether I am dealing with a positive or a negative ovary.

I think it is best to always examine the urine to see whether you have an alkaline reaction. for such urine always has a bad effect on the rabbit. You will get by without killing your rabbits. Occasionally we run across a toxic urine that will kill the rabbit in a very few minutes after injection. I have not been able to find out just the reason for this reaction.

DR. GEORGE F. KLUGH (Atlanta) : The main point I want to emphasize is getting a suitable rabbit. A rabbit that weighs three pounds. a three-months old rabbit, might be suitable and it might not. Rabbits vary in different breeds. You put a bigger burden on the test, if it is too young and immature. You have more development to produce in the ovary. The animal should be almost mature. Ordinarily, that is about a four-pound rabbit, and not less than four months old.

Another point I wanted to emphasize is the fact that 20 cc. given in two divided doses is too much. and you may in some conditions cause false positives.

I think if you use an animal with a suitable development, you do not have much trouble when looking for the ruptured follicle. The errors that workers have had with this test seem to me to have been due to using too young an animal in one case and too much urine in another case. You get too many false negatives if you use too young an animal, If you use too much urine you may get a false positive. I have never used more than 12 cc. in any of the tests, and have never had a false positive, and in using as much as 10 cc. in the proper sized rabbit I have not had false negatives. I have noticed that with the younger rabbits fewer follicles develop, because it takes more of the hormone to develop an immature ovary than it does one that is practically fully developed.

I want to thank the gentlemen for the discussion.

HARVEY G. BECK. Baltimore (*Journal A. M. A.,* Sept. 26, 1936), reports on a series of carefully studied cases of slow carbon monoxide asphyxiation. The symptoms exhibited have been correlated with the pathologic lesions produced in experimental animals and found at autopsy. The results establish the fact that slow carbon monoxide asphyxiation (anoxemia) produces a definite clinicopathologic entity despite views held to the contrary. The symptoms arise predominantly from organs rich in blood supply. thus demanding much oxygen. such as the central nervous system and the heart muscles. Owing to doubt and uncertainty as to the actual existence of the malady and a scant literature on the subject, the condition is not generally recognized by the profession and its importance has been underestimated. Since there is no medicinal remedy when the organic changes have once developed, treatment must be directed toward its prevention by proper public health measures.

ANTITOXIN TREATMENT OF MENINGOCOCCIC INFECTIONS AND MENINGITIS*

HOWARD J. MORRISON, M.D.
Savannah

Weischelbaum, in 1887, isolated and cultured the meningococcus and thus laid the foundation for the present etiologic conception of the disease. Jochmann initiated the clinical intrathecal use of an antiserum, evaluated earlier by animal experimentation by Kolle and Wassermann.

Flexner reviewed the entire subject of meningococcic meningitis in 1907-1908 and as the result of extensive laboratory and clinical investigations, he demonstrated the value of an antimeningitis serum in the treatment of the disease. He attributed the benefits of the serum clinically to its antibacterial qualities.

Through the next twenty-three years, none of the comprehensive reviews on meningococcic meningitis admitted the presence of an extracellular toxin. although Gordon and Murray agreed that an endotoxin was produced. This general belief led to the widespread use of an antibacterial serum. Murray, in 1929, stated: "No one has yet succeeded in demonstrating a soluble toxin in meningococcus cultures and all are ready to admit that such a toxin (extracellular) is not produced."

Efforts to associate any one type of meningococcus or any particular strain with various epidemics have not been successful. Also, it is generally agreed that the present polyvalent antibacterial serums are not wholly satisfactory. Wright showed in an outbreak observed by him that "A serum uniformly of the highest titer was not effective clinically." Hoyne has made similar observations more recently.

From the beginning of antiserum therapy of meningococcic meningitis, the serum was given by the intraspinal route until 1919 when Hoyne, Arkin, and Sherman reported a case treated by combined intravenous and intraspinal injections. Since the World War, the general method of administration has been to give the serum both intravenously and intraspinally for the first few days and if

*Read before the Medical Association of Georgia. Savannah, April 24, 1936.

any subsequent serum is needed, to give the remainder intraspinally. This trend of therapy has been due to the fact that meningococcic meningitis is recognized as a complication of a systemic disease. The term meningococcic meningitis should not be applied to all types of meningococcic infections any more than the term infantile paralysis should be applied to all forms of poliomyelitis. Meningococcic meningitis is the end result of many meningococcic infections just as infantile paralysis is the end result of many poliomyelitis infections. Because of this belief, a new term "Meningococcia" has been offered by Hoyne and with it a new classification for meningococcic infections:

(1) Meningococcic meningitis
(2) Meningococcemia with meningitis
(3) Meningococcemia without meningitis
(4) Meningococcus carriers.

Due to the widespread impression that the serious symptoms of meningococcus meningitis or meningococcemia are mainly the result of a toxemia, Ferry, Norton and Steele studied the properties of bouillon filtrates of the meningococcus and came to the following conclusions: (a) Bouillon filtrates from young cultures of the four recognized Gordon types of the meningococcus contain extracellular toxins specific to the four types as well as a toxin common to all types; (b) These toxins when injected individually into animals, develop specific antitoxins as well as some antitoxin of the other three types; (c) Animals injected with all four types of toxin at various times develop antitoxins specific to the individual type; (d) Convalescent serums possess neutralizing properties apparently specific toward these soluble toxins.

Ferry then showed that a meningococcus antitoxin, prepared by immunizing the horse with soluble specific toxins from all four Gordon types of the meningococcus, protected guinea pigs of 200 gram weight against fatal doses of the meningococcus, when the antitoxin was injected one to five hours before the culture was injected, when injected simultaneously with the culture, or when injected up to within three hours after the culture was given. Antimeningococcic serum, prepared according to the regulation methods prevailing at the present time, from the same strains

as the experimental antitoxin, when injected in the same size dose as the antitoxin failed to protect guinea pigs prophylactically against the fatal dose of the culture, while the antitoxin protected. Antimeningococcic serum when injected in the same size dose as the antitoxin failed to protect guinea pigs thereapeutically against the fatal dose of culture, while the antitoxin protected.

Ferry's next work was to corroborate the original findings of Flexner that experimental acute cerebrospinal meningitis can be produced in the monkey following the intraspinal inoculation of live meningococci. His further experiments on monkeys using the antimeningococcic serum and the meningococcic antitoxin showed: (a) antimeningococcic serum when injected intraperitoneally, following intraspinal inoculation with live meningococci, in doses comparable to those used with meningococcus antitoxin, did not prevent death from meningitis; (b) meningococcus toxin (extracellular) when injected intracisternally produced symptoms similar to those found in meningococcus cerebrospinal meningitis following inoculation with the live meningococcus intraspinally; (c) meningococcus antitoxin, when mixed with meningococcus toxin and injected intracisternally, had a very appreciable neutralizing effect on the toxin; (d) monkeys which had recovered from previous intracisternal injections of meningococcus toxin were protected against a fatal dose of live meningococcus culture.

Ferry concluded from his work that the symptoms of meningococcus cerebrospinal meningitis in laboratory animals are due in a large part to the action on the central nervous system of a soluble specific toxin elaborated by the meningococcus and that these symptoms can be modified or entirely prevented by the neutralization of this toxin by a specific antitoxin.

Ferry reported later that susceptible human beings can be immunized against meningococcus toxin as revealed by subsequent skin tests.

With this experimental background, the antitoxin was used clinically in the Children's Memorial Hospital, Cook County Contagious Hospital, and Municipal Contagious Disease Hospital, of Chicago, under the direction of

Dr. Archibald Hoyne and to a lesser extent in the Isolation Hospital of Memphis, under the direction of Dr. Gilbert Levy.

In every hospital antimeningococcic serum treated cases were used as a control. The patients receiving the antitoxin were selected only by reason of their not having had previous antimeningococcic serum. Irrespective of whether serum or antitoxin was used, the method of administration was uniform. When given intravenously as the initial dose, 105 cc. of antimeningococcic serum or 90 cc. of meningococcus antitoxin was diluted in 150 to 250 cc. of 10 per cent glucose, the solution being warmed and given by gravity, preferably by the drip method. Generally but one intravenous treatment is needed, except in the cases of uncomplicated meningococcemia, when intravenous therapy should be used entirely and used until the abatement of symptoms, referable to the disease. At the time of lumbar puncture, serum or antitoxin was given by gravity method in doses of 20 to 40 cc. daily until the fluid was clear and free from organisms. At such a time, the cell count of the spinal fluid is usually less than 100. In cases of a block in the spinal canal cisternal puncture was resorted to, both for drainage of fluid and for therapeutic administration. It is interesting to note that Hoyne had four cases of meningococcic infections that were treated solely with meningococcic antitoxin intravenously and that all of these patients recovered. Intramuscular administration was not used because of the serious nature of the disease.

The final data of Hoyne's investigations show that over a period of 18 months, 319 patients were treated, 217 receiving two well known standard brands of antimeningococcic serum with 100 deaths, showing a mortality rate of 46.1 per cent, and 102 cases receiving the experimental antitoxin with 20 deaths, showing a mortality of 20.6 per cent. Levy, in a small series of 24 cases treated with meningococcic antitoxin, had six deaths or a mortality of 25 per cent. His method of administration was much the same as Hoyne's. It is interesting to note that the mortality rate in Memphis over the nine year period prior to 1933 was 57.1 per cent. In a small series of 14 cases at the Children's Memorial Hospital, reported by Hoyne, two deaths occurred with a fatality rate of 14.3 per cent.

In addition to the marked reduction of the mortality rate, when antitoxin is used, other observations made seem pertinent. In no instance did an ocular or auditory complication develop after the institution of antitoxin therapy. The period of hospitalization for antitoxin treated patients averaged 16.2 days while those receiving antiserum averaged 18 days. Excluding 48 hour deaths, the mortality rate in the antitoxin treated cases was 9.6 per cent and in the antiserum treated cases was 29.6 per cent.

Attention should be called to the need of doing a skin sensitization test when antitoxin or antiserum is given intravenously and, in doubtful cases, a small amount of adrenalin may be given at the same time. Usually a serum reaction occurs at about the sixth or eighth day when it may be necessary to control the urticaria by means of adrenalin chloride.

Summary

1. The meningococcic antitoxin, prepared by injecting horses subcutaneously with increasing doses of the individual soluble toxins of the four types of meningococci, has a decided advantage over the antimeningococcic serum, prepared by injecting horses subcutaneously with increasing doses of the meningococcic organisms.

2. It is believed that as more antitoxin is given intravenously, less will have to be given intraspinally.

3. We may expect fewer complications from blindness and deafness when antitoxin is used.

4. Competent observers believe that the symptoms of meningococcus meningitis are due to the action on the central nervous system of a soluble specific toxin elaborated by the meningococcus.

5. Competent observers believe that the value of antimeningococcus serum is due to the amount of antitoxin it may happen to contain.

REFERENCES

1. Weischselbaum, A.: Ueber die Aetiologie der akuten Meningitis cerebrospinalis, Fortschr. d. Med. 5:573, 1887.
2. Jochmann, G.: Versuche zur Serodiagnostis und Serotherapie der epidemischen Genickstarr, Deutsche med. Wchnschr. 32:788, 1906.
3. Kolle, Wilhelm, and Wassermann, August: Versuche zur Gewinnung und Wertbestimmung eines Meningococcenserums, Deutsche med. Wchnschr. 32:609, 1906.
4. Flexner, Simon: Experimental Cerebrospinal Meningitis in Monkeys, J. Exper. Med. 9:142, 1907; Concerning a Serum Therapy for Experimental Infection with Diplococcus Intracellularis, ibid., p. 168 Flexner, Simon, and Jobling, J. W.: Serum

Treatment of Epidemic Cerebrospinal Meningitis, ibid., *10*;141, 1908; An Analysis of Four Hundred Cases of Epidemic Meningitis Treated with the Antimeningitis Serum, ibid., p. 690.
5. Gordon, M. H.: Cerebrospinal Fever, Medical Research Council, special report series, No. 50, 1920.
6. Murray, E. G. D.: The Meningococcus, Medical Research Council, special report series, No. 124, 1929.
7. Wright, J. S.: DeSanctis, A. G., and Sheplar, Adele: The Determination of the Value of Serum in the Treatment for Meningococcus Meningitis, Am. J. Dis. Child, *38*:730 (Oct.) 1929.
8. Ferry, N. S.: Norton, J. F.: and Steele, A. H.: Studies of the Properties of Bouillon Filtrates of the Meningococcus: Production of a Soluble Toxin, The J. of Immunology, Vol. XXI. No. 4 (Oct.) 1931.
9. Ferry, N. S.: Meningococcus Antitoxin, I. Prophylactic and Therapeutic Test on Guinea Pigs, the J. of Immunology, Vol. XXIII. No. 4 (Oct.) 1932.
10. Ferry, N. S.: Meningococcus Antitoxin, II. Therapeutic Tests on Monkeys, The J. of Immunology, Vol. XXIII. No. 4 (Oct.) 1932.
11. Ferry, N. S.: Meningococcus Toxin and Antitoxin, III. Further Tests on Monkeys, The J. of Immunology, Vol. XXVI. No. 2 (Feb.) 1934.
12. Ferry, N. S., and Schornack, P. J.: Meningococcus Toxin and Antitoxin, IV. Further Tests on Guinea Pigs and Rabbits, The J. of Immunology, Vol. XXVI. No. 2 (Feb.) 1934.
13. Ferry, N. S., and Steele, A. H.: Active Immunization with Meningococcus Toxin, The J. of the Am. Med. Assn. (Mar. 23) 1935, Vol. 104, pp. 983 and 984.
14. Hoyne, A. L.: Meningococcic Meningitis, A New Form of Therapy, The J. A. M. A. (Mar. 23) 1935, Vol. 104, pp. 980,983.
15. Hoyne, A. L.: Meningococcia (Meningococcic Infection), A New Remedy, Archives of Pediatrics (June) 1935.
16. Hoyne, A. L.: Meningococcic Meningitis, Importance of Intravenous Therapy, Illinois Med. Journal (Oct.) 1935.
17. Levy, Gilbert: Treatment of Meningitis, personal correspondence.
18. Hoyne, A. L.: Arkin, H. S. and Sherman, M. J.: Treatment of a Severe Case of Epidemic Meningitis by Combined Intravenous and Intraspinal Injections of Antimeningococcic Serum. J. A. M. A., *72*:22, 1918.

Discussion on Paper of Dr. Howard J. Morrison

DR. G. W. HOLMES CHENEY (Brunswick): Dr. Morrison has presented to us the experimental and clinical progress made in the treatment of meningococcic infection, especially meningitis. He has reviewed series of cases which help to show the relative efficiency of meningococcus antitoxin and antimeningococcic serum.

There are those who have not accepted, as yet, meningococcus antitoxin. We may mention Dr. Josephine B. Neal of the Department of Health, New York City. She writes: "I am unable to understand why an antitoxin, presumably prepared by injecting horses with the toxin, should have a particular effect on the meningococcus itself. There seems to be some difference of opinion in regard to the results of the agglutination test on the antitoxin. It seems to me that the best preparation would be a regular antibacterial serum with a good antitoxin content.' Dr. Neal's opinion is worthy of study and trial.

The progress made in improving antimeningococcus serum has been retarded, as there seems to be no reliable laboratory test to evaluate the therapeutic efficiency of a particular lot of serum. There is much speculation as to how it acts, and therefore a great need for an improved therapeutic agent in the treatment of meningococcus infection. Meningococcus antitoxin can be standardized, and its action is known.

Further work and time will be needed, but we feel that meningococcus antitoxin is an improved product. We do believe that a toxemia is predominant, and that antitoxin will control it more efficiently than any other known therapeutic agent. The cost of antitoxin and serum is the same.

Dr. Morrison's paper comes to us at an opportune time. With an increasing number of tourists each year,

we should have more infection and contagion, and cases of meningococcus infection will no doubt increase.

DR. HOWARD J. MORRISON (Savannah): Of course it is almost impossible to take up all of the controversies that do occur with the use of antitoxin over antiserum. Failures during the last 20 to 25 years in the treatment of meningococcic infection, particularly meningococcal meningitis, have disturbed the medical profession as to the efficacy of antimeningococcic serum. Antitoxin (meningococcic) apparently offers more hope.

It may be well to add that the general trend of therapy in meningococcal infections at the present time is toward the intravenous route rather than the intraspinal route. When antitoxin is given intravenously or when any horse serum is injected intravenously, it is quite necessary that the skin test be done on the individual before subjecting it to the therapy, because of the anaphylaxis that may occur. In any event, these patients always have delayed reaction, and it may be looked forward to as occurring between the sixth and tenth day, at which time they may run an elevation of temperature.

IN MEMORIAM*

A. J. MOONEY, M.D.
Statesboro

In keeping with a resolution passed by the Association a few years ago, your Committee on Necrology, at this time of the session when attendance is at its height, when old acquaintances are being renewed, when we look for familiar faces and handclasps of friends and fail to see them who were with us a short year ago, I will read to you the names of those who have passed to their eternal reward since our last session. Listen to the list of the honored: Anderson, James W., Gray, January 3, 1936, aged 70.

Austin, Guy Leslie. Pavo, December 11, 1935, aged 56.

Bailey, Eugene McKay, Acworth, March 2, 1936, aged 68.

Barron, John M. F., Milner, April 30, 1935, aged 78.

Brice, George P., Cumming, September 2, 1935, aged 75.

Campbell. John A., Nahunta, September 20, 1935, aged 51.

Clifton, Benjamin L., Millen, June 7, 1935, aged 77.

Coleman, Alexander Stuart Matheson, Douglas, November 15, 1935, aged 45.

Crane, Charles William, Augusta, April 1, 1936, aged 61.

Cranford, James Robert, Sasser, November 29, 1935, aged 65.

Drewry, T. Ellis, Griffin, March 18, 1936, aged 75.

Evans, William Walker, Blakely, May 10, 1935, aged 70.

Fincher, Edgar F., Atlanta, January 7, 1936, aged 66.

---

*Memorial address before the Medical Association of Georgia, Savannah, April 23, 1936.

Fullilove, Henry Marshall, Athens, November 17, 1935, aged 58.

Griffin, Archie, Valdosta, May 2, 1935, aged 65.

Griffin, William C., Cartersville, July 23, 1935, aged 80.

Harpe, Samuel Melvin, Calhoun, October 27, 1935, aged 72.

Henry, James Z., Ellenwood, March 20, 1936, aged 52.

Hinton, Charles Crawford, Macon, February 25, 1936, aged 48.

Hull, James Meriweather, Augusta, April 13, 1936, aged 77.

Joiner, Buford O'Neal, Tennille, June 16, 1935, aged 49.

Jones, Abram B., Tyrone, September 6, 1935, aged 59.

Jones, Francis Gilchrist, Atlanta, February 25, 1936, aged 50.

Kelly, John Oliver, Avera, October 31, 1935, aged 54.

Kemp, A. Pierce, Macon, January 13, 1936, aged 67.

King, James M., Metcalf, February 8, 1936, aged 78.

Lester, James A., Fayetteville, June 24, 1935, aged 65.

Lindsay, James Arthur, Cairo, February 8, 1936, aged 63.

Lovett, William Robert, Sylvania, November 11, 1935, aged 73.

Lyle, William Clifton, Carrollton, April 15, 1936, aged 65.

McClain, Marion Cicero, Tate, December 25, 1935, aged 76.

McDuffie, James Henry, Columbus, November 16, 1935, aged 76.

McMahan, John Walter, Alma, July 30, 1935, aged 60.

Miller, Robert Lee, Waynesboro, March 31, 1936, aged 66.

Nelson, G. W., Marshallville, February 26, 1936, aged 74.

Osborne, James C., Acworth, March 11, 1936, aged 70.

Peterson, Nichols, Tifton, March 13, 1936, aged 68.

Powell, John H., Atlanta, November 16, 1935, aged 66.

Prescott, Jesse P., Lake Park, April 4, 1936, aged 70.

Pumpelly, William Collins, Macon, September 18, 1935, aged 58.

Ridley, Robert Berrien, Atlanta, December 4, 1935, aged 56.

Sample, Robert L., Summit, March 12, 1936, aged 68.

Sigman, John Monroe, Macon, April 10, 1936, aged 56.

Simmons, Robert Olin, Rome, July 6, 1935, aged 52.

Tracy, John Lunsford, Sylvester, July 19, 1935, aged 61.

Waits, William J., Gray, April 25, 1935, aged 67.

Wall, Homer Augustus, Ochlochnee, January 27, 1936, aged 67.

Westmoreland, Willis F., Atlanta, December 4, 1935, aged 71.

White, John C., Atlanta, September 7, 1935, aged 76.

In passing, permit me to drop a verbal forget-me-not upon the memory of four of those who are so close to us on account of our former relation.

Willis F. Westmoreland: Professor of Surgery, doubtless at the time when lots of you graduated; Past President of the Medical Association of Georgia and member of the State Board of Health. He occupied an honored position called "orator" that was established in the State Association many years ago. His name adorns the diplomas which many of us hold.

Charles William Crane, of the University of Georgia Medical Department, a teacher who I am sure lots of you revere in memory.

William Clifton Lyle, for many years Secretary of the State Medical Association, formerly dean of the Medical Department of the University of Georgia.

And *J. M. Hull,* who taught lots of you diseases of the eye, ear, nose and throat. His name appears also on your diplomas.

As the great Ecclesiasticus wrote, "Or ever the silver chord be loosed or the golden bowl be broken; or the pitcher broken at the fountain; or the wheel broken at the cistern; then shall the dust return unto earth as it was and the spirit shall return unto God who gave it," so it is with our professional brethren who have passed on.

Some were of a ripe old age, others at the height of their careers and usefulness, others had just begun their life work of service.

How fitting it would be to chronicle for each of them the preparation for service, the outstanding qualifications of each, their various fields of activity, the medical sagas they have written and left behind to mark the blazing trail through the scientific medical and surgical fields through which they passed —glorious heritages to their living confreres, of the sick they had healed; of the lame they had caused to walk, of the pain they had alleviated, of the heartaches they had soothed, of the disconsolate who found solace in their sympathy and philosophy; of the homes where they had banished sadness and sorrow and brought gladness and joy; of the weak who had been made strong by their wisdom such as only a doctor can minister after a long philosophical study and understanding of the weaknesses and frailties of mankind; of the community leadership they had acquired through capability and respect of their fellow citizens; of the wonderful comfort brought to the spiritually convicted and penitent; how, through their life work and deeds of mercy, they followed in the footsteps of the Great Redeemer when He said, "Come unto me all you who labor and are heavy laden and I will give you rest"—how fitting it would be if such chronicle could be for each of them and their particular outstanding virtues, but such length would be superflous.

Their virtues exemplified while amongst us will furnish to us ideals for our guidance while we are still alive.

As Paul the Apostle spoke of the glory of the sun, moon and stars, and said that each star was different in its glory, so it is with the different virtues exemplified by our departed medical brethren.

Being philosophers, they must have had the fancies and temptations so necessary to the well-rounded life—resistance to develop strength; sorrows to make the joys sweeter; shadows to make the sunshine more welcome, and disappointments to develop stamina.

We are thankful for the ideals of the professional life they left us. A philosopher has said, "Ideals are like stars. You will not succeed in touching them with your hands, but like the seafaring man on the trackless waste of waters, you will choose them as your guides, and, following them, you will reach your destiny."

Man, for thousands of years, has endeavored to make a lasting memorial by his handiwork. He has erected monuments with their spires pointing to the heavens; with the labor of slaves he has endeavored to build a structure of stone and granite that would stand as a perpetual record of the might of man and as a marker for ages to come, but the remorseless tooth of time has brought them to an earthly level, and the sands of the desert and the storms of the heavenly elements have defaced them and all but covered them in obscurity. But the story of a well-lived life has survived and will continue long after the handiwork of man has gone.

Profiting by the beautiful virtues and ideals left us, let us choose them as our own, and, practicing them, live such lives of service that we also, familiar as we are with death, will not be afraid and will receive Him as a kind messenger sent to summon us after a life of usefulness on earth to a better life in accordance with the greater plan of the Almighty.

EARLY DIAGNOSIS OF TUMORS OF THE KIDNEY*

Early diagnosis of kidney tumors is usually not made. When *pain, bleeding* and an abdominal *tumor* are present the diagnosis is obvious; but the prognosis is bad, especially if the tumor is fixed. Early recognition offers the only hope of cure. At the present time a satisfactory pyelogram is the most reliable method of diagnosis.

The etiology of kidney neoplasms is as obscure as the cause of new-growths elsewhere. Chronic irritation due to infection has been suggested as a probable factor. Stones are present in about 15 per cent of the cases and it is highly probable that they play an important role. This lack of knowledge of the cause of neoplasms makes it necessary to correct all conditions that might give rise to irritation.

The three leading symptoms of renal tumors in the adult are: *hemorrhage, tumor* and *pain*. The hemorrhage may be intermittent or continuous, slight or massive, and secondary anemia may be marked. The tumor is usually a hard mass and can be felt in front and behind. It frequently reaches considerable size and may be movable or fixed, depending upon the size and surrounding adhesions. Pain, when present, is usually due to the pressure of the tumor and is dull in character. Only rarely is the pain acute; it is then due to infection, hemorrhage or a blood clot caught in the ureter, and radiates to the groin.

While *hemorrhage, tumor* and *pain* make the diagnosis obvious, they also indicate that the disease may be far advanced. The early occurrence of bleeding is a favorable factor, as it alarms the patient and should be a signal for a cystoscopic examination. The cystoscopic data are extremely significant because the patient may have a good functioning kidney in spite of the presence of the tumor.

The diagnosis is made from the history, physical examination, cystoscopy, renal function test, microscopic study of the urine and the pyelogram; not infrequently it is made at operation. *Pyelography* is the most valuable method of diagnosing early renal tumor

* Prepared for the Cancer Commission of the Medical Association of Georgia by Earl W. Floyd, M.D., and Jas. L. Pittman, M.D., Atlanta.

as well as the most accurate means now available for determining the condition of the tumor prior to operation. In practically every case it will show some renal deformity. Various deformities are produced by the different pathologic processes to which the kidney is heir and, of course, special study of these is necessary for a correct interpretation. In the very beginning of renal tumor the pyelogram shows a loss of normal cupping of the calices or a slight increase in the size of one or more of them, such as are found in tuberculous kidneys, hydronephrosis, pyonephrosis and cysts. Filling defects may be due to insufficient filling of the renal pelvis or to normal constrictions of the pelvis and calices and it is sometimes necessary to repeat the pyelogram before a correct diagnosis is made. After the tumor has advanced in the kidney it occasionally blocks the ureter and prevents the possibility of getting information by means of a pyelogram. An intravenous pyelogram frequently does not give sufficient information and a retrograde pyelogram must be performed.

The conditions confused with renal tumors are: (1) hydronephrosis, (2) polycystic kidney disease, and (3) blood clots. As a rule, hydronephrosis can be determined by cystoscopy, microscopic examination of urine, kidney function test and pyelogram. Since polycystic kidneys are bilateral, this condition may be ruled out by the same procedures, particularly regarding the function and pyelogram. Blood clots will sometimes cause an error in diagnosis, but they can be ruled out if the other methods of diagnosis are taken into consideration. Fragments of renal tumors occasionally are found in the urinary sediment and specimens should always be examined carefully for these fragments.

Metastasis in the epithelial growth takes place by way of the renal vein or the growth may extend directly by breaking through the capsule. X-ray study of a renal tumor is not complete unless roentgenograms of the chest and long bones, especially the femur, have been made to locate metastasis. The knowledge of the presence or absence of metastasis is of vital importance, not only in the diagnosis but also in the consideration of the type and kind of treatment to be recommended.

Nephrectomy offers the best hope of cure; particularly is this true of kidney tumors in adults. The embryonic types of tumors that occur in early childhood are radiosensitive. Frequently there is marked decrease in the size of these growths under radiation, but recurrence within a short time is the rule. Operative treatment is necessary after the institution of x-ray therapy; although this type of tumor undergoes regression following radiation, pathologic examination frequently shows remnants of neoplastic tissue left behind.

CRAWFORD W. LONG MEMORIAL PRIZE

Five copies of all papers read before the Eighty-Seventh Annual Session of the Medical Association of Georgia at Savannah, April 22, 23, 24, 1936, which contain original work by their authors should be submitted to the Chairman of the Crawford W. Long Memorial Prize Committee, Dr. William R. Dancy, 102-4 Jones Street, West, Savannah. The features of each article which the writer claims to be original should be stated in a letter addressed to the Committee and submitted with copies of the paper.

The Committee reserves the right to decline any paper and to withhold the prize unless it deems the manuscript worthy of the award.

Reprints of the papers published in the JOURNAL may be submitted. The authors of all papers who claim original work should forward copies to the Chairman without further delay.

INJURIES OF HAND: CLINICAL LECTURE AT KANSAS CITY SESSION

SUMNER L. KOCH, Chicago (*Journal A. M. A.*, Sept. 26, 1936), states that the arrest of hemorrhage, the treatment of shock, and the careful examination of the hand—not the wound—are the first steps in the care of an injured hand. The principles involved in the further treatment, as in the treatment of any compound injury, are care not to add injury to that which has already taken place, careful excision of hopelessly injured tissue, the use of a minimum amount of foreign material in the repair of the injured structures, closure of the open wound as soon as it can be done with safety, and rest until healing has taken place.

THE JOURNAL

OF THE

MEDICAL ASSOCIATION OF GEORGIA

Devoted to the Welfare of the Medical Association of Georgia

478 Peachtree Street, N. E., Atlanta, Ga.

OCTOBER, 1936

MALARIA

Now that the malaria season has reached its peak and its seasonal decline is before us, it may be well for each of us to think over our experiences with it during the present summer and to inquire very seriously how much progress we have made.

That malaria is a problem of vital importance to the State is a known fact. Not that the death rate itself is so great but that the amount of time which is lost through its ravages, the weakening of efficiency of a large agricultural population and the discouraging of new enterprises and new settlers are matters of great moment.

It is true that the whole State is not equally affected but the malaria zone extending across the State and lying immediately to the east of the geologic "fall-line" embraces a large area of the most fertile and valuable land in the State. Yet, the progress of this whole region, the earning capacity and activity of its inhabitants, is seriously impaired by the endemicity of this infection nor have we any reason to believe that this state of affairs will be greatly changed for a number of years to come.

An enormous amount of work in the line of drainage and filling has been done during the past few years—more this year than ever before—with the cooperation of the Federal Government, the advice and approval of the United States Public Health Service, and the persistent direction and encouragement of the State Board of Health. It will be at least a year or two before the full benefit of these important public works will be manifested and in the meantime, it is well to bear in mind that the continuous free intercommunication between the malarious and non-malarious sections of the State, because of improved roads and increased numbers of motor cars, may quite probably establish new foci of endemicity in Georgia, either by the trans-portation of infected individuals or by the transportation of infected anophelines. The great factor which makes for the continuance of a high malaria incidence is the number of latent or relapsing cases which are carried over through the winter to furnish a source of infection with the advent of the next spring.

Through some strange mental obliquity, little attention is paid to the presence among us of malaria carriers. Let the word go out that there is a typhoid carrier in a community or that there are diphtheria carriers in school and immediately the populace is agog. But everywhere throughout the malarial part of Georgia, carrier after carrier goes throughout the winter harboring enough infection to be a definite menace as soon as mosquitoes begin their work in the spring and but little thought or attention is given to the matter. There are few ways in which persistent attention to a malaria problem would be productive of better results than in a careful round-up of all suspected carriers and treating them to an extent which would render them innocuous.

It must be admitted that both the profession and the laity are at fault in permitting this state of affairs to exist. The doctor too frequently takes refuge behind the time-worn excuse that he is a busy practitioner and as soon as the patient is rid of the active paroxysms, gives only perfunctory advice as to what the subsequent management of the case should be, by which a cure rather than a temporary amelioration should be effected. Likewise, the patient, particularly those of lower intelligence and subject to great economic strain, feel that they must be back at work as soon as they can stand on their feet and do not subsequently return to the physician for further observation or instruction. In addition to this, a large percentage of the cases of malaria are self-treated and never see a doctor throughout the course of their illness; all of this in spite of the repeated information which has been given as to the "standard treatment" and as to the necessity of prolonged medication after the paroxysms shall have disappeared. A most excellent and convincing piece of work along this line was carried out by the State Board of Health under the direction of Dr. Daniel L. Seckinger, State Epidemiologist, in 1933 and 1934, in Calhoun County, the results of which were published in The American Journal of Tropical Medicine. November, 1935, under the title of "Atabrine and Plasmochin in the Treatment and Control of Malaria," a perusal of which would be most valuable to anyone unfamiliar with the article.

The physicians throughout the State should during this period of waning malaria seize every opportunity to impress upon their clientele and upon the public in general the chronicity of malaria and of the necessity of prolonged treatment by whatever means may seem most desirable. A careful attention to this most important matter should materially reduce the number of carriers in which the infection will survive until the next warm season.

EUGENE E. MURPHEY, M.D.

OBLIGATIONS TO OUR STATE MEDICAL ASSOCIATION

The State Medical Association is an organization which is a united society. As long as medicine was practiced by individuals in isolated communities progress was necessarily slow due to poor training and lack of information. Each physician was struggling in the twilight of medical knowledge brightened by an occasional ray of light furnished by word of mouth and observation. Efforts were directed almost entirely toward curative medicine with meager remedies. The coming of societies made it possible and finally necessary for doctors to attend meetings if they desired to keep abreast of progress and render helpful and faithful service to their patients. Many doctors in Georgia, though they have grown old, are still interested in their chosen work and are thus rendering helpful services because of our Association which furnishes a splendid JOURNAL each month filled with worth while information. Then, too, the annual meetings are occasions when speakers of world renown are presented who give us valuable information and renew in us desires to excel. This service can come only through personal contact and intimate acquaintance. It is an excellent post-graduate course brought to all of us without cost through our Association. Otherwise only a few could obtain it at great expense and loss of much time, and then would reach only a small per cent of our

people because this broad knowledge would not be—as it is now—common knowledge. As a matter of fact many doctors in Georgia without these helps would doubtless fall behind and possibly enter other fields of endeavor for which they had had no training and as a result fail, thus becoming unhappy. Organization, then, begets happiness.

It is awing to reflect as the crowds go by that each individual is influenced to a greater or lesser degree by some physician. If we keep our happiness we must divide it with our patients, some of whom have organic diseases to be eradicated or controlled while others present functional disturbances cared for only through adjusting attitudes toward problems in life which can be found and pointed out by doctors who are keeping up. Thus are sowed the seeds of kindness and happiness through knowledge made possible only through organized medicine. Without organization there can be no unity, nor will there be any official spokesman to present the claims of physicians as to their rights and privileges. It is true that what is best for the people will be best for the doctors in the long run, but the voices of physicians should be heard and must be considered in determining what is best for all concerned. Life must be made happy, safe and agreeable. This can be done only through organization.

To our Association we owe much for the many fine friendships, for without it they would never have had opportunities to form and grow to ripe maturities. Where county societies are active the members become acquainted and learn to respect and love one another despite their occasional differences. Unless they attend meetings they oftentimes do not know each other first hand and through exaggerated reports form wrong ideas and sometimes give utterances to unfair and unjust criticisms of their confreres which act on the one and react on the other, damaging all concerned. It may even dwarf communities through divisions that prevent pulling together. If you think you dislike someone, try getting acquainted. If you are not attending your county and state meetings, come in and pull or push. Fellowship, friendships and happiness, what a triad furnished so bountifully through our Medical Association!

Organized medicine helps by advancing science and dispelling ignorance. In our meetings and THE JOURNAL we can discuss quackery and learn that it is ignorance, part of which we must admit is ours. Cultists claim special knowledge in treating "nervous" people while some doctors have impatiently dismissed these sufferers as hysterical and advised them to forget it, as if their worries were not part of themselves. We must learn to teach these patients how to live with their neuroses and psychoses for they cannot live without them. Some will have to be referred to specialists before their tangled threads can be straightened out. Sympathetic understanding should come from the physician instead of slurs and abuse. This plan will increase the joy of living and save for the people millions of dollars annually which they are spending for self-medication and questionable advice. We have learned a great deal during this century, but there is much more to learn. Abuse is not the remedy. It will only retard development. Only sympathetic understanding and broad knowledge of human ills plus application of organized knowledge, which is in its final analysis, education, will suffice. If we learn we progress.

Public health was fostered by our organization and is a source of never-ending joy to our people. Through this agency comes the opportunity for physicians to render an unselfish service which private practice does not offer because the former is interested in prevention and the latter is concerned mainly in curative medicine. Private practice is necessarily limited while public health offers unlimited fields for all of us to render unselfish assistance to many who otherwise would suffer. Less suffering and more happiness, good fellowship and enduring friendships; increased knowledge and more useful and successful lives are made possible through THE MEDICAL ASSOCIATION OF GEORGIA. Surely obligations to our Association are indeed great.

J. A. REDFEARN, M.D.

"There is little or no therapeutic benefit in cash settlements paid to injured workmen who have traumatic neuroses." Carl Norcross, Ph.D., Rehabilitation Division, New York State Dept. of Education.

THE JOURNAL

Beginning with this issue of the JOURNAL an attempt has been made to improve the physical make-up of the publication. A better quality of paper is used with the hope that reading matter and illustrations will be easier for the eyes. The binding has been changed for the convenience of those who wish to file their journals in regular order. Four pages have been added to meet the increased demand for space.

From time to time, the Publication Committee and Editorial Staff have invited criticism of the JOURNAL. Many suggestions have been offered. For example, one critic would suggest leaving out of the publication certain advertisements while another would want to abolish the Woman's Auxiliary and avoid all mention of our good wives. Most commentators, however, evidently believe that the written word brings us "mind to mind" with each other and all exhibited kindness when making remarks concerning medical journals. Suffice it to say, an increasing number of physicians, nurses, public health workers, welfare workers and laymen believe in state medical journals.

"The[1] function of a state journal, when all is said and done, is not to publish the advances of pure science, not to advocate elaborate procedures possible only in expensively equipped hospitals, not to publish the discussions of the very rare conditions that are occasionally encountered in the great medical centers, nor to be an organ of any group of specialists. The functions of a state journal are to benefit the general practitioner by keeping him abreast of progress in clinical medicine and by allowing him to give other practitioners the benefit of his actual experience; and to keep the physicians of the state informed of the special problems that confront them, as in the passing of laws; and finally, to promote solidarity and friendship among the members of the Association by informing them of the doings of each other."

For many years there have been printed on the pages of the JOURNAL these words: "Devoted to the Welfare of the Medical Association of Georgia." Words more truthful, and perhaps more appropriate, would be: Devoted to the Welfare of All Georgians.

1. The Journal of the Medical Association of Georgia. Vol. XXIV, page 173. (May) 1935.

PITYRIASIS CAPITIS

Pityriasis capitis, a form of seborrheic dermatitis, is one of the most common diseases of man and at the same time one of the most responsive to good treatment.

Treatment of the scalp by laymen is rapidly developing into a lucrative business in this country, and represents only one of the many encroachments on the field of medicine. A great part of the responsibility for this condition must be assumed by the medical profession. We, as physicians, have failed to fulfill our obligation, if when consulted by patients about their scaling scalps or early loss of hair, either suggest some standard hair tonic or advise a reconciliation to a so-called inevitable hereditary alopecia.

Pityriasis capitis, the least severe phase of seborrheic dermatitis, has a particularly insidious onset, with no clinical signs of inflammation, but attention first being attracted to it by a thinning of the hair or a mildly itching sensation. Later, however, it manifests itself as a dry, branny desquamation beginning in small patches and rapidly involving the entire scalp with a profuse amount of fine powdery scales. There is a tendency for the hair in the affected areas to fall out, characteristically beginning on the vertex and frontal regions and progressively receding, commonly associated with premature alopecia in men. Treatment at this time can do much to preserve the remaining hair and encourage the regrowth of hair in follicles that have not already been destroyed.

The disease occurs in both sexes at all ages, perhaps more frequently in early adult life. Lack of good scalp hygiene and an oily or seborrheic type of skin are predisposing factors. In favor of the infectious nature of the disease are the many cases with a history of sudden onset following a visit to some hairdressing establishment, a permanent wave, or the use of another's comb or brush. The seborrheic scalp is an ideal culture media for such organisms as the flask bacillus of Unna and the pityrosporum of Macleod and Dowling.

Microscopically, even in the mildest grade of the affection, there is found an inflammatory infiltration about the papillary vessels, the ascending branches from the subpapillary plexus and along the hair follicles sufficient to account for the loss of hair and the interference with normal hair growth.

In the treatment it is best to avoid greasy ointments, patients objecting to the difficulty of their removal. Sulphur is the drug *par excellence* for this disease and should be used in a strength of from four to six per cent together with salicylic acid two to four per cent in a glyceride of starch base which, when properly made up, is a fine creamy mixture and is very easily shampooed from the scalp.

In the average case such a cream should be well massaged into the scalp for ten minutes, by the clock, nightly for one week and shampooed each following morning, using a mild soap. At the end of one week all the loose affected hair will have fallen out, the itching subsided and the scalp should be comparatively clean. The following week the same procedure should be carried out on alternate nights; then once weekly for the next four weeks, at the end of which time patients can be given a suitable lotion to be used once every two weeks or monthly as necessary.

For blonde or grey hair:

Mercury bichloride	0.2
Chloral hydrate	4.0
Glycerine	4.0 to 15.0
Alcohol	30.0
Rose water q.s ad.	120.0

For brunettes:

Resorcin	4.0
Tinct. Cantharides	25.0
Tinct. Capsicum	25.0
Oleum Ricini	8.0
Oleum Bergamot	2.0
Alcohol q.s. ad.	120.0

The above lotions may be altered to suit the individual, the amount of oil being increased or decreased as necessary.

Ultraviolet, air-cooled mercury quartz light, given in suberythema simulating doses, is also efficacious.

During the course of treatment, pure olive oil may be applied to the hair sufficient to overcome any excessive dryness. Patients should be instructed to sterilize their combs and brushes weekly, shampoo their scalps at least once a week and visit hair dressers who use sterile instruments. By so doing they will not only remain well, but materially prolong if not prevent a premature alopecia.

PHILIP H. NIPPERT, M.D.

CHANGING CONCEPTS IN RHINOLOGY

Research in rhinology has increased materially during the past decade. Many workers in this field have concentrated their efforts on the study of physics, physiology, biochemistry, histology, pathology and bacteriology rather than the improvement of surgical instruments and other mechanical procedures. Radical operative procedures are in many instances replaced by more conservative methods of treatment.

Goodale,[1] Foster,[2] Coakley[3] and Heetderks[4] have been interested in the physical effects of the nose on inspired and expired air as well as the effect on the nasal tissue of inspired air. Cone[5] has made exact studies of the variations in the temperature within the nose and has attempted to correlate his findings with clinical conditions. Proetz[6], McMurray[7] and Hunter[8] studied the air currents within the nose and the changing air pressure in the sinuses during respiration. Others[9] have studied the vasomotor effect in the nose after various external stimulants were applied. Bernheim and. Cohen[10] failed to establish scientific basis for correlation of the color of the nasal septum with specific diseases and disorders of metabolism.

Many workers[11][12][13] have interested themselves in minute study of the ciliated epithelium and mucus secretion in the nasal cavities, particularly with the view of obtaining a better understanding of infectious conditions and the reaction of the tissues to various drugs. Much of this research has been performed on human tissue which was kept alive in artificial media. Lierle and Moore[14] at the University of Iowa have investigated the action of the cilia in situ by means of transparent windows fixed over trephine openings in sinuses of animals, using special microscopes and lighting. Important are the cytologic studies of nasal and sinus secretions by Darling,[15] Watson-Williams,[16] Sewell[17] and others.

Bacteriologic studies of the secretions of the nose and sinuses have been continued and expanded by Ashjey and Frick[19] who are making an effort to evaluate the clinical pictures of various rhinologic conditions after studying the bacterial flora found at different times. Further study and progress is being made in allergy and many rhinologic problems certainly belong in this group when etiologic factors are considered. The hydrogen ion content, mineral content and the estimation of the total solids in secretions of the nose are receiving further study, as are many other subjects too numerous to mention.

TAYLOR S. BURGESS, M.D.

PELLAGRA

During the past few years the question of the etiology of pellagra has been reopened. The classic experiments of Goldberger and his associates seemed to establish the importance of vitamin B_2 deficiency, and for a time the cause of this disease seemed clear. The decade following Goldberger's announcement of the preventive and curative properties of substances rich in B_2 saw great advance in the field of prevention by adequate nutrition, but pellagra continued to occur with considerable frequency and yeast therapy of severe hospitalized cases proved vastly disappointing. Mortality rates in general hospitals, which had varied between 25 and 70 per cent, were reduced only 8 to 10 per cent by vitamin B_2 administration. Severely ill patients died, ferbrile or demented, without response to treatment. The incidence of peripheral and central nervous lesions was not materially influenced. In some localities, particularly in the North, increased consumption of alcoholic beverages of the most deleterious sort, may have played a part. Everywhere acute pellagra following severe acute alcoholism was notably intractable and was accompanied by an unusually high incidence of peripheral nervous involvement. In these cases especially, yeast therapy seemed inadequate.

To further complicate the picture, observers in widely separated places saw hospitalized pellagrins secure remission or apparent cure while being fed pellagra-producing diets, in some instances more deficient than that employed by Goldberger in his experiments.

Lowe, misled by the early resolution of skin lesions, maintained that hospitalization alone was sufficient to secure remission in many instances, provided the patients were given an ordinary diet. It must not be overlooked that so-called pellagra-producing diets were in many instances superior to the diet upon which the patients had been subsisting at home.

Following the demonstration by Minot and Murphy of the replacement effect of liver and liver extract in pernicious anemia, the further proof by Sturgis and Isaacs that desiccated pig's stomach contains an equally effective substance, and finally, the brilliant demonstration by Castle and his associates, that an intrinsic gastric defect, replaceable by normal gastric juice, is present in this disease, various observers sought to draw analogies between pernicious anemia and pellagra. Doubtless all were prompted by the fact that gastric anacidity is so commonly present in pellagra. Other features of the disease show a curious mingling of similarities and differences. Pernicious anemia is a disease of cold regions, its presenting symptoms referable to failure of normal erythropoiesis. Pellagra is predominantly a malady of temperate and subtropical zones, usually showing dermatitis and gastro-intestinal disorders as outstanding phenomena. Anemia is frequent but nearly always hypochromic and the bone marrow shows a type of reaction altogether different from that in Addisonian anemia. Lesions of the nervous system are common to both. Psychic disorders are frequent in pellagra; uncommon in pernicious anemia. Combined sclerosis is almost a part of the picture of pernicious anemia, but occurs in much fewer than half of pellagrins. Peripheral neuritis is present in a small number of patients with either disorder, perhaps more frequently in pellagra. Gastric dysfunction and glossitis are quite constantly present in both, although the bright red, slick, often fissured tongue of pellagra looks quite unlike the smooth, liver colored organ of pernicious anemia. Dyspepsia and diarrhea may be prominent features of either.

Boggs was perhaps the first to apply these analogies therapeutically. As he states, pellagrins on his service were fed liver empirically; later liver extract was given. As a result he reduced his mortality in a considerable series from 69 to 19.5 per cent. Almost simultaneously Spies was experimenting with liver extract, ventriculin and autoclaved yeast, all given in large amounts. Each of these substances produced rapid resolution of illness. When large quantities of liver extract were given, prolonged remission occurred.

Both Boggs and Spies suggested the presence of an intrinsic deficiency in pellagra; implying that liver and liver extract furnished the necessary combination of extrinsic and intrinsic factors to insure normal metabolism. More recently investigators of the University of Georgia School of Medicine have been able to produce remission or apparent cure of pellagra by administering normal gastric juice or an extract of pig's gastric mucosa to pellagrins maintained on a pellagra-producing diet. This additional evidence supports the hypothesis that pellagra is a conditioned deficiency, dependent on intrinsic as well as extrinsic defect. Such an hypothesis would explain the frequent therapeutic failure of yeast and the success of treatment with liver and liver extract, which contain the combination of extrinsic and intrinsic factors. It is doubtful, in fact most unlikely, that the intrinsic factors in pellagra and pernicious anemia are the same, the extrinsic factor in both is probably the B_2 complex.

From the therapeutic standpoint it is most strongly to be urged that all pellagrins be given the benefit of liver feeding or of large doses of liver extract administered over a period of two or three weeks.

V. P. SYDENSTRICKER, M.D.

The JOURNAL would like to record the scientific work of Georgia doctors. It earnestly requests, therefore, that each physician in the State who publishes a contribution in some other medical periodical submit an abstract of the article for these columns.

The Annual Conference of Secretaries of Constituent State Medical Associations of the American Medical Association will be held in the Assembly Room of the A. M. A. Building in Chicago, Monday and Tuesday, November 16 and 17. All officers of state associations are invited to attend the Conference. Any subject which it is desired to have discussed should be submitted in advance.

WOMAN'S AUXILIARY
OFFICERS, 1936-1937

President—Mrs. Wm. R. Dancy, Savannah.
President-Elect—Mrs. Ralph H. Chaney, Augusta.
First Vice-President—Mrs. B. H. Minchew, Waycross.
Second Vice-President—Mrs. Clarence L. Ayers, Toccoa.
Third Vice-President—Mrs. J. A. Redfearn, Albany.

Recording Secretary—Mrs. Warren A. Coleman, Eastman.
Corresponding Secretary—Mrs. Lee Howard, Savannah.
Treasurer—Mrs. W. A. Selman, Atlanta.
Historian—Mrs. Grady N. Coker, Canton.
Parliamentarian—Mrs. John E. Penland, Waycross.

COMMITTEE CHAIRMEN

Student Loan Fund
Mrs. Robert C. Pendergrass, Americus.
Health Films
Mrs. A. J. Mooney, Statesboro
Public Relations
Mrs. Wallace Bazemore, Macon.
Doctors' Day
Mrs. Ernest R. Harris, Winder.

Legislation
Mrs. Dan Y. Sage, 47 Inman Circle. Atlanta.
Press and Publicity
Mrs. J. Harry Rogers, 134 Huntington Rd., Atlanta.
Research in Romance of Medicine
Mrs. D. N. Thompson, Elberton.
Jane Todd Crawford Memorial
Mrs. Eustace A. Allen, 18 Collier Rd., Atlanta.

COMMITTEES

HEALTH EDUCATION

Chairman: Mrs. B. H. Minchew, 412 Williams Street, Waycross.
First District: Mrs. J. C. Metts, 735½ East Henry Street, Savannah.
Second District: Mrs. J. M. Barnett, Albany.
Third District: Mrs. J. Cox Wall, Eastman.
Fourth District: Mrs. R. S. O'Neal, LaGrange.
Sixth District: Mrs. Y. H. Yarbrough, Milledgeville.
Eighth District: Mrs. B. H. Minchew, 412 Williams Street, Waycross.
Ninth District: Mrs. F. B. Murphy, Canton.
Tenth District: Mrs. W. K. Philpot, 2151 Kings Highway, Augusta.

PUBLIC RELATIONS

Chairman: Mrs. Wallace Bazemore, 127 Beverly Place, Macon.
First District: Mrs. Walter E. Simmons. Metter.
Second District: Mrs. J. A. Redfearn, 527 Broad Avenue, Albany.
Third District: Mrs. B. W. Yawn, Eastman.
Fourth District: Mrs. Enoch Callaway, LaGrange.
Fifth District: Mrs. J. Bonar White, 769 Penn Avenue, N. E., Atlanta.
Sixth District: Mrs. Wallace Bazemore, 127 Beverly Place, Macon.
Eighth District: Mrs. John E. Penland, 912 Elizabeth Street, Waycross.
Ninth District: Mrs. E. H. Lamb, Cornelia.
Tenth District: Mrs. C. M. Burpee, 1127 Monte Sano Avenue, Augusta.

HYGEIA

Chairman: Mrs. Clarence L. Ayers. Toccoa.
First District: Mrs. L. A. DeLoach, 3402 Abercorn Street, Savannah.
Second District: Mrs. Carlton A. Fleming, Tifton.
Third District: Mrs. V. L. Harris. Pinehurst.
Fourth District: Mrs. H. H. Hammett, LaGrange.
Fifth District: Mrs. Leland G. Baggett, 79 Brighton Road. N. W., Atlanta.

Sixth District: Mrs. Walter E. Mobley, Massee Apartments, Macon.
Eighth District: Mrs. Kenneth McCullough, 907 Gilmore Street, Waycross.
Ninth District: Mrs. Clarence L. Ayers. Toccoa.
Tenth District: Mrs. J. C. Holliday, University Drive Athens.

PRESS AND PUBLICITY

Chairman: Mrs. J. Harry Rogers, 134 Huntington Road, N. W., Atlanta.
First District: Mrs. G. Hugo Johnson, 116 East Oglethorpe Avenue, Savannah.
Second District: Mrs. Alex Freeman, Albany.
Third District: Mrs. Marvin F. Haygood, P. O. Box 54, Chipley.
Fourth District: Mrs. W. R. McCall, 409 Hill Street. LaGrange.
Fifth District: Mrs. J. Harry Rogers, 134 Huntington Road, N. W., Atlanta.
Sixth District: Mrs. E. W. Allen, Allen's Invalid Home. Milledgeville.
Eighth District: Mrs. William Folks, Waycross.
Ninth District: Mrs. W. H. Garrison, Clarkesville.
Tenth District: Mrs. Robert C. McGahee, 2633 Raymond Avenue, Augusta.

LEGISLATION

Chairman: Mrs. Dan Y. Sage, 47 Inman Circle. Atlanta.
First District: Mrs. J. Wallace Daniel, Claxton.
Second District: Mrs. H. T. Edmondson. Moultrie.
Third District: Mrs. H. M. Tolleson, Eastman.
Fourth District: Mrs. J. C. Morgan, West Point.
Fifth District: Mrs. Dan Y. Sage, 47 Inman Circle Atlanta.
Sixth District: Mrs. Chas. C. Harrold, 550 Orange Street, Macon.
Eighth District: Mrs. W. F. Reavis, 1105 Satilla Boulevard, Waycross.
Ninth District: Mrs. Ralph Freeman, Hoschton.
Tenth District: Mrs. Stewart D. Brown, Royston.

(Continued on page 380)

GEORGIA DEPARTMENT OF PUBLIC HEALTH
T. F. ABERCROMBIE, M.D., *Director*

DEATHS AND CRUDE DEATH RATES

Crude rates by no means tell the whole story regarding the healthfulness of different localities. Race stock, occupations of the inhabitants, the sex and age distribution of the population, and the number of deaths of nonresidents are factors which must be considered before it can be determined that one state has a higher rate than another. But for comparing one area with another the crude death rates will suffice.

The number of deaths returned from Georgia for the year 1935 was 34,313, corresponding to a death rate of 11.3 per 1,000 population; this is 0.5 lower than the rate in 1934, which was 11.8.

The following death rates are per 100,000 population.

Typhoid and Paratyphoid Fever

The great decline in typhoid and paratyphoid fever rates in 1934 is a most glowing tribute to the efficiency of public health work. In 1935 there were 261 deaths corresponding to a death rate of only 8.6, whereas in 1934 the death rate was 10.5.

Malaria

Malaria is a term used somewhat loosely in some sections of the state, which undoubtedly has much to do with some of the higher rates recorded, especially in certain areas where certification is not always made by a physician. But accepting the certification as reported, the number of deaths from malaria in 1935 was 387 corresponding to a death rate of 12.8.

Smallpox

Smallpox for many years has been an important cause of death in Georgia. Since the first publication of our reports in 1920 it reached the highest point of 25 deaths in 1924. In the past five years there has not been over one death per year. In 1934 and 1935 there was only one death with a corresponding rate of 0.03.

Measles

Measles shows a downward trend, owing to the decrease in the epidemic of 1934. There were reported only 25 deaths in 1935 with a rate of 0.8 whereas in 1934 there were reported 540 deaths with a death rate of 18.0.

Scarlet Fever

Scarlet fever in 1935 shows an increase over 1934. Since the figures show for 1935, 23 deaths with a rate of 0.8 and for 1934 only 17 deaths with a rate of 0.6.

Whooping Cough

Whooping cough is decidedly a disease of very young children; in the registration area, in 1925, the number of deaths under three years of age formed more than 81 per cent of all deaths from this cause. In 1935 there were reported 194 deaths corresponding to a death rate of 4.9 and in 1934 there were 334 deaths with a death rate of 11.1.

Diphtheria

Diphtheria with the decrease in the rates from 1935 of 5.3 to the rate in 1921 of 14.3. This tribute to the progress of medicine is further shown in the reductions. In 1935 there were reported 161 deaths with a rate of 5.3 and in 1934 there were reported 188 deaths with a rate of 6.3.

Influenza and Pneumonia (all forms)

The death rate for these two causes shows an increase in the number and rate. In 1935 the number of deaths reported was 4,395 with a corresponding death rate of 144.9 and for 1934 they show 4,012 with a death rate of 134.3.

Tuberculosis (all forms)

Tuberculosis has shown a downward trend since 1928. We find that 1,731 deaths were reported for 1935 with a death rate of 57.1 and in 1934 we find 1,772 deaths with a rate of 58.9.

Cancer

Cancer with its annual increase in the number of deaths shows a decrease in 1935 over 1934. In 1935, 1,715 deaths were registered corresponding to a death rate of 56.6 and in 1934 1,762 deaths were registered with a rate of 58.6.

Pellagra

Pellagra has shown a decrease in the number and rate since 1929 of 871 deaths. In 1935 the number of deaths was 365, corresponding to a rate of 12.0 whereas in 1934 we had 351 deaths with a death rate of 11.7.

Cerebral Hemorrhage

This is one of the diseases that shows an increase in its death rate in 1935; 2,410 were registered in 1935 with a death rate of 79.5 and the number of deaths reported in 1934 was 2,310 with a rate of 76.8.

Heart Disease

Heart disease shows an increase in its annual rate of 1,923. We find that in 1935 heart disease registered 5,071 with a death rate of 167.3, whereas in 1934 5,019, a death rate of 166.9.

Nephritis

Nephritis in 1935 showed 3,155 deaths with a corresponding rate of 104.1. In 1934 it shows 3,301 with a death rate of 109.8.

Suicide

Suicide since 1920 has shown a decided increase in its death rates. In 1928 there were 128 deaths whereas in 1935 there were registered 300 deaths with a rate of 9.9 and in 1934, 297 deaths with a rate of 9.9.

Automobile Accidents

There has been a gradual increase since 1921 from 132 to 903 deaths in 1935. The death rate in 1935 was 29.8 and the deaths reported for 1934 were 774 with a rate of 25.7.

DEATHS AND CRUDE DEATH RATES PER 100,000 POPULATION FROM SPECIFIED CAUSES IN GEORGIA: 1934 and 1935

Cause of Death	Number 1935	Number 1934	Rate 1935	Rate 1934
ALL CAUSES	34,313	35,590	1132.4	1183.6
Typhoid Fever	261	316	8.6	10.5
Malaria	387	418	12.8	13.9
Smallpox	1	1	0.0	0.0
Measles	25	540	0.8	18.0
Scarlet Fever	23	17	0.8	0.6
Whooping Cough	149	334	4.9	11.1
Diphtheria	161	188	5.3	6.3
Influenza	1,357	1,009	44.8	33.6
Dysentery	163	219	5.4	7.3
Poliomyelitis	16	26	0.5	0.9
Lethargic Encephalitis	5	8	0.2	0.3
Meningococcus Meningitis	33	25	1.1	0.8
Tuberculosis (all forms)	1,731	1,772	57.1	58.9
Cancer	1,715	1,762	56.6	58.6
Diabetes Mellitus	388	389	12.8	12.9
Pellagra	365	351	12.0	11.7
Cerebral Hemorrhage	2,410	2,310	79.5	76.8
Heart Diseases	5,071	5,019	167.3	166.9
Pneumonia	3,035	3,030	100.2	100.8
Diarrhea and Enteritis—2 Yrs.	507	651	16.7	21.7
Cirrhosis of Liver	142	110	4.7	3.7
Nephritis	3,155	3,301	104.1	109.8
Puerperal Causes	458	505	15.1	16.8
Malformation and Early Infancy	1,736	1,904	57.3	63.3
Suicide	300	297	9.9	9.9
Homicide	661	720	21.8	23.9
Automobile Accidents	903	774	29.8	25.7
Other Accidents	1,525	1,477	50.3	49.1
Unknown or Ill-defined Causes	2,125	2,257	70.1	75.1
All Other Causes	5,505	5,860	181.7	194.9

BUTLER TOOMBS, Chief,
Bureau of Vital Statistics.

The Southern Medical Association will hold its Thirtieth Annual Meeting in Baltimore, Maryland, November 17-20, 1936. All members of the Medical Association of Georgia are invited to attend. The Seaboard Air Line Railway is booking reservations.

NEWS ITEMS

THE NINTH DISTRICT MEDICAL SOCIETY met in Newton and Ward Chapel, Gainesville, September 16th. Titles of scientific papers on the program were: "Fractures," Dr. Grady N. Coker, Canton: discussion led by Dr. J. H. Downey, Gainesville. "Uterine Hemorrhage," Dr. Geo. A. Traylor, Augusta, President-Elect of the Association; discussion led by Dr. J. K. Burns, Gainesville. Address by Dr. B. H. Minchew, Waycross, President of the Association. "The Doctor, His Town, His Patient," Hon. Henry H. Estes, Gainesville, President, Gainesville Chamber of Commerce.

DR. WARREN B. MATTHEWS, formerly Pathologist at the Wesley Memorial Hospital, Chicago, has been appointed Associate Professor of Pathology at Emory University School of Medicine, and Director of the Pathological Laboratory at Grady Hospital, Atlanta.

DR. W. R. CAMP, Fairburn, was host to the Fulton County Commissioners and a number of physicians at a fish fry at his lake six miles from Fairburn on September 3rd.

THE JOHN D. ARCHBOLD MEMORIAL HOSPITAL, Thomasville, has had its operating rooms air conditioned.

THE STAFF MEETING of the Georgia Baptist Hospital, Atlanta, was held on September 15th. Dinner was served in the Nurses' Home dining room.

THE FULTON COUNTY MEDICAL SOCIETY met at the Academy of Medicine, Atlanta, September 17th. Dr. Walter W. Daniel reported a case. "Pemphigus Neonatorum"; Dr. Stewart R. Roberts made a clinical talk. "Reversible Hypertrophy of the Heart in Myxedema"; Dr. J. G. McDaniel read a paper entitled, "A Comparative Study of Syphilitics and Non-Syphilitics on Fulton County Relief Rolls." The discussion was led by Dr. Martin T. Meyers, Dr. Edgar Boling and Dr. Jas. E. Paullin.

DR. HARRY L. ALLEN announces the opening of his office in Suite 610 Doctors' Building, 478 Peachtree Street, N. E., Atlanta, for the practice of general medicine and surgery.

DR. CHARLES ANDREWS has moved to Canton and assumed his duties as resident physician of the Coker Hospital.

THE BARTOW COUNTY MEDICAL SOCIETY met at the office of Dr. T. Lowry, Cartersville, on October 7th.

DR. OSCAR L. ROGERS, Sandersville, Washington County Commissioner of Health, spoke before a meeting of the Lions Club at Sandersville on September 2nd. He compared health conditions and statistics with those of fifteen years ago, and quoted figures to show the decrease in the mortality rates of 1920 and 1935 from tuberculosis, diphtheria, malaria, pellagra, smallpox and typhoid.

TERRELL COUNTY has entered a rural health conservation contest to be conducted by the U. S. Chamber of Commerce in cooperation with the American Public Health Association. The object is to assist in local health conservation. Physicians on the committee are as follows: Dr. Guy Chappell, Dawson, Chairman;

Dr. O. G. Cranford, Sasser; Dr. J. T. Arnold, Parrott; Dr. R. R. Holt, Parrott; Dr. R. E. Bowman, Bronwood.

DR. GUY G. LUNSFORD, Atlanta, Director of County Health Work with the State Department of Public Health, met with the Dougherty County Board of Health at Albany on September 3rd.

DR. J. COX WALL, Eastman, has begun work on the foundation for a brick building to be used as a hospital, according to announcement in the Eastman Times-Journal. It is to be equipped with the latest improved hospital accessories. Dr. N. L. Barker, Dr. I. J. Parkerson, Dr. Harold Peacock and Dr. B. W. Yawn will be associated with Dr. Wall.

DR. RALPH H. CHANEY, Augusta, spoke before a meeting of the Augusta Rotary Club on "A Few Highlights of Medical History," September 8th.

DR. C. F. HOLTON, Savannah, First Vice-President of the Association, has just returned from the Mayo Clinic, Rochester, Minnesota, and the Henry Ford Hospital, Detroit, Michigan, where he has been engaged in post-graduate work for several weeks.

THE THOMAS COUNTY MEDICAL SOCIETY met at the Archbold Memorial Hospital, Thomasville, September 16th. Dr. Chapman Q. Dykes, Carrabelle, Florida, read a paper entitled, "The Treatment of Pneumonia"; discussed by Dr. W. W. Jarrell, Dr. C. H. Ferguson, Dr. Arthur D. Little and Dr. Chas. H. Watt, all of Thomasville. Dr. S. E. Sanchez, Barwick, read a paper on "Cancer"; discussed by Doctors A. D. Little, Chas. H. Watt and C. H. Ferguson. Motion carried to ask Dr. C. K. Wall, Thomasville, to read his paper at the next regular meeting of the Society which was scheduled for this meeting and omitted on account of the absence of the author. Dr. Jas. N. Isler, Meigs, Vice-President, presided.

THE MUSCOGEE COUNTY MEDICAL SOCIETY met at the Ralston Hotel, Columbus, October 8th. Dr. V. P. Sydenstricker, Augusta, read a scientific paper. Addresses by Dr. B. H. Minchew, Waycross, and Dr. Geo. A. Traylor, Augusta, President and President-Elect, respectively, of the Association. Dinner was served in the hotel dining room.

THE MUSCOGEE COUNTY MEDICAL SOCIETY met at the Ralston Hotel, Columbus, on September 10th. Dr. Dan C. Elkin, Atlanta, read a paper entitled, "The Surgical Treatment of Tuberculosis"; Dr. Wm. C. Warren, Jr., Atlanta, "The Intracranial Complications of Otitis and Mastoiditis."

THE WILKES COUNTY MEDICAL SOCIETY met at the Washington General Hospital, Washington. The physicians of Greene, Lincoln, McDuffie, Oglethorpe and Taliaferro Counties were guests.

DR. WARD C. CURTIS, formerly of Roseville, Virginia, has moved to Toccoa and opened offices for the practice of medicine in the Franklin Building on Doyle Street.

DR. RICHARD B. WEEKS, Augusta, has been elected to fellowship in the American College of Surgeons.

THE WOMAN'S AUXILIARY entertained the members of the Jackson-Barrow Counties Medical Society to a picnic at the Riverside Swimming Pool, near Jefferson, on August 31st.

DR. O. B. BUSH, formerly in the Doctors' Building at 478 Peachtree Street, N. E., has moved his office to Suite 629 Candler Building, Atlanta.

THE SEVENTH DISTRICT MEDICAL SOCIETY met at the Marietta Golf Club, Marietta, September 30th. Titles of scientific papers on the program were: "Foreign Bodies in the Urinary Bladder," by Dr. John M. McGehee, Cedartown; discussed by Dr. J. W. Stanford, Cartersville, and Dr. J. L. Garrard, Rome. *Symposium on Syphilis*—"Congenital Syphilis," Dr. R. C. Maddox, Rome; discussed by Dr. R. W. Fowler, Marietta, and Dr. W. W. Anderson, Atlanta. "The Treatment of Early Syphilis," Dr. Fred H. Simonton, Chickamauga; discussed by Dr. J. C. Rollins, Dalton, and Dr. H. R. Perkins, Rockmart. "Tertiary Syphilis," Dr. D. B. Douglas, Trion; discussed by Dr. W. R. Richards, Calhoun, and Dr. J. H. Mull, Rome. "Cardiovascular Syphilis," Dr. Stewart R. Roberts, Atlanta; discussed by Dr. W. H. Perkinson, Marietta, and Dr. Carter Smith, Atlanta. "Syphilis of the Nervous System," Dr. Jas. N. Brawner, Smyrna; discussed by Dr. W. E. Wofford, Cartersville, and Dr. Richard B. Wilson, Atlanta. The Cobb County Medical Society entertained the members to a barbecue at 6:00 o'clock in the afternoon. Committee on Arrangements were: Dr. A. H. Fowler, Dr. W. M. Gober and Dr. C. D. Elder, all of Marietta. Officers of the Society are: Dr. P. O. Chaudron, Cedartown, President; Dr. N. A. Funderburk, Trion, President-Elect; and Dr. William Harbin, Jr., Rome, Secretary.

THE JOURNAL OFFICE has what it deems reliable information that there has been some one who attempted to put a fake insurance scheme over some of the Association's members in Burke County. You can always get information in reference to insurance companies authorized to do business in Georgia by writing to the Insurance Department, State Capitol, Atlanta.

THE SOUTHEASTERN DERMATOLOGICAL ASSOCIATION met in Atlanta on September 6th. The members of the Atlanta Dermatological Association gave a clinic composed of forty-five unusual problems in skin diseases. New officers of the Association are: Dr. Andrew L. Glaze, Birmingham, Ala., President; Dr. Herbert Alden, Atlanta, Secretary.

DR. AND MRS. J. B. JACKSON, Clarkesville, entertained the members of the Habersham County Medical Society and Auxiliary in their home on September 17th. A salad course with punch was served.

THE ATLANTA MEMBERS of the American Academy of Ophthalmology and Otolaryngology who attended the annual meeting at the Waldorf-Astoria Hotel, New York City, September 27th to October 2nd, inclusive, were: Dr. B. Russell Burke, Dr. W. E. Campbell, Dr. Grady E. Clay, Dr. Arthur G. Fort, Dr. Alton V. Hallum, Dr. Zach W. Jackson, Dr. Hugh M. Lokey, Dr. Wm. O. Martin and Dr. W C. Warren, Jr.

DR. GATES WAXELBAUM announces the opening of his offices in Suite 1114 Doctors' Building, 478 Peachtree Street, N. E., Atlanta, for the practice of general medicine.

DR. CHAS. A. GREER, Oglethorpe, was successful in his race for State Senator from the Thirteenth District in the Democratic primary held on September 9th.

DR. J. T. HOLT, Baxley, is the Democratic nominee from Appling County as representative in the Lower House of the 1937 session of the General Assembly of Georgia.

THE ATLANTA PSYCHOANALYTICAL SOCIETY gave its annual banquet at the Henry Grady Hotel, Atlanta, on October 2nd.

THE GEORGIA FEDERATION OF WOMEN'S CLUBS will distribute pamphlets prepared by the Cancer Commission of the Medical Association of Georgia, entitled, "The Prevention, Early Diagnosis and Treatment of Cancer and Precancerous Conditions." Educational meetings will be held in all Congressional Districts of the State under direct supervision of members of the Cancer Commission.

AT A MEETING OF HEALTH OFFICERS in Camilla on September 17th, quarantine regulations were adopted for Colquitt and Mitchell Counties as follows: "All cases of infantile paralysis and occupants of homes in which there are cases will be quarantined for fourteen days; all contacts will be quarantined for fourteen days from the time of the last contact; all children under sixteen years of age will be prohibited from attending schools, motion picture theaters or public gatherings and will not be allowed in stores." It was stated that the regulations were adopted to protect adjoining counties and communities and that no new cases of poliomyelitis had been reported.

THE FULTON COUNTY MEDICAL SOCIETY met at the Academy of Medicine, Atlanta, October 1st. Dr. J. K. Fancher presented a patient, "Complete Case of Hypotrichosis"; Dr. B. T. Beasley gave case report, "Arachnidism"; Dr. Lewis M. Gaines made a clinical talk on "Spinal Cord Changes in Pernicious Anemia—Demonstration of Patients"; Dr. M. Hines Roberts read a paper, "A Study of Mastoid Infection in Children." The discussion was led by Dr. Jas. J. Clark. Dr. L. D. Hoppe and Dr. Calhoun McDougall.

THE STAFF MEETING of Emory University Hospital, Atlanta, was held on October 5th. Dr. F. G. Hodgson read a paper entitled "Chronic Osteomyelitis"; discussed by Dr. Randolph Smith. Paper by Dr. Earl Floyd and Dr. Jas. L. Pittman. "Operations on the Single Kidney"; discussed by Dr. M. K. Bailey. Dr. John F. Denton read a paper, "Gangrene of the Rectum"; discussed by Dr. Geo. Eubanks.

THE COFFEE COUNTY MEDICAL SOCIETY met at Douglas on September 29th. T. S. Deen, Ph.G., read a paper entitled "The Practice of Pharmacy."

THE RANDOLPH COUNTY MEDICAL SOCIETY met at the Patterson Hospital, Cuthbert, on October 1st. Dr. T. F. Harper, Coleman, read a paper entitled, "Interesting Cases of Pellagra."

THE GEORGIA PEDIATRIC SOCIETY will meet in Atlanta, December 10th. Prominent speakers on the program are: Dr. John A. Toomey, Cleveland, Ohio, Associate Professor of Pediatrics at the Western Reserve University School of Medicine; Dr. Julius H. Hess. Chicago, Professor of Pediatrics at the University of Illinois College of Medicine; Dr. Henry F. Helmholz, Rochester, Minnesota, Chief in the Department of Pediatrics at Mayo Clinic; Dr. Wm. A. Mulherin. Augusta; Dr. Alfred A. Walker. Birmingham, Ala., and Dr. D. Lesesne Smith. Spartanburg, S. C. The members of the Scientific Committee are: Dr. Wm. Willis Anderson, Dr. W. L. Funkhouser, Dr. M. Hines Roberts and Dr. Joseph Yampolsky, all of Atlanta.

THE WARE COUNTY MEDICAL SOCIETY met in the Directors' Room of the Y. M. C. A. Building, Waycross, on October 7th. Dr. W. C. Hafford, Waycross, read a paper entitled, "Granuloma Genitalia Inguinal."

DR. D. HENRY POER, Atlanta, was elected President of the Atlanta Alumni Association of the Phi Delta Theta on September 29th.

DR. ALLEN E. HAUCK has been appointed resident physician at Emory University Hospital, Emory University.

DR. WILLIAM CARTER WATERS announces the removal of his office to Suite 303 Doctors' Building. 478 Peachtree Street, N. E., Atlanta.

THE EIGHTH DISTRICT MEDICAL SOCIETY met in the Elks Hall, Douglas, on October 13th. The scientific program consisted of an "Address" by Dr. B. H. Minchew, Waycross, President of the Association; paper entitled, 'Surgical Considerations—Case Report," Dr. W. W. Turner, Nashville; "Mortality Statistics," Dr. T. H. Johnston, Douglas; "Syphilis," Dr. S. Ross Brown. Atlanta, Assistant Chief; Division of Venereal Disease, State Board of Health; "Surgical Tuberculosis," Dr. R. L. Johnson, Waycross; "The Management of Fractures," Dr. Sage Harper, Ambrose; "Poliomyelitis," Dr. C. D. Bowdoin, Atlanta, Epidemiologist, State Board of Health; "The Present Status of Malaria and Its Treatment," Dr. H. M. Tolleson. Eastman. Dinner was served at the Doucoff Hotel. The members were guests of the Coffee County Medical Society.

DR. WARREN A. COLEMAN and Dr. H. M. Tolleson, Eastman, conducted thyroid clinics at the Coleman Sanatorium on September 22nd. Five patients with goiter were operated upon in the presence of a number of visiting physicians.

DR. WARREN A. COLEMAN, Eastman, with his family is visiting some of the principal cities of the East. While there, he will attend the meeting of the American College of Surgeons at Philadelphia, visit Johns Hopkins Hospital at Baltimore; and other hospitals and clinics in Boston and New York City.

THE STAFF MEETING of the Crawford W. Long Memorial Hospital, Atlanta, was held on October 8th. Dr. E. G. Ballenger. Dr. Omar F. Elder, and Dr.

Harold P. McDonald reported cases. "The Management of Carcinoma of the Prostate and Bladder."

THE DOWNEY HOSPITAL. Gainesville, will be enlarged and improved at an expense of $75,000.00 to $100,000.00 by its owners, Dr. J. H. Downey. Dr. J. K. Burns, Dr. E. W. Grove and Dr. C. D. Whelchel.

DR. THOS. G. RITCH, Jesup, is in Chicago taking post-graduate work in surgery at the Cook County Hospital. He will visit a number of other clinics and hospitals while there.

DR. ALEXANDER B. RUSSELL announces the opening of offices in the Peoples Bank Building, Winder. for the practice of medicine. He is a graduate of Emory University School of Medicine and served as an intern at Grady Hospital, Atlanta.

DR. WILLIAM R. DANCY. Savannah, Past President of the Medical Association of Georgia, addressed the surviving Confederate Veterans at a reunion held at Hotel Richmond. Augusta, October 6, 7, 8.

UNIVERSITY OF GEORGIA
SCHOOL OF MEDICINE

LABORATORY AND AUDITORIUM BUILDING

On September 22nd the Regents of the University System of Georgia let a contract to Wheatley and Mobley of Augusta, for the construction of a laboratory and auditorium building on the campus of the School of Medicine. Construction began September 30th. The new structure will house the departments of Physiology, Pharmacology and Biochemistry and an auditorium with a seating capacity of 350. The work must be completed by July 1, 1937. The cost will be between $70,000.00 and $75,000.00, unequipped.

The ground floor of the main medical school building has been renovated to house the department of Pathology in the north end and a beautifully appointed tavern type of dining-room in the south end. The entire third floor is now occupied by the department of Anatomy, Microscopic Anatomy having taken over the space formerly used by the department of Pathology.

Dr. Richard Torpin, formerly associated with Rush Medical College, has been made Associate Professor of Obstetrics and Gynecology and Chairman of the Department.

Dr. A. P. Briggs, formerly of St. Louis University Medical School, has been appointed Associate Professor of Biochemistry and of Medicine.

New research fellows are Dr. B. D. Bosworth, in medicine, and Dr. Warren Andrew, in anatomy.

By order of the Regents of the University System fourth year medical students were required to assist in making physical examinations of newly enrolled students in the various units over the State during September.

MEETING OF THE GEORGIA SECTION OF THE
SOUTHEASTERN SURGICAL CONGRESS

The Third Annual Clinical Congress will be held at
the Millen Hospital, Millen, Georgia, on Wednesday,
November 4, 1936. (Eastern standard time.)

Dr. T. C. Davison, Atlanta, Chairman.

Dr. Cleveland Thompson, Millen, will be host.

PROGRAM

10:00 A. M.

"Tumors of the Breast"
Dr. A. J. Mooney, Statesboro
Discussion to be opened by
Dr. E. A. Wilcox, Augusta

10:30 A. M.
"Injuries to the Lungs and Pleura"
Dr. Frank K. Boland, Atlanta
Discussion to be opened by
Dr. Fred B. Rawlings, Sandersville

11:00 A. M.
"Leg Ulcers"
Dr. Geo. A. Traylor, Augusta
Discussion to be opened by
Dr. C. E. Rushin, Atlanta

11:30 A. M.
"Operation for Kidney Stone"
Dr. Earl Floyd, Atlanta
Discussion to be opened by
Dr. Kenneth Hunt, Griffin

12:00 Noon
"Acute Abdominal Injury"
Dr. J. S. Turberville, Century, Fla.
Discussion to be opened by
Dr. Grady N. Coker, Canton

12:30 P. M.
Lunch—Courtesy of the Millen Hospital
"The Aims of the Southeastern Surgical Congress"
Dr. B. T. Beasley, Atlanta, Secretary

2:00 P. M.
"Hernias"
Dr. C. F. Holton, Savannah
Discussion to be opened by
Dr. C. B. Greer, Brunswick

2:30 P. M.
"Ureteral Stricture"
Dr. Wallace L. Bazemore, Macon
Discussion to be opened by
Dr. J. W. Shearouse, Savannah

3:00 P. M.
"Chronic Cholecystitis"
Dr. C. E. Wills, Washington
Discussion to be opened by
Dr. R. C. Franklin, Swainsboro

3:30 P. M.
"Industrial Injuries"
Dr. A. R. Rozar, Macon
Discussion to be opened by
Dr. Julian K. Quattlebaum, Savannah

This program will consist of presentation of patients
and case reports to be followed by discussions from the
floor. There will be no papers read.

BLOODPRESSURE, HOT DOGS AND MERRY-
GO-ROUNDS

The old-fashioned medicine man is slowly disappearing from sideshows and county fairs but today a new
charlatan is taking his place at beach resorts, fairs and
amusement parks. Equipped with a white coat, a steth-
oscope and a bloodpressure instrument, these operators
are capitalizing on the public's interest in bloodpressure.
Their main concern is collecting the ten or fifteen cents
they charge per 'patient.'

It is evident that bloodpressure readings taken by
such persons under such circumstances are of no value.
The "patient" is simply being bilked but the most
harmful part of this practice is the serious consequence
that may easily result in some cases regardless of whether
the information is erroneous or otherwise.

We are vigorously opposed to this misuse of medico-
scientific instruments, having gone on record with the
American Medical Association to this effect a year ago.
Moreover, we have refused to fill large orders for
Baumanometers to be used for such purposes.

This evil practice should be stopped and we would
appreciate your cooperation in reporting to us any
instance that comes to your attention—especially where
some definite harm has resulted to a patient.

W. A. Baum & Co., Inc., 460 West 34th Street,
New York, since 1916, originators and makers of
bloodpressure apparatus exclusively.

HEALTH AND SAFETY WORK OF THE
RED CROSS

From the inception of the Red Cross idea in the
mind of a young Swiss on the battlefield of Solferino,
down through the years, this worldwide volunteer
organization has had the cooperation and support of
the medical profession.

In expanding its services to include prompt assistance for victims of natural disasters and in promoting
health and safety through year-round programs of
public health nursing, instruction in first aid, in water
life saving and in home hygiene and care of the sick and
in its more recent establishment of highway emergency
first aid stations the American Red Cross has been aided
by the nation's foremost medical authorities, without
whose counsel and guidance little of lasting worth
could have been accomplished.

Through its public health nursing service the Red
Cross brings the visiting nurse to many small towns
and rural communities, where the number of physicians
and hospital facilities are at a minimum. Not only
through her nursing care, but also by her instruction to
mothers and girls in the community in health habits
and home hygiene does she assist the country doctor to
safeguard the health of his widely scattered practice.

Red Cross courses in first aid teach the layman how
to give emergency help to accident victims pending the
arrival of a physician. In the past quarter of a century
more than a million persons have received this instruction. In addition to saving many lives each year by
their prompt action in emergencies the layman first
aiders are doing much to promote safety in industry
and on the highways; for knowing the seriousness of

accidents in terms of suffering and time lost from work makes them more careful to avoid unnecessary hazards.

Like first aid, water life saving instruction has been developed by the Red Cross to meet a definite need. This effort has been responsible for an increased activity in healthful water sports throughout the nation, as well as to greatly reduce the percentage of drownings among bathers. So widespread have the life saving teachings been carried that today there is scarcely a public bathing place or youngsters' summer camp where swimmers are not watched over by a trained lifeguard.

All Red Cross services are supported by the annual membership dues of millions of Americans who join each year during the Roll Call, held from Armistice Day to Thanksgiving. Everyone is invited to have a part in the work of their Red Cross by enrolling in their local Chapter.

BALTIMORE
SOUTHERN MEDICAL ASSOCIATION
SEABOARD AIR LINE RAILWAY

In connection with the thirtieth annual meeting of the Southern Medical Association. Baltimore, Md., November 17th-20th, special air-conditioned sleeping cars will be operated via the Seaboard Air Line Railway as outlined on page VI of this issue quoting fares and schedules via Richmond, the home of the President, Dr. Frank M. Hodges.

The "Robert E. Lee" and the "Cotton States Special" are both fine completely air-conditioned trains affording convenient schedules to Baltimore combined with the latest modern travel comfort and Seaboard unexcelled dining car service. Special arrangements have also been made as you will note on page 34 September issue of the Southern Medical Journal for an "After Baltimore Cruise and Tour" down Chesapeake Bay to historic Virginia Peninsula, "The Cradle of the Nation," on "S. S. State of Maryland" of the Old Bay Line, owned and operated by the Seaboard Railway.

It is anticipated there will be a good attendance from the South, as a large number have already made Pullman reservations in the special sleepers, and in order that the Seaboard may provide sufficient Pullman cars it is urgently suggested that those who have not already made reservations communicate promptly with the office of Mr. H. E. Pleasants, Seaboard Railway, The 22 Marietta St. Bldg., Atlanta, Phone Walnut 2179, who will make necessary reservations and arrange at the proper time for delivery of rail and Pullman tickets to your office.

THE ANTAGONISTIC EFFECT OF METRAZOL TO SHOCK AND ANESTHETIC DEPRESSION
KARL SCHLAEPFER
(Anesth. & Anal., 15:202-206 (July-August) 1936)

Attention is called to the desirability of having some preparation on hand which would tend to restore normal cardio-respiratory function when shock or anesthetic depression occurs in surgical cases. Metrazol satisfies these requirements by its prompt, direct action, without an overstimulation of the circulation or respiration.

Since surgery is necessary in a great many patients who are "bad surgical risks" and it is desirable in other cases to shorten the period of post-operative depression, the effect of Metrazol was studied in both types of cases. In the first group, 1 or 2 cc. Metrazol were usually given both pre- and post-operatively at intervals of 1 to 2 hours. Normal saline and glucose were used in conjunction with Metrazol in a number of these cases and "often desperate cases responded to this combined treatment by lowered pulse rate and the respirations would become deeper and less frequent." The rapidity of the improvement could be regulated by shortening the intervals between the injections of Metrazol.

In the second group of cases, 2 cc. of Metrazol were given slowly, intravenously immediately after the operation if it was desirable to have the patient awake within the first hour. This was followed by a second dose within a half-hour which would bring about slow, complete awakening. When it was not necessary to obtain the prompt awakening which follows the intravenous injection of Metrazol, but merely to shorten the period of post-operative depression, one dose of 2 cc. of Metrazol was injected intramuscularly.

In summarizing his results Schlaepfer states: Metrazol is a useful adjunct to the surgical care of debilitated patients, to prevent or to overcome shock. In patients given avertin as a basal or complete surgical anesthetic Metrazol gives a striking effect. The period of post-operative hypnosis can be shortened to about one-fourth of the time usually noted."

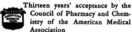

THE JOURNAL
OF THE
MEDICAL ASSOCIATION OF GEORGIA
DEVOTED TO THE WELFARE OF THE MEDICAL ASSOCIATION OF GEORGIA
PUBLISHED MONTHLY under direction of the Council

OFFICERS

B. H. MINCHEW, M.D., Waycross, President
GEO. A. TRAYLOR, M.D., Augusta, President-Elect
C. F. HOLTON, M.D., Savannah, First Vice-President
J. B. KAY, M.D., Byron, Second Vice-President
EDGAR D. SHANKS, M.D., Atlanta, Secretary-Treasurer
JOHN W. SIMMONS, M.D., Brunswick, Parliamentarian

PUBLICATION COMMITTEE

W. A. SELMAN, M.D., Atlanta, Chairman
CLEVELAND THOMPSON, M.D., Millen
EDGAR D. SHANKS, M.D., Atlanta

EDITOR
EDGAR D. SHANKS, M.D., Atlanta

ASSOCIATE EDITORS
L. MINOR BLACKFORD, M.D., Atlanta
T. C. DAVISON, M.D., Atlanta
DANIEL C. ELKIN, M.D., Atlanta
JACK C. NORRIS, M.D., Atlanta
CARTER SMITH, M.D., Atlanta
C. B. UPSHAW, M.D., Atlanta

BUSINESS MANAGER
H. L. ROWE, Atlanta

| Volume XXV | Atlanta, Ga., November, 1936 | Number 11 |

MEDICAL COLLEGES AND MEDICAL EDUCATION IN GEORGIA

At the close of the American Revolution there was, in the new State of Georgia, scarcely a doctor who had ever seen a cadaver or heard a medical lecture.[1] Medical education was obtained by apprenticeship to a "preceptor" for an indefinite length of time. The course of instruction consisted of reading the old medical books found about the house, compounding medicines from crude materials and making long night calls when the preceptor was "worn out." The principles of medicine were simple: bloodletting, blisters, purgatives and emetics.

Early in the nineteenth century medical societies were organized in several sections of the State. Their avowed purpose was the elevation of the medical profession and the protection of the people from the ravages of epidemic diseases which were accompanied by terrible loss of life, by industrial and commercial disaster, and by untold human suffering. Therefore, they had a large part in securing the legislative measures that raised the scholastic requirements for medical education, that drove out the army of quacks who infested the State. They had an important part also in the formation of the State Department of Health and the passage of public health laws. From these societies

evolved the regular medical colleges of Georgia.

In 1828, Dr. Milton Anthony, Dr. Lewis D. Ford and Dr. William R. Waring organized the Medical Academy of the State of Georgia[2] in Augusta. The following year the faculty was increased and the name changed to the Medical Institute of the State of Georgia, and a charter which gave the right to confer the degree of Doctor of Medicine was obtained from the Legislature. In 1833, the charter was amended and the name changed to the Medical College of Georgia. A year later a drive for funds resulted in an appropriation of $10,000 by the State, a gift of $5,000 from the city of Augusta, and contributions of varying sizes from a number of public spirited citizens. The total was a sum sufficient to permit the completion of the first unit of the school, providing lecture rooms and laboratories for anatomy, biology and chemistry. Thus, the first medical college in Georgia was launched. It has had an honorable and successful career. In 1911, the school property was conveyed to the State University and became the School of Medicine of the University of Georgia.

At the time of the organization of Medical College of Georgia the requirements for a medical degree were simple: the ability to read and write; a preliminary period spent with a preceptor; two courses of lectures of four months each, taken in separate years.

The faculty of the new college was dissatisfied with this condition. Accordingly, they addressed a letter to all the medical schools in the United States, requesting a conference in Washington, D. C., to study ways and means of increasing the length of the course and improving the quality of medical training. This attracted very little attention; so few replies were received that no conference was held. However, the effort was not lost, for Dr. James J. Walsh[3] states that this letter with its insistence on higher standards was the initial step in the founding of the American Medical Association, the greatest medical association in the world. It is gratifying to know that Georgia early saw the need and first had the courage to urge improvement.

In spite of the discouraging attitude of the other colleges, the faculty of the Medical College of Georgia increased the terms to six months; but in less than three years they found their lecture rooms practically empty. Georgia's students were going elsewhere. The College was compelled to return to its former program.

In 1838, a medical college was chartered in Savannah, but it did not begin to function until 1853.[4] "The first class was graduated in 1854, the epidemic year. Classes were graduated yearly until the War Between the States stopped all such activities. In 1865, the college was opened again and continued until 1881. . . . Differences arose in the medical faculty and another faculty was organized by Dr. H. L. Byrd in 1855, in the name of the Oglethorpe Medical College, and the first class was graduated in 1856. About four classes were graduated before the activities of this school were ended permanently by the war. . . . The faculty of the Savannah Medical College started and supported the Savannah Medical Journal; and the faculty of the Oglethorpe Medical College started and supported the Oglethorpe Medical and Surgical Journal. The latter journal died in 1860-61; the former was not published during the war, but resumed in 1865, and for a time was published by the Georgia Medical Society. The Savannah Medical College did its work partly in the Savannah Hospital and partly in a building built for them in part with State funds. . . . The building was used during the war for a soldiers' hospital, first by the Confederates and then by the Union troops, and later on was used as a marine hospital by Savannah. The Oglethorpe Medical College was conducted in a building in Yamacraw, a large residence which has since burned."[5]

During the period before the War Between the States there was a group—whether they had any fixed location we do not know—who called themselves the "Thomsonian College." They heaped abuse on the regular doctors and thus obtained a considerable following. Their system was practiced by a group of densely ignorant people and many lives were sacrificed in the name of "botanic medicine, steaming, etc." Dr. L. B. Grandy[1] quotes Dr. Milton Anthony as saying: "The degrading stain of Thomsonianism was a disgrace to the American character, the most stupendous system of quackery and the most insulting offering ever tendered to the understanding of a free and enlightened people." The college is listed in the American Medical Directory as having been located at Barbourville, but we are unable to find that there was ever such a town in the State.

In 1839, a medical college was chartered under the name of the Southern Botanico-Medical College. It functioned for a while in Forsyth; then, in 1846, moved to Macon and changed its name to the Reform Medical College of Georgia. In 1874, the name was again changed. It became the College of American Medicine and Surgery, and, in 1881, moved to Atlanta where it absorbed a medical college being conducted by Dr. S. F. Salter at the corner of Walton and Broad Streets. In 1884, it became the Georgia College of Eclectic Medicine and Surgery. The faculty made an honest effort to teach eclectic medicine. They were the first to extend their course of instruction to three and then to four years, but when the requirements and standards of medical education were raised by the American Medical Association they were compelled to suspend their work.

In the words of Omar Khayyam:

"The worldly hope men set their hearts upon
Turns ashes—or it prospers; and anon,
Like snow upon the desert's dusty face
Lighting a little hour or two—is gone."

There was at one time a medical college in Griffin and one in Dalton, but there are no data available by which we can describe their work. In 1866 Clark University (colored) secured a charter for a medical department, but it never functioned.

During the period from the close of the War Between the States and 1910 several medical colleges made flourishing attempts to establish themselves in Atlanta, which seemed to be a Mecca for commercialism in medical teaching as in industry. Under the stimulus of the American Medical Association and interested foundations which began to insist upon higher entrance requirements, better equipment, better instruction and full-time teachers in the fundamental branches, the State Medical Association secured the passage of laws for the protection of the people. As a result, these institutions closed their doors early in the twentieth century and only a few of their graduates are now active in the field of medicine.

Only two of the many medical colleges organized in Georgia are still functioning. One of these, the Emory University School of Medicine, had its origin in 1854 when Dr. John G. Westmoreland organized the Atlanta Medical College. In 1861 lectures were suspended and the building used as a hospital until the close of the war. The college was re-organized in 1866 with Dr. John G. Westmoreland again at its head.

Almost immediately after the Atlanta Medical College was organized in 1854 the faculty started a medical journal which attained considerable success. Later it suffered reverses and had its name and management changed several times, but it lived until the birth of our present splendid publication, the JOURNAL OF THE MEDICAL ASSOCIATION OF GEORGIA.

In 1879 the Southern Medical College was organized and ran as an active rival of the old school until 1898, when the demands for better medical education made it necessary to unite the two institutions. The new school was called the Atlanta College of Physicians and Surgeons.

In 1905 the Atlanta School of Medicine was organized and immediately became a creditable rival. To meet this competition the Atlanta College of Physicians and Surgeons erected new buildings and put in new equipment. Most important of all in the future development of the institution was their establishment in 1910 of full-time chairs in the sciences underlying the study of clinical medicine. To these chairs were called men who, by their training and the standard of their work, raised the general tone of the college and introduced the spirit of research in medicine.

Again, the faculties realized that consolidation was better than rivalry; so in 1913 the schools were united under the historic name, Atlanta Medical College, and soon achieved a recognized standard of merit. In 1915, further prestige and strength of organization were secured through a university connection. The Atlanta Medical College became the School of Medicine of Emory University and the graduates of the contributing colleges were accepted into the body of Emory alumni. Such was the fruition of the work of Dr. John G. Westmoreland and those who followed him—men of culture and refinement, honor and integrity, who left their influence for good on more than 3,000 alumni.

These alumni and the ones being added annually have lived up to their goodly heritage. They have given and are continuing to give unstinted service throughout the country, wherever they may have located. They are returning often to their Alma Mater—as to a preceptor—for further instruction, new methods, closer contact with the ever progressing science and art of medicine.

History moves in spirals—not circles. It comes back to the best that was in "the old days," but with the added height of accumulating knowledge. And so it is in the medical history of Georgia. In the past hundred years medical education left the preceptor, became organized and was standardized. Now, it has come back to the preceptor ideal, lifted up and re-vitalized by scientific principles, by hospital and laboratory facilities, and by the wider knowledge of the instructors who give tirelessly of their time and effort.

J. L. CAMPBELL, M.D.

REFERENCES

1. Grandy, L. B.: History of Medicine and Surgery in Georgia. Tr. M. A. Georgia, p. 193, 1895.
2. Foster, Eugene: The Medical Profession in Georgia, Memoirs of Georgia, Vol. II, subhead "Medical Schools", p. 148 (Sou. Historical Soc., 1895).
3. Walsh, J. J.: Encyclopedia Americana, Vol. 18, p. 543, 1921.
4. The F. W. P. very kindly detailed Geo. Raffalovich, Ph.D., to the work of collecting data for use in preparing this article. He has been most obliging in his efforts to place at my service all the material he had previously collected.
5. Quoted from personal letter from V. H. Bassett, Savannah, Ga. Sept. 24, 1936.

JOHN G. WESTMORELAND, M.D. (1816-1887)

Founder of the Atlanta Medical College, 1854; now the School of Medicine of Emory University.

Dr. Westmoreland organized the first Medical Society in Atlanta—the Brotherhood of Physicians. With his brother, Willis F., he founded Atlanta's first Medical Journal—The Atlanta Medical and Surgical Journal. He was a Confederate soldier and a Statesman, having served in the Legislature in 1856, where he secured an appropriation for the Medical College.

EMORY UNIVERSITY SCHOOL OF MEDICINE

Some years ago the JOURNAL recorded the history of the School of Medicine of the University of Georgia. In this issue an effort has been made to record the history of the School of Medicine of Emory University.

Medical education in this State has a long and honorable history. Since Oglethorpe came, in 1733, nineteen medical schools have functioned within the borders of Georgia. All of these schools have served their purpose; two, Emory and Georgia, have stood the test of time. With the advancement of all educational activities, medicine has now taken its place in the sciences. No longer is it fashionable or permissible to "read medicine"; indeed, with the State having only two medical schools and limited capacities for teaching, it is possible to make careful selection of prospective students.

The Council on Medical Education of the American Medical Association and the Association of American Medical Colleges regularly conduct surveys of all institutions with departments for teaching medicine. Seventy-seven institutions in the United States and ten in Canada are now listed by these organizations, and eighty-four have received the approval of the Council. These surveys together with the desire of all physicians to do their best in alleviating human suffering and in prolonging life, have gone far in promoting higher medical education.

Today Georgia has twenty-six hundred white physicians, the majority of whom are graduates of local institutions. All of them take pride in the growth and development of our two medical schools. Read this, the centenary number of the School of Medicine of Emory University, and place it with your prized possessions.

THE MEDICAL ASSOCIATION OF GEORGIA extends felicitations to the School of Medicine of Emory University. To the Centenary Committee representing the Medical School, Dr. J. L. Campbell, Chairman, Dr. Daniel C. Elkin and Dr. Glenville Giddings, and to various contributors, the Editorial Staff of the JOURNAL expresses thanks for these data.

EMORY UNIVERSITY SCHOOL OF MEDICINE*

Medical education in Atlanta is almost as old as the city itself, and the history of medical education in this city is to a large extent the history of Emory University's School of Medicine. In that institution the seeds planted by various groups of founders are coming to their full fruition.

In 1845, before Marthasville became Atlanta, the establishment of a medical college in the young and fast-growing city was discussed. In 1853 this talk was translated into action under the leadership of Dr. John G. Westmoreland. The Legislature granted a charter Feb. 14, 1854, for the Atlanta Medical College. Trustees named in the charter were L. C. Simpson, Jared I. Whitaker, John Collier, Hubbard Cozard, Daniel Hook, John L. Harris, William Herring, Green B. Haygood and James L. Calhoun. Seventy-eight students enrolled for the first course of lectures, running from May 1 to Sept. 1, 1855. Classes were held in the City Hall, located where the State Capitol now stands, and the introductory lecture was given by Dr. W. W. Flewellyn of Columbus.

The first faculty included M. G. Slaughter, Professor of Anatomy; J. W. Jones, Professor of the Principles and Practice of Medicine; Jesse Boring, Professor of Obstetrics and Diseases of Women and Children; W. F. Westmoreland, Professor of Principles and Practice of Surgery; J. E. Dubose, Professor of Physiology; G. T. Wilburn, Professor of Surgical and Pathological Anatomy; J. J. Roberts, Professor of Chemistry, and J. G. Westmoreland, Dean and Professor of Materia Medica and Therapeutics.

Dr. Westmoreland, who was elected Dean at the first meeting of the faculty, Jan. 31, 1855, was born in Monticello, Jasper County, Georgia, in 1816· He was educated in the Fayetteville Academy, read medicine with a neighboring country doctor and was graduated from the Medical College of Georgia at Augusta in March, 1843. He practiced medicine in Pike County before moving to Atlanta. The Atlanta Medical College was

largely his conception, and he was its Dean and Professor of Materia Medica and Therapeutics for at least 40 years, giving liberally of his time and money to the school. At one time he was elected a member of the Georgia House of Representatives for the sole purpose of seeking a donation from the State to help erect the Atlanta Medical College building. He succeeded in obtaining $15,000 on condition that the school agree to educate free one young man from each congressional district in the State.

Students attending the new medical school's first session were required to hear five lectures daily, beginning at eight in the morning and running until one in the afternoon. The instruction was illustrated with plates; demonstrations and models. There was one medical and one surgical clinic each week to provide practical instruction. Requirements for the degree of Doctor of Medicine were that the candidate be 21 years old, and of good moral character, that he complete three years of study, including two courses of lectures, and that he submit a thesis on some medical subject.

After three days of examinations at the end of the course, the faculty met to elect candidates for the degree. They used the blackball system. Four blackballs would definitely reject a student. Three blackballs would suspend him. Five white balls would elect him for the degree. Thirty-two students, who had come to the college from other medical schools, were graduated at the first commencement on Sept. 1, 1855.

Meantime, on June 21, 1855, a cornerstone was laid for the Medical College building on the present site of the Emory Division of Grady Hospital. H. D. Beman was orator of the occasion. The building was completed largely through the efforts of Dr. J. G. Westmoreland, who in addition to his duties as Dean, was serving as treasurer and as financial agent for building and equipping the College. The building was two stories high and contained eight rooms. These included three lecture rooms, an amphitheatre, and a dissecting room provided with skylights. It was completed for the opening of the second course of lectures in May, 1856. The structure was located on property given by Colonel L. P. Grant. He executed a deed to the property and

---

*Data for this article were taken from: The Founding and Early History of the Atlanta Medical College, Atlanta, 1854-1875, by F. Phinizy Calhoun, M.D. and A History of Emory University, 1836-1936, by H. M. Bullock.

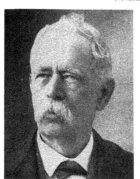

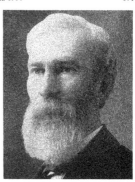

R. V. M. Miller, M.D. (1814-1896)

W. S. Armstrong, M.D. (1836-1896)

expressed a desire that it be used for educational purposes. In 1857 the immediate indebtedness of the College for the building and equipment was relieved by a grant of $15,000 from the Georgia Legislature.

In its first year the Medical College established the *Atlanta Medical and Surgical Journal* with Dr. J. P. Logan and Dean Westmoreland as editor and business manager, respectively. In 1857 the faculty elected Dr. J. P. Logan and Dr. Jesse Boring delegates to the American Medical Association meeting in Nashville, thus establishing the close relationships which have continued to the present time between the school and the Medical Association. About this time also the faculty indicated the esteem in which it held Dean Westmoreland by directing that his portrait be executed by "some competent artist" and placed in his classroom.

In 1858 the College established a dispensary with two physicians in charge. The College also had become a member of the American Medical College Association, which met at the same time as the American Medical Association, and the College regularly sent representatives to these meetings. The faculty was paid by dividing in shares the balance left from student fees after all running expenses had been paid. Each professor re-

ceived $778.85, in the spring of 1860, evidently for the work of the previous school year.

Oratory played a more important part in the curriculum than is the case nowadays. Among those who addressed the College at one time or another were Benjamin Hill, General John B. Gordon, Alexander Stephens, Dr. Robert Battey and Robert Toombs.

The year 1861 brought financial difficulties to the young medical college. There were few students and much difficulty in collecting fees. On Aug. 6, 1861 there was a faculty meeting. Minutes of this meeting were stopped in the midst of a sentence. There was no more classwork until after the war. The college building was converted into a hospital for the Confederate wounded. When General Sherman burned Atlanta the medical college building was saved by a stratagem of Dr. D'Alvigny, one of the professors. He plied the hospital employees with whisky, put them to bed, and persuaded Sherman's officers that the building was occupied by wounded. The building thus remained intact when the faculty met again on Aug. 16, 1865 to resume the work of the Medical College. Minutes of this meeting recorded the "profound gratitude to Almighty God that during the four years of bloody and desolating war, during which so many sad changes have oc-

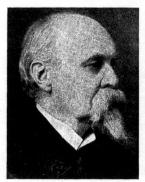

J. Scott Todd, M.D. (1847-1914)

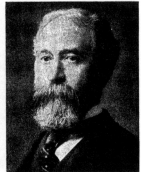

John G. Earnest, M.D. (1842-1932)

curred in every community and almost every family, every member of the faculty still lives, none having fallen by the casualties of war or otherwise."

Doctors were urgently needed throughout the South at this time and students could ill afford the time for two years' instruction. The faculty, therefore, decided on a winter term, in addition to the summer term which had previously been held, so that students might complete two courses of lectures within a calendar year.

Dr. Thomas S. Powell, as authorized agent for the faculty, in 1866, procured from the Mayor and City Council an appropriation of $5,000 in city bonds to be used for repairing the building and equipment which had been badly damaged during the war. This donation, however, became the topic of a heated controversy between groups centering around Dr. Powell on one hand and Dean Westmoreland on the other. Dr. Powell desired much of the money to be spent in connection with his work in obstetrics and diseases of women. But, contrary to his wishes, the money was spent in general repairs on the building and on the purchase of equipment. Subsequently charges of unprofessional conduct were discussed against Dr. Powell because he founded an institution called "The Ladies Home." The faculty finally stated it

could not hold any further connection with Dr. Powell and elected Dr. H. V. M. Miller of Rome to the chair of obstetrics. Dr. Powell carried his case to the Board of Trustees, who sided with him. This brought a split between the faculty and the trustees over the respective rights of the two bodies. Dr. Powell remained off the faculty and ten years later established the Southern Medical College, but that institution too was merged eventually into what now has become the Emory University School of Medicine.

Dr. Alexander Means, formerly President of Emory College, was President of the Atlanta Medical College faculty for many years, and Dr. J. G. Westmoreland served as Dean until 1868 when Jesse Boring was elected to that place. Dr. Westmoreland later became Dean again and served until the spring of 1874, when he was succeeded by V. H. Taliaferro from 1874-75 and J. T. Johnson from 1876 to 1880. In this era the professors were instructed to issue their own tickets to lectures, the tickets to cost $15 each. As there were eight professors, it is assumed the total tuition amounted to $120.

Dean Johnson improved the instruction by introducing special clinics for eye and ear work, diseases of women and venereal diseases, in addition to the regular medical and surgical clinics. Hospital accommodations

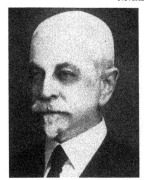

James B. Baird, M.D. (1849-1924)

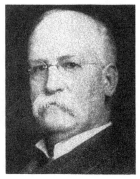

Abner W. Calhoun, M.D. (1845-1910)

also were being provided for a few patients. Since at this time there was agitation in Atlanta for the construction of a city hospital, the faculty petitioned the trustees to exert their influence to have the hospital built near the medical college as "no medical school at the present day can command public confidence without facilities more or less extensive for imparting practical instruction."

In 1873 the *Atlanta Medical and Surgical Journal*, which had been sold to Dr. John G. Westmoreland, was returned to the faculty of the Medical College to be conducted by them.

In May, 1874, a conference of Southern medical schools was called. W. F. Westmoreland was the delegate from the Atlanta Medical College. Dr. Westmoreland was instructed to support action "to elevate the standard and fees whenever her sister schools will justify the same . . ."

In June, 1874, Dr. James B. Baird was appointed to the position of lecturer upon diseases of the mind and nervous system.

The school was flourishing at this period, and had a growing student body. The length of the term was extended from sixteen to twenty weeks in 1879, and in 1889 the proctor happily reported that the faculty would receive $650 for that session. By 1893 the enrollment had reached 183 students, and

the work of the school had been much improved. Dr. H. V. M. Miller served as Dean, and Dr. W. S. Kendrick was proctor and secretary, from 1884 to 1896. At Dr. Miller's death, in 1896, Dr. Kendrick became Dean and continued in that office until he resigned in 1905.

The college had been empowered by charter in 1874 to offer courses in pharmacy, but it was not until the session of 1891-92 that instruction leading to the degree Doctor of Pharmacy was begun, with eleven students. Arrangements also were made a little later for students of the Atlanta Dental College to receive certain basic courses there. Through these years the college was gradually raising its standards. When the three-year requirement went into effect, the faculty worked out a more definitely graded system of instruction. The first year was devoted to the basic subjects, such as anatomy, materia medica, physiology, physics, chemistry, dissecting and histology. The second year included advanced courses in these subjects, the principles of surgery and medicine, clinical medicine and physical diagnosis, obstetrics and diseases of women and children, diseases of eye, ear and throat, and work in chemical and pathological laboratories. In the last year the student listened to lectures on the principles and practice of medicine, obstetrics and

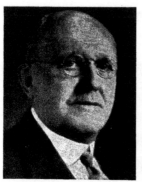 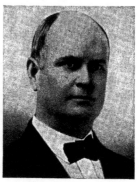

W. S. Elkin, M.D. (1858-)	Hunter P. Cooper, M.D. (1860-1906)

gynecology, operative surgery, regional anatomy, pathology, hygiene, medical jurisprudence, physical diagnosis, and eye, ear, and throat diseases. The students also attended general clinics and the bacteriological laboratory. Students in all classes were expected to attend the general clinics.

In 1898 the Atlanta Medical College was consolidated with the Southern Medical College to form the Atlanta College of Physicians and Surgeons.

The Southern Medical College had been established in 1878 by Dr. T. S. Powell, Dr. Robert C. Word and Dr. W. T. Goldsmith. It was the outgrowth of Dr. Powell's controversy over the city appropriation to the Atlanta Medical College and over his "Ladies Home." The Southern Medical College was chartered in 1878 with these trustees: T. S. Powell, R. C. Word, W. T. Goldsmith, D. A. H. Stephens, Judge S. B. Hoyt, G. T. Dodd, D. W. Lewis, A. F. Hurt, Rev. A. J. Battle, Rev. H. H. Parks, Rev. H. C. Hornaday, George M. McDowell, W. W. McAfee and Rev. J. J. Toons. The faculty elected in 1879 included A. S. Payne, William Rawlings, T. S. Powell, R. C. Word, G. M. McDowell, W. P. Nicolson, W. T. Goldsmith, H. F. Scott, G. G. Crawford, Lindsay Johnson, and later, Arthur G. Hobbs.

The building of the school was on what was then Porter Street, at what is now the corner of Equitable Place and Edgewood Avenue, in the rear of the Trust Company of Georgia building. The first session opened in Nov., 1879, with 64 students.

The Providence Infirmary was opened in 1880 by the Southern Medical College faculty. Covered walk-ways connected the college with the infirmary so that patients might be trundled back and forth for operations. Two years later, at Dr. Powell's suggestion, a group of Atlanta women organized the Ladies Hospital Association and held a fair. The proceeds were used to purchase the Central Hotel on Ivy Street and to equip it for hospital use.

Dr. Powell and his associates hoped to expand the Southern Medical College into a university. They opened a dental department in 1889 and contemplated the opening of pharmaceutical and law departments. There were more than 100 students at one time in the dental department, but the other contemplated departments did not materialize.

The Southern Medical College erected a new building on Butler Street in 1892. This structure was opposite Grady Hospital, then being constructed, and adjoined the building of the Atlanta Medical College. For six years

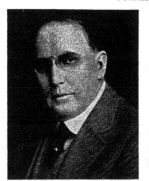

Wm. Perrin Nicolson, M.D. (1857-1928)

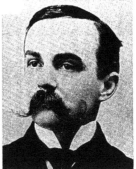

J. C. Olmsted, M.D. (1852-1928)

the two colleges operated as next-door neigh-bors and rivals. Animosities softened with time and it soon became apparent that one college would be stronger than two.

Dr. W. S. Elkin of the Southern Medical College proposed to Dr. W. S. Kendrick of the Atlanta Medical College about the first of March, 1898, that the two institutions merge. After much discussion a plan was worked out whereby a new school, styled the Atlanta College of Physicians and Surgeons, was established. The new institution assumed all property and obligations of the two col-leges, including the pharmaceutical depart-ment of one and the dental college of the other. Almost all members of the two fac-ulties became professors in the new college. Dr. W. S. Kendrick became Dean of the new college when the necessary charter changes were completed Nov. 9, 1898.

All instruction was given in the building of the former Atlanta Medical College, and the building of the Southern Medical College was closed. The new college opened its first year with an enrollment of 333, or only about fifteen short of the combined enroll-ments of the two old schools in the previous year. Of that number 214 were studying medicine, 88 dentistry, and 31 pharmacy. The commencement of 1900 was held at the Grand Opera House, now Loew's Grand Theater. Dean Kendrick announced the deci-sion of the faculty to require four courses of lectures for the degree, effective in 1901.

In 1903 Dr. Edward G. Jones was made proctor and registrar, relieving Dean Kendrick of much administrative detail. Two years later Dr. Jones sought to be assigned to the gynecologic clinic but was refused by a ma-jority of the faculty, and his place as registrar also was declared vacant. Dr. Kendrick de-clared he could not carry out his administra-tion of the school without Dr. Jones' assist-ance, so he too resigned. Dr. Jones and Dr. Kendrick then organized the Atlanta School of Medicine. This institution was later con-solidated with the College of Physicians and Surgeons.

. After Dr. Kendrick's resignation from the Atlanta College of Physicians and Surgeons his place as Dean was filled by Dr. W. S. El-kin. Before his resignation Dean Kendrick had advocated the building either of a new hospital or a new college building to provide more adequately for the enlarged attendance. Dr. A. W. Calhoun immediately pledged $10,000 toward the building project. Fac-ulty members and trustees raised the total pledged to $20,000. Dr. Calhoun's asso-ciates expressed their appreciation by naming

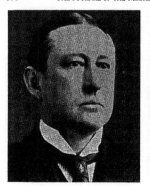

Willis F. Westmoreland, M.D. (1863-1935)

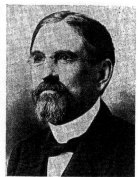

W. S. Kendrick, M.D. (1847-1918)

his chair the A. W. Calhoun Chair of Ophthalmology. Dean Elkin also gave $5,000.

Classes were transferred to the old Southern Medical College plant in Jan., 1906, to permit the wrecking of the old Atlanta Medical College building. Just a few days before the cornerstone was laid there was an announcement that Andrew Carnegie had given $10,000 to the building fund. The trustees established a chair to be known as the Andrew Carnegie Institute of Pathology. When the cornerstone was laid, April 6, 1906, word was passed among the faculty "that it would be appropriate for them to be present at the exercises, looking intelligent and cheerful, but poor." This must have presented an affecting picture, for Mr. Carnegie later increased his gift to $25,000. The new building was completed before the commencement of 1907. Dean Elkin pointed out in his annual report that the college then had five large buildings devoted to teaching medicine, dentistry, and pharmacy, representing an investment of about $250,000.

Full professorships at that time paid $300 for the year. Two members of the staff who carried extra duties received $500. The professors and other members of the teaching staff carried on regular medical practice in addition to their duties at the College. Dr.

J. Scott Todd, a most distinguished one-armed Confederate veteran, was Professor of Materia Medica and Therapeutics. Dr. James B. Baird, Sr., was Professor of the Principles and Practice of Medicine and was held in high esteem by the profession of the State. Dr. J. C. Olmsted, a gentleman of ante-bellum ancestry, added much zest to his lectures on clinical medicine by reminding the students that the time had passed when gentlemen could meet and settle their differences on the "field of honor." The first full-time technical man employed was Dr. H. F. Harris, who came from Jefferson Medical College to take the newly created chair of pathology and bacteriology in the fall of 1901.

Standards of the college continued to be raised from time to time. The old passing grade of 66-2/3 per cent had been raised to 70 per cent in the spring of 1899 and was raised to 75 per cent two years later. Throughout the period from 1907 to the merger with the Atlanta School of Medicine in 1913 there was a constant strengthening of academic standards. The teachers passed rules levying fines on themselves when they failed to appear for lectures. The equivalent of a first grade teacher's certificate was required for admission in the fall of 1908. This was raised to four years of high school work in the

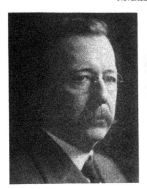 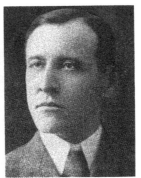

Geo. H. Noble, M.D. (1860-1932)

H. F. Harris, M.D. (1867-1926)

fall of 1912. A curriculum committee led by Dr. J. C. Johnson disclosed serious faults and urged reforms in 1908. It was suggested that a separate course be organized for each year and that the work be different and progressive throughout the departments, as students went from class to class. There was also a deficiency in practical training available for the students. Grady Hospital regulations were relaxed sufficiently at this time to permit one tour through the wards each day by an instructor-physician and a group of students. This was known as the Grady Ward Walk. In 1912 the Grady authorities consented to arrangements for more adequate bedside instruction.

The first fraternity, the Phi Chi, was organized in 1905, and the Clinical Medical Society was formed by the faculty in the following year. Faculty members, clinical assistants and senior students were eligible for membership.

Throughout the life of the College of Physicians and Surgeons, the Southern Dental College, under Dean S. W. Foster, and the Atlanta School of Pharmacy, under Dean George F. Payne, operated as almost independent enterprises. The School of Pharmacy was abolished in 1910. One of the reasons

was to provide more laboratory space for embryology, histology and neurology. In 1912 the desire of the College of Physicians and Surgeons to obtain a better rating led to negotiations for consolidation with the Atlanta School of Medicine.

Just six days after Dean Kendrick had resigned from the College of Physicians and Surgeons in 1905, a group of doctors in the office of Dr. E. C. Davis signed a paper pledging themselves to form a medical college. Signing the document were W. S. Kendrick, George H. Noble, E. G. Jones, E. C. Davis, J. M. Crawford, Stewart R. Roberts, Frank K. Boland and L. C. Fischer. On Dr. Kendrick's motion the college was called the Atlanta School of Medicine. Members of the faculty donated instruments and equipment. Arrangements were made to share the building of the Atlanta Dental School at Edgewood Avenue and Ivy Street. Within four weeks after the organization meeting, the school was in operation with 220 students drawn from eight Southern states.

The faculty decided that the term should run seven months instead of the customary six, and that four years of work would be required for the degree. The requirement for admission was the equivalent of a first-grade teacher's license.

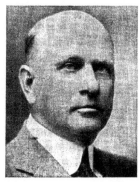

E. C. Thrash, M.D. (1867-1931)

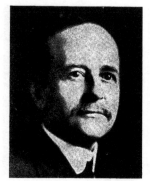

Floyd W. McRae, M.D. (1862-1921)

At the opening of the second session the school occupied a new four-story building at Luckie and Bartow streets. Provision was made for clinics, and a hospital annex was built at the personal expense of faculty members. Spurred on by rivalry with the College of Physicians and Surgeons, the new institution placed much emphasis on the quality of work and on bedside training. This training was not permitted by other hospitals, and hence was not available to the College of Physicians and Surgeons. The Atlanta School of Medicine also opened an obstetrical ward during the session of 1909-10 and this provided for practical work in that field.

The first published bulletin of the Atlanta School of Medicine listed as full professors Doctors W. S. Kendrick, J. M. Crawford, E. G. Jones, J. L. Campbell, R. T. Dorsey, and F. K. Boland, all of whom had formerly been associated with the College of Physicians and Surgeons. Other full professors were Doctors C. D. Hurt, G. H. Noble, E. C. Davis, E. C. Thrash, L. C. Fischer, Hansell Crenshaw and Stewart R. Roberts.

The increasing cost of equipment, the small tuition charges and the decreasing enrollments due to higher entrance requirements were making the proprietary medical schools less and less profitable. Meantime the Amer-

ican Medical Association and the Association of American Medical Colleges were fixing higher and higher standards. Endowments were required for those institutions which were to survive. In 1908 the faculty of the Atlanta School of Medicine sought affiliation with the University of Georgia. This movement was unsuccessful, but financial difficulties made the school receptive in 1913 to a proposal from the College of Physicians and Surgeons that the two institutions pool their resources.

One of the forces motivating this merger was the desire to secure approval of the Association of American Medical Colleges and the Council on Medical Education of the American Medical Association. The College of Physicians and Surgeons had adopted the 14-unit entrance requirement in 1912 and began correspondence with the Council on Medical Education, seeking the approval of that body. Dr. N. P. Colwell, of the Council, was of the opinion that if numerous improvements were made, the College might be given a Class A rating after another year, but that if the College of Physicians and Surgeons would merge with the School of Medicine, the consolidated institution could be placed in Class A at once. Articles of agreement were entered into by the two faculties on June 11, 1913 and

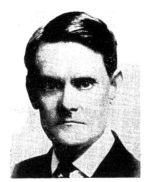

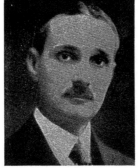

E. C. Davis, M.D. (1867-1931)   Edward G. Jones, M.D. (1873-1921)

the new charter for the Atlanta Medical College was issued Sept. 20, 1913. This returned to the institution the original name of the Atlanta Medical College and paved the way for it to become the medical school of Emory University.

Through the sessions of 1913-14 and 1914-15, under the leadership of Dean W. S. Elkin, the Atlanta Medical College made an effort to approximate the admission requirements for Class A medical colleges without losing too much patronage and income. The entrance requirement of one college year of biology, chemistry, physics, and a modern language was announced in 1914, but was not enforced fully until 1916. Since this produced a decrease in the freshman registration and it became apparent that the college could not survive without an endowment.

About this time plans were being made for the establishment of Emory University in Atlanta. Dean Elkin approached Asa G. Candler as to the possibility of making the Atlanta Medical College the medical department of the new University. It soon became obvious that a merger would be mutually advantageous to the Medical College and the University. The University, as its part, was to appropriate $250,000 to endow the

school, and was to build a new hospital in order to enlarge the teaching facilities. Trustees of the Atlanta Medical College were cordial in accepting the plan, and the entire holdings of the College were deeded to Emory University on June 28, 1915.

At first all instruction continued in the downtown plant, but in the fall of 1917 the freshman and sophomore years of medical instruction were moved to the new campus of Emory, while facilities for upperclassmen were greatly improved by the opening of the new J. J. Gray, Jr. Clinic Building on the downtown campus.

Dr. W. S. Elkin, who had been a faculty member of the old Southern Medical College, and who had been Dean of the Atlanta College of Physicians and Surgeons and of the Atlanta Medical College, continued to administer the affairs of the school in the University. The registration dropped sharply as more stringent entrance requirements became effective. The Bachelor of Science degree was given, beginning in 1915, to Emory students who completed two years of college work and two years of medical work. In 1921 the "combination course" was changed to three years of college and one year of medicine.

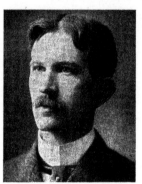

E. Bates Block, M.D. (1874-1932)

The entrance of the United States into the World War upset the routine of the medical school, as it did all educational institutions. By June, 1918, more than 47 professors and instructors had been commissioned in the Army or Navy, many of them for service with the Emory Unit, Base Hospital 43, which was organized in the summer of 1917 by Dr. E. C. Davis. This organization rendered notable service in France. At the time the Armistice was signed there were in the Unit 52 officers, 291 men, and 96 nurses, with 2,237 patients.

Abnormal post-war conditions brought financial difficulties to the School. Its deficit in 1918 was $19,000. Deficits continued until 1923-24 when the General Education Board made a series of appropriations for the School. These totalled about $140,000. Since these gifts ceased in 1928, the medical deficits have been met from the general funds of the University.

High standards have been maintained in the School. For a number of years the freshman enrollment has been limited to 60, and an improved basis of selection is reducing the number of those who fail to graduate. In 1922, largely through the generosity of Asa G. Candler, the new Wesley Memorial Hospital was opened on the University campus. It was not officially connected with the School until 1925, but the old Wesley Memorial Hospital had cooperated with the medical colleges from its inception. The hospital, established by the Methodist Church, was chartered in Nov., 1904, and was located at Auburn Avenue and Courtland Street. It continued to operate there until Dec., 1922, when the first units of the new hospital on the Emory campus were completed at a cost of $1,250,000. The operation of the hospital was taken over by the University in 1924, and in 1925 Wesley Memorial Hospital ceased its legal existence.

The school's downtown facilities were greatly improved by the conversion of the old building of the Atlanta College of Physicians and Surgeons into the Negro Division of Grady Hospital, under the control of the faculty of the School of Medicine for use in bedside instruction. There was further enlargement of hospital teaching facilities in 1931 when the white unit of Grady Hospital opened for teaching purposes its wards in general medicine, general surgery and obstetrics, and its dermatology clinic. Sixteen staff members from these departments were appointed to the faculty. A psychiatric clinic for negroes was opened in 1931, and in the same year provision was made for the study of abnormal cases at the Federal Penitentiary.

Dr. W. S. Elkin, after twenty years' service as Dean, was forced by ill health to resign in 1925. He was succeeded by Dr. Russell H. Oppenheimer, who the year before had become superintendent of Wesley Memorial Hospital. Dr. Oppenheimer continues to hold both positions. In addition to completing arrangements for more adequate hospital teaching, Dean Oppenheimer has modified the curriculum in conformity with newly developing ideas of medical education.

Clinical work and introduction to general medical topics has been introduced into the first two years of the curriculum, while the last two years have been given over almost entirely to clinical work. These changes were made after Dr. Oppenheimer had spent some time each year visiting leading medical schools, studying their curricula and preparing for the thoroughgoing reorganization which was put into effect in 1930.

GLENVILLE GIDDINGS, M.D.

DEPARTMENT OF GROSS ANATOMY

The Department of Gross Anatomy occupies the top floor of the John P. Scott Laboratory of the Anatomy Building on the University campus, having been moved there in 1917. Previously it had been located with all the other departments in the buildings of the Atlanta Medical College opposite Grady Hospital. On that site the medical course had been initiated with the study of anatomy by and from dissections since one year after the founding of the Atlanta Medical College in 1854 when Dr. Howell Nelson of New York was appointed the first Professor of Anatomy. For some reason his name appears for one year only and Dr. M. G. Slaughter, by some called the first Professor of Anatomy, held the post from 1855 until the suspension during the War Between the States (1861). With the re-opening in 1865, Dr. C. D. O'Keefe directed the work until 1872 when the place was filled by Dr. John Thad Johnson, who was also Dean.

Until near the end of Dr. Johnson's service, in 1889, there had been no anatomical law to protect the sanctity of cemeteries and to allow the use of the bodies of unclaimed paupers and criminals for the study of anatomy. Many stories are handed down of the arduous, thrilling and often unsuccessful attempts to secure suitable material for dissection by rifling new-made graves. Upon the Professor of Anatomy devolved this unpleasant duty for we are told that Doctor Slaughter frequently made long horse and buggy trips to bring in a corpse upon the seat beside him, preferably under cover of darkness. When Dr. W. S. Armstrong took charge of the department in 1889 the Anatomical Act had been in operation for two years and the announcements of that period state that the law was providing an abundance of material for dissection without the unpleasant necessity of desecrating burial places.

In 1896 Dr. Hunter P. Cooper succeeded Professor Armstrong and from 1898 until 1906 he remained as Professor equal in rank with Dr. W. Perrin Nicolson who had headed the anatomy department in the rival Southern Medical College during its entire existence (1878-1898), after which Dr. Nicolson was Professor of Anatomy in the merged school, The Atlanta College of Physicians and Surgeons, until 1910. Dr. Justin P. Grant then held the chair for two years, being succeeded in 1912 by Dr. James W. Papez who had come the previous year as his assistant. After the union with the Atlanta School of Medicine in which Dr. L. C. Fischer had been Professor of Anatomy (1905-1913), Dr. Papez continued in charge in the school under its reassumed title of Atlanta Medical College which name it retained when it became the Medical Department of Emory University in 1915. Under his guidance the work in anatomy was transferred to the present campus and was continued in the new laboratory buildings which were occupied in the autumn of 1917. After this date all the laboratory departments became more intimately a part of the University, eventually receiving some criticism as having acquired something of an academic flavor to the alleged detriment of the students who might enter the junior year with inadequate or delayed concepts of clinical medicine. When Dr. Papez left in 1920, Dr. P. E. Linebeck was designated Professor of Gross Anatomy during one year, being followed in the position by Hubert Sheppard, Ph.D., in 1921 and by the writer in 1923. Thus there have been a total of twelve incumbents with services ranging variously from one to thirty-two years.

Since the coming of Dr. Papez the professors have been full-time teachers who have given their entire interest to the study and teaching of anatomy. Before that it is probable that the professors were also engaged in private practice although one of the schools announced in 1898 that it would have salaried professors in the laboratory branches but twelve years later they announced the installation of such professors as if it had just been accomplished. If that is the case Dr. Grant may have been the first full-time Pro-

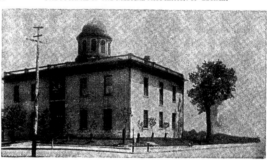

Atlanta Medical College, 1896

fessor of Anatomy. In the brief space allotted it is impossible to name all the assistants and demonstrators but many of the latter are still active as physicians of Atlanta. Among them are: Drs. J. L. Campbell, Frank K. Boland, W. A. Selman, W. E. Person, John F. Denton, C. E. Pattillo, Garnett W. Quillian, C. C. Aven, James R. McCord and M. W. McLarty. Besides the writer the present personnel consists of Dr. John Venable, Assistant Professor and Malcolm Gibson, A.M., Instructor, for the full-time staff; and Dr. Charles H. Mitchell, Instructor, who serves during laboratory hours.

The present quarters of the department are on the third floor of the Anatomy Building. This building is of modern fire-proof construction and it harmonizes architecturally with the other buildings of the campus. It provides a well lighted, clean and pleasant environment which is quite different from that found in most dissecting rooms seventy-five or even thirty years ago. The dissecting laboratory is a large room with windows on three sides which permit excellent ventilation and abundant light. Places for sixty students are provided at thirty tables whose tops are opaque, white plate glass. Improved facilities for lighting and other improvements have just been made. The offices and research rooms of the staff take up the remainder of this floor together with preparation and storage rooms as well as space for a number of museum specimens in cabinets. The lecture room

on the second floor is shared with the histology department. In the basement are the receiving and embalming room and the room where an ample supply of material for dissection is kept preserved for use as occasion demands and where the osteological specimens are prepared. All the rooms contain appropriate furniture and equipment but sufficient space is available for expansion so that needed instruments and materials can be accommodated as they may be secured.

In the surroundings described above the students and the staff cooperate in the study of the intricate structure of the human body. By gradual progressive separation of all its parts this marvelous mechanism is observed in all its actual, visible details. An understanding realization of the dynamic relationships of all the parts as components of a living, functioning organism is striven for by endeavoring to project, mentally, the dissected parts into a living being such as the student's own person or that of a patient by whom he may some day be called upon for diagnosis and treatment. In this way it is thought that the condemned "academic flavor" may be avoided. By word and lecture, by example and by citation of authoritative texts the teaching staff aid toward the attainment of this ideal understanding. Throughout its history that, essentially, has been the aim and ambition of the Anatomy Department of the Atlanta Medical College (the School of

Medicine of Emory University). From the time of the Revival of Learning after the Dark Ages it has been realized by medical teachers that successful medical training is based upon understanding of the structure and function of the human body and that such understanding can be gained only by actual observation of the structures themselves. Historical fact proves that excellence of medical training (and consequent practice) has been in direct ratio to intensity of anatomical dissection. So, recognizing that anatomy is part and parcel of all other studies in the medical course, it has continued to be the chief aim of the present departmental staff to aid the students by directing their efforts in making observations and in organizing and correlating these observations into an understanding of the structures of the living body. Thus, understanding and not mere memorizing is emphasized.

As time may be available from the principal aim the staff keep in touch with current work of other professional anatomists and engage in original investigation themselves in order to experience the stimulus which such work gives to their own enthusiasm in the study of anatomical structure. Some of these investigations that have been judged of value have been published from time to time. These articles include subjects in medical education, correlation of structure with function, reports and statistics of structural variations and descriptions of anomalies. The past achievements of the department in this regard are a matter of record in anatomical and medical journals. Space for citation of these is not available here. But the achievements springing from the chief aim are largely intangible and consist in the share of the anatomists in preparing the students for the remainder of their course and for their practical service to society as physicians and surgeons. This we believe to be of immeasurably greater value than all else as we visualize the thousands of doctors who have reflected credit upon their alma mater by the excellence of their professional service during the eight decades of her existence. Believing this we will continue to strive toward the objective of our aim.

HOMER BLINCOE, M.D.
Chairman.

DEPARTMENT OF HISTOLOGY

The Department of Histology, or Micro-anatomy as it should properly be designated since the subjects of embryology and neuro-anatomy are likewise given here, dates from 1916. Until this period these subjects were given in the general field along with gross anatomy. In 1916 a division was made in the Department of Anatomy and the Department of Micro-anatomy was begun, which confines its efforts to teaching the three subjects of histology, embryology and neuro-anatomy.

During the first several years the staff consisted of a full-time professor and a part-time technician. But as developments went on it became necessary to expand: a larger personnel was required to meet the improved type of work performed and teaching given. An assistant professor was added in the person of Dr. Charles W. Harwell, a graduate of the class of 1921 M, and who for a few years served as assistant to both departments. In 1923 Dr. Harwell joined the Micro-anatomy department as a full-time staff member. In a similar manner the technician served the two departments at first but such divided attention was not satisfactory to either, so a full-time technician was employed. In recent years the department has, therefore, enjoyed the benefits of a highly specialized micro-anatomy technic directed primarily toward slide accumulation, not a small part of which is preparing rare human embryos in serial section. The present status of the technic service in all its phases owes much to the faithful and efficient work of Mrs. Olive Russell.

In 1917 the laboratory divisions of the Medical School moved to their respective new quarters on the present Emory University campus. Micro-anatomy found a very comfortable and adequate adjustment on the second floor of the John P. Scott Anatomy Building. In this location there are facilities for the satisfactory functioning of all three courses given in the department — lecture room, student laboratory, preparation room, demonstration room, private research rooms, store and work rooms. In short, the housing requisites for the department have been very satisfactorily met. Other needs in the form of special appliances, instruments and departmental accessories still confront the organization but these will doubtless be added in time.

From the first the department has sought to develop a museum and collection of materials pertaining to micro-anatomical subjects. Students have been encouraged to conserve unique findings and specimens for permanent display. Some interesting and valuable material has been gathered. One special type of display article which has proven helpful to the students is that of the wax model. These models are genuinely and scientifically constructed replicas, greatly enlarged, of forms which are too small in themselves to be studied with the unaided eye. There is a small but valuable collection of these now available for use by the student. Museum cases and display tables have been gradually added to the equipment so that this unit is rapidly growing into an important part of the department's resources.

Yet, again, the growing demands of an increasing teaching efficiency brought about the establishment of a part-time undergraduate assistant. The first person to occupy this position was Dr. James Thoroughman, now with a missionary unit in China. He was followed by Dr. W. Mercer Moncrief, now practicing in Atlanta and he in turn was followed by Dr. Malcolm Cook. Dr. Cook is rapidly advancing to enviable esteem at the University of Minnesota. Still greater need of efficient teaching made it advisable to install a part-time graduate assistant in place of a student and the position is now occupied by such a person. The first to occupy this advanced position was Dr. P. L. Moon. He was followed by Dr. Edgar Boling, and the present occupant is Dr. A. Park McGinty.

The objective of the Micro-anatomy department is two-fold: first, there is the teaching of the students. In this function the effort is made to keep up-to-date with such ideas and practices in vogue in other similar laboratories over the country. Little time is devoted to the preparation of material by the student; just enough to acquaint him with the general idea of how much material is acquired. The very limited time available for these courses is utilized in bringing the student into as full and clear concept of the microscopic form as possible. He is urged to develop the habit of visualizing all his professional contacts, diagnostic, medical and surgical, in exact and minute form. While such minute and detailed dimension of the human body cannot be in the foreground of his later practical contacts, they should be woven into the fabric of his preparation. To the end, therefore, of obtaining an immediate and clear percept of the object with which he is dealing he asks three questions: First, what is this thing,—a gland, a muscle, a nerve, or a fascia? Next, what does it do by way of serving the body, its host,—digest food, absorb it, support an organ, or move a structure? Third, how does it carry on this function,—exactly, minutely? Pointedly, this is the gist of micro-anatomy.

The second objective in the department's functioning is that of investigation and original work. This field is kept keenly before the student but of course he is not required to exert himself personally in such lines. Yet there are in every class those who have not only the ability but the inclination for research and they are encouraged to develop such. The staff members, on the other hand, have been active along these lines all the while and their efforts have not been without fruitage. A number of papers have been published on some of the work done here. There are now four standard texts which quote data taken from one of these papers, the one pertaining to the taenia coli. The department also functioned a few years ago with a number of other laboratories in putting out an original Anatomy of the Rhesus monkey. Active work is now in progress on two lines of investigation, the area postrama of the floor of the fourth ventricle and the mechanism of double-visioning: one paper has been published on the latter subject.

P. E. LINEBACK, M.D., *Chairman.*

The law of worthy life is fundamentally the law of strife. It is only through labor and painful effort; by grim energy and resolute courage, that we move on to better things.—*Theodore Roosevelt.*

DEPARTMENT OF PHYSIOLOGY

The full significance of the changes that took place in the teaching of physiology at the time of reorganization of our School of Medicine in 1910, can best be understood in the light of the history of the development of medical physiology from the time of its inception in the early days of the republic. Only a broad outline of this interesting subject can be presented here.

The history of physiology in this country may be said to have had its beginning, according to Fulton, in 1789, with the establishment of a Chair of the Institutes of Medicine at the College of Philadelphia which, in 1791, merged with the University of Pennsylvania. The first incumbent of the chair was Caspar Wistar. He was succeeded by Benjamin Rush (1792), a distinguished physician and patriot whose interest in physiology dated from his student days at the University of Edinburgh as is shown by his graduation thesis which dealt with the physiology of digestion. A number of Rush's pupils followed in his steps and carried out experiments on this function which were embodied in their graduation theses (1803-1805). It is interesting to note that at this period William Beaumont was carrying out the experiments on gastric digestion which are the pride of early American physiology. At this time also, Robley Dunglison, Professor of Medicine at the University of Virginia, and subsequently at the Jefferson Medical College of Philadelphia, published a textbook of human physiology in two volumes (1832).

The arrival in New York of Brown-Séquard in 1852 stimulated the interest of the medical profession in physiology. On his third visit to the United States, this peripatetic physiologist was appointed Professor of the Institutes of Medicine at the Medical College of Virginia in Richmond. He was an active experimenter, intent on widening the boundaries of our knowledge of function, but aside from receiving little encouragement in his investigative work, stayed too short a time to build up a following. Other workers who contributed to the development of physiology in the early history of this subject in the United States were John C. Dalton and S. Weir Mitchell.

For a long time, the majority of the teachers of this subject were content with expository lectures, but a departure of the highest significance for the future was made by Bowditch when he established at the Harvard Medical School the first laboratory of physiology for the instruction of students (1871). Laboratories were subsequently organized in other schools. However, many of the medical schools of the period, and for many years after, had neither the means nor the inclination to establish expensive laboratories. The teachers were practitioners who undertook to instruct students for the income they derived, not only from the student fees, but also from what was called the "reflex" value of the position. Hence, the professorship of physiology and other scientific subjects was not considered particularly desirable. Under the conditions then prevailing, the establishment of a medical school by a group of clinicians was a profitable venture. It is not surprising, therefore, that according to Abraham Flexner the United States and Canada founded 450 medical schools in a little more than a century. Of these 155 were still in existence in 1910.

In the meantime, the organization in 1893 of the Johns Hopkins Medical School, with a provision for well equipped laboratories in charge of competent teachers giving their entire time to investigation and instruction, provided a new standard in medical education. It became increasingly evident that too many medical schools were not meeting modern requirements. In order to ascertain the facts, the Carnegie Foundation for the Advancement of Teaching undertook to carry out a study and publish a report on the schools of medicine of the United States and Canada.

At the time of the visit in Atlanta in 1909 of Abraham Flexner there were four medical schools in the city. The entrance requirements for each of these was designated as nominal. None of the schools had any teacher devoting full-time to the institution. The Atlanta College of Physicians and Surgeons organized in 1898 by a merger of the Atlanta Medical College and the Southern Medical College was "perhaps the best equipped of all the schools of its grade." It had good buildings and reasonably good

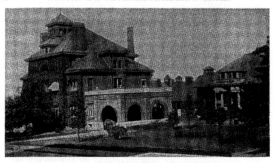

-Grady Hospital, 1906

laboratories of anatomy and pathology. There was no equipment worth speaking of for the teaching of physiology. Following the recommendations made by Mr. Flexner at the time of his visit the faculty decided to secure the services, among others, of a trained physiologist. This decision came in the summer of 1910.

Dr. H. F. Harris, who had been on the staff of the department of pathology at the Jefferson Medical College, and whom the writer had met at the time of one of his visits to Philadelphia, was kind enough to suggest the writer's name. After going over the school and conferring with the President of the College, Dr. W. F. Westmoreland and the Dean, Dr. W. S. Elkin, the writer accepted the offer to undertake the development of a department of physiology to meet modern requirements. As the equipment was insufficient, Dr. W. S. Elkin volunteered to supply the immediate needs of the department out of his own funds. It was then the middle of August. With the cooperation of supply dealers the laboratory was ready for work with the opening of the school in September. The only help available at that time was a young inexperienced assistant who, however, was also on a full-time basis. With the lack of proper preparation and indifferent discipline of the student body, the work of instruction was difficult. Since chemistry continued to be taught by a local practitioner,

and no attempt was made to instruct the students in physiological chemistry, the department of physiology organized a laboratory course dealing with the essentials of this subject. Later on, when a full-time professor of biochemistry was appointed the equipment was turned over to him. The author likewise recommended the organization of a separate course in pharmacology under the department of therapeutics. Dr. Hastings, who was instructor in physiology, gave the first laboratory course in pharmacodynamics.

The first years were exceedingly busy years. It was necessary for the staff not only to carry out the work of instruction in physiology and biochemistry, but to wire desks to supply current for its experimental work, improvise apparatus, draw charts, make lantern slides and conduct research work. At this time, the writer carried out an experimental investigation of the treatment of complete heart-block with Strophanthus. This work was done partly on man and partly on animals and was published in the Journal of Experimental Medicine. The writer also devised at this period a method for spinning the drum of a kymograph automatically which continues in use here and has been adopted in other laboratories. Experiments were also begun which led to the discovery of the function of the interauricular bundle. In spite of restricted means, the department managed to accumulate from year to year, reliable apparatus such

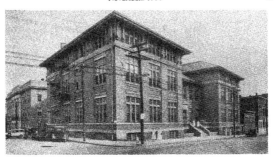

Emory University Division, Grady Hospital, 1936

as could be used not only in demonstrations but also in investigative work. The morale of succeeding classes gradually improved as it came to be realized that a reasonably high standard of scholarship and a correct attitude toward the work offered were expected.

Following a merger in 1913 of the Atlanta School of Medicine with the Atlanta College of Physicians and Surgeons the school resumed its original name of Atlanta Medical College and, as such, joined Emory University in 1915 to become its School of Medicine.

The decision to transfer the instruction of the first two years of medicine to the University campus necessitated the erection of laboratory buildings. The writer spent considerable time in planning the laboratories of physiology, giving special attention to devices for the distribution of different forms of electric current and of compressed air for artificial respiration. The furniture had to be carefully planned, including a special desk for each two students, animal tables, etc. The laboratories were now adequate for the needs of instruction and of the staff. From time to time special apparatus was secured to meet the growing demands of instruction and of investigation. As a consequence, the laboratories of physiology at Emory compare favorably with the better laboratories of the country, there being but few to excel them in facilities for the work of instruction. In the past decade, the size of the staff has been in-creased so as to make it possible to do work in keeping with present requirements. With the limited resources of the University the research activities of the department have been somewhat restricted, but in spite of this handicap it has been possible to carry on some investigative work. The department has published in recent years, among other things, the results of research on the distribution of the vagus fibers to the sino-auricular junction of the mammalian heart, the utilization of lactic acid by the heart muscle, the gaseous exchange of the heart, creatinuria induced by glucose and fructose, and is now engaged in a study of the metabolism of these two sugars.

In concluding this very brief recital of the development of physiology during the twenty-five years the writer has been with the school, he hopes that the future will have greater things in store, for the importance of physiology in medical thought cannot be over-emphasized. To quote Flexner in his epoch-making report: "Meanwhile, whatever its limitations, the physiological laboratory is of immense educational importance to the prospective physician. Physiology is, in a sense, the central discipline of the medical school. It is the business of the physician to restore normal functioning: normal functioning is thus his starting point in thought, his goal in action."

GEORGE BACHMANN, M.D.
Chairman.

DEPARTMENT OF PATHOLOGY AND BACTERIOLOGY

The Department of Pathology at Emory University incorporates the departments of Bacteriology and Clinical Laboratory Diagnosis. Therefore, medical teaching that in many medical schools is given in three departments is included in this one division. The personnel of the Department of Pathology include the following: Dr. Roy R. Kracke, Professor and Chairman of the Department, Dr. Warren Matthews, Associate Professor, Dr. Francis P. Parker, Assistant Professor, Dr. Elizabeth Gambrell, Instructor; Mrs. Hortense Garver, Assistant, and Miss Herma Barmettler, Technician and Secretary.

The Department of Pathology is also responsible for the laboratory activities of the associated University hospitals. All laboratory work in Emory University Hospital is operated under the supervision of the department as well as the laboratory of Grady Hospital. Since the resignation of Dr. Jack C. Norris, Dr. Warren Matthews has recently assumed direction of the laboratory at Grady Hospital.

The department is located on the first floor of the Anatomy Building on the University campus. It is well equipped for the teaching of the various courses, which include bacteriology and laboratory diagnosis in the fall of the year, and gross and microscopic tissue pathology in the winter and spring terms.

From eight to ten graduate students are in training in the department at all times. For the most part these are young women who ultimately go into the field of laboratory work in medicine.

During the last six years the chief research interest of the department has centered around the field of blood diseases. During this period nearly fifty papers have been published by the various medical journals; most of these in the field of hematology. At the present time two books are in preparation by the various members of the staff. These include a text-book of laboratory diagnosis in which there are twelve contributors from as many different medical schools. Also, the first American Atlas of Hematology will be off the press shortly, prepared by some of the departmental staff.

Research work goes on consistently on various subjects pertaining to the field of pathology and some of the staff members are in constant collaboration with other departments in scientific investigation.

Not less than ten exhibits have been prepared and shown at various medical meetings throughout the country in the last five or six years. The department has been awarded recognition in the form of certificates, gold medals, exhibit awards, etc., in every medical organization in which it has demonstrated its work, including the American Medical Association, American Society of Clinical Pathologists, Southern Medical Association and MEDICAL ASSOCIATION OF GEORGIA.

The most pressing need in the Department of Pathology at this time is increased physical facilities, preferably in the form of a new building, and increased income with particular reference to its personnel and supply budget. Even though trained personnel is available there is a certain point beyond which research activity cannot go unless ample supplies and equipment are available.

Naturally, it is the ambition of all members in the Department of Pathology, in common with other departments in the University, not only to train good physicians, well qualified for the practice of medicine, but also to firmly establish the standing and reputation of our school that it will rank in a class second to none.

ROY R. KRACKE, M.D.
Chairman

UNIVERSITY AFFILIATION OF MEDICAL SCHOOLS

Medical schools in this and other countries now spend from two to five times as much money as they receive from students tuition and fees. With increased demands for better laboratories, assistants for teaching and research, and the desire to attain and keep sacred their obligation to humanity, medical educators have been compelled to seek affiliation with well established institutions of learning. In this country such progress meant, in most instances, the affiliation of medical schools with universities.

In Georgia, as early as 1855, the Oglethorpe Medical College, operating in Savannah, sought affiliation with Emory College at Oxford. The trustees of Emory, however, were interested in other types of education and "respectfully declined" the request. Sixty years later the Atlanta Medical College became the School of Medicine of Emory University.

DEPARTMENT OF BIOCHEMISTRY

Under the direction of Dr. A. M. Muckenfuss this was the first department of the Medical School established on the Emory campus. He early began research on certain vitamins, but resigned in 1920 to accept other work.

The present staff consists of three full-time teachers and investigators, all members of Phi Beta Kappa and Ph.D. in training, with five or more years of experience in teaching.

The whole of the second floor of the Chemistry Building is used for this work in the Medical and Graduate schools. A small number of M.S. degrees are conferred annually, based on both theory and research.

approaches, including sulphur, iodine and similar studies.

A very hopeful avenue to greater speed as well as scope of research lies in the use of the new and marvelous magneto-optic apparatus built for us by Dr. F. Allison of Auburn, Ala., by which tests are now being made successfully which are one thousand times more sensitive than the spectrograph. Work has been in progress during the last four years to establish data through research on organic compounds so that service may be available for biochemical investigations. The reliability of the method has been confirmed by many tests, especially by 2300 photographs which will be published from his laboratory in October, 1936. None of the material is destroyed in testing by this method and one

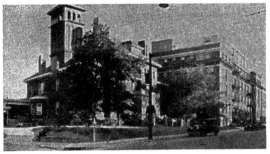

White Division, Grady Hospital, 1936

Many hundreds of hours have been spent in cooperation with the physicians of the hospitals with benefits to both phases of the work. It is hoped that a full-time chemist may soon be made available in the clinical work and thus integrate more closely the mutual services available from all concerned.

This department has had a small share in the research on the importance of metals in the diet which now loom so large in the present emphasis on the functions performed by metals in many physiologic processes both in plants and animals. But only a beginning has been made in this field. Other research has been done in metabolism along several

part in a million-million dilution is detectable. A former Atlanta chemist provided the funds to have the apparatus installed, though Dr. Allison would not accept compensation for his time and skill.

Reports from this department have been published in The Journal of Laboratory and Clinical Medicine; Science; Journal American Chemical Society et al. A clinical investigation of 140 cases has been reported and accepted for publication in a few weeks.

Our needs for future usefulness and expansion as well as more nearly complete cooperation with other departments are those common to nearly all such endeavors and it is hoped that additional funds in the form of endowment of fellowships and grants-in-aid may be made available to the department and to all others whose needs and purposes are potentially of such moment in the advance of pure and applied science for the benefit of all people now and later.

J. L. McGHEE, PH.D.
Chairman.

DEPARTMENT OF PHARMACOLOGY

Prior to June 1, 1915, when the Atlanta Medical College legally became the School of Medicine of Emory University, there had not been a separate department of pharmacology. However, the need for instruction in this, then relatively new, subject had been recognized and an attempt made to meet the need, for a short course in the subject was introduced into the curriculum as a part of the work in therapeutics. From the college bulletin of that year it appears that some space was provided in one of the buildings on Butler Street, in which some experiments were carried out by the students and a series of lectures was given by the instructor.

At the completion of the transfer, however, definite steps were taken toward the establishment of a separate department, when Dr. A. R. Bliss was called to Atlanta as the first Professor of Pharmacology. He organized the newly established department and, with the opening of the 1915-1916 session, began instruction in the first formal course in the subject ever given in the school. For two years the work was carried out at the plant on Butler Street, during which time the present medical buildings on the University campus in Druid Hills were being planned and constructed. With their completion in 1917, the instruction in the first two years, in the pre-clinical branches, was transferred to them, and thus to new and modernly equipped laboratories and class rooms.

Dr. Bliss remained at Emory as Professor of Pharmacology and Chairman of the department until his resignation in 1923. Dr. A. D. Bush was called from the University of North Dakota to fill the vacancy, but due to ill health he was forced to resign in 1928. The present incumbent, who had been Dr. Bush's assistant, was made acting chairman

of the department. At the present time the personnel consists of the chairman, his full-time assistant, a half-time student assistant and a full-time technician. The department is housed in the T. T. Fishburne Laboratory of the Physiology Building, occupying all of the first floor and a large part of the basement. While the staff and the physical equipment of the department are adequate for the effective teaching of the course in pharmacology, additions to both would materially aid in extensions and developments, which, under the existing circumstances, can be attained only slowly or not at all.

Since an appreciation and proper understanding of modern pharmacology depend upon a thorough grounding in physiology, the course logically follows the second year student's completion of the latter. One of the main objectives of the department is to approach and correlate the various aspects and divisions of the subject that the student will have, upon completion of the course, a well-rounded working knowledge of the entire field. This does not mean that the student is expected or required to have memorized a large body of unrelated facts, but rather that the facts as acquired will be so correlated that they fit nicely into the completed whole. By dwelling also on general principles the student comes to think of drugs and medicines from a true pharmacological viewpoint. Pharmacology, as all other medical sciences, is constantly changing in that new facts are being discovered about known drugs, new drugs are being prepared and some old drugs passing out of use. From this it is quite apparent that if the major objective was the mere acquisition of uncorrelated facts, the student a few years after leaving the course would be unprepared to solve the problems concerning the use of drugs as they arose. A training in proper and correct thinking will remain a part of an individual long after he has forgotten facts. Several factors, therefore, are considered of prime importance, namely: (1) Development in the student of the ability correctly to evaluate therapeutic claims made for drugs. The therapeutic use of a drug should rest upon the physiologic changes which it is capable of inducing in the animal organism; (2) acquisition of sufficient information about a drug, such as its

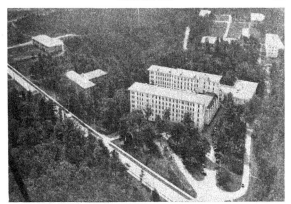

Section of Emory University Campus, 1936, Showing Emory University Hospital

correct name, the forms in which it is available, the methods of administering it, its dose, etc., that he will be adept in its prescription and its proper utilization in the treatment of disease; (3) learning the physiologic actions of a reasonable number of well established drugs, so that he may develop a truly scientific basis for their therapeutic use, and a sound skepticism concerning their therapeutic use not based upon experimental proof.

Because pharmacology is constantly changing, a course of instruction, if it meets the requirements, must be flexible. It would seem reasonable to assume that a course following a set plan year after year, would soon cease to be effective. Therefore, another objective of this department is to keep its course always flexible, to avoid becoming wedded to one certain way, and unhesitatingly to make a change when its need is recognized. At the present time the work is divided into two parts, didactic and laboratory, but at all times the two are closely correlated. The didactic work consists of a series of formal lectures over the actions of the more important drugs used in medicine, conferences and oral recitations which are quite informal and frequent written recitations. The students perform for themselves some of the laboratory exercises, but an increasing number of experiments are presented as demonstrations. Adequate practice in the construction of prescriptions and the prescribing of drugs is provided for throughout the course.

Research is considered an essential activity of the department personnel, and at all times problems which the limited budget and few workers permit, are being worked upon. The results of researches as reported in the current literature are closely followed and incorporated into the teaching.

EUGENE L. JACKSON, PH.C.
Chairman.

The country's educators should ponder on the problem that will confront them if the efforts of the protagonists of compulsory health insurance have their way, and such a form of delivering medical care to our people is thoughtlessly adopted.—*Medical News, Med. Soc. of State of N. Y.*

Will the physicians continue independent practitioners or job-holders as some predict?

TREND OF MEDICAL EDUCATION

A review of the teaching in the two clinical years of the Medical School during past years shows that the most notable change is the extensive development of practical instruction at the bedside of the patient. This change has been made at the expense of the older system of lectures and amphitheatre clinics, of which only a relatively few remain in the present curriculum. Those lectures which do remain have changed to a form of discussions between the instructor and the class and are designed to bring out fundamental principles involved in medicine, surgery, obstetrics and their sub-divisions.

In the present form of practical clinical instruction each class is divided into small groups who are assigned as "clinical clerks" to the medical, surgical, obstetric and special services of the hospital. On these services the student actually gets the history of the patient and does the usual physical and laboratory examinations. He then discusses the diagnosis and treatment with a member of the faculty. This discussion is either individual or in the presence of a group small enough to make a consideration of the patient's problem free and informal. The student follows the patient until dismissal or until the end of his clinical clerkship in any given service.

It is easy to see that this system places the student in exactly the same position in which he will find himself in future practice, so that the knowledge which he uses as a practitioner will be knowledge acquired as a student practitioner and not knowledge gained from an amphitheatre lecture. The idea can be illustrated by citing briefly the arrangements followed in one or two departments. In surgery, not only does the student do the history and physical examination and discuss the diagnosis and indicated treatment with a member of the faculty, but he also scrubs up and acts as an assistant in the operation. He studies the pathologic tissues removed at operation and discusses them with his group and the instructor. He follows and participates in the postoperative treatment of the patient and in other surgical procedures which are indicated.

The teaching of obstetrics is largely practical, — actual contact between student and patient. All normal cases are delivered by students in the hospital under supervision of capable instructors. The care of pregnant women is learned in the outpatient department where approximately three hundred women are under observation all of the time. Students take the histories, do the physical examination and outline the proper treatment under individual instruction from a member of the faculty.

Both the wards of the hospital and its outpatient department are used for clinical instruction. In the ward, the student studies that type of patient who requires hospitalization for diagnosis or treatment. It represents his future hospital practice. In the outpatient department he studies ambulatory patients. As he sees these patients on their subsequent visits he is able to watch the progress of their illness and determine the accuracy of his diagnosis and the effect of the treatment given. This work corresponds to the practice which he will carry on in his office.

If it were necessary to summarize the character of clinical instruction in the medical school at present, it probably could be best done by saying that the student learns by doing rather than by hearing.

RUSSELL H. OPPENHEIMER, M.D.
Dean.

What type of youth would be attracted to a medical career? After a difficult medical course of four years, and the necessary preparatory one, then the arduous post-graduate internship—to be qualified for what? A job, with a fixed income, with a definite number of assigned patients who, to follow the custom set in England, are not thoroughly examined even if there were time allowed to do it; fixed hours of work, perhaps a paid vacation, and at the end—a pension. A job-holder's career! A government employee with all that this implies!

Obviously such a system will attract quite a different type of man than was drawn into the present system, men who have won high renown and have given American medicine the high place it holds today.—*Medical News, Medical Society of the State of New York.*

Will not the emphasis in medical education also have to change? Will it not be necessary to train American medical officials rather than American doctors? We see a similar change in a trend in the field of nursing.

Individual endeavor brought astounding developments in medicine and attracted brilliant types of men. These men have been encouraged but not controlled by other agencies.

HYPERTENSION*

STEWART R. ROBERTS, M.D.
Atlanta

"What do you give for high blood pressure?" and "What do you do for high blood pressure?" are two common questions asked in present day medicine. The patient says: "I have high blood pressure and it goes up and down but the doctor says it stays too high." The surgeon asks whether he is justified in doing a major operation on a patient with normal kidneys but with high pressure. The applicant for insurance is abruptly refused his insurance because his pressure is above certain approved statistical tables for his age. The laity have learned that one with high pressure for many years is more apt than one with a normal pressure to have apoplexy, heart attacks, heart failure with dropsy and even kidney disease. *The Journal of the American Medical Association* averages from twenty to twenty-five new suggestions each year for the treatment of hypertension, and in addition numerous articles and abstracts on various phases of the subject. It is probably true that the average physician beset with hypertensive patients feels, of necessity, compelled to think more of therapeutics than of the origin, causes and nature of hypertension. It is a motley and difficult group whose functional and structural relations and progress constitute the signs and symptoms that we call hypertension, the hypertensive syndrome or the hypertensive symptom-complex. The wiser attitude is to consider the management of the patient with hypertension. This includes a consideration of his mental, emotional, instinctive and physical make up, which with his inheritance and habits, unite to form the larger living thing that we call the individual and his personality.

Essential hypertension is by far the most common type of chronic hypertension but there are other types, the causes of which are more difficult of diagnosis. Treatment demands that causes other than essential hypertension be carefully considered and ruled out before a final diagnosis of the essential variety is made. Among these are:

*From the Department of Internal Medicine, Emory University School of Medicine.

(1) Obstructing stone in the kidney or ureter which for some reason may raise the pressure to a chronic hypertensive state. I have seen two such cases with a drop, after the removal of the stone, to a high normal pressure. Chronic urinary obstruction is a general cause and is illustrated also by hypertrophy of the prostate, cystic disease of one or both kidneys and malignancy with metastases either in the kidneys or causing pressure upon the ureters. I saw one patient treated for essential hypertension; at autopsy we found a carcinoma of the uterus with metastases to the kidneys and other metastases causing pressure on the ureters. A pelvic examination had never been made.

(2) Acute or chronic glomerulonephritis, the association of renal hypertension and a true primary nephritis with the usual signs of decreased renal function, albumin, casts and blood in the urine, edema, anemia and enlarging heart. The blood pressure in the acute cases may rise with the urinary findings. Under 45 years of age this condition is usually a primary nephritis. After 45 essential hypertension may grade into the arteriosclerotic kidney with a final break into the findings of a chronic glomerulonephritis. Uremia rather than heart failure is the usual end of both types. The retinal arteries may present similar findings.

(3) Hypertension in pregnancy calls for an etiologic diagnosis of some importance. There are three probabilities: First, pregnancy may occur in the course of a rather early essential hypertension. The presence of hypertension before pregnancy, the absence of the renal findings of nephritis and the relative well being of the patient, are good points in favor of essential hypertension at an early age. Second, hypertension due to the glomerulonephritis of pregnancy reveals itself by the usual findings of nephritis, early and extreme edema, anemia, pallor and easy dyspnea. Third, hypertension associated with the toxemia of pregnancy, with albumin and casts in the urine but with no elevation of the blood urea or the total non-protein nitrogen of the blood. Hypertension here begins with a true spasm of the vessels well seen in the localized spasm and constrictions in the retinal arteries. This localization may be so extreme in the beginning as to present the appearance of a series of constrictures reminding one of sausage links. (Hallum's[2] paper is well worth while.) This condition probably is as clear an illustration of vasospasm as there is in medicine. The eclamptic convulsion may be the expression of advanced spasm in the brain (Cobb,[3] Spielmeyer[4]). Such hypertension seems not necessarily to start one on the way to essential hypertension. To one who would understand essential hypertension, the acute vasospasm of eclampsia is instructive. It shows what smooth muscle can do under stress.

(4) Hypertension due to arteriosclerosis calls for interpretation. Extreme sclerosis may exist with relatively normal pressures. Allbutt[5] long ago called this decrescent sclerosis. The arterial wall may thicken but the artery also lengthens through tortuosity and may in segments actually widen. Here is the union of structural sclerosis and normal blood pressure. But the real typical pressure of loss of elasticity and feeble power of recoil in the aorta has a common reading of a high systolic, a low diastolic and a high pulse pressure.

Such readings as 190/90 mm. Hg or 180/80 mm. Hg illustrate this well. Under the fluoroscope the aortas are usually dilated; this includes the ascending, transverse and descending segments just below the knob. From the left anterior oblique view the aortic window is narrowed. The great vessels at the second rib are widened. Functionally the recoil of the aortic wall is decreased due to the feebleness of the elastic tissues in the wall and degenerative structural changes. When the heart begins to fail, the systolic pressure begins to fall and at times the diastolic may rise slightly. Two clear interpretations seem of value here: (a) Systolic and pulse pressure hypertension with normal or relatively low diastolic pressure in individuals over 45 is usually associated with some loss of recoil and dilation of the thoracic aorta. Aortic incompetency, hyperthyroidism, extreme anemias, exercise and excitement should be ruled out of the picture. Such cases usually present increased dullness and a widened area on percussion of the upper third of the sternum. The heart assumes some of the work of propelling the blood formerly done by the recoil of the normal aorta. (b) Falling systolic and pulse pressures and a rising pulse rate are signs that heart failure is at hand even before edema occurs. Some degree of coronary sclerosis usually complicates the picture.

(5) Hypertension as one of the features of an over activity of the basophil cells of the anterior lobe of the pituitary gland leading to the formation of a small tumor called the basophil adenoma. Harvey Cushing[6] described this syndrome in 1932 and it is now called "Cushing's Syndrome." Boyd sums up the diagnostic picture as follows:

"(1) A rapidly acquired and usually painful adiposity, confined to the face, neck and trunk, and sparing the limbs. In one of Cushing's cases, a girl, aged 20 years, weighed 206 pounds. (2) A tendency to kyphosis. (3) Hirsutism of the face and trunk in females and preadolescent males. (4) Sexual dystrophy, shown by early amenorrhea in females and impotence in males. (5) A dusky or plethoric appearance of the skin. (6) A tendency to polycythemia. (7) Peculiar striations of the skin which give the abdominal wall, both male and female, an appearance of pregnancy. (8) Vascular hypertension. (9) Osteoporosis involving the vertebral column and long bones and causing pain in the back."

Such cases may occur without any demonstrable involvement of the pituitary, but rather with a tumor of the adrenal cortex, or a basophilic tumor of the pituitary may be associated with either hyperplasia or adenoma of the adrenal gland. Vernon E. Powell's[1] case was a girl of 22 with a pressure of 260/140 with amenorrhea. She apparently improved with three deep x-ray treatments.

(6) Adenoma of the adrenal cortex is associated with hypertension. As just noted, the clinical picture may not differ from that of a pituitary basophilic adenoma. There is evidence that there is a special hormone in the anterior lobe of the pituitary called the adreno-tropic hormone. These cases, while rare and difficult of certain diagnosis, are reported now from the different clinics.

(7) Coarctation of the aorta is associated with hypertension in the upper extremities. The systolic pressures are high, ranging from 140 mm. Hg upward. The pulse pressure is high as a result. One is amply repaid by studying this subject. L. Minor Blackford's[8] studies and those of Hamilton and Abbott[9] and Thomas Lewis[10] are well worth while. The pressing together or narrowing or what is even better, the stenosis of the aorta, occurs on the descending limb of the aortic arch beyond the origin of the left subclavian and at the insertion of the ductus arteriosus. The left ventricle discharges its systolic output against a stenotic obstruction and hypertrophy may result. The greatly dilated branches, chiefly of the subclavian arteries; namely, the scapular and internal mammary arteries, carry the blood in this round about way to the trunk and lower extremities. The patient may live to 40 or beyond. The pulsation in the femorals and below is feeble. It is not amiss to feel the femoral artery in each patient with hypertension, particularly in those under 40, and to watch for a bulging ascending aorta, a usually enlarged heart, forceful pulsations in the carotids even at rest, and large and tortuous vessels in the back and the axillary regions.

(8) Lead poisoning is usually associated with some degree of hypertension. Both the systolic and diastolic pressures are raised as a rule. Three factors may be at work here though certainly the causes of the rise in pressure would be difficult to prove in any given case. (1) Lead poisoning seems to cause a true vasospasm due to the direct action of lead on the intima. (2) Chronic changes in the vessel walls. (3) Changes in the kidney after the nature of a vascular nephritis with albumin and casts in the urine. Lead poisoning may occur without renal involvement but with rise in the pressure. A hypertension associated with a mild secondary anemia, one to two hundred stipled red cells per million erythrocytes, well demonstrated by Unna's methylene blue stain, the blue lead line on the gum margin and lead in the urine, prove the picture. "Lead follows calcium in storage and elimination" (Houston.[11]) The lead is driven back into the bones by food with a high calcium content and calcium lactate or gluconate. Collips Parathormone in 50 to 80 units daily may be used in extreme cases.

(9) Extreme degrees of heart block and complete block with dissociation of the ventricles may have high systolic and pulse pressures. A woman of 66 with 3 to 1 block had a pressure of 200/80 mm. Hg. Another of 64 with dissociation and a rate of 36 to 42 had a pressure of 260/70 mm. Hg. The slow rate with increased strength to each contraction and the increased output are factors. Widening of the great vessels and arteriosclerosis are other factors.

To interpret abnormal blood pressure, it is necessary to understand the applied physiology of normal blood pressure. And even normal pressure is an involved problem. Three pressures are taken with each reading: systolic, diastolic and pulse. How do they originate, what is their precise cause and limitation, and what their variation and control?

Blood pressure is the lateral or outward pressure exerted by the blood on the walls of the blood vessels. Cut an artery, and it spurts in diastole and spurts higher in systole. The lateral pressure varies from diastole to systole and back again in endless alternations. The diastolic pressure is the basic pressure; it is the lowest pressure during diastole of the heart. The systolic pressure is the maximum pressure during systole of the heart. The pulse pressure is the difference between the systolic and diastolic pressures. This makes it a mere subtraction, and as such it is useless for physiology and clinical use. It is rather a rough measure and indication of the stroke volume and the stroke value. It is the force of the left ventricle through the stroke volume as the latter is propelled into the aorta and added to the diastolic pressure, that gives the higher systolic pressure and reading. Blood pressure divisions are in terms of heart contraction, heart rest, and heart volume and force, as illustrated respectively by the systolic, diastolic and pulse pressures.

The heart then is the real source of blood pressure. Given a normal blood and blood volume, a normal vascular system with normal control and peripheral resistance, when the heart stops, the blood pressure ceases. The peripheral resistance, of which so much is written, exists functionally because of the heart, its stroke volume and stroke force. Evidence is afforded by the drop in pressure after coronary thrombosis, and the greater drop after rupture of the interventricular septum after infarction. At one end of the circulation is the heart that furnishes the force for pressure, at the periphery the arteriolar and capillary resistance against which the heart force expends itself. The systolic pressure is the stroke value of the left ventricle overcoming the diastolic pressure and propelling the blood. The latter includes also force to distend the elastic aorta. The diastolic pressure is a numerical statement of the peripheral resistance. The peripheral resistance involves several factors; the chief are the normal recoil of the elastic aorta, a normal blood, the integrity of the aortic valve, a normal tone of the resisting arterioles and a normal frictional resistance which includes the viscosity of the blood, the bore of the tubes and velocity of the flow.

All these factors and more are neither fixed nor static but are variable. Some of them vary in health and perhaps all of them vary in disease. Clinical illustrations are numerous. The venous return to the heart, the stroke volume, the dilation of the arterioles increase with exercise, hyperthyroidism and aortic regurgitation. Here the stroke value, the stroke volume, and the pulse pressure are increased. Hyperthyroidism increases the stroke volume with no increase, or perhaps a fall, in the diastolic pressure and a greatly increased pulse pressure. In mitral stenosis with the left ventricle delivering a smaller stroke volume, due to the mitral obstruction, pressure in the absence of other disease is usually low, averaging 100 to 110 mm. Hg. The relatively low blood pressure in aortic stenosis is due to two factors: first, the obstruction at the aortic opening and, second, some of the stroke value is expended in overcoming this obstruction before the blood even reaches the aorta to raise the diastolic pressure. With heart failure the stroke value fails in variable degree and the pulse pressure usually drops. A drop in pulse pressure means the systolic pressure is falling. In chronic hypertension, from any cause, the cardiac changes are so classic and common that they are easily recognized by the clinical eye. The strong stage, with slow pulse, a rise in pulse pressure proportionate to a healthy heart and the diastolic pressure, normal response to effort and full compensation. Second, the failing stage, slow, insidious, perhaps imperceptible in the beginning with dyspnea, dizziness, palpitation on effort, rapid pulse, failing heart and systolic pressure. And lastly, congestive heart failure with drop in systolic pressure because of primary drop in pulse pressure.

One outstanding fact about essential hypertension is that it begins in the arterioles of the periphery, then the innocent heart is drawn into the long struggle, and however bravely and long it responds to the overcoming of this vasospasm of the arterioles, it is ultimately doomed to failure and defeat.

Our imperfect knowledge of the causes of hypertension blur our efforts at its treatment. But somewhere between the vasomotor center in the fourth ventricle and such accumulated influences that play upon it as the respiratory center, the heart center, the hormones, oxygen and carbon dioxide supply, cerebral activity, psychic energy, the drive and influence of civilization, the influences of heredity and the increased tone of the arteries due to the over action of the vasomotor center, is developed this apparently untoward and ever increasing clinical entity that we call essential hypertension. One individual with fine brain, great drive, tremendous responsibility, friction, struggle, effort, disappointment, trouble, emotion and sometimes despair, at 66 maintains soft arteries and a normal blood pressure of 120/80 mm. Hg. The vasomotor nerves to the arterioles have never felt or been stimulated or clicked with a hyper-action of a vasomotor center. But another individual, leading the opposite kind of life, in pleasant places, a careful routine, no dissipation, apparently living a daily life that leads away from hypertension, will somehow have his vasomotor center increase its impulse to the vasomotor nerves and a mortal hypertension results. The explanation so far is lacking.

Treatment of Essential Hypertension

The limitations of treatment are well known. Essential hypertension is a chronic disease. Once begun its trend is high and for the life span. There are of course exceptions and qualifications. There is no drug that once and for all will break the grip of the vasomotor center on its subservient nerves and reduce a high pressure to a normal pressure. There is no method of living and no diet that will do this. The best we can do is to attempt to control the blood pressure with an attitude of mind, a poise, an external and internal calmness, reasonable food, sedative drugs and perhaps vasodilators from time to time. The treatment of essential hypertension is no simple matter. An inflamed appendix can be cut out and removed and the patient and the surgeon are through with it forever, but an essential hypertension is a functional evil of vascular mechanics that the victim has to live with and his physician has to do the best he can with. The following are guiding points:

1. Peace, poise and contentment of mind. Go slow and go easy each day. Avoid the drive toward a far-off triumph as riches, power, position and scholarship. Have a great faith. Be more content with life. And make less effort for the things of life. Do the day's work and after that one has only to live until bedtime.

2. Stabilize the emotions. Keep them under control. Every emotion, however good, is to be retained within the high inclosure of peace. This is a high art.

The emotions of happiness as well as the emotions of evil are to remain within reasonable bounds. Hypertension itself certainly stimulates the emotions, nervousness, anger, resentment, elation and sometimes consternation. "Let sleeping dogs lie." Close the back door. Be done with the past. Let your emotions sit on the front porch and look to the rising sun.

3. Put chains on the instinct. Leave fear and preservation to the gods. Be neither on the defensive nor on the offensive. One is a long time dead. And one is still alive. Be on good terms with the instinct of hunger. Do not worry about what you shall eat nor what you shall drink. The details are relatively unimportant. The quantity and the mass are very important. Slowly bring your weight to normal, if one is fat. Be reasonable at the table, not over active. Push your chair back after you have eaten to live. Seek pleasure elsewhere than at the table. Let the third instinct of sex be within reasonable bounds. Nature may aid you here anyway. Be more thinking and considerate of yourself and less instinctive.

4. Care for your body, not for your desires. The pressure falls during sleep and rest and before a good fire on a winter night. Go to bed sooner and go elsewhere less. A 20 minute warm tub bath at bedtime and a long night's sleep are hard to improve upon. A nap after lunch of 30 minutes to an hour, and train yourself to it, may cause a drop of 5 to 30 mm. from the morning tension. Walking is your best exercise, avoiding shortness of breath. Hurry and worry will undo all else. Horseback riding is not bad; lifting is. Something that soothes—an automobile ride, a book is another, a game is another. Open bowels daily, and drink water and eat fruits freely. If you can draw in some of your efforts, do so. Go home sooner and leave your work where you work. Tobacco is a vasoconstrictor and is to be avoided.

5. There are four drugs that appear useful. The most useful treatment is rarely mentioned. This is the example, the teaching, the strength, the influence and the psychotherapy of an understanding physician. He may not be able to reduce the patient's blood pressure to any great degree, but he can reduce the patient to that life of poise that will enable him to withstand his pressure. Sometimes this is more important than reducing the pressure, particularly if it is all that can be done. (a) A sedative is useful. Phenobarbital in half-grain doses at bedtime or after meals or after lunch and supper, or in larger individuals a grain at bedtime is a psychic sedative, slightly sleep producing, of several hours' influence and is invaluable. (b) Chloral hydrate in doses of 5 to 10 grains at bedtime or twice daily is useful for variable periods. It lacks the cumulative influence of the bromides and in these doses has no depressing influence upon the heart. (c) Of vasodilators there are two that are often of aid: erythrol tetranitrate in one-half grain doses (30 mg.), or nitroglycerin in 1/200 grain doses (0.3 mg.) are safe, can be taken for long periods and do permit some vasodilation. One of these may be given after breakfast and after supper, or once daily at bedtime. The nitroglycerin in this small dose is best given after meals. It does not cause headaches and it does take the edge off the tension of the circulation. Bleeding at

intervals aids some extreme cases. Finally, when the symptoms of an insidious heart strain begin, the activities and the efforts of the patient should be restricted to a smaller circle. As these increase the circle of activity decreases, until finally the third stage with heart failure demands a treatment for angina or for cardiac asthma or for congestive heart failure or for nephritis or for cerebral hemorrhage as indicated in the individual case.

REFERENCES

1. Powell, V. E.: Personal communication.
2. Hallum. A. V.: Eye Changes in Hypertensive Toxemias of Pregnancy. J. A. M. A., 106:1649-51, (May 9) 1936.
3. Cobb. Stanley: M. Clin. North America. 19:1583. 1936.
4. Spielmeyer: Arch. Neurol. & Psychiat.. 23:869, 1930.
5. Allbott, Clifford: Diseases of the Arteries. Vol. 1, page 10.
6. Cushing. Harvey: Basophil Adenoma. Bull. Johns Hopkins Hosp., 50:137, 1932.
7. Boyd, William: Pathology of Internal Diseases, ed. 2, Philadelphia: Lea & Febiger, 1934, p. 558.
8. Blackford. L. M.: Coarctation of Aorta. Arch. Int. Med., 41: 702, 1928.
9. Hamilton, W. F., and Abbott. M. E.: Coarctation of the Aorta of the Adult Type. Am. Heart. J., 3:381 and 574, 1928.
10. Lewis, T.: Material Relating to Coarctation of the Aorta of the Adult Type. Heart. 16:205, 1931.
11. Hoeston, W. R.: Art of Treatment. New York: Macmillan, 1936. page 265.

ARTERIOVENOUS ANEURYSM*

Daniel C. Elkin, M.D.
Atlanta

Aneurysmal swellings are for the most part due to true arterial dilatation, to a false aneurysm or pulsating hematoma, or to an arteriovenous communication. Their differentiation is important since the treatment of the latter is entirely different from the first two types. The diagnosis is not always easy, but as a rule it is characterized by a continuous bruit and thrill accentuated in systole, whereas in the spontaneous and false aneurysms there is a slight but distinct pause between the systolic and diastolic phases.

Fistulous communications between artery and vein comprise about one-fourth of all aneurysms of the peripheral vessels. In 104 operative cases in my own experience it occurred 28 times. It is usually the result of trauma but may rarely be congenital as it was in one patient of mine in whom a small communication existed between the common carotid and internal jugular vein (Fig. 3). The most common cause is a stab or bullet wound of an artery and vein which are closely incorporated in a common sheath. The femoral and carotid vessels are ideally situated in this respect and are the most commonly involved. However, any vessel may be the seat

*From the Department of Surgery, Emory University School of Medicine.

of the lesion, and in my patients it has been observed in the temporal, ophthalmic, subclavian, brachial, radial, digital and popliteal vessels.

William Hunter first described the condition in 1757.[1] He reported two instances of arteriovenous anastomosis in the brachial vessels produced by blood letting. He clearly recognized and accurately described the local clinical signs and stated that "blood passed immediately from the trunk of the artery into the trunk of the vein, and so back to the heart." In addition, he described the dilatation of the veins about the anastomosis and their pulsation, the dilatation of the artery above the lesion and its lessened size below it. Because the opening between the artery and vein was small, Hunter's two patients did not present, or he did not observe, the marked changes in the circulation which characterizes this condition.

Normally blood passes from the heart to artery, to capillary bed, to vein and back to the heart. If a fistula is present, the resistance is lowered and the blood is short-circuited from the artery directly to the vein without passing through the capillaries. The amount of blood so shunted into the vein and the effect upon the general circulation will be in direct proportion to the size of the fistula. In any event not all the blood will pass through the fistula but some will pass normally into the capillaries. Depending upon the size of the fistula, its location and duration, certain effects upon the heart, the blood pressure, the pulse rate, the peripheral circulation distal and proximal to the fistula, the surface temperature, and the collateral circulation have long been noted. Numerous clinical and experimental observations of this condition have been recorded in the literature since Hunter's observation, the chief contributors being Nicoladoni, Branham, Matas, Halsted, Reid and Holman.

The Effect on the Heart

Following the establishment of a fistula, the heart dilates and the extent of the dilatation will depend upon the size of the opening and its duration. In large fistulas the increase in the size of the heart takes place rapidly and eventually results in cardiac failure. The exact mechanism responsible for the dilatation and hypertrophy are not known, but follow-

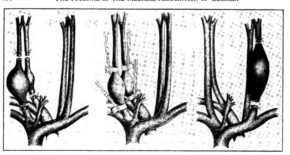

FIG. 1.
Arteriovenous fistula, right common carotid—internal jugular, caused by stab wound. Treated by quadruple ligation and excision. Recovery.

FIG. 2.
Arteriovenous fistula, right common carotid—internal jugular. Treated by temporary ligation and excision of fistula and closure of wounds in artery and vein. Recovery.

FIG. 3.
Congenital arteriovenous fistula, left common carotid—internal jugular. Treated by excision of vein and suture of wound in artery. Recovery.

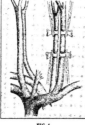
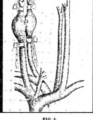
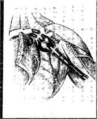

FIG. 4.
Arteriovenous fistula, left common carotid—internal jugular. Treated by temporary ligation and closure of wounds in artery and vein. Recovery.

FIG. 5.
Arteriovenous fistula, right common carotid. Treated by temporary ligation and closure of wounds in artery and vein. Recovery.

FIG. 6.
Arteriovenous fistula, left axillary from bullet wound. Treated by quadruple ligation and excision. Recovery.

ing excision of the communication the heart soon returns to its normal sizè (Fig. 23). Holman[2] has shown in arteriovenous communications experimentally produced that there is an actual increase in the blood volume, and it has long been observed clinically that there is an increase in the pulse rate. With the closure of the fistula the blood volume and the pulse rate return to normal limits. There is likewise an increase in cardiac output, which returns to normal with closure of the communication. This increase in cardiac output,

the tachycardia and the increased blood volume are due to the imposition on the heart of additional peripheral system, and the dilatation and hypertrophy are probably the result of the increased work the heart is called upon to perform. Reid[3] believes that other factors may be responsible, and calls attention to the fact that "cardiac changes are always associated with dilatation of the proximal portion of the involved artery." He also pointed out that "demand of the part beyond it (i. e., the fistula) for a better blood

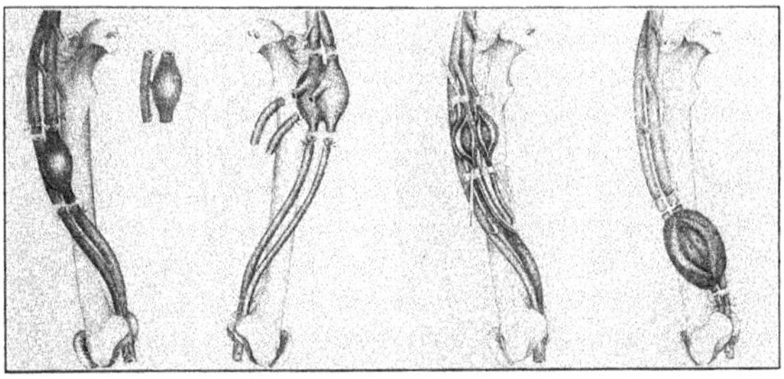

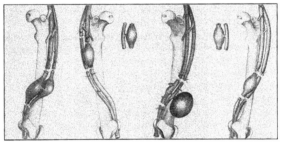

FIG. 7.
Arteriovenous fistula, right femoral, from bullet wound. Treated by quadruple ligation and excision. Recovery.

FIG. 8.
Arteriovenous fistula, left femoral. Treated by quadruple ligation and excision and ligation of profunda artery and vein. Recovery.

FIG. 9.
Arteriovenous fistula, profunda femoris. Treated by temporary ligation and closure of the openings in artery and vein. Recovery.

FIG. 10.
Arteriovenous fistula, right femoral. Treated by quadruple ligation and excision. Recovery.

FIG. 11.
Arteriovenous fistula, left femoral. Treated by quadruple ligation and excision. Recovery.

FIG. 12.
Arteriovenous fistula, right femoral. Treated by quadruple ligation and excision. Recovery.

FIG. 13.
Arteriovenous fistula, left femoral with secondary arterial aneurysm. Treated by quadruple ligation and excision and excision of the aneurysm. Recovery.

FIG. 14.
Arteriovenous fistula, right femoral. Treated by quadruple ligation and excision. Recovery.

supply may also be a factor in increasing the pulse rate."

Effect on the Blood Pressure and Pulse Rate

Holman has shown that following the experimental production of a fistula in a dog, there is a marked drop in the blood pressure and an increase in the pulse rate. The blood pressure returns to normal within a few days but a slight acceleration in the pulse rate remains. Immediate blood pressure changes have not been noted in clinical cases but the same phenomena of falling blood pressure and increased pulse rate probably occur. When seen weeks or years after the production of the fistula the patient's blood pressure is usually within normal limits. If the communication is closed by pressure there is an immediate rise in the systolic pressure, together with a slowing of the pulse. Both of these phenomena are temporary and persist for only a few seconds. The explanation for the rise in pressure is that with closure of the fistula the peripheral

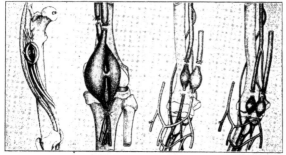

FIG. 15.
Arteriovenous fistula, profunda femoris. Treated by proximal ligation of artery and vein. Improvement but recurrence of aneurysm.

FIG. 16.
Arteriovenous fistula, right popliteal. Treated by quadruple ligation and excision. Recovery, but patient developed a spontaneous aneurysm of the femoral artery three years later.

FIG. 17.
Arteriovenous fistula, right brachial. Treated by quadruple ligation and excision. Recovery.

FIG. 18.
Arteriovenous fistula, right brachial. Treated by quadruple ligation and excision. Recovery.

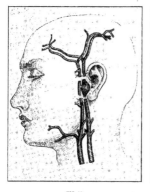
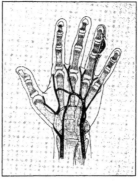

FIG. 19.
Arteriovenous fistula, right temporal. Treated by quadruple ligation and excision. Recovery.

FIG. 20.
Arteriovenous fistula, digital. Treated by quadruple ligation and excision. Recovery.

resistance is raised since the blood is shunted through the capillary bed. The drop in pulse rate is probably brought about through the reflex vagal action when the pressure rises in the aorta. Lewis and Drury[4] found that it was abolished by atropinization, but I have not been able to abolish it, although I have tried to do so in five instances by giving one-thirtieth grain of atropine. This drop in pulse rate is characteristic of arteriovenous fistula

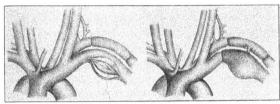

FIG. 21.
Arteriovenous fistula, left subclavian. Treated by ligation of artery and closure of wounds in artery and vein and obliteration of venous sac. Recovery.

FIG. 22.
Arteriovenous fistula, left subclavian. Patient died suddenly on the operating table when the artery and vein were ligated, probably due to acute cardiac failure.

and is of diagnostic value since it does not occur when blood is occluded from a spontaneous or traumatic aneurysm. The phenomenon was first described by Nicoladoni[5] in 1875, and later, but independently, by Branbam[6] in 1890.

Effect on the Blood Vessels

William Hunter noted that the artery proximal to the fistula was enlarged but that distal to the fistula it was smaller than normal. He also mentioned the enlargement of the veins. This observation has been confirmed many times and occurs almost invariably if the fistula is large. The arterial dilatation may extend as far back as the heart, but the venous enlargement is most marked near the fistula, both proximal and distal to it. It is probably due, as Holman[2] thinks, to the "greatly increased blood mass which accumulates in the shorter circuit by virtue of the decreased peripheral resistance at the site of the fistula." The dilatation of the veins is due to the increased pressure in them. Reid[3] is of the opinion that the arterial enlargement is due to degenerative changes plus the increased work and stress thrown upon the vessels. This arterial degeneration may lead to the formation of a spontaneous aneurysm as occurred to two of my patients. In one (Fig. 13) an aneurysm developed near the site of a femoral arterial fistula and eventually ruptured. In another (Fig. 16) an aneurysm developed in the femoral artery three years after excision of an arteriovenous fistula of the popliteal vessels.

Effect on the Collateral Circulation

There is no condition which produces such collateral circulation as an arteriovenous aneu-

rysm. However, this circulation is for the most part useless since most of the blood in the collateral vessels passes back through the fistula without nourishing the part beyond. The amount of collateral circulation will depend on the size of the opening and upon its duration. Fistulas of long standing usually produce a network of vessels about the fistula which make the operation extremely difficult and tedious. While this circulation is of little value when the fistula is open, it means that the operation can be done without the fear of producing gangrene, provided sufficient length of time is allowed for the development of the circulation. The collateral circulation is so great that the surface temperature in the part beyond is usually raised above that of the normal corresponding part when the fistula is excised. For example, the circulation in the foot after excision of a popliteal aneurysm is as good, or even better, than that of the opposite foot.

Treatment

The effect on the heart, general circulation and the part affected, demands that an arteriovenous fistula be eliminated. The manner of obliteration is of importance because if the operation is incompletely done, recurrence is sure to take place. The time of operation is likewise of importance. In general it should be as early as possible after collateral circulation has been established. This, as a rule, will not be more than two or three months and by that time the wound causing the fistula will have completely healed and the danger of infection will have passed.

On theoretical grounds it would seem best to repair the opening in both the artery and

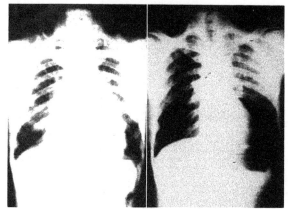

FIG. 23a.   FIG. 23b.
Teleoroentgenograms of patient shown in Fig. 7. Note cardiac hypertrophy with return of heart to normal size
one month after operation

vein but this is technically difficult and with such a procedure there is always the liability of a recurrence. Since the collateral circulation is of such abundance, quadruple ligation of the artery and vein with complete excision is the method of choice.

The operation should be carried out with the greatest care because of the large number of vessels and because their thinness and friability may lead to uncontrollable hemorrhage. With the obliteration of the fistula a sudden load is thrown upon the heart because of the increased blood volume. This may lead to sudden heart failure and death, as happened in one of my cases (Fig. 22). This eventuality may be overcome if, as Holman suggested, venesection be performed at the time of operation and 500 cc. to 1,000 cc. of blood withdrawn. Because of cardiac damage the patient should have a long period of rest following operation.

Conclusions

1. Fistulous communications between artery and vein comprise about one-fourth of all aneurysms of the peripheral vessels.

2. Unlike true aneurysms, arteriovenous communications produce effects upon the heart, general circulation and the part involved, which are dangerous or even fatal.

3. Differentiation from other types is important because of the difference in treatment.

4. The fistula should be obliterated, preferably by quadruple ligation and excision as soon as sufficient collateral circulation has developed to nourish the part.

BIBLIOGRAPHY

1. Hunter, William: Med. Obs. Soc. Phys., London, 1:323, 1757.
2. Holman, Emil: The Recognition and Treatment of Arteriovenous Communications, Internat. Clin., 4:154, 1934.
3. Reid, Mont. R.: Abnormal Arteriovenous Communications. Acquired and Congenital, Arch. Surg., 11:25, 1925.
4. Lewis, Thomas, and Drury, A. N.: Observations Relating to Arteriovenous Aneurysms, Heart, 10:301, 1923.
5. Nicoladoni, quoted by Lewis, Dean: Lancet, 2:621, 1930.
6. Branham, H. M.: Aneurysmal Varix of the Femoral Artery and Vein Following a Gunshot Wound, Internat. J. Surg., 3:250, 1890.

One looks on at the busy clinic with its not-so-poor looking, able-to-buy-lottery-tickets clientele, and at the long lines of that clientele's waiting cars stretching for blocks on every side of the hospital. One shudders a bit.

The scene changes and we look into the empty private offices of the same clinic doctors.—*Medical Times*, *Sept. 1936*.

THE CONSERVATIVE MANAGE-
MENT OF ECLAMPSIA*

E. D. COLVIN, M.D.
R. A. BARTHOLOMEW, M.D.
Atlanta

In Georgia, 438 women died of puerperal causes during 1935. It is a shameful fact that 142, or 32.4 per cent, of these deaths were complicated by eclamptic toxemia.

In an investigation of deaths in eclamptic women, by the Committee on Maternal Mortaliay of the State Medical Association, the following facts deserve attention: Sixty-nine per cent of the women were less than 26 years of age; 76 per cent were pregnant for the first time; 87 per cent had reached the eighth month of gestation; 19 per cent died undelivered; 62 per cent started into labor spontaneously; 68 per cent had received no prenatal care or instructions; 58 per cent died in their homes and 38 per cent were delivered by some form of operative procedure. The fetal mortality was 45 per cent.

With the above facts in mind, we must confess that our entire set-up for providing maternal care to the women of our State is inadequate.

Why do so many women die of eclampsia? The disease is of unknown etiology, yet enough is known of its clinical features to make it almost preventable and to a certain extent controllable. The statistics reported from well-organized obstetric clinics prove this claim. The chief reasons for such a high death rate in this State are:

1. There is poor cooperation on the part of the laity, due to a lack of appreciation of the importance of prenatal care.

2. The medical profession fails too often to discover the onset of pre-eclampsia, on account of indifferent prenatal supervision and a failure to manage it intelligently after it has been discovered.

3. Too frequently pregnancies or labors, complicated by toxemia, are terminated by operative interference.

4. We are in need of adherence to a more uniform, standardized, conservative treatment for pre-eclampsia and eclampsia.

*From the Department of Obstetrics, Emory University School of Medicine, Emory University.

Without lay cooperation the profession can make little headway in its efforts to lower the mortality of eclampsia. The public must be more strongly urged to seek and insist on proper prenatal care. It becomes our duty to impress upon the public the importance of this care through education and establishment of more prenatal clinics.

Too often there is a lack of understanding of just what is necessary in rendering prenatal care, and a lack of willingness and conscientious effort in carrying it out. A physician must be able to recognize the symptoms and signs of developing toxemia. He should spare no time in close observation of its course, once it has manifested itself. At the crossroads he must be capable and willing to choose the right course of management.

Without a doubt, many patients with preeclampsia have been permitted to develop eclampsia while the attendants hopefully pursued a course of watchful expectancy. Often we place entirely too much emphasis on the life of an unborn, premature fetus, in attempting to carry a pre-eclamptic mother nearer to term. Its life is always problematic, and still more so if the mother should develop eclampsia. On the other hand, there are still some physicians who, with scapel and instruments in hand, cannot be impressed with the known fact that toxemic patients are not good surgical risks. Time after time, the Committee on Maternal Mortality of the MEDICAL ASSOCIATION OF GEORGIA reviewed the records of women in the throes of convulsions,—in shock, who were rushed into nearby hospitals and immediately delivered by cesarean section. Some of them 'lived; too many of them died.

An enormous volume of literature has developed on the treatment of eclampsia. The death rate remains too high, though considerable reduction has been brought about by the gradual abandonment of operative procedures and the substitution of a conservative type of therapy. The average maternal mortality is still about 20 per cent; for the fetus 20 to 30 per cent. In the mother it is far lower when she is delivered prior to the onset of convulsions.

The ideal management of eclampsia should begin during the prenatal stage of pregnancy. In severe, or rapidly advancing toxemias, labor should be induced prior to the onset of convulsions. The presence of convulsions greatly increase the mortality and complicates the management of the condition.

The cardinal manifestations of toxemia of pregnancy and the order of their appearance are listed below. The appearance of any one, or combination of these symptoms and signs, should tell the attendant that "something is wrong" and attract his attention to a careful study and observation of the patient.

1. *Elevation of Blood Pressure*—The earliest sign of a developing toxemia is usually an elevation of the diastolic level. At this time or within a short while the systolic pressure begins to rise. As a rule, the systolic elevation is much more rapid in ascent, but is followed by a gradual rise of the diastolic pressure. The rise may be slow and constant over a period of several weeks; in other patients it may come with great speed, an increase of 30 to 40 mm. in systolic and 10 to 20 mm. in diastolic pressure within one week.

The presence of a gradual elevation or persistent high diastolic blood pressure during the last two months of pregnancy is sufficient reason to suspect developing toxemia. It should serve as an indication for more frequent observations, to determine if and when labor should be induced.

2. *Urinary Changes*—Some degree of albuminuria is a fairly constant finding in the presence of pre-eclampsia. As a rule, it appears as a faint trace shortly after the beginning of the elevation of the blood pressure. It varies from a faint trace in early toxemia to a degree of boiling solid in advanced toxemia. The change from a cloudy to a flocculent precipitate usually indicates that the toxemia is approaching dangerous ground. In general, the amount of albumin rises in direct ratio to the elevation of the blood pressure. Albuminuria, in the presence of an elevating blood pressure, is always indicative of the onset of toxemia. The amount of urine voided is usually decreased. It may contain casts, especially in the presence of chronic nephritis.

3. *Edema or Swelling*—When swelling of the lower extremities is present upon arising in the morning and extends well up the legs, it usually is an indication of the presence of a toxemia, rather than a manifestation of pressure from the enlarging uterus. This is especially true when the edema affects the upper part of the body—the hands and face. The amount of edema is not a fair index to the degree of toxemia present. Occasionally there are cases of severe toxemia in which little or no edema is present.

4. *Rapid Gain of Weight*—This is due largely to the accumulation of fluids in the edematous tissues and to a lack of dietary control. A too rapid gain of weight during the last two months of pregnancy should arouse suspicion of impending toxemia.

5. *Headache*—This symptom usually develops after the blood pressure has become elevated and a heavy trace of albumin has appeared in the urine. It is usually the symptom that causes the unattended patient to seek the attention of a physician. Its presence, in late pregnancy, warrants further investigation as to the presence of toxemia.

Space will not permit a discussion of other important clinical, laboratory and retinal symptoms and signs associated with pre-eclampsia. More will be accomplished by stressing the early symptoms and signs of toxemia at a time when eclampsia may be prevented than by emphasizing its terminal ones, at a time when convulsions handicap our efforts.

A pregnant woman should be examined by her physician at least once a month during the first seven months, and every two weeks during the remainder of her pregnancy. The appearance of any one of the above-mentioned symptoms and signs is evidence of beginning toxemia and is an indication for more frequent observations — three to five day intervals if necessary.

Some patients with toxemia, if treated early by rest, diet and measures to increase elimination, will show a reduction of the blood pressure, a decrease in the degree of albuminuria and edema along with a disappearance of symptoms. This type of patient should be kept under careful observation and may be permitted to continue her pregnancy. If the signs and symptoms do not abate under this plan of treatment—and in the great majority they do not—a different type of therapy must be instituted.

It is often difficult to designate the exact time when the pregnancy must be terminated. One must consider carefully the degree of severity of each of the signs and symptoms. As a rule, a systolic pressure of 150 mm. or a diastolic pressure of 95 mm. necessitate a termination of the pregnancy. A rising blood pressure, accompanied by an increasing albuminuria, persistent edema and headache, in spite of expectant treatment, indicates that the toxemia is increasing. Time must not be lost in getting the patient into labor, otherwise convulsions may occur. Many times a sympathetic attendant will delay the induction of labor, hoping to obtain a more mature fetus. If convulsions develop during this time, he has gambled and will often lose both mother and baby. If she survive, her vascular system, kidneys and other vital tissues have possibly been permanently damaged by the presence of the toxins within her system.

In the presence of eclamptic convulsions, the management of the condition is much more complicated. Treatment is based upon the following essentials, listed in the order of their need: 1. The patient must be protected from body injury during periods of convulsions and unconsciousness; 2. the convulsions must be controlled; 3. labor must be induced if not already established; 4. toxins must be diluted and eliminated; and finally, 5. supportive treatment, particularly to the heart, must be maintained.

From the Obstetrical Clinic of Dr. James R. McCord, in the Emory University Colored Division of Grady Hospital, there comes the report of only ten deaths in the treatment of 148 consecutive patients with eclampsia—a remarkably low mortality rate of 6.7 per cent. This therapy, a conservative one, consists of the use of morphine, magnesium sulphate and intravenous glucose solution, followed by the induction of labor if it has not already begun.

From Dr. McCord's report, certain outstanding facts warrant our consideration. They serve as an example to illustrate what could be accomplished throughout this State if we, as physicians, would follow this technic. Analysis of his report shows that 123 patients, or 86 per cent, delivered spontaneously. Only two cesarean sections were performed. Both of these were done prior to Jan., 1928, and for indications other than the toxemia. Eighteen forceps operations, including fourteen low, and four mid types, were performed, and all except two, for definite indications other than the eclampsia.

Seventy-six per cent of the babies were alive when discharged from the hospital. This fact supports McCord's opinion that eclamptics too often are subjected to dangerous and unnecessary operative risks in the interest of the baby. However, he states that 24 per cent of these were premature infants and that an increased neonatal or infant mortality would be expected in this group of babies.

The technic of the morphine, magnesium sulphate and glucose treatment of eclampsia is as follows: As soon as the eclamptic patient is seen, disregard temporarily the fact that she is pregnant. First, give a quarter or half grain of morphine sulphate hypodermically, ac-cording to the size of the woman and the severity of the convulsions. An attendant, constantly at her side, protects her tongue and prevents body injury during convulsions. Immediately following the morphine, give 20 cc. of 10 per cent solution of magnesium sulphate intravenously. Repeat this every hour until the convulsions are controlled. Usually by the time the second or third dose of magnesium sulphate has been given, the convulsions will have ceased. Thereafter, additional doses of 20 cc. of the 10 per cent solution of magnesium sulphate are given deep in the gluteal muscles at intervals of one to two hours. Very rarely does an eclamptic require the upper limit of six or seven doses of magnesium sulphate within twenty-four hours before the convulsions are controlled.

Magnesium sulphate, obtainable in 20 cc. ampules of 10 per cent strength, can be secured from all reliable pharmaceutical firms. It is inexpensive, does not deteriorate and can be carried in one's bag. It is the sheet anchor in the treatment of eclampsia through its action as a sedative to involuntary muscle fibers; in removing fluid from the edematous brain, thus diminishing the coma; in drawing fluids from the water-logged tissues, and increasing the elimination through the kidneys.

As soon as the convulsions are controlled, 300 cc. of 25 per cent glucose solution are given intravenously and this should be repeated every eight hours until the patient is definitely improved. The water used must be freshly distilled and the solution injected very slowly, otherwise a reaction may occur. Today, glucose in varying strengths can be purchased in 500 to 1,000 cc. ampules, ready for intravenous use.

If freshly distilled water or the large ampules are not obtainable, it is best to give the ampule of concentrated glucose (25 Gm. of glucose in 50 cc. of distilled water) directly into the vein without diluting it, and immediately thereafter give saline or 2 per cent glucose solution subcutaneously in 500 to 1,000 cc. injections. Fluids should be given by mouth or per rectum if the patient becomes conscious.

After the convulsions have been controlled, the induction of labor is the next important consideration. A safe, simple and most dependable way of inducing labor is by artificially rupturing the membranes. This must be done according to thorough antiseptic technic, bearing in mind that toxemia renders the patient more susceptible to infection. The vulva is shaved and thoroughly cleansed and the examining finger of the gloved hand pushed through the cervix, stripping the membranes from around the internal os. This procedure stimulates contractions and aids in the formation of a sac of fluid which is easier to rupture. By means of an amnion trocar, a dressing forceps or an open safety pin with bent point, the membranes are artificially ruptured. The presenting part is lifted slightly at intervals to permit 300 or 400 cc. of amniotic fluid to escape. The finger, held in the cervical canal during this time, prevents a gush of fluid and lessens the possibility of prolapse of a loop of cord. Following the rupture of the membranes, the patient is treated as a case of normal labor.

With the convulsions controlled, the magnesium sulphate is continued as indicated—not at hourly intervals. The glucose solution is given intravenously every eight hours until the convulsions are controlled and the patient's condition definitely improved. Fluids can be continued as previously mentioned.

As labor nears the end, the woman is given every chance to deliver spontaneously. Anesthesia should be very light. Operative interference should be withheld until definite indications arise. Fortunately, eclamptics usually have good uterine contractions and the duration of labor is usually less than is the average.

This method will save maternal lives. It can be used in the home as well as in hospital deliveries. Morphine and magnesium sulphate can be carried in the obstetric kit. Ampules of concentrated glucose can always be secured, if it is not possible to secure fresh distilled water for making solutions. Concentrated solutions of glucose must not be given outside of the vein.

This method is not always the easy way out of the difficulty and is not the short route, as compared with cesarean section, but it is simple and safer for the future as well as the present pregnancy. Any form of treatment of eclampsia that yields a maternal mortality rate of 6.7 per cent is well worth adoption. Without a doubt, this management of eclampsia would lower the maternal mortality of our State more than 25 per cent.

1040 Ponce de Leon Ave., N. E.

FACULTY—EMORY UNIVERSITY SCHOOL OF MEDICINE, 1936

W. LLOYD ADAMS	GEORGE W. FULLER
HERBERT S. ALDEN	WILLIAM L. FUNKHOUSER
EUSTACE A. ALLEN	ELIZABETH GAMBRELL
GORDON G. ALLISON	HORTENSE GARVER
WILLIAM W. ANDERSON	JAMES GASTON GAY
WILLIAM B. ARMSTRONG	T. BOLLING GAY
GEORGE BACHMANN	IRA M. GIBSON
M. K. BAILEY	GLENVILLE GIDDINGS
POPE BAKER	LAUREN H. GOLDSMITH
WILLIAM L. BALLENGER	WILLIAM S. GOLDSMITH
EVART A. BANCKER	WALTER C. GOODPASTURE
FORREST M. BARFIELD	EDGAR H. GREENE
HUGH H. BARFIELD	LON W. GROVE
CRAWFORD F. BARNETT	HOWARD HAILEY
RUDOLPH A. BARTHOLOMEW	JOHN HALDI
C. R. F. BEALL	CHARLES E. HALL, JR.
LEE BIVINGS	ALTON V. HALLUM
L. MINOR BLACKFORD	J. FLETCHER HANSON
CORBETT BLALOCK	MILLER T. HARRISON
HOMER BLINCOE	CHARLES W. HARWELL
FRANK K. BOLAND	EMMETT D. HIGHSMITH
F. KELLS BOLAND	JOSEPH H. HINES
EDGAR BOLING	FRED G. HODGSON
HAROLD M. BOWCOCK	LEWIS D. HOPPE
BENJAMIN H. BOYD	CHAMPNEYS H. HOLMES
JAMES N. BRAWNER, JR.	WALTER R. HOLMES
WILLIAM W. BRYAN	PATRICK M. HOWARD
ALLEN H. BUNCE	CONWAY HUNTER
TAYLOR S. BURGESS	EUGENE L. JACKSON
B. RUSSELL BURKE	ZACK W. JACKSON
EDWIN S. BYRD	JACK W. JONES
T. LUTHER BYRD	WILLIAM H. KISER, JR.
ABNER W. CALHOUN	GEORGE F. KLUGH, JR.
PHINIZY CALHOUN	ROY R. KRACKE
JAMES L. CAMPBELL	CLARENCE LAWS
DONALD F. CATHCART	ROY S. LEADINGHAM
AMEY CHAPPELL	GEORGE T. LEWIS
LEROY CHILDS	ALBERT O. LINCH
JAMES J. CLARK	PAUL E. LINEBACK
GRADY E. CLAY	MASON I. LOWANCE
BENJAMIN H. CLIFTON	ROBERT G. MCALILEY
HUGH COCHRAN	JAMES A. MCALLISTER
EMMETT D. COLVIN	JAMES R. MCCORD
ERNEST S. COLVIN	JAMES G. MCDANIEL
HERSCHEL C. CRAWFORD	CALHOUN MCDOUGALL
JOHN B. CROSS	WILLIAM L. MCDOUGALL
CHARLES W. DANIELS	JOSEPH L. MCGHEE
TOM FORREST DAVENPORT	A. PARK MCGINTY
HAL M. DAVISON	FLOYD W. MCRAE
THOMAS C. DAVISON	JAMES D. MARTIN, JR.
JOHN F. DENTON	JAMES J. MARTIN
J. HARRIS DEW	WILLIAM O. MARTIN
ROGER W. DICKSON	JOSEPH C. MASSEE
AVARY M. DIMMOCK	FREDERIC R. MINNICH
WARREN S. DOROUGH	WILLIAM R. MINNICH
MARK S. DOUGHERTY	CHARLES H. MITCHELL
WILLIAM M. DUNN	WILLIAM E. MITCHELL
DANIEL C. ELKIN	J. MERRELL MONFORT
MURDOCK EQUEN	S. LESLIE MORRIS
FRANK L. ESKRIDGE	HUGH G. MOSLEY
GEORGE F. EUBANKS	LEWIE H. MUSE
JAMES K. FANCHER	DEWEY T. NABORS
IRA A. FERGUSON	PHILIP H. NIPPERT
EDGAR F. FINCHER	GEORGE H. NOBLE
JOHN B. FITTS	JACK C. NORRIS

BOMAR A. OLDS
RUSSELL H. OPPENHEIMER
CHARLES H. PAINE
EVANGELINE PAPAGEORGE
FRANCIS P. PARKER
JAMES E. PAULLIN
SAMUEL W. PERRY
WELDON E. PERSON
HAYWARD S. PHILLIPS
D. HENRY POER
VERNON E. POWELL
MARION C. PRUITT
JOSEPH C. READ
HERBERT L. REYNOLDS
KEITH C. RICE
JEFFERSON L. RICHARDSON
JULIAN G. RILEY
CHARLES W. ROBERTS
M. HINES ROBERTS
STEWART R. ROBERTS
WILL ROBERTS
LISLE B. ROBINSON
CHARLES E. RUSHIN
H. CLIFF SAULS

WILLIAM A. SELMAN
EDGAR D. SHANKS
CARTER SMITH
LEWIS M. SMITH
RANDOLPH SMITH
WILLIAM A. SMITH
CECIL STOCKARD
CYRUS W. STRICKLER
CYRUS W. STRICKLER, JR.
COSBY SWANSON
HERBERT L. TREUSCH
WILLIAM H. TRIMBLE
CHARLES B. UPSHAW
EBERT VAN BUREN
JOHN VENABLE
GREEN D. WARREN
WILLIAM C. WARREN, JR.
J. CALVIN WEAVER
GEORGE A. WILLIAMS
RICHARD B. WILSON
R. HUGH WOOD
EDWARD S. WRIGHT
JOSEPH YAMPOLSKY
W. WALTER YOUNG

WANTED

A Used Static Machine in Good Condition. Moderately Priced. Give Description and Price. Write "C" care of THE JOURNAL.

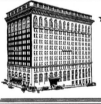

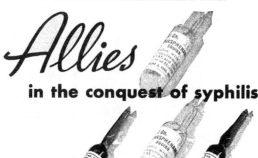

THE JOURNAL
OF THE
MEDICAL ASSOCIATION OF GEORGIA

DEVOTED TO THE WELFARE OF THE MEDICAL ASSOCIATION OF GEORGIA
PUBLISHED MONTHLY under direction of the Council

| Volume XXV | Atlanta, Ga., December, 1936 | Number 12 |

CHRONIC ARTHRITIS AND FIBROSITIS*

HAL M. DAVISON, M.D.
MASON I. LOWANCE, M.D.
CRAWFORD F. BARNETT, M.D.
Atlanta

Chronic arthritis has a low mortality rate, a little over one per one hundred thousand. Yet it is the greatest single cause of disability in temperate climates, and produces more prolonged suffering and greater economic loss than any other chronic disease.

A survey by the Metropolitan Life Insurance Company has shown[1] that 164.4 persons per hundred thousand suffer from some form of rheumatism, comprising nine per cent of all diseases recorded. This survey found only one-half as many cases of tuberculosis as of rheumatism, two-fifths as many cases of cerebral hemorrhage, and one-tenth as many of cancer.

From the standpoint both of human suffering and of economic loss, the duration of chronic arthritis is important. The average duration of illness from tuberculosis is three years, and from carcinoma only half that long, but the disability and suffering caused by chronic arthritis may last twenty or thirty years, or even longer. The estimated economic loss per year in the United States caused by chronic arthritis is two hundred million dollars. The human suffering to which this money loss is incident can not be estimated.

For a long time the treatment of arthritis was regarded as hopeless, but there has developed over the past few years a new interest and a brighter outlook. Pemberton et al.[2] state that, under the treatment outlined in their article, over 80 per cent of all patients with chronic arthritis should im-

prove, and Wyatt[3] states that 90 per cent of all patients can be helped.

In this paper we will limit our discussion to the chronic arthritides, and will use the classification adopted in 1928 by the American Committee for the Control of Rheumatism[5]:

CLASSIFICATION	Synonyms[a]
Atrophic Arthritis	Chronic proliferative,[a] Rheumatoid (British Ministry of Health and International League for the Control of Rheumatism) Infectious Still's disease (in childhood).
Hypertrophic Arthritis	Chronic degenerative,[a] Osteo-arthritis (British Ministry of Health and the International League for the Control of Rheumatism) Spondylitis
Fibrositis	Myositis Muscular rheumatism Torticollis Lumbago

The pathologic changes in the development of atrophic arthritis may be divided into several different processes which may take place separately or conjointly.

1. The synovial membrane of the joint takes on the property of marked proliferation, produces a layer of granulation tissue which extends over the margins of the articular cartilage as a pannus layer.

2. At the same time, there is a proliferation of the perichondrium of the articular cartilage.

These two processes may destroy and absorb part or all of the articular cartilage, leaving in its place a thick layer of fibrous tissue.

3. In the marrow spaces beneath the joint surfaces, there is a proliferation of connective tissue with the formation of vascular granulation tissue, which undermines and destroys the articular cartilage from below.

*Read before the Medical Association of Georgia, Savannah, April 23, 1936.

4. Following this process, there may be a proliferation of the endosteum of the marrow spaces, with the formation of new trabeculae which extend upward with the granulation tissue of the marrow into the cartilage of the joint surface, and form new bone.

These processes may affect both joint surfaces, and fuse, causing ankylosis of the joint. If the process in the synovial membrane predominates, fibrous ankylosis results; if the process from the marrow predominates, the result is bony ankylosis.

Following this partial or complete ankylosis, the bones become lighter and the trabeculae smaller and less numerous, due to disuse of the joint; therefore, the term *atrophic arthritis*.

In atrophic arthritis and Still's disease, there are at times found subcutaneous nodules varying from 2 mm. to 2 cm. in diameter.[6] These nodules are very similar to, if not identical with, those found in rheumatic fever, and suggest a relationship between these diseases. These nodules are most often found on the dorsal surface of the forearm but may be found in other parts of the body, especially on the hands, knees, over the sacrum, and in the scalp.

The pathologic changes in hypertrophic arthritis begin with a fibrillation of the cartilaginous matrix, followed by a splitting and softening of the articular cartilage. This finally causes erosion, resulting in exposure of the underlying bone. The process is usually localized, but may be general and extend over the entire joint surface. On the opposite joint surface there occurs a compensatory overgrowth to keep the joint surfaces in contact. At the junction of the capsule and cartilage there may be increased activity of the perichondrium, resulting in the formation of new cartilage or bone in the form of lipping or of Heberden's nodes. The denuded bone becomes dense and highly polished, and is described as *eburnated* bone.

Beneath the joint there is a diminution of trabeculae and at times the formation of small mucoid cysts. The synovial membrane is usually thickened, at times forming villous granulations which may calcify and break off to form osteophytes.

While motion may be painful and markedly limited, the process in hypertrophic arthritis never continues to the point of complete ankylosis.

The pathologic process in chronic fibrositis begins with a localized cellular infiltration, together with a serous or serofibrinous exudate in the fibrous tissue and between the muscle bundles. Later, new fibrous tissue forms, which contracts and causes circumscribed or diffuse indurations. Pressure may interfere with circulation and cause atrophy of the muscles involved and replacement by fibrous tissue.[8]

Diagnosis

Atrophic arthritis most frequently occurs between the ages of fifteen and fifty, in long, thin individuals who are often undernourished and anemic.

The process usually begins with a bilateral, symmetric involvement of the smaller joints of the hands and feet, producing a fusiform enlargement of the phalanges. There are pain and stiffness in the morning, which disappear upon activity. The pains may be migratory. The patient complains of headache, malaise and anorexia, and there is usually a slight fever.

The skin is atrophic, glossy, and the extremities are cold and clammy. The process is progressive and may spread to any joint. There is limitation of joint movements, with pain, stiffness and swelling. Muscular atrophy appears early, and continues in proportion to the duration and extent of the disease. The condition may remain static, or may progressively advance to the stage of marked deformity and complete ankylosis. In females there may be marked improvement during pregnancy with continuance of symptoms after delivery.

Laboratory Findings

There is usually an anemia and a slight leukocytosis. The blood sedimentation rate is usually 30 mm. or more in one hour.[9] The glucose tolerance test in a large percentage of cases shows a retarded elimination of glucose from the blood, the blood glucose in some cases reaching 250 mg. per cent. This is supposed to be caused by changes in the smaller blood vessels and arterioles in the muscles and in and about the joints, retarding the utilization of blood glucose by the muscles.

NORMAL JOINT
DIAGRAM OF VERTICAL SECTION

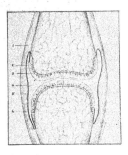

KEY: 1. Fibrous Capsule; 2 Articular Cartilage; 3. Zone of Provisional Calcification; 4. Joint Cavity; 5. Synovial Membrane; 6. Trabeculae.

Fig. 1

HYPERTROPHIC ARTHRITIS
DIAGRAM OF DISEASED JOINT

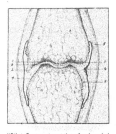

KEY: 1. Erosion of cartilage to eburnated bone on articular surface; 2. Lipping-new growth of bone at periphery of joint 3. Eburnated bone due to endosteal thickening of original trabeculae; 4. Cartilage shows only at margins of joint 5. Moderate thickening of capsule; 6. Synovial membrane thickened with granulation tissue, which calcifies.

Fig. 2

The blood serum usually shows a positive agglutination test in a high titre to several different strains of hemolytic streptococci.[10] The histamine reaction is delayed or absent.

Hypertrophic arthritis occurs most frequently after the age of forty-five, or in women after the menopause. The patient is usually well developed, healthy, and often obese.

The onset is gradual, and there are no migratory pains. The joint involvement is often asymmetric, and the process as a whole is less generalized than in the atrophic type. The larger, weight-bearing joints, most often the knees, are affected early. In the beginning, there is slight enlargement of the joints, which may later increase, the joint becoming irregular in shape. Heberden's nodes are often found. Ankylosis is rare, and never complete.

The muscles and skin rarely show changes. There is no fever, seldom any blood changes; the agglutination tests are negative; the sedimentation rate is usually 20 mm. or less in one hour, and there is usually no change from the normal glucose tolerance curve.

In gout, or chronic metabolic arthritis, the attacks in a large percentage of cases, begin with pain or swelling in one or both great toes. The typical patient is in middle life, and gives a history of a high purine diet and a moderate but chronic use of alcohol. There is usually a history of recurrent joint symptoms, with complete remission between attacks. Later, other joints of the lower extremities and joints of the hands become involved, and tophi are present in the toes, fingers, ears and about the olecranon bursae.

In almost all cases there is an increase of uric acid in the blood, impairment of renal function, and x-ray examination shows "punched out" areas about the affected joints.

Symptoms are usually relieved quickly by placing the patient on a diet low in purines and free of alcohol. The administration of Colchicum and salicylates hastens recovery.

Chronic mixed arthritis occurs not infrequently. Usually there are found hypertrophic changes in the knees, lower extremities, or spine, while atrophic changes are found in the upper extremities. In some patients a hypertrophic arthritis is imposed on a preceding atrophic arthritis in the same joint.

Tuberculous arthritis most often simulates atrophic arthritis, but the involvement is usually confined to one large, weight-bearing joint, and the process is usually slow.

The sedimentation rate is rarely above 15 mm. to 20 mm. in one hour, and the tuberculin test is usually positive. Examination of the joint fluid for tubercle bacilli, guinea pig injection, or biopsy may be necessary to establish definitely the diagnosis.

In *gonococcic arthritis*, there is usually a demonstrable gonococcic infection in the patient or history of a recent infection. A large joint is usually involved alone at first, though the process may spread later to other joints. The onset is sudden, the temperature higher, and the pain greater than in cases of atrophic arthritis.

Intermittent hydrorthrosis is characterized by a periodic effusion into a joint cavity, usually the knee, and most often the right one. It may last four or five days, with intervals of about twelve days between attacks. The cause is unknown, but trauma appears to play a part. Certain cases are apparently allergic, possibly caused by sensitization to foods.

In *acute rheumatic fever*, the onset is as a rule much more acute than that of atrophic arthritis. There is usually a history of acute infection just prior to attacks. Symptoms tend to migrate from joint to joint, but the affected joints in most cases are not those initially affected by atrophic arthritis, nor are there the typical fusiform changes of the phalanges. The fever is higher, and there is a tendency to cardiac involvement. The disease runs a course of about four weeks, and leaves no permanent signs in the joints. Salicylates are of marked value in the treatment.

Joint involvement of specific origin, such as hemophilic arthritis, suppurative arthritis (pneumococcic, staphylococcic, streptococcic), typhoid arthritis, luetic arthritis, may be diagnosed by history and laboratory findings and treated accordingly.

Etiology

Since there are great differences in the pathologic changes in atrophic and hypertrophic arthritis, it is likely that distinctly different causative factors must be involved. Etiologic factors may be primary or secondary.

Secondary etiologic factors in both types:

Heredity: Heredity apparently plays but little part.

Sex: More females than males suffer from atrophic arthritis, with an approximate ratio of two to one.

In hypertrophic arthritis the sex incidence is about equal.

Mental factors: Attacks of either type of arthritis often appear after psychic or emotional upsets.

Endocrines: In some cases, disturbance of various endocrines appear to predispose to arthritic attacks. Hypothyroidism and the changes of the menopause appear to play a part in the causation of hypertrophic arthritis. Hyperthyroidism seems to be a factor in some cases of atrophic arthritis.

Physical agents: Fatigue, trauma and chronic exposure to wet and cold play a part.

Mechanical factors: Obesity, faulty posture, occupational injuries and prolonged or repeated strain on special joints predispose to hypertrophic arthritis.

Age: Senile changes produce alteration in the blood supply, cause undernutrition of joint structures, thereby predisposing to hypertrophic arthritis.

Primary Causes

In atrophic arthritis, the tissue reactions are inflammatory in nature, and therefore presumably infectious in origin.[10 11 12 13 14 15] It is impossible to review in this paper the enormous volume of literature on the subject. Practically all investigators agree, however, that the process is infectious in origin, focal infections being responsible in the great majority of cases. The reports of observers vary as to the percentage of sources of the infection from different parts of the body, but all agree that infected tonsils rank first, and infection about the teeth, either apical abscess or pyorrhea, second. Other sources of infection are the sinuses, the colon, the gallbladder, the prostate and seminal vesicles, the cervix and uterus, the pharynx, the middle

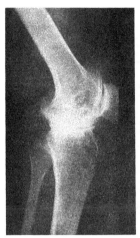

Fig. 3
Atrophic arthritis of knee joint.

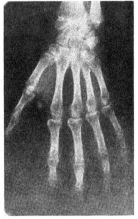

Fig. 4
Atrophic arthritis of hand.

ear, the appendix, the fallopian tubes, the kidneys (pyelitis), and diverticula of the colon. Often two or more foci are active causes at the same time.

Much experimental work has been done in an effort to determine the organisms responsible for this type of rheumatism. Many different strains of streptococci have been cultivated from the foci of infection, from the blood of the patients, from glands found near affected joints, and from the joints themselves[16 17 18 19 20]. Many workers have found that the blood serum of these patients agglutinates many different strains of streptococci in a high titre, there being no specificity for any one strain. Opinions and findings vary, but the evidence is in favor of the idea that different strains of streptococcus viridins and streptococcus hemolyticus probably cause atrophic arthritis.

Zinsser[21] believes that acute rheumatic fever, atrophic arthritis and fibrositis are all allergic reactions caused by sensitization to

the bacterial antigens, disintegration products form foci of infection. Freiburg and Dorst[22] believe that there is an infectious arthritis with bacteria active in the joints, and that there also exists an allergic arthritis produced by sensitivity to bacterial products from distant foci in the body and without active organisms in the joints.

In chronic hypertrophic arthritis, the changes are primarily degenerative in character, presumably caused by changes occurring with age and affecting the nutrition of joint structures. Some[23] have advanced evidence to show that bacteria also play a role in the production of this type of arthritis. Others[24] have called attention to the frequent occurrence of amebic dysentery in these patients. The most accepted etiologic theory, however, is that the pathologic changes are produced by trauma to the weight-bearing joints from obesity, together with the accessory cause of arterial aging, altered blood supply, lowered nutrition to joint structures, colonic toxemia, endocrine disturbance[25] and, possibly infection.

Patients who have never shown evidence of arthritis may have joint involvement during the period of immobilization in casts or splints. This involvement may not be confined to the joint immobilized, but may include other joints in the same extremity. In other words, inactivity of joints tends to favor the development of the disease.[33] The appearance of the joints involved is similar to that described under atrophic arthritis, but lipping and proliferation of bone do occur, so the process may be classified as a mixed type of arthritis. This condition is practically never seen in patients under twenty years of age, but occurs with increasing frequency in proportion to the age of the patient. We have seen a similar condition occurring in hemiplegic joints.

The majority of opinions favor the theory of the infectious origin of fibrositis, identical with that of atrophic arthritis.[3 36] Other theories are that certain apparently fibrositic manifestations, especially lumbago, may be gout[37 38], that fibrositis may be toxic in origin, caused by toxins absorbed from the bowels or from infectious foci, and that the fibrositis is caused by histamine absorbed from the intestines.

TREATMENT

Preventive Measures

1. Education of the public in relation to:
   (a) The economic and social importance of chronic arthritis.
   (b) Predisposing factors, their removal and prevention:
   Mental hygiene, physical hygiene, unnecessary exposure, prompt relief of effects of necessary exposure, proper air and sun; dry, properly heated dwellings; care of the teeth, prompt treatment of infections, care of the colon, proper diet, especially in middle life, maintenance of proper weight, proper posture.
2. Industrial hygiene leading to the prevention of unnecessary chronic trauma to joints and of unnecessary exposure in work.

Early Diagnosis

Wyatt[3] makes the statement that of all the factors entering into the successful treatment of the chronic arthritides, early diagnosis is the most important. The length of time allowed to elapse between the onset of symptoms and the beginning of treatment will greatly influence the result of any therapy applied. Early diagnoses are dependent upon careful histories and examinations, including thorough physical examinations with such laboratory and x-ray examinations as may be necessary.

Removal of Causes

The causes of chronic arthritis may be divided into *bacterial, chemical or metabolic,* and *mechanical.*

There seems little doubt that the chief cause of atrophic arthritis is bacterial infection, and the experience of many physicians proves that the early removal of foci of infection effects a cure in a large percentage of cases, at times without other treatment. In hypertrophic arthritis this is seldom the case. Removal of infectious foci seldom affects to any marked degree the course of the disease and other treatment is necessary. However, frank foci of infection should always be removed when possible, even in gout, because of the effect on the general health of the patient, and because infection may be the provocative factor in the beginning of any type of arthritis.

Focal infections in the tonsils and about the teeth are by far more important than all others. The history of repeated infections in the tonsils, enlarged tonsils, congestion of the pillars or of the tonsils themselves, the presence of bacteria or pus in the crypts, and enlargement of the associated lymph glands are said to be aids in the diagnosis of infected tonsils. It is our impression from numerous examinations of tonsils before and after operation that there is no sure way of diagnosing infection in a tonsil, and that in cases of atrophic arthritis all tonsils should be removed, but that in all other types of chronic arthritis, they should not be removed unless the preponderance of evidence indicates actual infection.

Focal infections about the teeth can usually be demonstrated by a careful examination by a competent dentist or by x-ray. At times, small infected areas behind a tooth root may not be diagnosed by x-ray. A tooth with more than one root will at times give a "live" reaction, though one of the nerves may be dead and a definite infection exist.

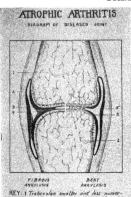

KEY: 1 Trabeculae smaller and less numerous than in normal bone; 2. Capsule slightly thickened; 3. Pannus of granulation tissue arising from synovial membrane. 4 Fibrous adhesions partially obliterating joint cavity; 5. Bony adhesions, cartilage entirely disappeared.

Fig. 5

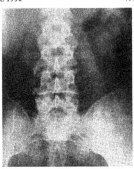

Fig. 6
Hypertrophic arthritis of spine.

Non-vital teeth with a partially and therefore improperly filled root canal are always a possible source of infection, even when no x-ray evidence of infection is presented. Teeth about which absorption of the alveolar process by pyorrhea has advanced beyond the bifurcation of the roots always hold the possibility of active infection. Wholesale extraction of teeth is never indicated, but in the case of the teeth, as with the tonsils, proven infection should always be eradicated for the benefit of the patient's general health, and in all cases of atrophic arthritis, all suspicious teeth should be sacrificed.

All other possible foci of infection, in addition to teeth and tonsils, should be sought and eradicated.

It must be said that some cases of all types of arthritis do recover at times in the presence of focal infection, and other cases recover in which no focus of infection was ever demonstrated.[29] It is evident, therefore, that increasing the general body resistance, making the general health better, and

the use of other therapeutic measures may be efficacious.

The removal of chemical or metabolic causes of chronic arthritis consists mainly of dieting, of the care of the colon, and the treatment of concurrent endocrine disorders. These will be more fully discussed later.

The removal of mechanical factors is of most importance in hypertrophic arthritis, and consists mainly of the treatment of obesity, the elimination of injuries to the joint structures, especially those occasioned by repeated occupational strains, and of postural correction, with special reference to flat feet.

Other Measures

Diet. It has been shown that in patients with atrophic arthritis, glucose is not removed from the blood as rapidly as in normal individuals. Cases of hypertrophic arthritis are often overweight.[4] Clinically, all cases of chronic arthritis usually feel better and improve faster on a restricted caloric intake.[3] Ordinarily, about 30 calories per kilogram of body weight give the proper amount of food. However, the total amount of food and the type of food must be prepared according to the patient's individual requirements. Every diet should produce enough residue for normal bowel movements, should provide a balance of the alkali-ash foods with the acid-ash foods, enough carbohydrates to prevent acidosis, and should contain the caloric requirement for the height, weight, and habits of the patient, the proper amounts of protein, mineral salts, water, and vitamins.

Cases of hypertrophic arthritis usually require but little meat, but cases of atrophic arthritis, so frequently anemic, should be given meat.

In the beginning of treatment, the diet may have to be more restricted for one or two weeks, but the average diet may be summarized as follows:

Protein, 0.75 Gm. per kilogram of body weight.

Vegetables, 5 per cent and 10 per cent (but no 20 per cent) in fairly large amounts, cooked, and raw, served as salads as desired.

Fruits, melons and berries (except bananas) in moderate amounts three times a day.

One small slice of whole wheat bread, or one roll, or one bran muffin, or the equivalent in crackers three times a day.

No sugar nor sweets.

The rest of the caloric requirement is made up of fat—butter, cream, milk, buttermilk and olive oil.

The diet should be varied so that the patient will not tire of it.

Specimen Meals

Morning—One egg or bacon
    Muffin or toast
    Butter
    Weak tea or decaffeinized coffee
    Cream, if desired
    Saccharin for sweetening

Noon—Soup
    Two vegetables
    Green salad, with dressing
    Bread or muffin or crackers
    Fruit
    Milk

Night—Soup
    Meat or fish
    Green salad with dressing
    Fruit
    Bread or roll or muffin, toasted, if desired
    Butter
    Cheese
    Milk or decaffeinized coffee with cream.

Extra vitamins may be added in the form of ABD capsules, yeast, or cod liver oil. Dreyer and Reed[20] have reported cases of chronic arthritis of both types treated successfully by the administration of massive doses of vitamin D, 200,000 to 1,000,000 units per day. We have had no experience with this method of treatment.

Vaccines are useful with the atrophic type only.[21,22] From the available literature and from our own experience, we believe that the best results are obtained by the intravenous administration of vaccines from mixed strains of streptococci. Doses are given at weekly intervals, fifty to one hundred million at the first dose, and the dose increased each time by one hundred million, if no marked reaction occurs. Five or more injections are given, the maximum dose being eight hundred million. When this dose is reached, it may be repeated twice at intervals of fifteen days.

The Colon. The treatment of constipation and the correction of toxemia caused by absorption from the colon are important. These should be corrected by the use of diet as outlined, and the judicious use of some combination of the following:

Mineral oil, agar agar, psyllium seed, saraka, regulin, and the like.

Breathing exercises, abdominal exercise, and abdominal massage will also help.

Colonic irrigations of normal saline or of 5 per cent sodium bicarbonate solution are useful for some patients, but should not be used too often nor too long.

Pemberton[9] describes the characteristic colon of the arthritic:

"The colon is of greater caliber than normal, of greater length, more convoluted, and reduplications are present. There is usually delayed emptying and ileo-cecal regurgitation. After treatment, the appearance of the colon often returns to normal."

Drug Therapy. The use of morphine or other narcotics for the relief of pain is not advisable, because of the chronicity of the disease. The salicylates are useful in some cases, and aspirin in doses of five to ten grains is probably the best. Aspirin apparently possesses the property of increasing blood circulation about the affected areas. For this same purpose, Pemberton[9] advises the use of small doses of erythrol tetranitrate, beginning with 1/12 grain and gradually increasing to 1/4 grain three times a day. Iodine in the form of potassium iodide or tincture of iodine, ten drops in milk three times a day, has been used to advantage.

Arsenic in the form of Fowler's solution, sodium cacodylate intravenously, or small doses of neoarsphenamine, has been of great assistance.

Strychnine (elixir of iron, quinine, and strychnine phosphates) in small doses is used as a general tonic and to increase tonicity of muscles and to prevent atrophy.

In the presence of anemia, liver extract should be given by injection to prevent the necessity of giving large doses of liver and meat by mouth. Excessive meat in the diet appears in some cases to have caused hypertrophic changes in cases originally of the atrophic type.

Endocrine Therapy. The administration of thyroid extract, one grain of the American product three times a day, has been helpful in some cases, especially of the hypertrophic type.[33] Atrophic arthritis occurs at times in connection with hyperthyroidism. For this reason, the basal metabolic rate of patients with atrophic arthritis should be determined before thyroid is administered.

The administration of ovarian extracts or of follicular hormones is indicated in case of hypertrophic arthritis occurring at the menopause.

Sulphur. Injections of colloidal sulphur [34 35 36 37 38 39 40] are used in the treatment of both types of arthritis, and seem to be equally efficacious in each. No contraindications to its use are reported. Following these injections there have developed in some cases one or more of the following: Urticaria, a scarlatiform rash, nausea, vomiting, abdominal cramps, diarrhea, anorexia, severe weakness, headache, nervousness, muscle soreness, and insomnia. Two of our patients complained of so much pain from the intravenous injection that we were forced to confine their injections to the intramuscular method.

For the past few months we have used sulfur diasporal, the aqueous solution for intravenous injection and the oily solution for intramuscular injection. Different authors advocate various technic of administration. One physician[33] has given alternating doses, intravenous and intramuscular, six doses a week, and continues until improvement results. He has given as high as seventy doses to individual patients, with no complications.

We usually give doses of 10 mg. to 20 mg. intravenously, and of 20 mg. intramuscularly. We begin with small doses, and increase if there are no untoward symptoms, and if improvement does not show on the smaller dosage. Three courses of ten injections each, one injection every day or every second day, are given at intervals of two or three weeks.

We wish only to mention here the treatment of chronic arthritis by the use of bee venom and by gold salts. We have not employed these preparations in the treatment of our arthritic cases, but the reader is referred to the excellent book by Beck on *Bee Venom Therapy*[52] and to an article by Pemberton[53] on the use of the gold preparations.

Mechanotherapy and Physiotherapy. Iontophoresis of choline derivatives or of histamine[41 42 43] is of special help in fibrositis and atrophic arthritis, and may also be helpful in some cases of hypertrophic arthritis. The galvanic current is used to introduce these substances into the tissues through the intact skin. We have used histamine iontophoresis in a number of cases, with success in most of them.

(Other physicians have tried the injection of histamine for arthritis, and report excellent results.)

Other measures we have found of help are the electric bakers, the infra-red lamp, diathermy through affected joints and for fibrositis, and the ultraviolet light in atrophic arthritis.[44 45 46] Sun baths are better than the ultraviolet lamp, and some of our patients who have not improved at home have been advised to go to a warmer climate where they may take sun baths and avoid cold and humidity.

Of all forms of physiotherapy used for the treatment of arthritis, we believe that fever therapy is the best.[47 48 49 50] In the last three years we have treated 188 cases of chronic arthritis of both types with the hyperpyrexator, a cabinet type of machine. Other therapeutic measures, as indicated in each case, have been employed adjunctively, and excellent results have been obtained in about 35 per cent of the cases, and fair results in 40 per cent more.

Other measures useful and necessary are massage, passive motion, properly limited exercise for the individual patient, and rest as needed.

Many of our cases have been treated in conjunction with orthopedic surgeons, who have instituted proper orthopedic measures as necessary.

Conclusion

In closing, we wish to emphasize the following:

1. Seventy-five per cent or more of patients suffering from chronic arthritis and fibrositis may now be greatly helped or cured by proper treatment.

2. Early diagnosis and early treatment are necessary to obtain the best results, but no patient should be dismissed as hopeless until all appropriate measures have been tried. Total or partial relief from pain and increased mobility of joints may often be obtained in severe and long standing cases.

3. Each patient should be carefully studied to make an accurate diagnosis and to determine etiologic factors. The treatment must be individualized according to findings, and changed as indicated during the course of the disease.

4. Close cooperation of orthopedic surgeon, physiotherapist and internist is necessary to produce the best results.

BIBLIOGRAPHY

1. Dublin, Louis I.: Chronic Arthritis and Rheumatoid Conditions. (Chapter I. B. L. Wyatt). William Wood and Company, New York. 1933.
2. Pemberton, Ralph, and Bach. T. F.: A Brief Review of the Treatment of Chronic Arthritis. Med. Clin. of N. A. 18:107 (July) 1934.
3. Wyatt, B. L.: Chronic Arthritis and Fibrositis. William Wood and Company, New York. 1933.
4. Hall, Francis C., and Myers. Walter K.: Diet in Chronic Arthritis. Arch. Int. Med. 55:403-410 (March) 1935.
5. Exhibit on Rheumatism. Prepared by the American Committee for the Control of Rheumatism, and exhibited before the A. M. A., Cleveland. 1934. Published by A. M. A.
6. Dawson, M., and Boots, R.: Nodules in Chronic Arthritis. Am. Jour. Path. 8:283. 1932.
7. Clawson B. J., and Wetherby, M.: Subcutaneous Nodules in Rheumatoid Arthritis. J. A. M. A. 95:1894. 1930.
8. Llewellyn, L. J., and Jones, A. B.: Fibrositis. William Heineman, London. 1915.
9. Pemberton, Ralph: Arthritis and Rheumatoid Conditions. Lea and Febiger, Philadelphia. 1935.
10. Cecil, R. L., Nichols, E. E., and Stainsby, W. J.: The Etiology of Rheumatoid Arthritis. Am. Jour. Med. Sci. 181:12. 1931.
11. Rosenow, E. C.: The Relation of Dental Infection to Systemic Disease. Dental Cosmos 59:485-491, 1917.
12. Nakamura, T.: Focal Infection and Elective Localization in Ulcer of Stomach and in Arthritis. Ann. Surg. 79:29-43. (Jan.) 1924.
13. Rosenow, E. C.: Cataphoretic Velocity of Streptococci as Isolated in Studies of Arthritis. Arch. Int. Med. 51:377, 1933.
14. Haden, R. L.: Elective Localization of Streptococci. South. M. J. 19:253-260 (April) 1926.
15. Hench. P. S.: Bauer. Walter; Fletcher, A. A.; Ghrist, David; Hall. Francis: and White, Preston: The Present Status of the Problem of "Rheumatism": A Review of Recent American and English Literature on "Rheumatism" and Arthritis. (In three parts). Ann. Int. Med. 8:10, 1315; Ibid. 8:11, 1495; Ibid. 8:12, 1673. 1935.
16. Forkner, C. E., Shands, A. R., and Poston, M. A.: Synovial Fluid in Chronic Arthritis; Bacteriology and Cytology. Arch. Int. Med. 42:675-702, (Nov.) 1928.
17. Key, J. A., and Dorst, S. E.: The Allergic Joint. J. Lab. and Clin. Med. 15:1109-1116, (Aug.) 1930.
18. Cecil, R. L., Nichols, E. E., and Stainsby, W. J.: Bacteriology of Blood and Joints in Chronic Infectious Arthritis. Arch. Int. Med. 43:571, 1929.
19. Dawson, M. H. Olmstead, M., and Boots, R. H.: Agglutination Reactions in Rheumatoid Arthritis. J. Immunol. 23:187, 1932.
20. Nichols, E. E., and Stainsby, W. J.: Further Studies on the Agglutination Reactions in Chronic Arthritis. J. Clin. Inv. 12:505, 1933.
21. Zinsser, H.: The Bacteriology of Rheumatic Fever and the Allergic Hypothesis. Arch. Int. Med. 42:301, 1928.
22. Freiberg J. A., and Dorst. S. E.: The Allergic Joint. J. Lab. and Clin. Med. 15:1109-1116, (Aug.) 1930.
23. Crowe, H. W.: Bacteriology and Surgery of Chronic Arthritis and Rheumatism. 'Oxford Medical Publications. 1927.
24. Barrow, J. V., and Armstrong, E. L.: Intestinal Protozoa and Chronic Disease with Especial Reference to Chronic Arthritis. J. Iowa M. Soc. 15:553-558, (Oct.) 1925; also in Illinois M. J. 47:427-432, (June) 1925.
25. Fisher, A. G. T.: Hunterian Lecture (abridged) on Osteoarthritis: Pathology, Aetiology, and Principles of Surgical Treatment. Lancet 2:1.6, (July 1) 1922.
26. Rosenow. E. C.: Relations of, and the Lesions Produced by, Various Forms of Streptococci, with Special Reference to Arthritis. J. A. M. A. 61:2007-2008, (Nov. 29) 1913.
27. Llewellyn. L. J.: Aspects of Rheumatism and Gout. Their Nature, Prevention, and Control. W. Heineman, London. 1927.
28. Albee, F. H.: Myofascitis from an Orthopedic Standpoint. J. A. M. A. 91:1364-1370, (Nov. 3) 1928.
29. Pemberton, Ralph; Buckman, T. E.; Foster, G. L.; Robertson. J. W., and Tompkins. E. H.: Studies on Arthritis in the Army, based on 400 Cases. Arch. Int. Med. 25:231, 335, 1920.
30. Dreyer, L., and Reed, C. I.: Treatment of Arthritis with Massive Doses of Vitamin D. Arch. Phys. Ther., X-ray, Rad.: 16:537,540, (Sept.) 1935.
31. Clawson. B. J., and Wetherby, M.: An Experimental Basis for Intravenous Vaccine Therapy in Chronic Arthritis, with a Summary of Results Obtained in Patients. Ann. Int. Med. 9:12, (June) 1935.
32. Buckley, C. W.: The Causes and Treatment of Arthritis. Brit. M. J. 3819:469, (Mar. 17) 1934.
33. Duncan, W. S.: Relationship of Thyroid Disease to Chronic Non-Specific Arthritis. J. A. M. A. 99:1239, 1932.
34. Todd, A. T.: Chronic Rheumatism. Brit. M J. 1:1048-1051, (June 11) 1927.
35. Cohen, David: Personal Communication. (Louisville, Ky.) 1936.
36. Senturia, B. D.: 'Results of Treatment of Chronic Arthritis and Rheumatoid Conditions with Colloidal Sulphur. J. Bone and Joint Surg. 16:1;118,125, (Jan.) 1934.
37. Woldenberg. S. C.: The Treatment of Arthritis with Colloidal Sulphur: report of 250 Cases. South. M. J. 28:875-881, (Oct.) 1935.
38. Cawadias, A. P.: Rheumatoid Arthritis: Its Causation and Treatment. Brit. M. J. 2:602-603, (Oct. 3) 1925.
39. Cawadias, A. P.: Sulphur Metabolism in Arthritis Deformans. Lancet 1:1283-1285, (June 18) 1927.
40. Wheldon, T. G., and Rolland. J. M.: The Use of Colloidal Sulphur in the Treatment of Arthritis. J. Bone and Joint Surg. 15:1, 94-97, (Jan.) 1933.
41. Klinge, D. H.: Treatment of Myositis. Arthritis, and Disturbance of Peripheral Circulation with Histamine by Cataphoresis. Arch. Surg. 29:138, 1934.
42. Shanson, B., and Eastwood, C. G.: The Use and Action of Histamine in Rheumatism. Lancet 1:1226-1228, 1934.
43. Kovacs. J.: Iontophoresis of Acetyl-beta-methyl-choline Chloride in the Treatment of Chronic Arthritis and Peripheral Vascular Disease. Am. J. Med. Sci. 188:32. 1934.
44. Telling, W. H. M.: The Clinical Importance of Fibrositis in General Practice. Brit. M. J. 3874:689, (April 6) 1935.
45. Hunter, Chas.: Fibrositis (Myalgia. Chronic Muscular Rheumatism). Canad. M. A. J. 16:1319-1324, (Nov.) 1926.
46. Kovacs, Richard: Physical Therapy in Chronic Arthritis. Med. Jour. and Ret. 138:372-374; (Nov. 15) 1933; 398-400, (Dec. 6) 1933.
47. Davison, H. M., and Lowance, M. I.: The Treatment of Arthritis with the Clark Hyperpyrexiator. Med. World, (Dec. 7) 1933.
48. Davison, H. M.: Lowance. M. I., and Barnett, C. F.: Hyperpyrexia in General Medicine. Clin. Med. and Surg. 42:11, 545-552, (Nov.) 1935.
49. Davison. H. M.: Lowance. M. I., and Barnett, C. F.: Hyperpyrexia: An Evaluation of Its Use in Office Practice. Med. Rec. 143:5;253, (March 18) 1936.
50. Hench. P. S.; Slocumb. C. H., and Popp, W. C.: Fever Therapy: Results for Gonorrheal Arthritis. Chronic Infectious (Atrophic) Arthritis. and Other Forms of "Rheumatism". J. A. M. A. 104:20;1779, (May 18) 1935.
51. Bock, B. F.: Bee Venom Therapy. D. Appleton-Century Co., New York. 1935.
52. Pemberton, H. S.: One Hundred Cases of Chronic Arthritis Treated by Gold. Lancet 228:1057, (May 4) 1935.
53. Ely, L. W., and Mensor, M. C.: Studies on the Immobilization of the Normal Joints. Surg., Gynec. and Obst. 57:212-215, (Aug.) 1933.

Discussion on Paper of Drs. Hal M. Davison, Mason I. Lowance and Crawford F. Barnett

DR. ERNEST F. WAHL (Thomasville) : I am sorry Dr. Davison was not able to cover everything in his paper. The manuscript leaves very little to be said.

Of great interest to the practicing physician is the

periodicity of the attacks of chronic arthritis. They will come without any known cause, and quite often disappear without any known cause. The habit of these attacks of clearing up by themselves makes one wonder at times whether their treatment is having any effect or whether it was just time for it to disappear. Many of these patients with fibrositis go to a physician with an abdominal complaint, or at least thinking that they have a disease of some of the abdominal organs. We have had many come thinking they had appendicitis because they had pain in the right lower quadrant of the abdomen, when it was simply a spastic muscle from the myositis, and on closer questioning, asking the patient to observe symptoms more closely, we found it was only a muscle soreness and was associated with a sort of freezing up of the muscles of the posterior area as well. The symptoms cleared up on exercise.

I do not believe there is any one cause of hypertrophic arthritis. It comes at a time when a great many things have happened to the individual, both in the way of overwork, stress, strain, bad eating habits, and repeated attacks of various types of infection, possibly chronic constipation, intestinal disorder for twenty to forty years, and there is no way to evaluate all of those effects on the body. I believe when we get the manifestations of arthritis at that time, we are getting the end result of a very long process. If that is true, there is little wonder that some of them do not respond any better than they do to treatment.

DR. JAMES E. PAULLIN (Atlanta): The interesting paper of the authors raises for discussion the important question of the prevalence of various types of arthritis. The American Society for the Study and Control of Rheumatism is devoting a considerable amount of time and research in an effort to solve some of the problems concerning this prevalent and crippling disease. I do not believe that there is yet any unanimity of opinion as to whether there are really two different types of arthritis, that is, one cannot say positively that all types of the disease commonly called rheumatism can be separated into the atrophic and hypertrophic varieties. When one studies closely the pathologic lesions of rheumatism it is observed that a single joint may show pathologic characteristics of the lesion described as occurring in atrophic arthritis and, at the same time, in a different part of the joint, the pathologic lesion which is typical of that described as occurring in hypertrophic arthritis. Not all workers are agreed in accepting the streptococcus as the organism which causes the lesions in atrophic arthritis or chronic infectious arthritis. It is true that serologic studies of the blood in the majority of patients with atrophic arthritis show agglutination phenomena for this organism, but despite this fact considerable more study must be devoted to this problem and more convincing evidence must be submitted before one can say that the streptococcus is the organism producing this disease.

As Dr. Davison has brought out in his paper, in one type of arthritis, the atrophic variety, the pathologic process begins in the synovial membrane. It is an inflammatory, proliferative, progressive disease from the beginning. In the so-called hypertrophic variety of arthritis the lesion is not so acute. It is more of a chronic condition which does not produce any considerable amount of crippling. As to whether the two processes are the same but differ in degree cannot, at this time, be definitely stated. Atrophic arthritis begins as a rule at an earlier age period, whereas the hypertrophic variety usually starts late in life and is usually associated with other degenerative diseases.

I am sorry that the doctor did not have sufficient time in his paper to enter into a discussion of the various problems concerned in the treatment of this disease. There are so many fads and so many fancied facts in regard to treating arthritis, and there are so many so-called specific remedies which are frequently advocated as being of benefit in relieving these sufferers that a discussion of this problem would be most valuable. We must appreciate the fact that all patients with arthritis go through periods of remission and periods of exacerbation and we must not be led, because of the nature of the disease, to assume that the remission which occurs during treatment is entirely the result of our therapeutic efforts.

DR. J. L. CAMPBELL (Atlanta): I am not competent to discuss this subject from a medical viewpoint. I only want to call your attention to its prevalence and the large percentage of permanent disability caused by it. In 1929 a survey of chronic diseases was made in Massachusetts. From this survey it was found that among the four million population of the state 138,000 persons had some form of rheumatism, 5,600 of whom were totally disabled. The average life of the rheumatic patient is about 14 years. The first ten years, one is partially disabled, but the last four years means total disability and helplessness. Therefore, it seems to me that the younger men entering the field of internal medicine should devote much time and attention to its study.

Dr. Davison and his group are doing good work. I know, however, the results are discouraging at the present, but it is to be hoped that in the no distant future that success may be attained.

DR. HAL M. DAVISON (Atlanta): I thank the gentlemen for their discussion. In closing, I wish to call your attention to the fact that over 75 per cent of our cases of arthritis have received enough relief from their symptoms to make the treatment worth while.

We believe that early diagnosis and early treatment are necessary to obtain the best results. We have many different forms of treatment available, so that we may try various forms of therapy, if our first is not efficacious. In most of our cases, we have used the hyperpyrexator together with some other type of treatment. The use of sulphur has not given us the percentage of relief that is reported in the literature. When an article reports 100 per cent success with any treatment, we must reserve our opinion until we test it for ourselves.

The Minnesota State Medical Association, through its Committee on Public Policy and Legislation, reaffirms its belief in the general principles of the traditions of medical practice and makes suggestions to facilitate an orderly administration of medical relief.

THE JOURNAL

OF THE

MEDICAL ASSOCIATION OF GEORGIA

Devoted to the Welfare of the Medical Association of Georgia

478 Peachtree Street, N. E., Atlanta, Ga.

DECEMBER, 1936

THE GEORGIA WORKMEN'S COMPENSATION ACT

The Georgia Workmen's Compensation Act provides, among other things, necessary medical attention for injured employees for a period not to exceed thirty days, and a maximum allowance of one hundred dollars to cover medical, surgical and hospital expense.

Surgeons of experience know the fallacy of expecting a fractured femur, simple or compound, to heal within thirty days. They know the difficulty in effecting a surgical cure for hernia where the hospitalization, anaesthesia, assistant's and surgeon's fees all are to come out of the sum of one hundred dollars. The average cost of hospitalizing a white patient in Georgia is over four dollars per day. It is important that hernia patients be kept in bed for not less than two weeks following the operation and should remain under observation another six weeks. When the hospital and other expenses are paid there remains practically nothing of the one hundred dollars to pay the surgeon for his time and skill. Compound fractures require prolonged hospitalization and often surgical operations to restore the injured patient to the point where he becomes a wage earner and provider for his family. It is ridiculous to think that this desirable end can be achieved within thirty days, and at a total cost of one hundred dollars. As it now stands in this State, the industrial surgeon must continue to treat these cases of severe injuries for weeks or even months after the thirty day limit has expired, gratuitously, and unless the insurance carrier makes some extra provision covering excess medical and hospital expense, then usually his entire treatment is without remuneration.

Comparison in the provisions of the Act in Georgia and other states follow:

California: Reasonable medical, surgical and hospital treatment.

Colorado: Reasonable medical, surgical and hospital treatment for four months. Maximum five hundred dollars. No time limit in the case of hernia.

Delaware: Maximum one hundred and fifty dollars. Board may increase time and amount.

Florida: Medical, surgical and hospital service as process of recovery may require.

Illinois: Medical, surgical and hospital service as reasonably required to effect a cure.

Kentucky: Reasonable medical, surgical and hospital service for ninety days.

Louisiana: Reasonable medical, surgical and hospital service, maximum two hundred and fifty dollars.

Maryland: Maximum five hundred dollars.

Michigan: Reasonable medical and hospital service for ninety days.

Missouri: Medical, surgical and hospital treatment as reasonably required for ninety days, not over seven hundred and fifty dollars, longer in cases requiring specialized or surgical treatment at discretion of the board.

Montana: Reasonable aid for six months. Maximum three hundred dollars. Special operating fee of one hundred dollars in case of hernia.

Nevada: Reasonable medical, surgical and hospital treatment for six months which may be extended an additional year by Commission.

New Jersey: Reasonable medical and hospital service. Special operating fee of one hundred fifty dollars in case of hernia.

New Mexico: Reasonable medical and hospital service. Maximum three hundred and fifty dollars. Special operating fee of seventy-five dollars in case of hernia.

New York: Such medical, surgical and hospital service as nature of injury requires. Charges limited to prevailing rates.

North Carolina: Reasonable medical, surgical and hospital service, not exceeding ten weeks and such additional time as Commission may decide.

Ohio: Maximum two hundred dollars, except in unusual cases.

Oregon: Maximum two hundred and fifty dollars. Commission may allow additional service.

Pennsylvania: Reasonable medical, surgical and hospital service for thirty days. Maximum one hundred dollars, *except* in hospital cases.

Rhode Island: Eight weeks. Maximum one hundred and fifty dollars.

South Dakota: Twelve weeks. Maximum two hundred dollars.

Utah: Reasonable medical and hospital service. Maximum five hundred dollars, more if found necessary.

Virginia: Necessary medical, surgical and hospital service for sixty days or one hundred and eighty days at order of Commission. Charges limited to prevailing rates.

West Virginia: Reasonable medical, surgical and hospital aid. Maximum eight hundred dollars.

United States Longshoremen: Such medical, surgical and hospital service as nature of injury requires. Charges limited to prevailing rates.

It may be seen from the foregoing data that most of the states recognize the importance of "reasonable" medical, surgical and hospital service. The doctors of Georgia are reasonable in their charges and conscientious in their work. There are few doctors in this State who will cease treating an injured person after the thirty day limit has expired even though they know that they will not be paid for such service.

It is time for the Legislature of Georgia to take cognizance of these facts and amend the industrial act to permit "reasonable" charges and a "reasonable" period of treatment. When this is accomplished the injured employee and the people who render him service during his illness will receive due consideration.

NEWS ITEMS

DR GLENVILLE GIDDINGS, Atlanta, is the third to have his name inscribed on the Hardman Loving Cup. Copy of the inscription follows:

"Doctor Glenville Giddings
818 Doctors Building
Atlanta, Georgia
for experimentation and study of
'Certain Observations on
the Physiology of Sleep'
Eighty-Seventh Annual Session
Medical Association of Georgia
Savannah, Georgia
April 21-24, 1936."

Dr. Roy R. Kracke, Emory University, was the first, and Dr. James A. Redfearn, Albany, second.

THE GEORGIA MEDICAL SOCIETY (Chatham County, Savannah) met on October 13th. Dr. Lee Howard read a paper entitled, "Blood Count Versus Blood Studies"; Dr. John W. Daniel reported a case, "The Use of Protamine-Insulinate."

THE FIFTH DISTRICT MEDICAL SOCIETY met at the Academy of Medicine, Atlanta, on October 15th. The program consisted of: "Address" by Dr. B. H. Minchew, Waycross, President of the Association; "Address," Dr. Geo. A. Traylor, Augusta, President-Elect of the Association. Dr. Jos. Earle Moore, Johns Hopkins University, Baltimore, Maryland, spoke on "The Management of the Wassermann-Fast Patient"; Dr. Wm. A. Smith, Atlanta, read a paper entitled, "Quinine Treatment of Myotonia Congenita" and gave a moving picture demonstration of a case; discussion was led by Dr. Richard B. Wilson, Atlanta. Dr. Joseph Yampolsky, Atlanta, read a paper, "The Use of Stovarsol and Stovarsol and Bismuth in the Treatment of Syphilis in Children"; discussion was led by Dr. Donald F. Cathcart and Dr. J. H. Lange, both of Atlanta.

DR. S. ROSS BROWN, Atlanta, gave a lecture in the school auditorium at Lawrenceville on "Venereal Diseases," October 14th.

DR. H. G. HUEY, Homerville, has been reappointed for a four year term on the State Board of Medical Examiners. Dr. Harold F. McDuffie, Atlanta, was appointed to fill an unexpired three year term on the Board.

THE SECOND DISTRICT MEDICAL SOCIETY met at Hotel Colquitt, Moultrie, on October 8th. Speakers on the program were: Dr. Roy A. Hill, Thomasville; Dr. Jas. R. Paulk, Moultrie; Dr. A. B. Jones, Quitman; Dr. J. V. Rogers, Cairo; Dr. J. R. McMichael, Quitman; Dr. D. Henry Poer, Atlanta; and Dr. C. W. Strickler, Atlanta. Dr. J. E. Lanier, Moultrie, was toastmaster at the banquet.

DR. WM. J. HUSON, formerly of Augusta, has moved to Covington. The Covington News announces that he is building a hospital.

DR. LEWIS H. ODEN, JR., Blackshear, has been appointed physician for Pierce County.

DR. A. B. DANIEL, formerly with the Central of Georgia Railway Hospital at Savannah, has returned to Claxton and associated with his father, Dr. J. Wallace Daniel, in the practice of medicine.

THE JACKSON-BARROW COUNTIES MEDICAL SOCIETY met at the Winder Hotel, Winder, on October 5th. Dr. W. L. Mathews, Winder, read a paper on the "Various Causes of Backache."

DR. H. L. TIPPINS, Baxley, has just returned from Chicago where he took post-graduate work for six weeks in pediatrics.

THE GEORGIA UROLOGICAL ASSOCIATION met at Hotel Dempsey, Macon, October 29th. Titles of papers on the scientific program were: "Surgery of the Ureter—Lantern Slides and Motion Pictures," Dr. Robert B. McIver, Jacksonville, Fla.; "Non-Shadow Casting Renal and Ureteral Calculi—Lantern Slides," Dr. J. C. Pennington and Dr. Earl C. Lowry, Nashville, Tenn.; "History of Urology in Georgia," Dr. Stephen T. Brown, Atlanta; "Urinary Antiseptics," Dr. H. W. E. Walther, New Orleans, La. Members were served a Dutch luncheon at Hotel Dempsey. Officers of the Association are: Dr. J. C. Keaton, Albany, President; Dr. Earl Floyd, Atlanta, President-Elect; Dr. W. E. Upchurch, Atlanta, Secretary-Treasurer.

THE ASSOCIATION OF AMERICAN MEDICAL COLLEGES met at Emory University, October 26, 27, 28. Speakers on the program and titles of their addresses were: Dr. J. N. Baker, Montgomery, Ala., "The Need for Closer Integration of the Agencies Interested in Medical Education and Licensure"; Dr. E. E. Reinke, Nashville, Tenn., "Liberal Values in Premedical Education"; Dr. Ralph J. Gilmore, Denver, Colo., "Liberal Arts Background for Medicine"; Dr. Frank L. Babbott, Jr., Brooklyn, N. Y., "What Medical Colleges Expect Hospitals to Do to Continue Education of the Intern"; Dr. C. W. Munger, Valhalla, New York, "The Continued Education of the Medical Student During His Internship." Atlanta physicians who engaged in the discussion, "TEACHING OBJECTIVES AND METHODS IN EMORY UNIVER-

SITY SCHOOL OF MEDICINE" and their respective subjects were: Dr. Dan C. Elkin, "Surgery"; Dr. R. A. Bartholomew, "Obstetrics"; Dr. R. H. Oppenheimer, "Medicine"; Dr. M. Hines Roberts, "Pediatrics"; Dr. W. W. Young, "Psychiatry." The program for the final day of the meeting was devoted to a symposium on "INTEGRATION OF THE MEDICAL CURRICULUM." Individual subjects for the various speakers were: "The Integration of the Medical Curriculum in the Preclinical Years," Dr. Geo. S. Eadie, Durham, N. C.; "Self Help in the Teaching of Pathology," Dr. William Boyd, Winnepeg, Canada; "The Integration of Clinical Medicine with the Preclinical Sciences," Dr. J. C. Meakins, Montreal, Canada; "The Value and the Need of Coordination in the Teaching of Surgery," Dr. Alton Ochsner, New Orleans, La.; "Tendencies in Medical Practice—A Study of the 1930 Graduates," Dr. H. G. Weiskotten, Syracuse, N. Y.

THE NEW BROOKS COUNTY HOSPITAL at Quitman opened recently. It has been stated that the institution has been filled almost to capacity since its dedication.

A CHEST CLINIC was conducted at Moultrie on October 28th by members of the Colquitt County Medical Society and the State Board of Health.

DR. A. PARK MCGINTY announces the opening of offices in Suite 511 Doctors' Building, 478 Peachtree Street, N. E., Atlanta. He was formerly engaged as instructor in internal medicine at the University of Michigan Medical School, Ann Arbor.

A LIST OF CITIES IN GEORGIA with hospitals in each approved by the American College of Surgeons, follows: ALBANY—Phoeby Putney Memorial Hospital; ATHENS—Athens General Hospital; ATLANTA—Albert Steiner Clinic, Crawford W. Long Memorial Hospital, Georgia Baptist Hospital, Grady Memorial Hospital, Henrietta Egleston Hospital, Piedmont Hospital, St. Joseph's Infirmary, United States Penitentiary Hospital, Veterans Administration Hospital, Emory University Hospital, Scottish Rite Hospital and Fort McPherson Station Hospital; AUGUSTA—University Hospital, Veterans' Administration Hospital, and Wilhenford Hospital; COLUMBUS—City Hospital; CUTHBERT—Patterson Hospital; EASTMAN—Coleman Sanitarium; FORT BENNING—Station Hospital; FORT OGLETHORPE—Station Hospital; GAINESVILLE—Downey Hospital; MACON—Macon Hospital, Middle Georgia Sanatorium, and Oglethorpe Private Infirmary; MILLEDGEVILLE—Milledgeville City Hospital; MILLEN—Millen Hospital; PLAINS—Wise Sanitarium; ROME—Harbin Hospital and McCall Hospital; SAVANNAH—Central of Georgia Railway Hospital, Charity Hospital, St. Joseph's Hospital, United States Marine Hospital, and Warren A. Candler Hospital; THOMASVILLE—John D. Archbold Memorial Hospital; VALDOSTA—Little-Griffin Private Hospital; WARM SPRINGS—Georgia Warm Springs Foundation; WAYCROSS—Atlantic Coast Line R. R. Hospital and Ware County Hospital.

THE STATE BOARD OF MEDICAL EXAMINERS met at the State Capitol, Atlanta, on October 13 and 14. Applicants for licenses examined were: Harry L. Allan, Atlanta; Seth M. Beale, Elkin, N. C.; Stuart Pitner Vandiviere, Brundidge, Ala. Reciprocity licenses were granted to the following: Zia M. Bagdadi, Augusta; Dritz Albert Brink, Blackshear; Thomas Sterling Clairborne, Boston, Mass.; Jack Galin, Gilman, Ill.; Z. H. McKinney, Deepstep; and Richard Turpin, Augusta. Members of the Board present were: Dr. J. O. Elrod, Forsyth; Dr. J. L. Howell, Atlanta; Dr. H. G. Huey, Homelville; Dr. C. F. Griffith, Griffin; Dr. J. W. Palmer, Ailey; Dr. D. T. Rankin, Alto; Dr. Luke Robinson, Covington; and Dr. Harold F. McDuffie, Atlanta. Officers elected for the ensuing year are: Dr. J. L. Howell, Atlanta, President; Dr. D. T. Rankin, Alto, Vice-President.

DR. R. C. FRANKLIN, Swainsboro, attended the International Medical Assembly of the Interstate Postgraduate Medical Association of North America at St. Paul, Minnesota, October 12-16.

DR. BRUCE THREATTE, Columbus; Dr. W. L. Pomeroy, Waycross, and H. A. Seaman, Waycross, were elected to fellowship in the American College of Surgeons.

DR. AND MRS. O. N. HARDEN, Cornelia, entertained the members of the Habersham County Medical Society and Auxiliary at their home on October 8th.

DR. C. O. WILLIAMS, West Point; Dr. Hal C. Miller, Atlanta; Dr. A. A. Morrison, Dr. W. A. Norton and Dr. E. J. Whelan, all of Savannah, attended the recent annual session of the Clinical Congress of the American College of Surgeons at Philadelphia, Pa.

THE GEORGIA SECTION of The Southeastern Surgical Congress met at the Millen Hospital, Millen, on November 4th. The scientific program consisted of titles for papers as follows: "Tumors of the Breasts," Dr. A. J. Mooney, Statesboro; "Injuries to the Lungs and Pleura," Dr. Frank K. Boland, Atlanta; "Leg Ulcers," Dr. Geo. A. Traylor, Augusta; "Operation for Kidney Stone," Dr. Earl Floyd, Atlanta; "Acute Abdominal Injury," Dr. J. S. Turberville, Century, Fla.; "Hernias," Dr. C. F. Holton, Savannah; "Ureteral Stricture," Wallace L. Bazemore, Macon; "Chronic Cholecystitis," Dr. C. E. Wills, Washington; "Industrial Injuries," Dr. A. R. Rozar, Macon. Discussions on the various papers were led by: Dr. E. A. Wilcox, Augusta; Dr. F. B. Rawlings, Sandersville; Dr. C. E. Rushin, Atlanta; Dr. Kenneth Hunt, Griffin; Dr. Grady Coker, Canton; Dr. C. B. Greer, Brunswick; Dr. J. W. Shearouse, Savannah; Dr. R. C. Franklin, Swainsboro; Dr. Julian K. Quattlebaum, Savannah. Lunch was served at the Millen Hospital. Dr. B. T. Beasley, Atlanta, Secretary of the Congress, spoke on the "Aims of the Southeastern Surgical Congress."

THE STAFF MEETING of St. Joseph's Infirmary, Atlanta, was held on October 27th.

THE GEORGIA MEDICAL SOCIETY, Savannah, met on October 26th. Dr. Robert L. Rhodes, Augusta, read a paper entitled, "Carcinoma of the Gallbladder with Discussion of the Bilary Problem"; the discussion was led by Dr. J. K. Quattlebaum and Dr. J. L. Elliott, both of Savannah. Dr. J. L. Elliott reported a case, "Ovarian Cyst of Unusual Proportions."

DR. B. T. BEASLEY announces the removal of his offices to Suite 701, Hurt Building, Atlanta.

THE STATE BOARD OF HEALTH is promoting an extensive venereal disease program which includes venereal disease treatment clinics in thirteen Georgia Counties as follows: Bibb, Chatham, Clarke, DeKalb, Dougherty, Floyd, Fulton, Glynn, Lowndes, Muscogee, Richmond, Walker and Ware.

DR. WILLIAM PERRIN NICOLSON, Atlanta, announced that the Society of Clinical Surgeons presented a bronze plaque of Dr. Crawford W. Long to the Royal College of Surgeons at Edinburgh, Scotland.

DR. AND MRS. E. B. DAVIS, Byromville, entertained numbers of friends in their home at 'Hillcrest" on their twenty-fifth wedding anniversary, October 19th.

DR. JOHN W. ODEN, Milledgeville, has been re-elected Superintendent of the Milledgeville State Hospital for a term of two years.

DR. JAS. E. PAULLIN, Atlanta, was elected President of the American Clinical and Climatological Association at its annual meeting in Richmond, Va., October 27th.

THE GEORGIA MEDICAL SOCIETY, Savannah, met on November 10th. Dr. T. H. D. Griffitts, Malaria Research Laboratory, U. S. P. H. S., read a paper entitled, "Malaria—Some Comments on the Past and Future"; Dr S. E. Wilson reported a case, "Foreign Body in the Bladder." Refreshments were served.

THE STAFF MEETING of Emory University Hospital was held on November 1st. Dr. F. Kells Boland reported a case, "Uterine Sarcoma"; Dr. Stewart R. Roberts, "Amebiasis Associated with Tuberculosis"; discussed by Dr. Daniel C. Elkin and Dr. Roy R. Kracke; Dr. Ed S. Wright reported a case, "Chronic Mastoiditis."

THE RANDOLPH COUNTY MEDICAL SOCIETY met at the Patterson Hospital, Cuthbert, November 5th. Dr. J. C. Patterson was the principal speaker.

DR. FREDRIC R. MINNICH announces the removal of his office to Suite 511 Doctors' Building, 478 Peachtree Street, N. E., Atlanta.

THE MACON MEDICAL SOCIETY of Bibb County met at Ridley Hall, Macon, on November 3rd. Dr. A. R. Rozar read a paper on "Appendicitis."

DR. AND MRS. PAUL MCGEE, Waycross, entertained the members of the Ware County Medical Society in their home on November 4th. Chicken supper was served. Dr. Lewis H. Oden, Jr., Blackshear, read a scientific paper.

DR. H. C. ATKINSON, Macon, has just returned from Philadelphia where he has been for several weeks taking post-graduate study in diagnosis and internal medicine.

THE AMERICAN MEDICAL ASSOCIATION, Chicago, announces that all applications for space in the Scientific Exhibit for its 88th Annual Session to be held at Atlantic City, New Jersey, June 7-11, 1937, must be submitted before February 1, 1937. "The exhibits will be placed, as far as possible, in groups corresponding to the sections of the Scientific Assembly." Applications may be sent to section representatives, or to the Director, Scientific Exhibit, American Medical Association, 535 North Dearborn Street, Chicago, Ill.

THE FULTON COUNTY MEDICAL SOCIETY met at the Academy of Medicine, Atlanta, November 5th. Dr. Everett L. Bishop reported a case, "Adamantinoma of the Tibia"; Dr. Richard B. Wilson, case, "Multiple Gliomas of the Brain"; Dr. A. J. Ayers made a clinical talk, "One Hour Two-Dose Glucose Tolerance Test (Exton)"; Dr. Amey Chappell and Dr. Lee Bivings, paper, "Blood Studies on Negro Women During Pregnancy." The discussion was led by Dr. C. B. Upshaw, Dr. E. D. Colvin and Dr. Geo. F. Klugh.

THE STAFF MEETING of the Crawford W. Long Memorial Hospital, Atlanta, was held on November 12th. Dr. Frank K. Boland reported a case, "Surgical Treatment of Tuberculosis—with Moving Pictures."

THE CENTENNIAL CELEBRATION of Emory University was held in the Glenn Memorial Auditorium at Emory University, December 4th to 13th, inclusive.

DR. EDGAR G. BALLENGER, Atlanta, spoke on the "Treatment of. Gonorrhea" before the Southeastern Branch Society of the American Urological Society at Charlotte, N. C., December 4th. Dr. Earl Floyd, Atlanta, is Secretary-Treasurer; Dr. Stephen T. Brown, member of the Executive Committee.

DR. R. H. FIKE, Atlanta, spoke before a meeting of the Cartersville Rotary Club on "The Number of Deaths from Cancer in America Last Year," November 4th.

DR. THOS. B. PHINIZY, Augusta, Acting Richmond County Commissioner of 'Health, in a statement published in the Augusta Herald, in part says: "The presence of mosquitoes, malaria and pest in Augusta and in her immediate vicinity, has been less than at any time within my memory. This is based on personal observation and on the number of mosquito complaints received in the offices of the health department. This condition, I believe, is due to the vast amount of drainage work in the vicinity of Augusta and to better mosquito control measures. In spite of the relative lack of mosquitoes the incidence of malaria is rising."

THE JACKSON-BARROW COUNTIES MEDICAL SOCIETY met in the offices of Dr. C. B. Almand and Dr. S. T. Ross, Winder, on November 2nd. Dr. W. T. Randolph, Winder, read a paper entitled, "Therapeutic Measures in the Treatment of Malaria." Dr. Grady

N. Coker, Canton, Councilor for the Ninth District, spoke on "Medical Societies."

THE THIRD DISTRICT MEDICAL SOCIETY met at Fitzgerald on November 11th. Titles of papers on the scientific program were: "The Practical Approach to the Diagnosis of Organic Heart Disease," by Dr. W. Edward Storey, Columbus; discussed by Dr. P. L. Williams, Cordele, and Dr. W. G. Elliott, Cuthbert. "The Treatment of Bronchial Asthma," Dr. L. E. Abram, Fitzgerald; discussed by Dr. M. L. Malloy, Vienna, and Dr. J. Fred Adams, Montezuma. "The Conservative Treatment of Acute Mastoiditis," Dr. J. B. Thompson, Columbus; discussed by Dr. S. A. Scruggs, Americus, and Dr. T. E. Bradley, Fitzgerald. Report by Dr. J. C. Patterson, Cuthbert, Councilor for the Third District.

THE GEORGIA MEDICAL SOCIETY, Savannah, met on November 24th. Dr. V. P. Sydenstricker, Augusta, read a paper on "Pellagra." Dr. Lloyd Boggs from Chunju Mission Hospital, Korea, spoke on his experiences in Korea, China.

THE REGULAR STAFF MEETING of St. Joseph's Infirmary, Atlanta, was held on November 24th. Dr. H. W. Jernigan reported a case of "Multiple Fractures with Recovery"; Dr. D. Henry Poer and William Kiser, case, "An Unusually Interesting Congenital Anomaly of the Intestinal Tract."

DR. J. COX WALL, Eastman, and associates announce the opening of The Clinic at Eastman on November 26th. Associated with Dr. Wall are: Dr. N. L. Barker, Dr. I. J. Parkerson and B. W. Yawn.

THE STATE BOARD OF CONTROL announces the re-election of Dr. John W. Oden, Superintendent of the Milledgeville State Hospital, and members of the medical staff as follows: Dr. S. A. Anderson, Dr. L. A. Bailey, Dr. Wm. A. Bostwick, Dr. R. W. Bradford, Dr. G. K. Cornwell, Dr. C. G. Cox, Dr. Geo. L. Echols, Dr. J. I. Garrard, Dr. Franklin P. Holder, Dr. R. V. Lamar, Dr. L. P. Longino, Dr. J. D. Wiley, Dr. Y. H. Yarbrough.

DR. GEORGE A. ANDREWS has returned to Trion and reopened his office for the diagnosis and treatment of diseases of the eye, ear, nose and throat; after spending four months in government work at the Veterans' Administration Facility, St. Cloud, Minnesota.

DR. W. P. SMITH, JR., formerly with the Emory University Hospital, has opened offices at 319 Church Street, Decatur.

DR. W. R. MCCOY AND DR. C. L. DAVIS, both of Alma, entertained the members of the Coffee County Medical Society at a barbecue dinner on November 24th. Instead of a scientific program, those present engaged in a discussion of "Medical Jurisprudence."

THE SOUTHERN MEDICAL ASSOCIATION, headquarters in Birmingham, Alabama, he'd its annual meeting in Baltimore, November 17-20. Officers elected for the ensuing year were: Dr. Frank K. Boland, Atlanta, President-elect; Dr. Sidney M. Miller, Baltimore, First Vice-President; Dr. Leander A. Riely, Oklahoma City, Okla., Second Vice-President; Mr. C. P. Loranz, re-elected Secretary-Manager for a term of five years. Dr. Roy R. Kracke, Emory University, Secretary of the Committee on Pathology; Dr. J. H. Kite, Atlanta, Secretary of the Committee on Bone and Joint Surgery. SCIENTIFIC EXHIBITS BY GEORGIA PHYSICIANS AND SUBJECTS were: "Chest," Dr. Wm. Willis Anderson, Atlanta; "Hematology," Dr. Roy R. Kracke, Emory University; "Idiopathic Thrombopenic Purpura," Dr. Lon Grove, Atlanta; "Plastic Surgery," Dr. W. G. Hamm, Atlanta; "Neoplastic Diseases," Dr. Jack W. Jones, Atlanta; "Gynecology," Dr. Jas. N. Brawner, Jr., Atlanta; "Industrial Medicine and Public Health," Dr. E. D. Colvin, Atlanta (Maternal Mortality in Georgia in 1935); "Genito-Urinary Diseases, Dr. Earl Floyd and Dr. Jas. L. Pittman, Atlanta; "Central Nervous System," Dr. Edgar F. Fincher, Jr., Atlanta; "Cardiovascular Diseases," Dr. H. C. Sauls and Dr. Carter Smith, Atlanta; (Clinical and Electro-Cardiac Studies in Coronary Occlusion), Dr. L. Minor Blackford, Atlanta (Syphilitic Aortic Insufficiency, Review of 210 Cases) ; "Ophthalmology," Dr. Grady E. Clay and Dr. J. Mason Baird, Atlanta; "Orthopedic Surgery," Dr. Lawson Thornton and Dr. Calvin Sandison, Atlanta. MOVING PICTURE DEMONSTRATIONS by Georgia Physicians were: "Fifty Fractures of Neck of Femur Treated Immediately with Smith-Petersen Nail," Dr. Lawson Thornton and Dr. Calvin Sandison, Atlanta; "Subtotal Thyroidectomy for Exophthalmic Goiter" and "Total Thyroidectomy for Nodular Toxic Goiter," Dr. D. Henry Poer, Atlanta; "Outline of Treatment of Burns," Dr. J. D. Martin, Jr., Atlanta. PHYSICIANS ON SCIENTIFIC PROGRAM: Dr. V. P. Sydenstricker and Dr. John W. Thomas, Augusta, paper, "Certain Etiological Factors in Pellagra"; Dr. Jas. E. Paullin, Atlanta, discussed, "The Treatment of Endemic Pellagra"; Dr. Jack C. Norris, Atlanta, discussed, "Embolism of the Pulmonary Artery"; Dr. Joseph Yampolsky, Atlanta, paper, "A Comparative Study of the Use of Stovarsol and Stovarsol with Bismuth in Syphilis in Children"; Dr. M. Hines Roberts, Atlanta, paper, "A Study of Mastoid Infection in Children—Lantern Slides"; Dr. Everett L. Bishop, Atlanta, paper, "Adamantinoma of the Tibia—Lantern Slides"; Dr. Everett S. Sanderson, Augusta, paper, "Cultivation of Ducrey's Bacillus and Preparation of an Antigen for Intracutaneous Diagnosis of Chranceroidal Infection"; Dr. W. W. Young, Atlanta, paper, "Mental Hygiene in Changing Times"; Dr. V. P. Sydenstricker, Augusta, discussed, "The Bone Changes in Sickle Cell Anemia"; Dr. Jack W. Jones, Atlanta, paper, "Autohemotherapy in Dermatology"; Dr. Howard Hailey, Atlanta, discussed, "Radiation Therapy of Carbuncles"; Dr. Samuel F. Rosen, Savannah, paper, "Unusual Reaction from Thyroid Vaccine Administered Intravenously in Psoriasis—Lantern Slides"; Dr. D. Henry Poer, Atlanta, paper, "Newer Methods of Diagnosis and Treatment of Thyroid Disorders"; Dr. Daniel C. Elkin, Atlanta, paper, "Thyroidectomy—Factors Influencing the Mortality"; Dr. Robert L.

Rhodes, Augusta, paper, "Carcinoma of the Gallbladder"; Dr. J. H. Kite, Atlanta, discussed, "Arthrodesis of Knee with an Intramedullary Peg"; Dr. Lawson Thornton, Atlanta, paper, "Fracture Service in a Small General Hospital"; Dr. Olin S. Cofer, Atlanta, paper, "Treatment of Procidentia Uteri by the Vaginal Route—Lantern Slides"; Dr. Jno. W. Turner, Atlanta, discussed, "Treatment of Procidentia Uteri by the Vaginal Route"; Dr. Amey Chappell and Dr. F. Lee Bivings, Atlanta, paper, "Anemia and Pregnancy — A Three Year Study on Negro Women"; Dr. E. D. Colvin, Atlanta, discussed, "Anemia and Pregnancy — A Three Year Study on Negro Women"; Dr. Earl Floyd and Dr. Jas. L. Pittman, Atlanta, paper, "Malignant Tumors of Adult Kidney"; Dr. Edgar G. Ballenger, Atlanta, discussed, "Patent Urachus"; Dr. Montague L. Boyd, Atlanta, discussed, "Management of the Atonic Bladder Due to Obstruction of the Vesical Neck"; Dr. J. R. Garner, Atlanta, discussed, "The Doctor in Court"; Dr. Stewart R. Roberts, Atlanta, paper, "Cardiovascular Renal Disease"; Dr. V. P. Sydenstricker, Augusta, discussed, "Cardiovascular Renal Disease"; Dr. Henry M. Michel, Augusta, discussed, "Fractures of the Os Calcis"; Dr. Edgar F. Fincher, Jr., Atlanta, discussed, "Pyogenic Meningitis of Otitic Origin"; Dr. Murdock Equen and Dr. Frank Nueffer, Atlanta, paper, "Total Laryngectomy as an Approach to Esophageal Carcinoma—Recovery"; Dr. Dunbar Roy, Atlanta, "Clinical Observations of the Eustachian Tube"; Dr. J. Calhoun McDougall, Atlanta, discussed, "The Evaluation of Hearing Aides"; Dr. Grady E. Clay, Atlanta, paper, "Interesting Lesions of the Fundus Oculi"; Dr. Hal M. Davison, Atlanta, discussed, "Food Allergens—A Statistical Analysis of Fifty Cases Relative to the Genetic Classification of Foods"; Dr. E. D. Colvin, Atlanta, paper, "Maternal Mortality in Georgia During 1935"; Dr. T. F. Abercrombie, Atlanta, discussed, "Maternal Mortality in Georgia During 1935." MEMBERS FROM GEORGIA WHO REGISTERED: Adams, Chas. C., Augusta; Ainsworth, Harry, Thomasville; Alden, Herbert S, Atlanta; Allen, E. W., Milledgeville; Anderson, Wm. Willis, Atlanta; Arnold, J. T., Parrott; Atkinson, H. C., Macon; Aven, C. C., Atlanta; Ayers, A. J., Atlanta; Ballenger, E. G., Atlanta; Barrow, Craig, Savannah; Bashinski, Benj., Macon; Beasley, B. T., Atlanta; Bradley, R. H., Chatsworth; Bishop, Everett L., Atlanta; Bivings, W. T., Atlanta; Blackmar, Francis B., Columbus; Blanchard, Mercer, Columbus; Boland, F. K., Atlanta; Bowdoin, Chas., Atlanta; Bradley, D. M., Waycross; Brawner, Jas. N., Atlanta; Bray, S. E., Savannah; Brim, J. C., Pelham; Broaddrick, G. L., Dalton; Broderick, J. Reid, Savannah; Byrd, T. L., Atlanta; Calhoun, A. W., Atlanta; Calhoun, F. P., Atlanta; Cary, R. F., Dawson; Chappell, Amey, Atlanta; Childs, J. R., Atlanta; Clay, Grady E., Atlanta; Clements, H. W., Adel; Cline, B. McH., Atlanta; Cofer, Olin S., Atlanta; Colvin, E. D., Atlanta; Copeland, H. J., Griffin; Cousins, W. L., Atlanta; Cranston, W. J., Augusta; Crawford, H. C., Atlanta; Daniel, Chas. H., College Park; Davison, Hal M., Atlanta; Derrick, H. C., Oglethorpe; Dexter, C. A., Columbus; Dykes, A. N., Columbus; Edgerton, M. T., Jr., Atlanta; Elrod, J. O., Forsyth; Equen,

Murdock, Atlanta; Faggart, G. H., Savannah; Fincher, E. F., Jr., Atlanta; Fitts, J. B., Atlanta; Fort, M. A., Bainbridge; Fuller, G. W., Atlanta; Funkhouser, Wm. L., Atlanta; Gaines, Lewis M., Atlanta; Garner, Jas. R., Atlanta; Goolsby, R. C., Jr., Macon; Grove, L. W., Atlanta; Hailey, Howard, Atlanta; Hamm, W. G., Atlanta; Hanner, J. P., Atlanta; Harbin, Lester, Rome; Harbin, W. P., Rome; Harrell, H. P., Augusta; Harrold, Thos., Macon; Hesse, H. W., Savannah; Holmes, L. P., Augusta; Howard, Lee, Savannah; Irvin, H. L., Dalton; Irvin, I. W., Albany; Jackson, R. L., Atlanta; Jarrell, W. W., Thomasville; Johnson, Raymond L., Waycross; Kandel, H. M., Savannah; Kay, Jas. B., Byron; Keen, O. F., Macon; Kelley, D. C., Lawrenceville; Kite, J. H., Decatur; Knowles, Fred L., Savannah; Kracke, Roy R., Emory University; Laws, Clarence L., Atlanta; Lee, Lawrence, Savannah; Little, A. G., Valdosta; Maner, E. N., Savannah; Massenburg, G. Y., Macon; McCoy, W. R., Alma; McDougall, J. C., Atlanta; McGee, H. H., Savannah; McMichael, J. R., Quitman; McRae, Floyd W., Atlanta; Meeks, D. H., Nicholls; Metts, J. C., Savannah; Michel, H. M., Augusta; Minchew, B. H., Waycross; Mixson, W. D., Waycross; Morrison, H. J., Savannah; Neill, F. K., Albany; Norris, Jack C., Atlanta; Oppenheimer, R. H., Emory University; Palmer, J. W., Ailey; Parker, F. P., Atlanta; Paullin, Jas. E., Atlanta; Peacock, J. H., Atlanta; Phinizy, Thos. B., Augusta; Pittman, C. S., Tifton; Pittman, Jas. L., Atlanta; Poer, D. Henry, Atlanta; Primrose, A. C., Americus; Pruitt, Marion C., Atlanta; Revell, S. T. R., Louisville; Richardson, R. W., Macon; Roberts, M. Hines, Atlanta; Roberts, Stewart R., Atlanta; Rosen, S. F., Savannah; Rosenberg, H. J., Atlanta; Sanderson, E. S., Augusta; Sauls, H. C., Atlanta; Saye, E. B., Macon; Scott, W. M., Milledgeville; Shanks, Edgar D., Atlanta; Sherman, J. H., Augusta; Smith, S. H., Atlanta; Smith, S. S., Athens; Starr, Trammell, Dalton; Sandison, J. Calvin, Atlanta; Schley, Francis B., Columbus; Selman, W. A., Atlanta; Shields, H. F., Chickamauga; Smith, M. R., Cordele; Sweet, Mary F., Decatur; Standifer, J. G., Blakely; Sydenstricker, V. P., Augusta; Talmadge, Harry E., Athens; Thomas, D. R., Jr., Augusta; Thomas, J. W., Augusta; Thurmond, A. G., Waynesboro; Thurmond, J. W., Augusta; Traylor, Geo. A., Augusta; Turner, John W., Atlanta; Waring, A. J., Savannah; Watson, O. O., Macon; West, C. M., Atlanta; Wheat, R. F., Bainbridge; Wilcox, E. A., Augusta; Williams, L. W., Savannah; Williams, W. J., Augusta; Willis, L. W., Bainbridge; Wright, P. B., Augusta; Yampolsky, Joseph, Atlanta; Young, W. W., Atlanta. Names of members who registered on November 17th and 20th are not available.

DR. C. F. HOLTON, Savannah, has been appointed to the official staff of our next Governor, Hon. E. D. Rivers of Lakeland.

THE WARE COUNTY MEDICAL SOCIETY met at the Okefenokee Golf Club on December 2nd. Dr. W. F. Reavis and Dr. L. W. Pierce, Waycross, were hosts at a turkey and barbecue dinner. Officers were elected for the ensuing year.

THE GEORGIA MEDICAL SOCIETY, Savannah, met on November 24th. A resolution in reference to the Workmen's Compensation Act was adopted as follows: "At a meeting of the special committee appointed by the Society it was agreed to recommend that a motion be passed by the Georgia Medical Society stating that it is the consensus of opinion of the Society that the present Workmen's Compensation Act is unfair to the doctor and to the patient in limiting the period of treatment to 30 days and the maximum medical and hospital charges to $100. It was also recommended that the secretary of the Society write to the Senator and Representatives of the First District and also to the Secretary of the State Association asking them to urge an extension of the time limit of treatment to 90 days and to increase the medical and hospital expense to a maximum of $250."

DR. EDGAR D. SHANKS, Atlanta, Secretary-Treasurer of the Association, attended the Conference of Secretaries of State Medical Associations in the Assembly Room of the American Medical Association Building, Chicago, November 16-17. The Conference is sponsored by the A. M. A. Dr. Allen H. Bunce, Atlanta, member of the Board of Trustees of the A. M. A., attended meetings of the Trustees on November 13-14, and the Conference of Secretaries on the 16th and 17th.

THE RANDOLPH COUNTY MEDICAL SOCIETY met at the Patterson Hospital, Cuthbert, on December 3rd. Dr. F. S. Rogers, Coleman, read a paper entitled "Coronary Occlusion."

THE SIXTH DISTRICT MEDICAL SOCIETY met in Ridley Hall, Macon, December 2nd. Titles of papers on the scientific program were: "The Acute Abdomen," by Dr. E. B. Claxton, Dublin; "The Anemias of Infancy and Childhood," Dr. Wm. C. Boswell, Macon; "X-Ray Therapy in Carcinoma of the Breast," Dr. Thomas Harrold, Macon; "What Public Health Means to the General Practitioner," Dr. O. H. Cheek, Dublin; "Spinal Anesthesia," Dr. W. M. Scott, Milledgeville; "Practical Points in the Treatment of Congestive Heart Failure," Dr. James A. Fountain, Macon. Other speakers on the program were: Dr. B. H. Minchew, Waycross, President of the Association; Dr. H. G. Weaver, Macon, Councilor of the Sixth District.

DR. AND MRS. ROBERT B. LAMB, Demorest, entertained the members of the Habersham County Medical Society and Auxiliary in their home on November 12th.

DR. R. P. MORROW, West Point, is taking postgraduate work at Tulane University of Louisiana School of Medicine, New Orleans.

THE FULTON COUNTY MEDICAL SOCIETY met at the Academy of Medicine, 38 Prescott Street, N. E., Atlanta, December 3rd. Dr. John R. Walker reported a case, "Removal of Dermoid Cyst Attached to Urinary Bladder"; Dr. Stacy C. Howell read a paper, "Action of Epinephrine on the Diseased Human Eye"; Dr. Dan C. Elkin, paper, "Treatment of Wounds of the Heart."

DR. N. B. BATEMAN AND DR. SAMUEL Y. BROWN announce their association in the practice of medicine and surgery. Suite 523 Candler Building, Atlanta.

THE ASSOCIATION of the Seaboard Air Line Railway Surgeons held its Twenty-Fourth Annual Session at Havana, Cuba, December 2-4. Dr. H. W. Birdsong, Athens, reported a case, "Spinal Cord Injury"; Dr. H. A. Smith, Americus, discussed, "Radical Treatment of the Enormous and the Non-Discernible Types of Inguinal Hernia." The official banquet was held in the Banquet Hall of the Sevilla-Biltmore Hotel on December 6th. Many sight-seeing tours were available for the attending physicians. Dr. J. W. Palmer, Ailey, is Secretary-Treasurer of the Association.

THE GEORGIA MEDICAL SOCIETY, Savannah, held its regular meeting on December 8th. The program consisted of annual reports of officers and chairmen of committees. Officers were elected for 1937.

DR. J. H. HAMMOND, LaFayette, was entertained on his eightieth birthday at dinner in the home of Dr. and Mrs. Richard C. Shepherd of LaFayette. He was honored with congratulations from many acquaintances.

DR. CHARLES W. REID, Pelham, has completed a half century practicing medicine in Mitchell and adjoining counties. He is 78 years of age. His daughter, Mrs. John Monaghan, presented the Tallulah Falls School with a $2,000.00 perpetual scholarship in honor of Dr. Reid. He has never owned an automobile or used one in his practice.

DR. JAMES J. CLARK, Atlanta, was elected President of the medical staff of Emory University Hospital; Dr. I. A. Ferguson, Atlanta, Vice-President; Dr. H. H. Allen, Decatur, re-elected Secretary-Treasurer.

THE GEORGIA PEDIATRIC SOCIETY held its meetings at the Biltmore Hotel and Academy of Medicine, Atlanta, on December 10th. Speakers included: Dr. Julius Hess, University of Illinois College of Medicine, Chicago; Dr. John A. Toomey, Western Reserve University School of Medicine, Cleveland, Ohio; Dr. Henry F. Helmholz, Mayo Clinic, Rochester, Minn.

DR. KIRK SHEPARD announces the opening of his office in Suite 618 Doctors Building, 478 Peachtree Street, N. E., Atlanta, for the practice of surgery, gynecology and obstetrics.

DR. HARRY T. HARPER, JR., formerly on the staff of the University Hospital, Augusta, has removed to Eastman and will be associated with Dr. Warren A. Coleman and others at the Coleman Sanatorium in the practice of cardiology.

THE Macon Medical Society of Bibb County held its annual banquet at the New-Yorker on December 15th. Officers for the ensuing year were installed.

OBITUARY

Dr. J. Beal Powers, Macon: Emory University School of Medicine, Emory University; aged 74; died at his home on September 16, 1936. He had been in ill health for about one year and was forced to abandon his practice on that account. Dr. Powers was quite popular among his acquaintance and clientele and a valuable citizen. Surviving him are his widow, three daughters. Mrs. H. B. Smith, Jacksonville, Georgia; Mrs. L. T. Wilt, Macon; and Miss Lucile Powers, Macon. Funeral services were conducted from the Mount Zion Baptist church, Loraine. Burial was in the churchyard.

Dr. William P. Williams, Blackshear; member; Bellevue Hospital Medical College, New York City, 1888; aged 69; died at a Waycross hospital on September 24, 1936. He was an outstanding physician of Pierce County and a member of a pioneer family. His father. Dr. Benjamin F. Williams, was a delegate to the first Constitutional Convention in Georgia and one of the first two settlers of Waycross. Dr. Williams was physician for Blackshear and Pierce County. He was a member of the Ware County Medical Society, Knights of Pythias and Presbyterian church. Funeral services were conducted from the Blackshear Presbyterian church. Burial was in the city cemetery.

Dr. Jarrell N. Hogg, Macon: Emory University School of Medicine, 1879; aged 83; died at the home of his daughter, Mrs. Allen J. Smith, Macon, on September 28, 1936. He was born and reared in West Point and resided there until he retired from active practice of medicine 17 years ago. Dr. Hogg was a useful citizen, active in civic and religious affairs. He was a member of the Masonic lodge and the Methodist church. Surviving him are three daughters. Mrs. Allen J. Smith, Macon; Mrs. Harry Hatch, Los Angeles, Cal., and Mrs. Leslie George, Perry, Florida; one son. Jarrell N. Hogg, Jr., Macon. Funeral services were conducted from the home of his daughter. Mrs. Smith, by Rev. Randolph Clairborne. Burial was in West Point cemetery.

Dr. Lonie W. Hodges, Gainesville; member; University of Georgia School of Medicine, 1897; aged 60; died of coronary thrombosis in his office on September 29, 1936. He was a native of Walton County, practiced medicine in Winder for many years and moved to Gainesville eighteen years ago. Dr. Hodges limited his practice to ophthalmology, otology, laryngology and rhinology. He had an extensive practice and maintained offices in Winder and Gainesville. People who knew Dr. Hodges believed in him and trusted him. He was a member of the Hall County Medical Society, Ninth District Medical Society, Southern Medical Association and the First Christian church at Winder. Surviving him are his widow; one sister, Mrs. Ossie Lanier, Bogart; two brothers, J. N. Hodges, Monroe, and Henry Hodges, Watkinsville. Funeral services were conducted from the First Christian church of Winder by Rev. W. A. Foster and Rev. R. Q. Leavell. Interment was in Rose Hill cemetery at Winder. Members of the Ninth District Medical Society formed an honorary escort.

Dr. Robert L. McMichael, Buena Vista: Atlanta College of Physicians and Surgeons, Atlanta, 1900; aged 65; died at his home after a long illness on October 1, 1936. He was an active and successful practitioner for more than twenty-five years and until he was disabled. Dr. McMichael was held in high esteem by many acquaintances. Surviving him are his widow;

five daughters. Mrs. Miller R. Bell, Milledgeville; Mrs. Carey Owen Pickard, Memphis, Tenn.; Misses Marjorie and Gladys McMichael, Buena Vista; one son. Robert L. McMichael, Atlanta. Funeral services were conducted from the Methodist church by Rev. J. W. Lilley. Burial was in Buena Vista cemetery.

Dr. David M. Wheelis, Columbus; Southern Medical College, Atlanta, 1887; aged 74; died at his home. 3401 Hamilton Road, on October 9, 1936. He was a native of Chambers County, Alabama. Dr. Wheelis was a prominent physician in Muscogee County until forced to retire about ten years ago on account of ill health. He was a member of the Methodist church. Surviving him are his widow; three daughters. Mrs. C. N. Campbell, Decatur, Ala.; Mrs. O. J. Gaudray and Mrs. L. C. Jones, both of Columbus. Funeral services were conducted from the chapel of Britton & Dobbs by Rev. N. M. Lovein. Burial was in Riverdale cemetery.

Dr. William Isham Hailey, Hartwell; member; Louisville Medical College, Louisville, Ky., 1893; aged 66; died at his home after a long illness, on October 15, 1936. He was one of the leading citizens of Hart County, prominent physician and surgeon with an extensive practice in Hart and adjoining counties. Dr. Hailey was one time President of the Hartwell Board of Education, and Mayor of Hartwell, Chairman of the Hart County Democratic Executive Committee, member of the State Board of Health when the State Tuberculosis Sanatorium at Alto was built and served on the Building Committee. Dr. Hailey was liberal in his support of civic and religious organizations. He was a prominent physician and surgeon and gave unstintingly of his time and professional skill to the rich and destitute when his services were needed. Dr. Hailey was a member of the Hart County Medical Society and the Baptist church. Surviving him are his widow; seven sons. Dr. J. Henry Hailey, Dr. Isham B. Hailey and Frank E. Hailey, Hartwell; Dr. Howard Hailey, Atlanta; Dr. Rucker M. Hailey, Miami, Fla.; Dr. Hugh E. Hailey, New York City. Rev. Rufus D. Hodges conducted the funeral services. Burial was in the city cemetery.

Dr. Wallace W. Norris, Atlanta: University of the South Medical Department. Sewanee, Tenn., 1905; aged 65; died at his home, 545 Oakland Avenue, October 19, 1936. He was a native of Meriwether County. Dr. Norris was a prominent physician and had practiced medicine in Atlanta for thirty years. He was a member and deacon of the Capitol Avenue Baptist church. Surviving him are his widow, one sister and two brothers. Rev. W. H. Major conducted the funeral services from the Capitol Avenue Baptist church. Interment was in Oakland cemetery.

Dr. Nathaniel Hooks Lozier, Sandersville; member; University of Georgia School of Medicine. Augusta, 1914; aged 46; died in an Atlanta hospital after an illness of short duration, on October 2, 1936. He was born and reared at Warthen and began practice there, then moved to Sandersville. Dr. Lozier received his literary education at Mercer University. He was a prominent physician and owner of a large tract of farming land. Dr. Lozier was charitable and one of the State's best citizens. Surviving him are his widow; two daughters, Miss Mary Lozier, Atlanta, and Miss Martha Lozier, Sandersville; two brothers and two sisters.

Dr. John B. Weldon, Inman; Atlanta College of Physicians and Surgeons, Atlanta, 1906; aged 52; died at his home on October 23, 1936. Many warm personal friends held Dr. Weldon in high esteem. He was a member of the Inman Methodist church. Rev. Mr. Stone conducted the funeral services from the Inman Methodist church. Burial was in the Inman cemetery.

Dr. Frank Lee Cato, Leslie; member; Jefferson Medical College of Philadelphia, Pa., 1887; aged 73; died at his home on October 23, 1936. He received his literary education at Mercer University, Macon. Dr. Cato before he retired had an extensive practice in Sumter and adjoining counties. Surviving him are his widow and one son, Dr. Frank Cato, New Orleans. La. Funeral services were conducted from the Leslie Baptist church. Burial was in the village cemetery.

Dr. Willis W. Rutland, LaGrange; Southern Medical College, Atlanta, 1889; aged 73; died at a private hospital on October 24, 1936. He was born and reared in Chambers County, Alabama. His life and work have been useful for the promotion of the welfare of his home community, and lasting friendships were acquired by his untiring and skilful medical care of his patients. Dr. Rutland was a member of the Odd Fellows, Masons and the United Congregational Christian church. Surviving him are his widow; three daughters, Mrs. Tom Garrett, LaGrange; Mrs. R. H. Wade, Cochran; Mrs. W. C. Page, Ashboro, N. C.; two sons, Dr. S. C. Rutland, LaGrange, and D. A. Rutland, Bryn Mawr, Pa. Funeral services were conducted by Rev. J. H. Knight from the residence. Interment was in Shadow Lawn cemetery. Members of the Troup County Medical Society formed an honorary escort.

Dr. William Washington Liles, Gainesville; member; Georgia College of Eclectic Medicine and Surgery, Atlanta, 1899; aged 61; died at his home on November 6, 1936. He was a native of Hall County and had resided there all his life, except, while in literary and medical schools. Dr. Liles began the practice of medicine at Flowery Branch, Hall County, later removed to Gainesville. He served as county physician for twelve years. He was affable, accommodating, and served his clientele in a most pleasing manner. Dr. Liles was a successful physician and one of the State's most useful citizens. He was a member of the Hall County Medical Society, Ninth District Medical Society and the Methodist church. Surviving him are his widow; one daughter, Miss Annie Maude Liles; two sons, T. E. Liles, Gainesville, and Alton G. Liles, Buford. Rev. Gresham with Rev. Jones conducted the funeral services from the Central Baptist church. Burial was in Alta Vista cemetery.

Dr. Harvey W. Smith, Atlanta; Georgia College of Eclectic Medicine and Surgery, Atlanta, 1899; aged 72; died of heart disease in Miami, Fla., November 8, 1936. He was a native of Sumter County. Dr. Smith had been a resident of Atlanta for seventeen years and an active and successful physician until he retired on account of ill health. He was active in civic and religious affairs and a member of the Trinity Avenue Methodist church. Surviving him is his son, George T. Smith, Albany.

Dr. Lee L. Robinson, Boston; Georgia College of Eclectic Medicine and Surgery, Atlanta, 1893; aged 64; died at his home, after a long illness, on November 5, 1936. He practiced at Valdosta for many years, later at Quitman, then moved to Boston. Dr. Robinson was an affable and congenial gentleman, public spirited and had many friends. Surviving him are his son, L. L. Robinson, Jr., Miami, Fla.; two sisters, Mrs. J. P. Wade, Camilla, and Mrs. M. E. Wade, Brooks County; one brother, J. G. Robinson, Oakland, Fla. Funeral services were conducted at the graveside and interment in the Robinson cemetery in Brooks County.

Dr. Luther Asbury DeLoach, Savannah; member; Atlanta College of Physicians and Surgeons, Atlanta, 1905; aged 53; died at his home on November 22, 1936. He was born in Liberty County. After receiving his degree in medicine, he practiced at Glennville, Tattnall County, until sixteen years ago and removed to Savannah. Dr. DeLoach served as Councilman and as Mayor of Glennville while residing there. He was active in professional, civic and religious affairs. Dr. DeLoach was a member of the Georgia Medical Society, American Medical Association, Kiwanis Club and the First Baptist church in which he served as deacon for a number of years. He had many personal friends and was one of the State's best citizens. Surviving him are his widow; one son, Laurence DeLoach; one daughter, Mrs. Cloyce W. Harty, all of Savannah. Funeral services were conducted from the First Baptist church by Dr. Arthur Jackson. Interment was in Bonaventure cemetery. Officers and deacons of the First Baptist church with members of the Georgia Medical Society were honorary pallbearers.

BOOK REVIEWS

Endocrinology in Modern Practice. By William Wolf, M.D., M.S., Ph.D. 1,018 pages, 252 illustrations. W. B. Saunders Co., 1936. This volume is one of the most complete endocrine treatises recently published. It is flavored with occasional unproved theories but in the main is reliable and interesting reading. There are 36 chapters, divided into three groups: (1) The Endocrines. (2) The Endocrine Aspects of Non-endocrine disorders. (3) Endocrine Diagnosis.

Chief among its virtues are the numerous tables at the end of each chapter, summarizing the essentials of diagnosis of the disorders of each of the endocrine glands. Another valuable and unusual feature is the classification and description of endocrine disorders under each of the various specialties.

The author has attempted to encourage the physician, whether general practitioner or specialist, to think along endocrine lines. There are numerous illustrations, most of which are excellent. A diagram illustrating the interaction—stimulation and antagonism—of the various endocrines is printed in colors.

The section on Diagnosis illustrates the multitudinous laboratory tests and procedures which have developed in this field as well as the special type of history taking and physical examination for glandular stigmata. The author has accomplished a prodigious task well.   J. K. FANCHER, M.D.

SYPHILIS AND ITS TREATMENT: By WILLIAM A. HINTON, M.D. The Macmillan Monographs, Pages 321. Price $3.50; The Macmillan Company, New York, 1936.

Dr. Hinton still holds that mercury is most valuable in the treatment and should not be abandoned. He believes that syphilis is a likely cause of delayed union in fractures of the long bones. He does not believe that the provocative dose of arsphenamine is of value, as repeated Wassermanns will also usually eventually show a positive. He attaches less importance to repeated spinal punctures than most medical authorities have done in recent years. He minimizes the importance of treating apparently latent syphilis, though he must know that at this stage visceral changes are being wrought that can not be remedied when they become clinically manifest. Moreover, the reviewer can not see the rationale of limiting a syphilitic patient to "four to six cigarettes a day."

Although this book is a model of condensation, it runs counter to so many principles of syphilotherapy that seem to have been established in recent years that its value is questionable. However, most general practitioners, who must from the nature of things handle the majority of cases of syphilis, do not succeed in treating the patient recently infected with syphilis as thoroughly as Dr. Hinton advises (which is much less than Stokes, Moore and other prominent syphilologists insist upon). If the general practitioner after reading this book will insist upon his patients receiving as much treatment as is advised therein, the book will have justified itself.—L.M.B.

THE MEDICAL AND ORTHOPEDIC MANAGEMENT OF CHRONIC ARTHRITIS: By RALPH PEMBERTON and ROBERT B. OSGOOD. The Macmillan Co., New York. Price $5.00.

Chronic arthritis causes a great deal of suffering and an immense economic loss. Cases last such a long time, respond so poorly to any specific medicine that both the patient and the doctor become discouraged.

This book is the result of years of careful study by two eminent authorities on rheumatic conditions. They are both active workers on both American and International Committees for the control of Rheumatism. They know their subject and they are not discouraged —in fact this book is the most optimistic of any book I have seen on the subject. They claim that much can be done for even the worst cases of chronic arthritis. This is just the kind of a book that a physician should read who has to treat arthritis. They have given fair consideration to all methods of treatment—drugs, vaccines, physical therapy are all discussed. Then they give a rational method of handling these cases. They know good results can be obtained, for they have obtained them and they tell one in detail how these patients can be relieved.

FRED G. HODGSON, M.D.

DISABILITY EVALUATIONS: By EARL D. MCBRIDE, Assistant Professor of Orthopedic Surgery, University of Oklahoma School of Medicine (Lippincott).

Those of us who do a considerable volume of industrial surgery are often embarrassed by questions from attorneys or industrial commissioners as to what percentage of disability exists because of the permanent loss of a finger or toe or ankylosis of some minor joint. Upon such estimations compensation is granted and it is seldom indeed that two doctors arrive at the same conclusion in a given case.

In Dr. McBride's book DISABILITY EVALUATIONS he has carefully taken up this question and formulated a method through which such evaluations can be correctly arrived at. This feature alone warrants this

book being on the desk of every industrial surgeon and also commends itself to the attention of insurance adjusters and lawyers who try cases before industrial commissions, and to the commissioners themselves.

The book is profusely illustrated with photographs, x-ray studies and drawings. The function of the various parts of the anatomy is carefully considered and there are many complete tables scientifically worked up to enable the busy surgeon to prepare himself for the proper answers to cross-examination by attorneys both friendly and otherwise.

One interesting feature of the book is the complete table covering the compensation laws of the various states of the Union and Canada. It is quite interesting to note the difference in funds allowed for medical and hospitalization in the various states.

In addition to the purely statistical features of the book Dr. McBride has masterfully presented the subject of fractures, back injuries and nerve injuries. This makes it a handy reference from an orthopedic standpoint as his presentation of etiology, treatment and prognosis of these injuries is thoroughly sound.

The only criticism to be found in the volume is that Dr. McBride has a tendency to think in terms of higher mathematics and it is the writer's opinion that most doctors who have a successful industrial practice have been away from school so long they have forgotten all they knew of trigonometry and other branches of mathematics and therefore will find it difficult to follow Dr. McBride in some of his deductions.

C. F. HOLTON, M.D.

THE STOMACH AND DUODENUM: By EUSTERMAN AND BALFOUR. W. B. Saunders Company, Philadelphia, pp. 956, price $10.00.

This book is by far the best of similarly written books that I have read. The subject matter is covered very thoroughly from several different points of view, but nevertheless, there is very little unwarranted repetition and the work gives one an excellent idea of the subject.

The illustrations are good, the descriptions of surgical indications and procedures are excellent and the chapter on "Applied Physiology of the Stomach and Duodenum," gives one an entirely new concept of just what is taking place and allows him to apply treatment on a rational basis.

I. A. FERGUSON, M.D.

THE CLINICAL USE OF DIGITALIS: By DREW LUTEN, A.B., M.D., Associate Professor of Clinical Medicine, Washington University School of Medicine; Physician to Barnes Hospital, Saint Louis. 226 pages. Price $3.50. Springfield and Baltimore: Charles C. Thomas, 1936.

In 1785, the great Withering announced his experience with foxglove in the treatment of dropsy. The careful clinical study of his patients had enabled him to lay down the fundamentals in the proper use of digitalis. Unfortunately the furor attending its introduction led to the widespread and indiscriminate use of the drug—for a number of years it was used as a specific in the treatment of tuberculosis—with of course its subsequent virtual abandonment.

Mackenzie, though it is hard to find fault with this great figure, announced that the benefit of digitalis was a result of the slowing of the pulse, and that it was of greatest value in the treatment of auricular fibrillation with a rapid ventricular rate and congestive failure. His distinguished successor, Thomas Lewis, has so greatly emphasized this aspect of digitalis therapy that there has been a tendency, particularly abroad, to consider digitalis of no benefit except in such cases. However, the result of extensive experimentation both on animals and humans and of clinical observation, much of which we are proud to observe has been done in the United States, has brought us back to the sound position announced by Withering nine years after the Declaration of Independence.

Luten has summarized the study of digitalis to date in a short and wholly admirable book. Thoroughly scientific, this book is yet not encumbered with many graphic records that tend to bewilder the man not specially trained in cardiology.

It is strange how 151 years of study has brought us back to the clinical principles enunciated by Withering: Digitalis is still the sheet anchor in the treatment of heart failure regardless of its cause. Thirty grains of the dried leaf (of high grade) is still more than enough to digitalize almost all patients, and will produce signs of poisoning in many of them. Poisoning is not desirable. The optimal maintenance dosage can only be determined by a method of trial and error.

Every physician who treats patients with congestive heart failure will be able to do so better and with more assurance after careful study of this book. He will also be interested in seeing how the most recent scientific investigations have lent support to the practical principles laid down so long ago by that master clinician.

L.M.B.

COUNTIES REPORTING FOR 1937

Hall County Medical Society

The Hall County Medical Society announces the following officers for 1937:

President—H. H. Lancaster, Clermont
Vice-President—B. B. Davis, Gainesville
Secretary-Treasurer—Hartwell Joiner, Gainesville
Delegate—W. C. Kennedy, Talmo
Alternate Delegate—J. L. Meeks, Gainesville
Censors—J. H. Downey, J. K. Burns and Hartwell Joiner, all of Gainesville.

Macon Medical Society of Bibb County

The Macon Medical Society of Bibb County reports the following officers for 1937:

President—W. L. Bazemore, Macon
President-Elect—W. R. Golsan, Macon
Vice-President—H. C. Atkinson, Macon
Secretary-Treasurer—W. Chas. Boswell, Macon
Librarian—W. E. Mobley, Macon
Delegate—A. R. Rozar, Macon
Delegate—H. C. Atkinson, Macon
Alternate Delegate—Alvin E. Siegel, Macon
Alternate Delegate—W. W. Chrisman, Macon.

Colquitt County Medical Society

The Colquitt County Medical Society announces the following officers for 1937:

President—W. R. McGinty, Moultrie
Vice-President—W. L. Bennett, Moultrie
Secretary-Treasurer—R. M. Joiner, Moultrie
Delegate—C. C. Brannen, Moultrie
Alternate Delegate—J. R. Paulk, Moultrie.

Tri County Medical Society
(Calhoun, Early and Miller)

The Tri County Medical Society announces the following officers for 1937:

President—R. R. Bridges, Leary.
Vice-President—J. S. Beard, Edison.
Secretary-Treasurer—J. G. Standifer, Blakely.
Delegate—Holt Darden, Blakely.
Alternate Delegate—J. G. Standifer, Blakely.

Taliaferro County Medical Society

The Taliaferro County Medical Society announces the following officers for 1937:

President—T. C. Nash, Philomath.
Secretary-Treasurer—Jno. A. Rhodes, Crawfordville.
Delegate—T. C. Nash, Philomath.

Spalding County Medical Society

The Spalding County Medical Society announces the following officers for 1937:

President—Geo. L. Walker, Griffin.
Vice-President—D. L. Head, Zebulon.
Secretary-Treasurer—H. J. Copeland, Griffin.
Delegate—A. H. Frye, Griffin.
Alternate Delegate—W. C. Miles, Griffin.

HONOR ROLL FOR 1936

1. Randolph County, Dr. W. G. Elliott, Cuthbert, October 30, 1935.
2. Dougherty County, Dr. I. M. Lucas, Albany, December 27, 1935.
3. Monroe County, Dr. G. H. Alexander, Forsyth, February 14, 1936.
4. Hancock County, Dr. H. L. Earl, Sparta, February 25, 1936.
5. Elbert County, Dr. A. S. Johnson, Elberton, March 6, 1936.
6. Worth County, Dr. G. S. Sumner, Sylvester, March 12, 1936.
7. Rockdale County, Dr. H. E. Griggs, Conyers, March 21, 1936.
8. Morgan County, Dr. W. C. McGeary, Madison, March 30, 1936.
9. Turner County, Dr. J. H. Baxter, Ashburn, March 30, 1936.
10. Ware County, Dr. Kenneth McCullough, Waycross, March 30, 1936.
11. Georgia Medical Society (Chatham County), Dr. Otto W. Schwalb, Savannah, April 17, 1936.

HONOR ROLL FOR 1937

1. Randolph County, Dr. W. G. Elliott, Cuthbert, September 28, 1936.
2. Dougherty County, Dr. I. M. Lucas, Albany, December 12, 1936.

Directory
of the
Medical Association of Georgia
for 1936

Names of all Members and Officers are published as corrected by Secretaries of County Societies.

ALTAMAHA
(Appling County)
Officer
Secretary-Treasurer .... Holt, J. T.
Members
Branch, W. D., Baxley
Holt, J. T., Baxley
Kennedy, F. D., Baxley
McCracken, H. C., Baxley
Overstreet, E. J., Baxley
Powell, W. H., Hazlehurst

BALDWIN COUNTY
Officers
President .... Anderson, S. A.
Vice-President .... Bailey, L. A.
Secretary-Treasurer .... Fulghum, Chas. B.
Delegate .... Binion, Richard
Alternate Delegate .... Evans. R. E.
Members
Allen, E. W., Milledgeville
Allen, H. D., Jr., Milledgeville
Anderson, S. A., Milledgeville
Bailey, L. A., Milledgeville
Binion, Richard, Milledgeville
Bostick, W. A., Hardwick
Bradford, R. W., Milledgeville
Corswell, Gibson K., Milledgeville
Cox, C. G., Milledgeville
Echols, Geo. L., Milledgeville
Evans, R. E., Milledgeville
Fulghum, Chas. B., Milledgeville
Garrard, J. I., Hardwick
Hall, T. M., Milledgeville (Hon.)
Holder, F. P., Jr., Milledgeville
Jordan, William, Milledgeville
Longino, L. P., Hardwick
Miles, W. G., Milledgeville
Moran, O. F., Milledgeville
Oden, John W., Milledgeville
Sanchez, A. S., Eatonton
Scott, W. M., Milledgeville
Smith, J. P., Eutaw, Ala.
Wheeler, G. A., Milledgeville (Hon.)
Wiley, John D., Milledgeville
Woods, O. C., Milledgeville
Yarbrough, Y. H., Milledgeville

BARTOW COUNTY
Officers
President .... Wofford, W. E.
Vice-President .... Stanford, J. W.
Secretary-Treasurer .... Lowry, T.
Delegate .... Lowry, T.
Alternate Delegate ...... Wofford, W. E.
Members
Adair, R. E., Cartersville
Bowdoin, C. D., State Capitol, Atlanta
Bowdoin, J. P., State Capitol, Atlanta
Bradford, H. B., Pine Log
Burton, R. E., Kingston
Horton, A. L., Cartersville
Howell, S. M., Cartersville
Lowry, T., Cartersville
McGowan, H. S., Cartersville
Shamblin, A. C., Cartersville
Stanford, J. W., Cartersville
Wofford, W. E., Cartersville

BEN HILL
Officers
President .... Willis, G. W.
Vice-President .... McMillan, J. E.
Secretary-Treasurer .... Osborne, L. S.
Delegate .... Abram, Lewis
Alternate Delegate .... Dorminy, E. J.
Members
Abram, Lewis, Fitzgerald
Bradley, T. B., Fitzgerald
Coffee, W. P., Fitzgerald
Dorminy, E. J., Fitzgerald
Frazier, J. L., Fitzgerald (Asso.)
Harper, A., Wray
McMillan, J. E., Fitzgerald

Osborne, L. S., Fitzgerald (Hon.)
Ward, Frank, Fitzgerald (Asso.)
Ware, D. B., Fitzgerald
Ware, R. M., Fitzgerald
Wilcox, C. H., Fitzgerald
Willis, G. W., Ocilla

BIBB COUNTY
Officers
President .... Corn, Ernest
President-Elect .... Bazemore, W. L.
Vice-President .... Hall, John I.
Secretary-Treasurer .... Golsan. W. R.
Delegate .... Kay, Jas. B.
Delegate .... Weaver, O. H.
Members
Adams, I. H., Georgia Casualty Bldg.,
   Macon
Aldrich, Fred N., Georgia Casualty Bldg.-
   Macon
Anderson, C. L., 700 Spring St., Macon
Anderson, J. C., Georgia Casualty Bldg.
   Macon
Applewhite, J. D., 720 New Street, Macon
Atkinson, H. C., 700 Spring St., Macon
Bashinski, Benj., 700 Spring St., Macon
Bazemore, Wallace L., Georgia Casualty
   Bldg., Macon
Boswell, Wm. Chas., Georgia Casualty Bldg.,
   Macon
Brown, J. P., Middle Georgia Sanatorium.
   Macon
Camp, J. A., Roberta
Christman, W. W., 700 Spring St., Macon
Clay, J. Emory, The Clinic, Macon
Coleman, Y. K., 124 Hardeman Ave., Macon
Corn, Ernest, 700 Spring St., Macon
Cowart, J. W., Walden (Hon.)
Daniel, Orman, First Nat'l Bank & Trust
   Co. Bldg., Macon
Derry, H. P., 664 College St., Macon
   (Hon.)
Dove, W. B., Grand Bldg., Macon
DuPree, G. W., Gordon
Evans, A. P., Pinehurst
Farmer, C. Hall, The Clinic, Macon
Fountain, J. A., Georgia Casualty Bldg.,
   Macon
Gewinner, N. G., 1205 Vineville Ave.,
   Macon (Hon.)
Golsan, W. R., Georgia Casualty Bldg.,
   Macon
Goolsby, R. Cullen, Jr., 700 Spring St.,
   Macon
Gortin, B. S., 636 Orange St., Macon
Greene, B. W., Bibb Bldg., Macon -
Hall, J. I., Georgia Casualty Bldg., Macon
Hall, T. H., 617 Mulberry St., Macon
Harrold, C. C., 700 Spring St., Macon
Harrold, Thos., 700 Spring St., Macon
Haslem, J. E., Fort Valley
Hembree, J. A., Company 3404, C.C.C.,
   Ramsour, N. C.
Hinton, C. C., 700 Spring St., Macon
   (Deceased)
Holmes, J. P., Georgia Casualty Bldg.,
   Macon
Hurley, T. A., The Clinic, Macon
Johnson, J. E. L., Roberta
Kay, J. B., Byron
Keen, O. F., Oglethorpe Infirmary, Macon
Kemp, Paul S., Georgia Casualty Bldg.,
   Macon
King, J. L., Georgia Casualty Bldg., Macon
Martin, J. P., 403 Cherry St., Macon
Massenburg, G. Y., The Clinic, Macon
McAfee, L. C., Bibb Bldg., Macon
McLaughlin, C. K., The Clinic, Macon
McMichael, V. H., 122 DeSoto Place, Ma-
   con (Hon.)
Meriwether, W. W., Georgia Casualty Bldg.,
   Macon
Millen, G. T., First Nat'l Bank & Trust
   Co. Bldg., Macon (Hon.)
Mobley, W. E., 700 Spring St., Macon

Moses, Harry, Bibb Bldg., Macon
Newman, W. A., 700 Spring St., Macon
Newton, R. G., Georgia Casualty Bldg.,
   Macon
Palmer, S. B., Georgia Casualty Bldg.,
   Macon
Penington, C. L., 700 Spring St., Macon
Phillips, A. M., Georgia Casualty Bldg.,
   Macon
Porch, Leon D., Georgia Casualty Bldg.,
   Macon
Rawls, Lewis L., Georgia Casualty Bldg.,
   Macon
Richardson, C. H., 700 Spring St., Macon
Richardson, R. W., Georgia Casualty Bldg.-
   Macon
Ridley, C. L., Macon Hospital, Macon
Rogers, T. E. 700 Spring St., Macon
Ross, J. T., First Nat'l Bank & Trust Co.
   Bldg., Macon (Hon.)
Ross, Thos. L., 700 Spring St., Macon
Rotar, A. R., Oglethorpe Infirmary, Macon
Rubin, S. N., Grand Bldg., Macon
Saye, E. B., Macon Hospital, Macon
Siegel, Alvin E., Georgia Casualty Bldg.,
   Macon
Smisson, Roy C., Fort Valley
Smith, Horace D., Veterans' Administra-
   tion Facility, Los Angeles, Cal.
Smith, J. Allen, 700 Spring St., Macon
Suarez, Raymond, Georgia Casualty Bldg.,
   Macon
Swilling, Evelyn, Georgia Casualty Bldg.,
   Macon
Thompson, O. R., 700 Spring St., Macon
Vinson, Frank, Fort Valley
Walker, D. D., 700 Spring St., Macon
Ware, Ford, Georgia Casualty Bldg., Macon
Wasden, C. N., Georgia Casualty Bldg.,
   Macon
Watson, O. O., The Clinic, Macon
Weaver, H. G., 700 Spring St., Macon
Weaver, Olin H., 700 Spring St., Macon
Williams, W. A., Georgia Casualty Bldg.,
   Macon
Zachary, J. D., Gray

BLUE RIDGE SOCIETY
Officers
President .... Daves, J. M.
Vice-President .... Prince, E. L.
Secretary-Treasurer .... Crawford, C. B.
Delegate .... Watkins, E. W.
Members
Chastain, W. C., Ellijay
Crawford, C. B., Blue Ridge
Daves, J. M., Blue Ridge
Duckett, A. W., Blue Ridge
Prince, E. L., Morganton
Rogers, W. H., Young Cane
Tankersley, J. S., Ellijay
Watkins, E. W., Ellijay

BROOKS COUNTY
Officer
Secretary-Treasurer ...... Jones, A. B., Jr.
Members
Clower, R. J., Morven
Groover, M. E., Quitman
Jelks, E. L., Quitman
Jones, A. B., Jr., Quitman
McMichael, J. R., Quitman
Moye, T. R., Quitman
Smith, L. A., Quitman

BULLOCH-CANDLER-EVANS
COUNTIES
Officer
Secretary-Treasurer ...... Simmons, W. E.
Members
Cone, R. L., Statesboro
Deal, J. W., Claxton
Deal, B. A., Statesboro
Ellis, S. T., Claxton
Floyd, W. E., Statesboro

Jones, D. B., Metter
Kennedy, R. L., Metter
Kennedy, W. D., Metter
McElveen, J. M., Brooklet
Mooney, A. J., Statesboro
Olliff, H. H., Register
Simmons, W. E., Metter
Stapleton, C. B., Groveland
Temples, Leo G., State Board of Health,
State Capitol, Atlanta
Watkins, E. C., Brooklet

BURKE COUNTY
Officers
President..............Byne, J. M., Jr.
Vice-President..........Lowe, W. R.
Secretary-Treasurer.....Thurmond, A. G.
Delegate..............McCarver, W. C.
Members
Bargeron, E. A., Waynesboro
Bent, H. F., Midville
Byne, J. M., Jr., Waynesboro
Byne, J. M., Sr., Waynesboro
Daniel, Byron, Sardis
Hillis, W. W., Sardis
Lewis, J. B., Waynesboro
Lowe, W. R., Midville
McCarver, W. C., Vidette
Miller, R. L., Waynesboro (Deceased)
Thurmond, A. G., Waynesboro

BUTTS COUNTY
Officer
Secretary-Treasurer......Hammond, R. L.
Members
Akin, B. F., Jackson
Hammond, Robert L., Jackson

CARROLL COUNTY
Officers
President ....Spruell, T. M.
Vice-President........Goodwyn, H. J.
Secretary-Treasurer....Reese, D. S.
Delegate.............Scales, S. F.
Members
Barker, H. L., Carrollton
Baskin, C. L., Bremen
Burgess, P. L., Bowdon, R. 1
Pitts, C. C., Carrollton
Goodwyn, H. J., Carrollton
Hogue, W. L., Villa Rica
Hulsey, J. M., Villa Rica
King, O. D., Bremen
Kirby, E. G., Bowdon
Lyle, W. C., Carrollton (Deceased)
Nutt, J. J., Bowdon, R. 1
Powell, B. C., Villa Rica
Powell, John E., Villa Rica
Reese, D. S., Carrollton
Roberts, O. W., Carrollton
Scales, S. F., Carrollton. R. 1
Smith, W. P., Bowdon
Spruell, T. M., Temple
Styles, O. R., Bowdon
Thomasson, W. E., Carrollton
Wilson, L. E., Bowdon

GEORGIA MEDICAL SOCIETY
(Chatham County)
Officers
President ....Holton, C. F.
President-Elect........Paggart, G. H.
Vice-President.........Bray, S. E.
Secretary-Treasurer....Schwalb, O. W.
Delegate..............Metts, J. C.
Delegate..............Morrison, A. A.
Alternate Delegate.....Morrison, H. J.
Alternate Delegate.....Quattlebaum, J. K.
Members
Anderson, J. J., DeRenne Apartments,
Savannah
Baker, J. O., 126 East Oglethorpe Ave.,
Savannah
Barrow, Craig, Chippewa Square, Savannah
Bassett, V. H., City Hall, Savannah
Bedingfield, W. O., 7 West Gordon St.,
Savannah
Blake, H. H., 408 Abercorn St., Savannah
Blitch, J. R., Ellabell (Hon.)
Bray, S. E., DeRenne Apartments, Savannah
Broderick, J. R., 415 Abercorn St.,
Savannah
Brown, C. T., Guyton
Brown, W. E., 12 East Taylor St., Savannah
Charlton, T. J., 220 East Oglethorpe Ave.,
Savannah
Chisholm, J. F., 512 Abercorn St.,
Savannah
Chisholm, J. F., Jr., 512 Abercorn St.,
Savannah
Cole, W. A., 24 East Taylor St., Savannah
Corson, E. R., 10 West Jones St.,
Savannah (Hon.)
Crawford, W. B., 14 East Taylor St.,

Savannah
Crawford, W. B., Jr., 14 East Taylor St.,
Savannah
Dancy, Wm. R., 104 West Jones St.,
Savannah
Daniel, Jno. W., 14 East Jones St.,
Savannah
Daniel, Jno. W., Jr., 114 East Jones St.,
Savannah
deCaradeuc, St. J. R., DeRenne Apts.,
Savannah
DeLoach, L. A., 118 West Jones St.,
Savannah (Deceased)
Demmond, E. C., DeRenne Apartments,
Savannah
Drane, Robert, DeRenne Apartments,
Savannah
Dunn, L. B., 201 East York St., Savannah
Eberhardt, J. P., U. S. Marine Hospital,
Savannah
Edwards, D. B., 606 Drayton St., Savannah
Egan, M. J., 210 East Liberty St.,
Savannah
Egloff, G. E., 215 East Gaston St.,
Savannah
Elliott, J. L., Hotel DeSoto, Savannah
Epting, M. J., 20 East Jones St., Savannah
Exley, H. T., 116 East Jones St., Savannah
Faggart, G. H., 18 West Oglethorpe Ave.,
Savannah
Freedman, L. M., 350 Bull St., Savannah
Gleaton, E. N., 210 East Gaston St.,
Savannah
Graham, R. E., 9 West Gordon St.,
Savannah
Harris, R. V., American Bldg., Savannah
Hesse, H. W., 112 East Jones St., Savannah
Holton, C. F., DeRenne Apartments,
Savannah
Howard, Lee, DeRenne Apartments,
Savannah
Iseman, C., 105 East Jones St., Savannah
Johnson, G. H., 116 East Oglethorpe Ave.,
Savannah
Jones, Jabez, DeRenne Apartments, Savannah
Jones, J. P., 109 East Jones St., Savannah
Kandel, H. M., 432 Abercorn St., Savannah
King, Ruskin, 201 East Hall St., Savannah
Lang, G. H., 204 East Liberty St., Savannah
Lattimore, Ralston, 2 East Jones St.,
Savannah
Lee, Lawrence, DeRenne Apartments,
Savannah
Levington, H. L., 209 East Gaston St.,
Savannah
Long, W. V., Hotel DeSoto, Savannah
Manor, E. N., 247 Bull St., Savannah
Martin, R. V., 109 West Jones St.,
Savannah
Maseaud, M. A., Pineora
McGee, H. H., 346 Bull St., Savannah
Metts, Jas. C., 427 Bull St., Savannah
Morrison, A. A., 108 East Jones St.,
Savannah
Morrison, H. J., 427 Bull St., Savannah
Myers, W. M., 402 Drayton St., Savannah
Neville, R. L., 718 Drayton St., Savannah
Norton, W. A., 105 East Oglethorpe Ave.,
Savannah
Oliver, R. L., Port Wentworth, Savannah
Olmstead, G. T., 22 East Taylor St.,
Savannah
O'Neill, J. C., 202 East Liberty St.,
Savannah
Osborne, E. S., 19 East Jones St., Savannah
Peterson, T. A., 7 West Gordon St.,
Savannah
Pinholster, J. H., 4 West Liberty St.,
Savannah
Quattlebaum, J. K., 3 West Perry St.,
Savannah
Rabhan, L. J., 314 East Gaston St.,
Savannah
Redmond, C. G., 707 Barnard St., Savannah
Righton, H. Y., 101 East Waldburg St.,
Savannah
Riner, C. R., 627 Wocomaw Ave.,
Columbia, S. C.
Rosen, Samuel F., 4 East Jones St.,
Savannah
Sanford, Shelton P., U. S. Marine Hospital,
Savannah
Schwalb, Otto W., 1½ East Gordon St.,
Savannah
Sharpley, H. F., DeRenne Apartments,
Savannah
Sharpley, J. G., Central of Georgia Rail-
way Hospital, Savannah
Shaw, W., 124 East Oglethorpe Ave.,
Savannah
Sheppuse, William, 14 East Taylor St.,
Savannah
Thomas, M. R., 202 East Oglethorpe Ave.,
Savannah

Touchton, G. L., 144 Bull St., Savannah
Train, J. K., 1107 Bull St., Savannah
Usher, Chas., 6 East Liberty St., Savannah
Usher, J. A., 1302 Bull St., Savannah
Waring, A. J., DeRenne Apartments,
Savannah
Waring, T. P., DeRenne Apartments,
Savannah
Whelan, E. J., 14 West Jones St., Savannah
Williams, L. W., 107 East Jones St.,
Savannah
Wilson, S. E., 12 West Jones St., Savannah
Wilson, W. S., 221 East Jones St.,
Savannah (Hon.)

CHATTOOGA COUNTY
Officers
President ....Talley, R. E.
Vice-President.........Brown, H. D.
Secretary-Treasurer....Smith, Isman
Delegate..............Little, R. N.
Alternate Delegate ....Funderburk, N. A.
Members
Andrews, G. A., Trion
Brown, H. D., Summerville
Bryant, W. J., Summerville (Hon.)
Douglas, D. B., Trion
Funderburk, N. A., Trion
Hair, W. B., Summerville
Little, R. N., Summerville
Rodgers, J., Trion
Shamblin, B. F., Lyerly (Hon.)
Smith, Inman, Trion
Smith, J. A., Lyerly (Hon.)
Talley, R. E., Trion
Wood, M. N., Valdosta (Hon.)

CHEROKEE COUNTY
Officers
President ....Moore, R. M.
Vice-President.........Coker, N. J.
Secretary-Treasurer....Brooks, Geo. C.
Delegate..............Pettit, J. T.
Alternate Delegate ....Turk, J. P.
Members
Atherton, H. G., Jasper
Boring, J. R., Canton
Brooks, Geo. C., Canton
Coker, G. N., Canton
Coker, N. J., Canton
Hendrix, M. G., Ball Ground
McClain, M. C., Marble Hill (Hon.)
(Deceased)
Moore, R. M., Waleska (Hon.)
Murphy, P. B., Philippi, W. Va.
Pettit, J. T., Canton
Robinson, G. G., Tate
Roper, C. J., Jasper
Turk, J. P., Nelson
Vansant, T. J., Woodstock

CLARKE COUNTY
Officers
President ....Gholston, W. D.
Vice-President.........Davis, J. W.
Secretary-Treasurer....Simpson, Jno. A.
Delegate..............Harris, H B.
Alternate Delegate ....Bryant, C. H
Members
Banister, H. G., Ila
Birdsong, H. W., Athens
Brown, R. K., Athens
Brown, W. W., Athens
Bryant, C. H., Comer
Cabaniss, W. H., Athens
Coile, F. W., Winterville
Davis, J. W., Athens
Dickens, C. H., Madison
Florence, Loren, Athens
Gerdine, Linton, Athens
Gholston, W. D., Danielsville
Goss, R. M., Athens
Harris, H. B., Athens
Holliday, Henry C., Athens
Hubert, M. A., Athens
Kelly, Geo. W., Carlton
McKinney, J. C., Athens
Middlebrooks, C. O., Athens
Moss, W. L., Athens
Reynolds, H. I., Athens
Simpson, Jno. A., Athens
Smith, S. S., Athens
Talmadge, Harry, Athens
Veale, Emory O., Arnoldsville
Westbrook, R. J., Ila
Wheichel, G. O., Athens
Whitley, L. L., Crawford

CLAYTON-FAYETTE COUNTIES
Officers
President ....Seawright, E. C.
Vice-President.........Wallis, J. R.
Secretary-Treasurer....Bussey, T. J.
Delegate..............Chambers, J. A. S.

Alternate Delegate ...... Kemper, H. D.
Members
Ballard, I. W., Forest Park
Busey, T. J., Fayetteville
Chambers, J. A. S., Inman
Henry, J. Z., Ellenwood (Hon.)
(Deceased)
Kemper, H. D., Jonesboro
Seawright, E. C., Fayetteville
Wallis, J. R., Lovejoy

COBB COUNTY
Officers
President..........Crawley, W. G., Jr.
Vice-President.........Mitchell, W. C.
Secretary-Treasurer.......Terry, H. B.
Delegate.........Perkinson. W. H.
Alternate Delegate .... Gober, W. Mayes
Members
Bagley, D. A., Austell
Bailey, E. M., Acworth (Deceased)
Crawley, W. G., Jr., Acworth
Elder, C. D., Marietta
Ellis, J. W., Kennesaw
Fowler, A. H., Smyrna
Fowler, R. W., Marietta
Gober, W. Mayes, Marietta
Hagood, G. F., Marietta
Kemp, W. M., Marietta (Hon.)
Lester, J. B., Marietta
Middlebrooks, J. D., Powder Springs (Hon.)
Mitchell, W. C., Smyrna
Perkinson, W. H., Marietta
Terry, H. B., Acworth

COFFEE COUNTY
Officers
President............Crovatt, J. G.
Secretary-Treasurer....Johnston, T. H.
Delegate.........Harper, Sage
Alternate Delegate......Clark, T. H.
Members
Clark, T. H., Douglas
Crovatt, J. G., Douglas
Dismuke, H. L., Ocilla
Harper, Sage, Wray
Johnston, T. H., Douglas
McElroy, S. L., Ocilla
Meeks, D. H., Nicholls (Hon.)
Moorman, I. W., Douglas
Quillian, B. O., Douglas
Shellhouse, L. H., Willacoochee
Sibbett, Wm. A., Douglas (Hon.)
Smith, J. R., St. Simons Island (Hon.)
Wallace, J. W., Douglas

COLQUITT COUNTY
Officers
President............Chesnutt, T. H.
Vice-President ....Edmondson, H. T.
Secretary-Treasurer.......Joiner, R. M.
Delegate.........Brannen, C. C.
Alternate Delegate ....McGinty, W. R.
Members
Bennett, W. L., Moultrie
Brannen, C. C., Moultrie
Chesnutt, T. H., Moultrie
Edmondson, H. T., Moultrie
Funderburke, A. G., Moultrie
Joiner, R. M., Moultrie
Lanier, J. E., Moultrie
McGehee, Henry M., Moultrie
McGinty, W. R., Moultrie
Paulk, J. R., Moultrie
Slocumb, C. B., Doerun
Whittendale, W. H., Norman Park
Woodall, J. B., Moultrie
Wright, J. J. C., Doerun

COWETA COUNTY
Officers
President...........Tanner, W. H.
Secretary-Treasurer ....Cochran, M. F.
Members
Bailey, T. S., Newnan
Barge, A. A., Newnan (Hon.)
Cochran, M. F., Newnan
McDonald, R. H., Newnan
Peniston, Joe B., Newnan
Tanner, W. H., Newnan, R. 3
Woodroof, Wm. L., Newnan

CRISP COUNTY
Officers
President............McArthur, T. J.
Vice-President..........Williams, H. J.
Secretary-Treasurer ......Wooten, L. O.
Delegate.........Adams, Chas.
Members
Adams, Charles, Cordele
Dorminy, J. N., Cordele (Hon.)
Flournoy, H. C., Warwick
Harvard, V. O., Arabi

McArthur, T. J., Cordele (Hon.)
Smith, M. R., Cordele
Whelchel, A. J., Cordele
Williams, H. J., Cordele
Williams, L. E., Cordele
Williams, P. L., Cordele
Wooten, L. O., Cordele

DECATUR-SEMINOLE COUNTIES
Officers
President............Smith, E. C.
Vice-President..........Chason, Thos.
Secretary-Treasurer.......Ehrlich, M. A.
Delegate.........Ehrlich, M. A.
Alternate Delegate ....Wheat, R. F.
Members
Alford, A. E. B., Bainbridge
Bridges, R. L. Z., Brinson
Chason, Gordon, Bainbridge
Chason, Thos., Donalsonville
Ehrlich, M. A., Bainbridge
Ehrlich, Sigo, Bainbridge
Fort, M. A., Bainbridge
Jenkins, H. B., Donalsonville
Smith, E. C., Donalsonville
Welch, Carl B., Attapulgus
Wheat, R. F., Bainbridge
Whittle, Wm. E., Iron City
Wilkinson, W. L., Bainbridge
Willis, L. W., Bainbridge

DeKALB COUNTY
Officers
Secretary-Treasurer........Ansley, H. G.
Delegate.........Ansley, H. G.
Members
Allgood, C. L., Scottdale
Andrews, W. W., Tucker
Ansley, H. G., 131 Clairmont Ave. Decatur
Blincoe, Homer, P. O. Box 789, Emory University
Evans, J. R., 120 Clairmont Ave., Decatur
McCurdy, W. T. Sr., Stone Mountain
Stewart, Thos. W., Lithonia
Sweet, Mary F., Agnes Scott College, Decatur
Watkins, A. R., Chamblee
Webb, Wm. A., Lithonia
Wilson, B. V., Decatur Bank & Trust Co. Bldg., Decatur

DOOLY COUNTY
Officers
President............Mobley, H. A.
Secretary-Treasurer........Malloy, M. L.
Delegate.........Davis, E. B.
Members
Daves, V. C., Vienna
Davis, E. B., Byromville
Harris, V. L., Pinehurst
Malloy, Martin L., Vienna
Mobley, H. A., Vienna
Rose, J. R., Unadilla

DOUGHERTY COUNTY
Officers
President............Freeman, A. R.
Vice-President..........Thomas, F. E.
Secretary-Treasurer........Lucas, I. M.
Delegate.........McKemie, H. M.
Alternate Delegate ....Thomas, F. E.
Members
Bacon, A. S., Albany
Barnett, J. M., Albany
Cook, W. S., Albany
Freeman, Alex R., Albany
Hilsman, A. H., Albany
Irvin, I. W., Albany
Keaton, J. C., Albany
Lucas, I. M., Albany
McDowell, Thos. C., Albany (Hon.)
McKemie, H. M., Albany
Neill, F. K., Albany
Redfearn, J. A., Albany
Robinson, Hugo, Albany
Ryan, W. P., Albany
Sapp, E. E., Albany
Thomas, Frank E., Albany
Thomas, H. R., Albany
Tye, J. P., Albany
Welch, Leonard E., Albany (Hon.)

DOUGLAS COUNTY
Officers
President ....Vansant, C. V.
Secretary-Treasurer......Hamilton, R. E.
Delegate.........Vansant, C. V.
Members
Hamilton, R. E., Douglasville
Vansant, C. V., Douglasville

ELBERT COUNTY
Officers
President...........Johnson, J. E., Jr.

Vice-President.........Johnson, W. A.
Secretary-Treasurer........Johnson, A. S.
Delegate.........Thompson, D. N.
Alternate Delegate ....Smith, A. C.
Members
Adams, F. L., Elberton, R.F.D. (Hon.)
Bailey, D. V., Elberton
Gaines, T. H., Elberton, R.F.D.
Johnson, A. S., Elberton
Johnson, J. E., Elberton
Johnson, J. E., Jr., Elberton
Johnson, W. A., Elberton
Mattox, B. B., Elberton
Smith, A. C., Elberton
Smith, F. A., Elberton
Thompson, D. N., Elberton
Ward, G. A., Elberton, R. 1

EMANUEL COUNTY
Officers
President...........Chandler. J. H.
Vice-President..........Franklin. R. C.
Secretary-Treasurer.......Franklin. R. C.
Delegate.........Powell. C. C.
Members
Brown, R. G., Graymont
Chandler, J. H., Swainsboro
Franklin, R. C., Swainsboro
Franklin, V. E., Graymont
Powell, C. E., Swainsboro
Sample, R. L., Summit (Deceased)
Smith, Claud, Swainsboro
Smith, D. D., Swainsboro
Smith, G. L., Swainsboro (Hon.)
Warren, E. L., Valley View Sanatorium, Patterson, N. J.
Youmans, S. S., Oak Park

FLOYD COUNTY
Officers
President ....Garrard, J. L.
Vice-President..........Harbin, R. M., Jr.
Secretary-Treasurer.....Johnson, Ralph N.
Delegate.........Harbin, W. P., Jr.
Members
Archer, E. B., Rome
Banister, W. G., Rome
Borders, W. A., Armuchee
Chandler, J. L., Rome
Cheney, J. N., Silver Creek
Conner, J. C., Cave Springs
Cox, R. P., Rome
Dellinger, A. H., Rome
Elmore, B. V., Rome
Garrard, J. L., Rome
Gilbert, Warren, Rome
Harbin, Lester, Rome
Harbin, R. M., Jr., Rome
Harbin, R. M., Sr., Rome
Harbin, W. P., Jr., Rome
Harbin, W. P. Sr., Rome
Johnson, Ralph N., Rome
Lewis, W. H., Rome
Maddox, R. C., Rome
McArthur, C. H., Rome (Hon.)
McCall, J. T., Rome
McCord. M. M., Rome
McCord, Ralph, Rome
Methvin, S. R., Lindale
Moore, Clifford, Lindale
Moss, T. H., Rome
Mull, J. H., Rome
Routledge, A. F., Rome
Sewell, W. A., Rome
Shaw, W. J., Rome (Hon.)
Smith, G. B., Rome

FORSYTH COUNTY
Officer
Secretary-Treasurer ....Lipscomb, W. E.
Members
Lipscomb, W. E., Cumming
Mashburn, Marcus, Cumming
Tribble, P. W., Cumming

FRANKLIN COUNTY
Officers
President............Brown, S. D.
Secretary-Treasurer........Smith, B. T.
Members
Brown, J. R., Lavonia
Brown, S. D., Royston
Freeman, J. M., Lavonia (Deceased)
McCrary, H. L., Royston
McCrary, J. O., Royston
McCrary, W. M., Carnesville
Pool, H. T., Lavonia
Ridgway, Edwin R., Royston
Ridgway, O. T., Royston
Smith, B. T., Carnesville

FULTON COUNTY
Officers
President............Clay, Grady E.

President-Elect.............Sauls. H. C.
Vice-President.............Eubanks. G. F.
Secretary-Treasurer........Harrison. M. T.
Delegate...................Aven. C. C.
Delegate...................Davison. T. C.
Delegate...................Fincher. E. F., Jr.
Delegate...................Greene. Ed. H.
Delegate...................Strickler, C. W.

Members

Abercrombie. T. F.. State Capitol. Atlanta
Adams, C. M.. 23 West Paces Ferry Road. Atlanta
Adams. C. R., 840 Gordon St., S. W. Atlanta
Adams. H. M. S.. Candler Bldg.. Atlanta
Agnor. Elbert B.. Grady Hospital. Atlanta (Asso.)
Aiken, W. S.. First Nat'l Bank Bldg.. Atlanta
Alden. H. S.. Medical Arts Bldg.. Atlanta
Allen. E. A.. Candler Bldg.. Atlanta
Allison. Gordon G.. Haas-Howell Bldg.. Atlanta
Almand. C. A.. 717 Brookridge Drive. N. E.. Atlanta
Anderson. Geo. M.. 607 Lee St., S. W.. Atlanta
Anderson, Wm. Willis. 478 Peachtree St.. N. E.. Atlanta
Armstrong. T. B.. Candler Bldg.. Atlanta
Armstrong. W. B.. 478 Peachtree St.. N. E.. Atlanta
Arnold. W. A.. Atlanta Nat'l Bank Bldg.. Atlanta
Artaud. F. E.. P. O. Box 234. New Port Richey. Fla. (Asso.)
Artega. Oliver. Atlanta Nat'l Bank Bldg.. Atlanta
Arthur, J. F.. 105 Forest Ave:. N. E.. Atlanta
Asher. Wm. T.. 780 Ponce de Leon Ave.. N. E.. Atlanta
Askew. H. H.. Candler Bldg.. Atlanta
Atkins. F. M.. 478 Peachtree St.. N. E.. Atlanta
Avary. A.. Soldiers Home, Atlanta (Hon.)
Avary. J. C.. 969 West Peachtree St.. N. W.. Atlanta
Aven. C. C.. Medical Arts Bldg.. Atlanta
Ayers. A. J.. Medical Arts Bldg.. Atlanta
Ayer. G. D.. 152 Forrest Ave.. N. E.. Atlanta
Baggett. L. G.. 478 Peachtree St.. N. E.. Atlanta
Bailey. M. K.. Medical Arts Bldg.. Atlanta
Baird. Jas. B.. Medical Arts Bldg.. Atlanta
Baird. J. Mason. Medical Arts Bldg.. Atlanta
Baker. Luther P.. Atlanta Nat'l Bank Bldg.. Atlanta
Baker. W. Pope. 157 Forrest Ave.. N. E.. Atlanta
Ballenger. E. G.. Healey Bldg.. Atlanta
Ballenger. W. L.. 478 Peachtree St., N. E.. Atlanta
Bancker. E. A.. Jr.. 478 Peachtree St.. N. E.. Atlanta
Barber. W. E.. 1031 Springdale Road. N. E.. Atlanta (Asso.)
Barber. F. M.. 10 Pryor St. Bldg.. Atlanta
Barfield. Hugh H.. 478 Peachtree St., N. E.. Atlanta
Barfield. J. R.. 592 Clifton Road. N. E.. Atlanta
Barnett. Crawford F.. Jr.. 478 Peachtree St.. N. E.. Atlanta
Barnett. S. T.. 26 Linden Ave.. N. E. Atlanta (Hon.)
Barnett. S. T., Jr.. 26 Linden Ave.. N. E. Atlanta
Bartholomew. R. A.. 1040·Ponce de Leon Ave.. N. E.. Atlanta
Bateman. N. B.. Jr.. Candler Bldg.. Atlanta
Beasley. B. T.. Hurt Bldg.. Atlanta
Bell. Kenneth R.. Fort McPherson (Asso.)
Benson. M. T.. Medical Arts Bldg.. Atlanta
Benson. M. T.. Jr.. Medical Arts Bldg.. Atlanta
Berger. Louis. 116 Brown Place. S. W.. Atlanta
Bibb. L. B.. P. O. Bldg.. Atlanta (Asso.)
Bishop. Everett L.. Medical Arts Bldg.. Atlanta
Bivings. F. Lee. Exchange Bldg.. Atlanta
Bivings. Wm. Troy. Jr.. Exchange Bldg.. Atlanta
Bivings. Wm. Troy. Exchange Bldg.. Atlanta
Blackford. L. Minor. 104 Ponce de·Leon Ave.. N. E.. Atlanta
Blackman. W. W.. 418 Capitol Ave.. S. E.. Atlanta
Blalock. Jno. C.. Medical Arts Bldg.. Atlanta

Blandford. W. C.. Candler Bldg.. Atlanta
Bleich. J. K.. 478 Peachtree St.. N. E.. Atlanta
Boland. Chas. G.. 157 Forrest Ave.. N. E.. Atlanta
Boland. Frank K.. 478 Peachtree St.. N. E.. Atlanta
Boland. F. Kelis. Jr.. 478 Peachtree St.. N. E.. Atlanta
Boling. Edgar. 478 Peachtree St.. N. E.. Atlanta
Bourbon. Rollo F.. Fort McPherson (Asso.)
Bowcock. Chas. M.. 132 West Wesley Ave.. N. W.. Atlanta
Bowcock. H. M.. 478 Peachtree St.. N. E.. Atlanta
Bowie. Clyde H.. Grady Hospital. Atlanta (Asso.)
Boyd. Ben H.. Grant Bldg.. Atlanta
Boyd. M. L.. 563 Capitol Ave.. S. W.. Atlanta
Boynton. C. E.. 118 Forrest Ave.. N. E.. Atlanta
Bradford. Jos. H.. Battle Hill Sanatorium. Atlanta
Brannen. Cliff. Wm. Oliver Bldg.. Atlanta
Brawner. A. F.. Smyrna
Brawner. Jas. N.. 2800 Peachtree Road. Atlanta
Brawner. Jas. N.. Jr.. 478 Peachtree St.. N. E.. Atlanta
Brawner. L. E.. Medical Arts Bldg.. Atlanta
Brown. S. Ross. 11 Hunter St.. S. W.. Atlanta
Brown. S. T.. Medical Arts Bldg.. Atlanta
Brown. Samuel Y.. 478 Peachtree St.. N. E.. Atlanta
Bryan. Wm. W.. Grady Hospital. Atlanta
Bucknell. Howard. East Hampton. Long Island. N. Y.
Bullard. T. P.. Palmetto
Bunce. Allen H.. 139 Forrest Ave.. N. E.. Atlanta
Busch. J. C.. Anderson Ave.. S. W.. Atlanta
Burgess. Taylor S.. Medical Arts Bldg.. Atlanta
Burke. B. Russell. 478 Peachtree St.. N. E.. Atlanta
Bush. O. B.. Candler Bldg.. Atlanta
Butner. J. Hendrick. 73 Eleventh St.. N. E.. Atlanta
Byram. Jas. H.. Grand Theater Bldg.. Atlanta
Byrd. Edwin S.. 478 Peachtree St.. N. E.. Atlanta
Byrd. T. L.. 478 Peachtree St.. N. E.. Atlanta
Calhoun. F. P.. 478 Peachtree St.. N. E.. Atlanta
Callaway. J. T.. 1514 Rogers Ave.. S. W.. Atlanta (Asso.)
Camp. E. W.. Jr.. Grady Hospital. Atlanta (Asso.)
Camp. R. T.. Fairburn
Camp. W. R.. Fairburn (Hon.)
Campbell. J. L.. 478 Peachtree St.. N.·E:. Atlanta (Hon.)
Campbell. W. E.. Jr.. Medical Arts Bldg.. Atlanta
Carothers. J. B.. 105 Forrest Ave.. N. E.. Atlanta
Cathcart. Don F.. 478 Peachtree St.. N. E.. Atlanta
Carron. I. T.. Candler Bldg.. Atlanta
Champion. W. L.. Grant Bldg.. Atlanta
Chappell. Amey. 478 Peachtree St.. N. E.. Atlanta
Chester. Jno. B.. Fort McPherson (Asso.)
Childs. J. R.. Medical Arts Bldg.. Atlanta
Childs. L. W.. Grant Bldg.. Atlanta
Clark. Jno. A.. P. O. Bldg.. Atlanta (Asso.)
Clark. J. J.. 478 Peachtree St.. N. E.. Atlanta
Clarke. M. L. B.. Candler Bldg.. Atlanta
Clay. Grady E.. Medical Arts Bldg.. Atlanta
Clifton. Ben H.. 478 Peachtree St.. N. E.. Atlanta
Cline. B. McH.. Grand Theater Bldg.. Atlanta
Cochran. Hugh. Medical Arts Bldg.. Atlanta
Cofer. Olin S.. 478 Peachtree St.. N. E.. Atlanta
Cole. G. C.. 907 Marietta St.. N. W.. Atlanta (Hon.)
Collier. T. J.. 1781 Peachtree St.. N. E.. Atlanta
Collier. Thos. W.. Main St.. College Park
Colvin. E. D.. 1040 Ponce de Leon Ave.. N. E.. Atlanta
Colvin. B. S.. Healey Bldg.. Atlanta
Combs. J. A.. 478 Peachtree St.. N. E.. Atlanta
Compton. Henry T.. Georgia School of Technology. Atlanta
Conner. Homer L.. Fort McPherson (Asso.)

Cooke. Virgil C.. Healey Bldg.. Atlanta
Cooper. Geo.. Jr.. Emory University Hospital. Emory University (Asso.)
Copeloff. M. B.. Grant Bldg.. Atlanta
Corley. F. L.. Atlanta Nat'l Bank Bldg.. Atlanta
Cousins. W. L.. Candler Bldg.. Atlanta
Cowan. Z. S.. Grand Theater Bldg.. Atlanta
Crawford. Clyde L.. 26 Linden Ave.. N. E.. Atlanta
Crawford. H. C.. 478 Peachtree St.. N. E.. Atlanta
Crawford. J. H.. Grant Bldg.. Atlanta
Cross. Jno. B.. Medical Arts Bldg.. Atlanta
Curtis. Walker L.. College Park
Dabney. W. C.. 73 Eleventh St.. N. E.. Atlanta
Daly. Leo P.. Medical Arts Bldg.. Atlanta
Daly. R. R.. Georgia Savings Bank Bldg.. Atlanta (Hon.)
Daniel. Chas. H.. College Park
Daniel. W. W.. Georgia Savings Bank Bldg.. Atlanta
Daniels. C. W.. 152 Forrest Ave.. N. E.. Atlanta
Davenport. T. P.. 104 Ponce de Leon Ave.. N. E. Atlanta
Davis. J. E.. Grand Theater Bldg.. Atlanta
Davis. S. C.. 309 Peachtree Battle Ave.. R. 6. Atlanta
Davis. Wm. B.. College Park
Davison. Hal M.. 478 Peachtree St.. N. E.. Atlanta
Davison. T. C.. 478 Peachtree St.. N. E.. Atlanta
DeLoach. A. G.. Citizens & Southern Nat'l Bank Bldg.. Atlanta
Dimmark. Leila. 1051 Hudson Drive. N. E.. Atlanta
Denit. Guy B.. P. O. Bldg.. Atlanta (Asso.)
Denton. J. F.. 478 Peachtree St.. N. E.. Atlanta
Dew'. J. Harris. 126 Forrest Ave.. N. E.. Atlanta
Dickson. Roger W.. 33 Ponce de Leon Ave.. N. E.. Atlanta
Dimmock. A. M.. Hurt Bldg.. Atlanta
Dismukes. Jackson B.. Fort McPherson (Asso.)
Donaldson. H. R.. Grant Bldg.. Atlanta
Donough. M. S.. 478 Peachtree St.. N. E.. Atlanta
Dorsey. R. T.. 26 Linden Ave.. N. B.. Atlanta
Dougherty. Mark S.. 139 Forrest ·Ave.. N. E.. Atlanta
Duncan. John B.. First Nat'l Bank Bldg.. Atlanta
Dunn. W. M.. Candler Bldg.. Atlanta
DuVall. W. B.. 26 Linden Ave.. N. E.. Atlanta
Eberhart. Chas. A.. Medical Arts Bldg.. Atlanta
Edgerton. M. T.. Candler Bldg.. Atlanta
Elder. Or·F.:· Healey Bldg.. Atlanta
Elkin. Dan C.. 478 Peachtree St.. N. E.. Atlanta
Elkin. W. S.. 478 Peachtree St.. N.·E.. Atlanta (Hon.)
Emery. W. B.. Candler Bldg.. Atlanta
Equen. Murdock S.. 104 Ponce de Leon Ave.. N. E.. Atlanta
Eskridge. Frank. 744 West Peachtree St.. N. W.. Atlanta
Etheridge. J. H.. Atlanta Nat'l Bank Bldg.. Atlanta
Eubanks. Geo. F.. 478 Peachtree St.. N. E.. Atlanta
Ezzard. Thos. M.. Roswell
Fancher. J. K.. Medical Arts Bldg.. Atlanta
Fanning. ·O. O.. Grand Bldg.. Atlanta
Ferguson. I. A.. 478 Peachtree St.. N. E.. Atlanta
Fincher. Ed. F.. Jr.. Medical Arts Bldg.. Atlanta
Fincher. L. C.. 35 Linden Ave.. N. E.. Atlanta
Fitts. Jno. B.. Medical Arts Bldg.. Atlanta
Flowers. A. P.. Medical Arts Bldg.. Atlanta
Floyd. Earl H.. 478 Peachtree St.. N. E.. Atlanta
Floyd. J. T.. Medical Arts Bldg.. Atlanta
Fort. Arthur G.. 478 Peachtree St.. N. E.. Atlanta
Fort. Lynn. Jr.. Medical Arts Bldg.. Atlanta
Foster. K. E.. College Park
Foster. Maude E.. Hurt Bldg.. Atlanta
Fowler. Clarence D.. Henrietta Egglestoni Hospital. Atlanta (Asso.)
Fowler. M. F.. Grant Bldg.. Atlanta
Freeman. J. F.. 986 Hemphill Ave.. N. W.. Atlanta

Fuller, Geo. W., 478 Peachtree St., N. E.,
Atlanta
Fuller, J. R., Citizens & Southern Nat'l
Bank Bldg., Atlanta
Funkt, John, 712 Durant Place, N. E.,
Atlanta
Funkhouser, W. L., 33 Ponce de Leon Ave.,
N. E., Atlanta
Fuqua, E. F., 986 Hemphill Ave., N. W.,
Atlanta
Gaines, L. M., 478 Peachtree St., N. E.,
Atlanta
Gardner, W. A., Stone Mountain
Garner, John P., Medical Arts Bldg., Atlanta
Garner, J. R., 4 Hunter St., S. E., Atlanta
Garver, Carl C., 121 Clairmont Ave.,
Decatur
Gaussemel, S. D., 478 Peachtree St., N. E.,
Atlanta
Gay, J. G., 104 Ponce de Leon Ave., N. E.,
Atlanta
Gay, T. Bolling, Medical Arts Bldg., Atlanta
Giarratano, Jerome F., Federal Prison Hos-
pital, Atlanta (Asso.)
Gibson, Eugene P., College Park
Giddings, C. G., 478 Peachtree St., N. E.,
Atlanta (Hon.)
Giddings, Glenville, 478 Peachtree St.,
N. E., Atlanta
Gilbert, W. L., County Courthouse, Atlanta
Glenn, Wadley R., Grady Hospital, Atlanta
(Asso.)
Goldsmith, W. S., Hurt Bldg., Atlanta
Goodpasture, W. C., Medical Arts Bldg.,
Atlanta
Goodwyn, Thos. P., 478 Peachtree St.,
N. E., Atlanta
Graydon, E. L., Candler Bldg., Atlanta
Greene, Edgar H., 478 Peachtree St., N. E.,
Atlanta
Griffin, Claude, Medical Arts Bldg., Atlanta
Grove, L. W., Medical Arts Bldg., Atlanta
Guffin, T. F., East Point
Guthrie, N. J., Medical Arts Bldg., Atlanta
(Asso.)
Hailey, Howard, Candler Bldg., Atlanta
Hailey, Hugh, Grady Hospital, Atlanta
(Asso.)
Hall, C. J., Jr., Candler Bldg., Atlanta
Hall, O. D., Georgia Baptist Hospital,
Atlanta
Hallum, Alton V., 478 Peachtree St., N. E.,
Atlanta
Hames, F. W., Candler Bldg., Atlanta
Hamm, W. G., Medical Arts Bldg., Atlanta
Hancock, T. H., 320 Crew St., S. W.,
Atlanta (Hon.)
Hanner, Jas P., Medical Arts Bldg., Atlanta
Hanson, A. F., Masonic Temple, Decatur
Hardin, L. Sage, Medical Arts Bldg., Atlanta
Harrison, M. T., Medical Arts Bldg., Atlanta
Hauck, Allen E., Emory University Hos-
pital, Emory University
Henry, J. Lamont, Grady Hospital, Atlanta
(Asso.)
Hewell, Guy C., 33 Ponce de Leon Ave.,
N. E., Atlanta
Heyser, D. T., 190 Boulevard, S. E., Atlanta
Highsmith, E. D., Trust Co. of Georgia
Bldg., Atlanta
Hill, O. Reed, Henrietta Egleston Hospital,
Atlanta (Asso.)
Hines, J. H., Grady Hospital, Atlanta
Hobby, A. Worth, Medical Arts Bldg.,
Atlanta
Hodges, J. H., Hapeville
Hodges, W. A., 492 Page Ave., N. E.,
Atlanta
Hodgson, F. G., Medical Arts Bldg., Atlanta
Hoke, Michael, 551 Capitol Ave., S. W.,
Atlanta
Holden, F. C., Candler Bldg., Atlanta
Holloway, Geo. A., Grand Theater Bldg.,
Atlanta
Holmes, C. H., 478 Peachtree St., N. E.,
Atlanta
Holmes, W. R., Jr., 478 Peachtree St.,
N. E., Atlanta
Holtzelaw, Morris R., Grady Hospital,
Atlanta (Asso.)
Hoppe, L. D., Medical Arts Bldg., Atlanta
Horton, B. E., Atlanta Nat'l Bank Bldg.,
Atlanta
Howard, P. M., College Park
Howell, J. L., Medical Arts Bldg., Atlanta
Howell, Stacy C., 144 Ponce de Leon Ave.,
N. E., Atlanta
Hudson, O. H., Atlanta Nat'l Bank Bldg.,
Atlanta
Huguley, G. P., 126 Forrest Ave., N. E.,
Atlanta
Hull, Marion McH., 573 West Peachtree St.,
N. E., Atlanta
Hunter, C. W., 744 West Peachtree St.,
N. W., Atlanta

Hurt, J. S., 478 Peachtree St., N. E.,
Atlanta
Hutchins, J. T., 1704 Lakewood Ave., S. E.,
Atlanta
Hutto, Wm. E., Haas-Howell Bldg., Atlanta
Ivey, John C., Georgia Savings Bank Bldg.,
Atlanta
Jackson, Zach W., 478 Peachtree St., N. E.,
Atlanta
Jenkins, M. K., Hurt Bldg., Atlanta
Jennings, Jas. L., 1704 Lakewood Ave.,
S. E., Atlanta
Jernigan, H. W., 478 Peachtree St., N. E.,
Atlanta
Johnson, J. C., 478 Peachtree St., N. E.,
Atlanta
Johnson, McClaren, 478 Peachtree St., N.
E., Atlanta
Johnson, Trimble, 478 Peachtree St., N. E.,
Atlanta
Johnston, J. F., P. O. Bldg., Atlanta
(Asso.)
Jones, Jack W., Medical Arts Bldg., Atlanta
Kahn, Samuel, 929 North Highland Ave.,
N. E., Atlanta
Kallus, Edward J., Fort McPherson (Asso.)
Kane, Thos. M., Grand Theater Bldg.,
Atlanta
Kea, V. B., Grand Theater Bldg., Atlanta
Kelley, L. H., 478 Peachtree St., N. E.,
Atlanta
Kelley, W. A., 478 Peachtree St., N. E.,
Atlanta
Kemper, C. G., 478 Peachtree St., N. E.,
Atlanta
Kendrick, Douglas B., Jr., Station Hospital,
Fort McPherson (Asso.)
Kennedy, J. P., City Hall, Atlanta
Keramidas, Theo. C., Grady Hospital, Atlanta
(Asso.)
Key, Claude T., 78 Ellis St., N. E., Atlanta
Kirkland, S. A., 478 Peachtree St., N. E.,
Atlanta
Kiser, W. H., Jr., 104 Ponce de Leon Ave.,
N. E., Atlanta
Kite, J. H., 478 Peachtree St., N. E.,
Atlanta
Klugh, Geo F., 139 Forrest Ave., N. E.,
Atlanta
Klugh, Geo. F., Jr., 139 Forrest Ave.,
N. E., Atlanta
Kracke, Roy R., Anatomy Bldg., Emory
University
Krafts, H. N., Candler Bldg., Atlanta
Lake, Wm. F., Medical Arts Bldg., Atlanta
Landham, J. W., 139 Forrest Ave., N. E.,
Atlanta
Lange, John H., Jr., Grady Hospital, Atlanta
(Asso.)
Lawrence, C. E., Candler Bldg., Atlanta
Laws, C. L., Medical Arts Bldg., Atlanta
Ledingham, R. S., Medical Arts Bldg.,
Atlanta
Lee, C. A., Citizens & Southern Nat'l Bank
Bldg., Atlanta
Linch, A. O., 157 Forrest Ave., N. E.,
Atlanta
Lokey, M. H., Medical Arts Bldg., Atlanta
Longino, D. R., Medical Arts Bldg., Atlanta
Longino, T. D., 106 Montgomery Ferry
Drive, N. E., Atlanta
Lowance, Mason L., 478 Peachtree St.,
N. E., Atlanta
Lyon, G. T., 745 Marietta St., N. W.,
Atlanta
Malone, O. T., 157 Forrest Ave., N. E.,
Atlanta
Manget, A. D., 139 Forrest Ave., N. E.,
Atlanta
Martin, J. D., Jr., 478 Peachtree St., N. E.,
Atlanta
Martin, J. J., 478 Peachtree St., N. E.,
Atlanta
Martin, Wm. O., Jr., 478 Peachtree St.,
N. E., Atlanta
Mashburn, Chas. M., 139 Forrest Ave., N.
E., Atlanta
Masses, A. C., 478 Peachtree St., N. E.,
Atlanta
Matthews, Lawrence P., Grady Hospital,
Atlanta (Asso.)
Matthews, O. H., 139 Forrest Ave., N. E.,
Atlanta
Maulding, Homer R., Georgia Baptist Hos-
pital, Atlanta (Asso.)
Mayo, John R. S., Fort McPherson
Atlanta (Asso.)
Meyers, Martin T., Medical Arts Bldg.,
Atlanta
Miller, H. C., 478 Peachtree St., N. E.
Atlanta
Mims, C., Mortgage Guarantee Bldg.,
Atlanta

Minnich, Fred R., 478 Peachtree St., N. E.,
Atlanta
Minnich, Wm. R., Medical Arts Bldg.,
Atlanta
Minor, Henry W., 157 Forrest Ave., N. E.,
Atlanta
Mitchell, Chas. H., Medical Arts Bldg.,
Atlanta
Mitchell, Marvin A., 478 Peachtree St.,
N. E., Atlanta
Mitchell, Wm. E., Medical Arts Bldg.,
Atlanta
Mizell, G. C., 126 Forrest Ave., N. E.,
Atlanta
Monfort, J. M., 478 Peachtree St., N. E.,
Atlanta
Moon, P. L., Atlanta Nat'l Bank Bldg.,
Atlanta
Morris, J. L., Alpharetta
Morris, S. L., Jr., 573 West Peachtree St.,
N. W., Atlanta
Murray, Geo. M., 139 Forrest Ave., N. E.,
Atlanta
Muse, L. H., Medical Arts Bldg., Atlanta
Myers, Guy A., Grady Hospital, Atlanta
McAliley, R. G., 104 Ponce de Leon Ave.,
N. E., Atlanta
McAllister, J. A., 126 Wesley Ave., N. E.,
Atlanta (Hon.)
McCall, Jno. T., Jr., Piedmont Hospital,
Atlanta (Asso.)
McCay, C. G., Atlanta Nat'l Bank Bldg.,
Atlanta
McCord, J. R., 50 Armstrong St., N. E.,
Atlanta
McDaniel, J. G., Grand Theater Bldg.,
Atlanta
McDonald, H. P., Healey Bldg., Atlanta
McDonald, Paul, Bolton
McDougall, J. C., Medical Arts Bldg.,
Atlanta
McDougall, W. L., 478 Peachtree St, N. E.,
Atlanta
McGarity, Jas. A., Augusta
McGeachy, Thos. E., 121 Clairmont Ave.,
Decatur
McGee, Roy W., Ben Hill
McGinty, A. Park, 478 Peachtree St., N. E.,
Atlanta
McLarty, M. W., Atlanta Nat'l Bank Bldg.,
Atlanta
McRae, F. W., Jr., Medical Arts Bldg.,
Atlanta
Nabors, Dewey T., Wm. Oliver Bldg.,
Atlanta
Nall, Jas. D., 500 Chestnut St., N. W.,
Atlanta
Neel, M. M., Volunteer Bldg., Atlanta
Nellans, C. T., 139 Forrest Ave., N. E.,
Atlanta
Nelson, R. M., Grand Theater Bldg., Atlanta
(Hon.)
Nettle, F. C., Candler Bldg., Atlanta
Newberry, R. E., Candler Bldg., Atlanta
Nicholson, J. H., Healey Bldg., Atlanta
Nicolson, Wm. Perrin, Jr., 478 Peachtree
St., N. E., Atlanta
Nippert, Philip H., 478 Peachtree St., N.
E., Atlanta
Noble, G. H., Jr., 478 Peachtree St., N. E.,
Atlanta
Norris, Jack C., 478 Peachtree St., N. E.,
Atlanta
Nuckolls, John Bond, Grady Hospital,
Atlanta (Asso.)
Olds, Bomar, Medical Arts Bldg., Atlanta
Oppenheimer, R. H., 50 Armstrong St.,
N. E., Atlanta
Osborne, C. V., 427½ Moreland Ave.,
N. E., Atlanta
Owensby, N. M., Medical Arts Bldg.,
Atlanta
Paine, C. H., 123 Forrest Ave., N. E.,
Atlanta
Parham, LeRoy G., Medical Arts Bldg.,
Atlanta
Patton, Lewis S., Southern Mutual Bldg.,
Athens
Paullin, Jas. E., Medical Arts Bldg., Atlanta
Pentecost, M. P., 478 Peachtree St., N. E.,
Atlanta
Perry, Samuel W., 478 Peachtree St., N. E.,
Atlanta
Person, W. J., Candler Bldg., Atlanta
Petrie, Eleanor B., 304 Walton Drive,
Atlanta
Petrie, Lester M., 103 Sycamore St., Decatur
Phillips, H. S., Medical Arts Bldg., Atlanta
Pinson, C. H., Hapeville
Pittman, Jas. Lee, Jr., 478 Peachtree St.,
Atlanta
Poer, D. Henry, Medical Arts Bldg., Atlanta
Powell, V. E., 768 Juniper St., N. E.,
Atlanta

Preston, Jno. F., Jr., Piedmont Hospital, Atlanta (Asso.)
Pruitt, M. C., Medical Arts Bldg., Atlanta
Quillian, G. W., 1254 Peachtree Road, Apt. A2, Atlanta (Asso.)
Quillian, Wm. B., Jr., Grady Hospital, Atlanta (Asso.)
Quillian, W. E., Medical Arts Bldg., Atlanta
Ragan, W. B., Jr., 25 Third St., N. E., Atlanta
Rawister, Hubert, Candler Annex, Atlanta
Rayle, Albert A., 478 Peachtree St., N. E., Atlanta
Read, Joseph C., Medical Arts Bldg., Atlanta
Redd, S. C., 157 Forrest Ave., N. E., Atlanta
Reed, Clinton, Candler Bldg., Atlanta
Register, D. W., 850 Briarcliff Road, Apt. 6, Atlanta (Asso.)
Reynolds, H. L., 478 Peachtree St., N. E., Atlanta
Rhodes, C. A., Atlanta Nat'l Bank Bldg., Atlanta
Rice, Keith C., Medical Arts Bldg., Atlanta
Ridley, H. W. Grant Bldg., Atlanta
Riley, J. G., Grant Bldg., Atlanta
Roberts, C. W., 26 Linden Ave., N. E., Atlanta
Roberts, J. Will, 478 Peachtree St., N. E., Atlanta
Roberts, M. Hinet, 104 Ponce de Leon Ave., N. E., Atlanta
Roberts, Stewart R., 768 Juniper St., N. E., Atlanta
Robinson, L. B., 35 Fourth St., N. E., Atlanta
Robinson, W. C., Atlanta Nat'l Bank Bldg., Atlanta (Hon.)
Rogers, J. Harry, 478 Peachtree St., N. E., Atlanta
Rosenberg, H. J., 478 Peachtree St., N. E., Atlanta
Rouglin, L. C., Candler Bldg., Atlanta
Roy, Dunbar, Grand Theater Bldg., Atlanta (Hon.)
Rudder, Fred, Fort McPherson (Asso.)
Rush, Gus Adolphus, Jr., Emory University Hospital, Emory University (Asso.)
Rushin, C. E., 478 Peachtree St., N. E., Atlanta
Sage, D. Yu, Medical Arts Bldg., Atlanta
Sanders, A. S., 139 Forrest Ave., N. E., Atlanta
Sandlinn, J. Calvin, 478 Peachtree St., N. E., Atlanta
Sauls, H. C., Medical Arts Bldg., Atlanta
Schneider, J. F., Route 4, Box 286, Atlanta
Sellers, T. F., State Capitol, Atlanta
Selman, W. A., 157 Forrest Ave., N. E., Atlanta
Sharkleford, B. L., Medical Arts Bldg., Atlanta
Shallenberger, W. F., 33 Ponce de Leon Ave., N. E., Atlanta
Shanks, Edgar D., 478 Peachtree St., N. E., Atlanta
Sinkon, S. J., Candler Bldg., Atlanta
Sloan, W. P., Candler Bldg., Atlanta
Smith, Archibald, First Nat'l Bank Bldg., Atlanta
Smith, Carter, Medical Arts Bldg., Atlanta
Smith, Lewis M., Medical Arts Bldg., Atlanta
Smith, Linton, 427½ Moreland Ave., N. E., Atlanta
Smith, M. F., Grand Theater Bldg., Atlanta
Smith, Simon H., 478 Peachtree St., N. E., Atlanta
Smith, Wm. A., Medical Arts Bldg., Atlanta
Smith, W. P., Jr., 319 Church St., Decatur (Asso.)
Smith, W. Randolph, 478 Peachtree St., N. E., Atlanta
Sommerfeld, J. E., 360 Ponce de Leon Ave., N. E., Atlanta (Hon.)
Spaulding, Wm. L., Fort McPherson, (Asso.)
Spearman, G. F., Medical Arts Bldg., Atlanta
Stamps, Samuel, Candler Bldg., Atlanta
Staton, T. R., 478 Peachtree St., N. E., Atlanta
Stephens, R. G., Candler Bldg., Atlanta
Stewart, Calvin B., 904 Peachtree St., N. E., Atlanta
Stewart, J. C., 1308 Stewart Ave., Atlanta
Stirling, A. W., Baldwin Heights, Baldwin
Stockard, Cecil, Candler Bldg., Atlanta
Strickler, C. W., 123 Forrest Ave., N. E., Atlanta
Strickler, C. W., Jr., 123 Forrest Ave., N. E. Atlanta
Swanson, Cosby, 478 Peachtree St., N. E., Atlanta

Swint, R. C., 1811 North Rock Springs Road, Atlanta
Taranto, Morris B., Grant Bldg., Atlanta
Tasker, Arthur N., Fort McPherson (Asso.)
Thomas, Elzie B., 153 Lakeview Ave., N. E., Atlanta
Thompson, D. O., Grant Bldg., Atlanta
Thomason, J. W., P. O. Box 204, East Point
Thomason, W. L., Candler Bldg., Atlanta
Thomson, J. D., 158 Forrest Ave., N. E., Atlanta
Thornton, Lawson, 478 Peachtree St., N. E., Atlanta
Tidmore, T. L., 858 Adair St., N. E., Atlanta
Timberlake, G. B., Candler Bldg., Atlanta
Toepel, Theo., Candler Bldg., Atlanta (Hon.)
Trimble, Geo. C., East Point (Hon.)
Trimble, W. H., Medical Arts Bldg., Atlanta
Turk, L. N., Jr., Candler Bldg., Atlanta
Turner, J. W., 151 Ponce de Leon Ave., N. E., Atlanta
Upchurch, Wilborn E., 478 Peachtree St., N. E., Atlanta
Uphaw, C. B., 33 Ponce de Leon Ave., N. E., Atlanta
Van Buren, E., 768 Juniper St., N. E., Atlanta
Van Dyke, A. H., Grant Bldg., Atlanta
Van Hook, Riley C., Jr., Piedmont Hospital, Atlanta (Asso.)
Vinson, C. D., 72 Anniston Ave., S. E., Atlanta
Vinson, Luther M., 478 Peachtree St., N. E., Atlanta
Visanska, Samuel A., 820 Ponce de Leon Ave., N. E. Atlanta (Asso.)
Walker, E. Y., Medical Arts Bldg., Atlanta
Walker, Jno. R., 152 Forrest Ave., N. E., Atlanta
Walton, Jno. M., Grant Bldg., Atlanta
Ward, Emmett, Medical Arts Bldg., Atlanta
Warner, W. P., Jr., Piedmont Hospital, Atlanta
Warnock, C. Murray, Crawford W. Long Memorial Hospital, Atlanta (Asso.)
Warren, W. C., Jr., 478 Peachtree St., N. E., Atlanta
Warren, W. C., 478 Peachtree St., N. E., Atlanta
Waters, Wm. G., Jr., 478 Peachtree St., N. E., Atlanta
Waxelbaum, G. J., 478 Peachtree St., N. E., Atlanta
Weaver, J. Calvin, 78 Ellis St., N. E., Atlanta
Wells, W. F., Medical Arts Bldg., Atlanta
West, C. M., Candler Bldg., Atlanta
Whitworth, Clyde W., Grady Hospital, Atlanta (Asso.)
Wiggins, L. W., P. O. Box 4124, Atlanta
Williams, E. C., Georgia Baptist Hospital, Atlanta (Asso.)
Williams, Geo. A., Medical Arts Bldg., Atlanta
Willingham, T. I., Medical Arts Bldg., Atlanta
Wilson, R. B., 478 Peachtree St., N. E., Atlanta
Withers, Samuel M., Piedmont Hospital, Atlanta
Woods, C. B., Fort McPherson (Asso.)
Wood, R. Hugh, 478 Peachtree St., N. E., Atlanta
Wright, E. S., Medical Arts Bldg., Atlanta
Yampolsky, Joseph, 478 Peachtree St., N. E., Atlanta
York, Jesse H., Medical Arts Bldg., Atlanta
Young, W. W., 478 Peachtree St., N. E., Atlanta

GLYNN COUNTY
Officers
President............Simmons, J. W.
Vice-President...........Harrell, J. P.
Secretary-Treasurer........Willis, T. V.
Delegate................Greer, C. B.
Members
Avera, J. B., Brunswick
Branham, H. M., Brunswick
Burford, Robert S., Brunswick
Chesry, G. W. H., Brunswick
Conn, Webb, Brunswick
Egbert, E. H., St. Simons Island
Fishburne, C. C., Darien
Greer, C. B., Brunswick
Harrell, J. P., Brunswick
Simmons, J. W., Brunswick
Vermilye, John H., Whipple, Arizona

Willis, Tom Van, Brunswick
Winchester, M. E., Brunswick

GORDON COUNTY
Officers
President.................Barnett, W. R.
Secretary-Treasurer.......Johnston, Z. V.
Delegate..................Johnston, Z. V.
Alternate Delegate........Barnett, W. R.
Members
Acree, M. A. Calhoun
Banks, Geo. T., Fairmount
Barnett, W. R., Calhoun
Billings, J. E., Fairmount
Boerders, D. J., Calhoun, R. 2
Fite, B. W., Resaca
Hall, W. D., Calhoun
Johnston, Z. V., Calhoun
Parham, J. B., Calhoun
Richards, W. R., Calhoun

GRADY COUNTY
Officers
President...............Reynolds, A. B.
Secretary-Treasurer.......Rogers, J. V.
Delegate.................Rogers, J. V.
Members
Clower, Eugene, Cairo (Hon.) (Deceased)
Rehberg, A. W., Cairo
Reynolds, A. B., Cairo
Rogers, J. V., Cairo
Walker, W. A., Cairo (Hon.)
Warnell, J. B., Cairo

GREENE COUNTY
Officers
President...............Adams, E. G.
Secretary-Treasurer.....Gheesling, Goodwin
Members
Adams, E. G., Greensboro
Cheves, Harry L., Union Point
Gheesling, Goodwin, Greensboro

GWINNETT COUNTY
Officer
Secretary-Treasurer.......Williams, A. D.
Members
Hinton, W. T., Dacula
Hutchins, W. J., Buford
Kelley, D. C., Lawrenceville
Orr, A. C., Buford
Puett, W. W., Norcross
Williams, A. D., Lawrenceville

HABERSHAM COUNTY
Officers
President...............Lamb, R. B.
Vice-President...........Crow, H. E.
Secretary-Treasurer......Harden, O. N.
Delegate................Harden, O. N.
Members
Barrett, Clara, State Capitol, Atlanta
Brabson, T. H., Cornelia
Collins, Katherine R., Turnerville (Hon.)
Crow, H. E., Alto
Duckett, P. Y., Cornelia (Hon.)
Garrison, D. H., Clarkesville
Garrison, W. H., Clarkesville
Harden, O. N., Cornelia
Hardman, C. T., Tallulah Falls
Jackson, J. B., Clarkesville
Lamb, E. H., Cornelia
Lamb, R. B., Demorest
Rankin, D. T., Alto
Roberts, B. J., Cornelia
Schenck, H. C., State Capitol, Atlanta

HALL COUNTY
Officers
President...............Grove, E. W.
Vice-President..........Hulsey, J. M
Secretary-Treasurer......Joiner, Hartwell
Delegate................Downey, J. H.
Alternate Delegate......Rogers, R. L.
Members
Barker, Hampton E., Dahlonega
Burns, J. K., Jr., Gainesville
Butler, C. G., Gainesville
Cagle, W. D., Gainesville
Chandler, B. B., Gainesville
Cheek, Pratt, Gainesville
Davis, B. B., Gainesville
Downey, J. H., Gainesville
Garner, W. R., Gainesville
Grove, E. W., Gainesville
Hulsey, J. M., Buford
Hutchins, J. W., Buford
Hodges, L. W., Gainesville (Deceased)
Joiner, Hartwell, Gainesville
Kennedy, W. C. Talmo
Lancaster, H. H., Clermont
Liles, W. W., Gainesville (Deceased)
Meeks, J. L., Gainesville
Neal, L. G., Cleveland

Palmour, W. A., Gainesville
Phillips, H. K., Cleveland
Rogers, R. L., Gainesville
Tilthaw, H. S., Gainesville
Ward, Eugene L., New Holland
Wellborn, C. J., Gainesville
West, S. A., Dahlonega
Whelchel, C. D., Gainesville

HANCOCK COUNTY
Officers
President.............Darden, Horace
Secretary-Treasurer.........Earl, H. L.
Delegate............Jernigan, C. S.
Alternate Delegate......Hutchings, E. H.
Members
Darden, Horace, Sparta
Earl, H. L., Sparta
Hutchings, Ernest H., Sparta
Jernigan, C. S., Sparta

HARRIS COUNTY
Officer
Secretary-Treasurer.......Haygood, M. F.
Members
Bussey, Benj. N., Waverly Hall
Haygood, M. F., Iowa State Department of
Health, Des Moines, Iowa
Stinson, Forrest C., Waverly Hall

HART COUNTY
Officers
President..............Jenkins, J. I.
Vice-President...........Teasley, B. C.
Secretary-Treasurer.......Meredith, A. O.
Members
Harper, G. T., Dewey Rose, R. 2
Jenkins, A. J., Hartwell
Jenkins, J. L., Hartwell, R. 1
Meredith, A. O., Hartwell
Teasley, B. C., Hartwell
Teasley, Harry E., Hartwell

HENRY COUNTY
Officers
President................Tye, R. L.
Secretary-Treasurer.........Ellis, H. C.
Delegate................Smith, J. G.
Members
Carmichael, W. W., Hampton (Hon.)
Colvin, E. G., Locust Grove
Crawford, R. L., Locust Grove
Ellis, H. C., McDonough
Harper, J. W., Hampton
Smith, J. G., McDonough
Tye, R. L., McDonough

HOUSTON-PEACH COUNTIES
Officers
President................Story, J. W.
Vice-President...........Evans, H. E.
Secretary-Treasurer.......Cater, R. L.
Members
Cater, R. L., Perry
Evans, H. E., Perry
Story, J. W., Perry

JACKSON-BARROW COUNTIES
Officers
President................Lord, C. B.
Vice-President..........Almand, C. B.
Secretary-Treasurer.......Stovall, J. T.
Delegate...............Almand, C. B.
Alternate Delegate.......Scoggins, P. T.
Members
Adams, R. P., Winder (Hon.)
Allen, L. C., Hoschton
Allen, M. B., Hoschton
Almand, C. B., Winder
Freeman, Ralph, Hoschton
Hardman, L. G., Commerce
Harris, E. R., Winder
Lord, C. B., Jefferson
Mathews, W. L., Winder
McDonald, E. M., Winder
Randolph, W. T., Winder
Rogers, A. A., Commerce
Ross, S. T., Winder
Stovall, J. T., Jefferson

JASPER COUNTY
Officer
Secretary-Treasurer......Lancaster, E. M.
Members
Anderson, J. F., Hillsboro (Hon.)
Belcher, F. S., Monticello
Lancaster, E. M., Shady Dale
Pittard, L. Y., Monticello

JEFFERSON COUNTY
Officers
President...............Pilcher, J. J.
Vice-President........Carpenter, G. L.

Secretary-Treasurer......Revell, S. T. R.
Delegate..............Revell, S. T. R.
Members
Bryson, L. R., Louisville
Carpenter, Geo. L., Wrens
Ketchin, B. C., Louisville
Lewis, J. R., Louisville
Peacock, J. D., Wadley
Pilcher, Jno. J., Wrens
Revell, S. T. R., Louisville

JENKINS COUNTY
Officers
President...............Lee, H. G.
Vice-President..........Mulkey, Q. A.
Secretary-Treasurer.......Thompson, C.
Delegate..............Thompson, C.
Members
Jones, J. M., Thrift (Asso.)
Lee, H. G., Millen
Lunsford, G. G., State Capitol, Atlanta
Mulkey, A. P., Millen
Mulkey, Q. A., Millen
Senn, H. B., Millen
Thompson, C., Millen

LAMAR COUNTY
Officers
President.............Pritchett, D. W.
Secretary-Treasurer......Traylor, S. B.
Members
Corry, J. A., Barnesville
Jackson, J. H., Barnesville
Pritchett, D. W., Barnesville
Traylor, S. B., Barnesville
Willis, C. H., Barnesville

LAURENS COUNTY
Officers
President..............Cheek, O. H.
Vice-President.........Coleman, A. T.
Secretary-Treasurer.......Ferrell, R. G., Jr.
Delegate..............Hodges, C. A.
Members
Barton, J. J., Dublin
Bedingfield, W. B., Rentz
Bell, Jno. A., Dublin
Benson, R. S., Alamo, R. 1
Carter, J. G, Jr., Scott
Cheek, O. H., Dublin
Claxton, E. B., Dublin
Coleman, A. T., Dublin
Ferrell, R. G., Jr., Dublin
Hicks, Chas. L., Dublin
Hodges, C. A., Dublin
New, J. E., Dexter
Thompson, W. C., Dublin
Ware, A. D., Toombsboro

LOWNDES COUNTY
(South Georgia Medical Society)
(Berrien, Clinch, Cook, Echols,
Lanier and Lowndes)
Officers
President.............Clements, H. W.
Vice-President..........Smith, L. A.
Secretary-Treasurer.....Hutchinson, L. R.
Delegate..............Crozier, G. T.
Alternate Delegate.......Saunders, A. F.
Members
Askew, P. H., Nashville
Askew, P. H., Jr., Nashville
Clements, H. W., Adel
Crozier, G. T., Valdosta
Elder, E. B., Erlanger Hospital, Chatta-
nooga, Tenn.
Parhar, M. B., Valdosta
Giddens, C. C., Valdosta
Hutchinson, L. R., Adel
Johnson, A. M., Valdosta
Little, A. G., Valdosta
Mixson, Joyce, Valdosta
Mixson, J. P., Valdosta
Owens, B. G., Valdosta
Quillian, E. P., Clyattville
Ring, L. J., Lenox
Saunders, A. F., Valdosta
Shepard, W. M., Adel
Smith, J. M., Valdosta
Smith, L. A., Quitman
Smith, T. H., Valdosta
Talbot, T. M., Valdosta (Hon.)
Thomas, F. H., Valdosta
Thompson, E. F., Nashville
Turner, W. V., Nashville
Williams, T. C., Valdosta

MACON COUNTY
Officers
President.............Frederick, D. B.
Vice-President..........Savage, C. P.
Secretary-Treasurer.......Adams, Thos. M.
Delegate.............Adams, Thos. M.

Alternate Delegate........Greer, Chas. A.
Members
Adams, J. Fred, Montezuma
Adams, Thos M., Montezuma
Derrick, H. C., Oglethorpe
Frederick, D. B., Marshallville
Greer, Chas. A., Oglethorpe
Lightner, L. L., Ideal
Mullino, F. M., Montezuma
Nelson, G. W., Marshallville (Hon.)
(Deceased)
Savage, C. P., Montezuma

McDUFFIE COUNTY
Officers
President..............Churchill, C. W.
Vice-President..........Riley, B. F., Jr.
Secretary-Treasurer.......Wilson, J. R.
Delegate..............Wilson, J. R.
Members
Churchill, C. W., Thomson
Riley, B. F., Jr., Thomson
Wilson, J. R., Thomson

MERIWETHER COUNTY
Officers
President..............Jackson, T. W.
Vice-President..........Bennett, V. H.
Secretary-Treasurer.......Gilbert, R. B.
Delegate..............Gilbert, R. B.
Alternate Delegate........Allen, W. P.
Members
Allen, W. P., Woodbury
Bennett, V. H., Gay
Copeland, Benj. H., Shiloh
Dixon, J. L., Woodbury
Ellis, W. P., Chipley
Gilbert, R. B., Greenville
Jackson, J. J., Manchester
Jackson, T. W., Manchester
Johnson, J. A., Manchester
Kirkland, W. P., Manchester
Peeler, J. E., Woodland
Rhyne, W. P., Warm Springs

MITCHELL COUNTY
Officer
Secretary-Treasurer.......Stevenson, C. A.
Members
Belcher, D. P., Pelham
Brim, J. C., Pelham
Mobley, J. W., Jr., Pelham
Reid, C. W., Pelham
Roles, C. L., Camilla
Stevenson, C. A., Camilla

MONROE COUNTY
Officers
President................Smith, W. J.
Vice-President..........Elrod, J. O.
Secretary-Treasurer.....Alexander, G. H.
Members
Alexander, G. H., Forsyth
Elrod, J. O., Forsyth
Goolsby, R. C., Sr., Forsyth
Smith, B. L., Forsyth
Smith, W. J., Juliette

MONTGOMERY COUNTY
Member
Palmer, J. W., Ailey

MORGAN COUNTY
Officers
President.............Fambrough, W. M.
Vice-President..........Carter, D. M.
Secretary-Treasurer.......McGeary, W. C.
Delegate..............Porter, J. L.
Members
Carter, D. M., Madison
Fambrough, W. M., Bostwick
McGeary, W. C., Madison
Porter, J. L., Rutledge
Prior, Felix M., Apalachee (Hon.)

MUSCOGEE COUNTY
Officers
President..............Walker, Jno. E.
Vice-President..........Spikes, J. L.
Secretary-Treasurer.......Cook, Wm. C.
Delegate..............Schley, Francis B.
Alternate Delegate.......Jenkins, W. F.
Members
Akamatsu, Geo. T., City Hospital, Columbus
(Asso.)
Armstrong, G. E., Fort Benning (Asso.)
Baier, Geo. F., III, Fort Benning (Asso.)
Baird, A. M., Doctors Bldg., Columbus
(Deceased)
Baker, E. L., Doctors Bldg., Columbus
Barry, Wm. E., Fort Benning (Asso.)
Bauchspies, Rollin L., Fort Benning (Asso.)
Berry, Arthur N., Murrah Bldg., Columbus

Blanchard, Mercer, Swift-Kyle Bldg., Columbus
Blackmar, Francis B., Swift-Kyle Bldg., Columbus
Bracher, Allen N., Fort Benning (Asso.)
Brannon, O. C., Murrah Bldg., Columbus
Brooks, H. W., Buena Vista
Brummette, Jas. S., Fort Benning (Asso.)
Bush, John, 313 Fourteenth St., Columbus
Carter, C. B., 1545 Third Ave., Columbus
Chaney, Thos. M., Fort Benning (Asso.)
Cirlot, J. S., Fort Benning (Asso.)
Cook, Wm. C., Swift-Kyle Bldg., Columbus
Cooke, W. L., Doctors Bldg., Columbus
Dexter, C. A., Murrah Bldg., Columbus
Dillard, Guy J., Murrah Bldg., Columbus
Duckworth, Jas. W., Fort Benning
Columbus (Asso.)
Dykes, A. N., 1229 Second Ave., Columbus
Gaston, Joseph H., Doctors Bldg., Columbus
Gilliam, O. D., Doctors Bldg., Columbus
Graham, O. L., Fort Benning (Asso.)
Hall, M. W., Fort Benning (Asso.)
Hesner, Geo. E., Fort Benning (Asso.)
Howard, Jas. W., Fort Benning (Asso.)
Jenkins, W. F., City Hospital, Columbus
Johnson, C. D., Murrah Bldg., Columbus
Johnson, J. H., Murrah Bldg., Columbus
Jordan, W. P., Doctors Bldg., Columbus
Kinberger, Albert G., Fort Benning (Asso.)
Kusmirz, Morris J., City Hospital, Columbus (Asso.)
Lanahan, C. R., Fort Benning (Asso.)
Levine, H. A., City Hospital, Columbus (Asso.)
Mahaney, J. D., Woolworth Bldg., Columbus
Mayhew, W. E., Swift-Kyle Bldg., Columbus
McDuffie, J. H., Jr., Masonic Temple, Columbus
Moses, Alice, 1413 Second Ave., Columbus
Murray, G. S., Swift-Kyle Bldg., Columbus
Murray, O. B., City Hospital, Columbus (Asso.)
North, W. D., Fort Benning (Asso.)
Peacock, C. A., Murrah Bldg., Columbus
Qualls, Guy L., Fort Benning (Asso.)
Rea, R. P., Fort Benning (Asso.)
Reiber, Martin R., Fort Benning (Asso.)
Schley, Francis B., Swift-Kyle Bldg., Columbus
Smith, L. L., Fort Benning (Asso.)
Smith, W. A., Fort Benning (Asso.)
Spikes, J. L., Doctors Bldg., Columbus
Stammeil, Chas. A., Fort Benning (Asso.)
Stapleton, J. L., 1229 Second Ave., Columbus
Stevens, J. H., City Hospital, Columbus (Asso.)
Storey, W. E., Swift-Kyle Bldg., Columbus
Thompson, J. B., Swift-Kyle Bldg., Columbus
Threatte, Bruce, Swift-Kyle Bldg., Columbus
Walker, Jno. E., Masonic Temple, Columbus
Willis, J. N., Swift-Kyle Bldg., Columbus
Wilson, Frank W., Fort Benning (Asso.)
Wise, J. H., Swift-Kyle Bldg., Columbus
Wooldridge, J. C., Murrah Bldg., Columbus
Youmans, J. R., 1140½ Broad St., Columbus
Young, Chas. T., Fort Benning (Asso.)
Young, S. E., Midland

NEWTON COUNTY
Officer
Secretary-Treasurer . . . . Travis, W. D.
Members
Baxley, W. W., Porterdale
Palmer, Clarence B., Covington
Sams, J. J., Covington
Travis, W. D., Covington
Walters, S. L., Covington
Wilson, Pleas, Newborn

OCMULGEE SOCIETY
(Bleckley, Dodge, Pulaski)
Officers
President . . . . Massey, W. F.
Secretary-Treasurer . . . . . . Parkerson, I. J.
Delegate . . . . Bush, A. R.
Alternate Delegate . . . . Parkerson, I. J.
Members
Barker, Jno. L., Eastman (Hon.)
Brown, E. C., Hawkinsville
Bush, Albert R., Hawkinsville
Coleman, W. A., Eastman
Harris, E. C., Bibb Bldg., Macon
Massey, W. F., Chester
Parkerson, I. J., Eastman
Pirkle, W. H., Cochran
Powell, Jno. F., Gresston (Hon.)
Smith, J. M., Eastman
Tolleson, H. M., Eastman
Wall, J. C., Eastman

Whipple, R. L., Cochran
Williamson, J. G., Rhine
Yawn, B. W., Eastman

POLK COUNTY
Officers
President . . . . Whitely, S. L.
Vice-President . . . . Wood, C. V.
Secretary-Treasurer . . . . . McGehee, Jno. M.
Delegate . . . . Good, Jno. W.
Alternate Delegate . . . . Wood, C. V.
Members
Chapman, W. A., Cedartown (Hon.)
Chaudron, P. O., Cedartown
Cooper, J. J., Cedartown
Goldin, Robert B., Rockmart
Good, Jno. W., Cedartown
Lucas, W. H., Cedartown
McBryde, T. B., Rockmart
McGehee, Jno. M., Cedartown
Peek, C. W., Cedartown
Perkins, Henry R., Rockmart
White, Geo. M., Rockmart
Whitely, S. L., Cedartown
Wood, C. V., Cedartown

PUTNAM COUNTY
Officers
President . . . . Griffith, E. F.
Secretary-Treasurer . . . . . . Clodfelter, T. C.
Members
Clodfelter, Thos. C., Eatonton
Griffith, E. F., Eatonton

RABUN COUNTY
Officers
President . . . . Dover, J. C.
Secretary-Treasurer . . . . Green, J. A.
Delegate . . . . Dover, J. C.
Alternate Delegate . . . . Green, J. A.
Members
Dover, J. C., Clayton
Green, J. A., Clayton

RANDOLPH COUNTY
Officers
President . . . . Garry, Loren, Jr.
Vice-President . . . . McCurdy, E. C.
Secretary-Treasurer . . . . Elliott, W. G.
Delegate . . . . Elliott, W. G.
Alternate Delegate . . . . Harper, T. F.
Members
Baldwin, J. O., Fort Gaines
Binion, W. W., Benevolence (Hon.)
Carter, Geo. Bluffton (Hon.)
Crook, W. W., Cuthbert
Elliott, W. G., Cuthbert
Gary, Loren, Georgetown
Gary, Loren, Jr., Shellman
Harper, T. F., Coleman
Martin, P. M., Shellman
Massengale, Leonard R., Cuthbert
McCurdy, E. C., Shellman
Patterson, J. C., Cuthbert
Rogers, F. S., Coleman
Sasers, Annette McD., Cuthbert (Hon.)
Shelly, W. P., Albany (Hon.)
Weathers, A. F., Shellman
Wimberly, William, Fort Gaines (Hon.)

RICHMOND COUNTY
Officers
President . . . . Fund, Edgar R.
Vice-President . . . . Sherman, J. H.
Secretary-Treasurer . . . . . . McGahee, R. C.
Delegate . . . . Kelly, G. L.
Delegate . . . . Chaney, R. H.
Alternate Delegate . . . . . . Cranston, W. J.
Alternate Delegate . . . . . . Davidson, A. A.
Members
Agee, M. P., Southern Finance Bldg., Augusta
Akerman, Joseph, 831 Fifteenth St., Augusta
Armstrong, E. S., 1345 Greene St., Augusta
Battey, Colden R., 638 Greene St., Augusta
Battey, W. W., Jr., 428 Sixth St., Augusta
Bedingfield, W. R., Southern Finance Bldg., Augusta
Berr, C. M., University Hospital, Augusta
Bernard, G. T., 203 Thirteenth St., Augusta
Blanchard, C. A., 926 Broad St., Augusta
Blanchard, P. G., Appling
Brittingham, Jno. W., 1345 Greene St., Augusta
Brown, T. P., Marion Bldg., Augusta
Bryans, L. C., Southern Finance Bldg., Augusta
Burdashaw, J. F., Johnson Bldg., Augusta
Burpee, C. M., University Hospital, Augusta
Butler, J. H., Southern Finance Bldg., Augusta
Callison, H. Grady, Department of Health, Columbia, S. C.
Chiney, Ralph H., 1001 Greene St., Augusta

Crane, C. W., 1345 Greene St., Augusta
Cranston, W. J., Southern Finance Bldg., Augusta
Crichton, Robert B., 434 Broad St., Augusta
Davidson, A. A., 1116 Greene St., Augusta
Eve, H. J., 619 Greene St., Augusta
Gibson, C., Thomson
Goodrich, W. H., Southern Finance Bldg., Augusta
Goodwin, T. W., 1345 Greene St., Augusta
Gray, J. D., 1345 Greene St., Augusta
Harrell, H. P., Southern Finance Bldg., Augusta
Henry, C. G., Southern Finance Bldg., Augusta
Hensley, E. A., Gibson
Holmes, L. P., Southern Finance Bldg., Augusta
Kelly, G. Lombard, Medical College, Augusta
Kershaw, Marie M., Southern Finance Bldg., Augusta
Kilpatrick, A. J., 407 Seventh St., Augusta
Kilpatrick, Chas. M., 1345 Greene St., Augusta
Ler, F. Lansing, Southern Finance Bldg., Augusta
Levy, M. S., Southern Finance Bldg., Augusta
Lewis, S. J., Southern Finance Bldg., Augusta
Mathews, W. E., Southern Finance Bldg., Augusta
May, E. R., Lincolnton
McGahee, R. C., 1345 Greene St., Augusta
Mealing, H. G., Southern Finance Bldg., Augusta
Michel, H. M., Southern Finance Bldg., Augusta
Mountain, G. W., 2612 Walton Way, Augusta
Mulherin, P. X., 1001 Greene St., Augusta
Mulherin, Philip A., 1001 Greene St., Augusta
Mulherin, Wm. A., 1001 Greene St., Augusta
Murphey, Eugene E., 432 Telfair St., Augusta
Norvell, J. T., Southern Finance Bldg., Augusta
Page, Hugh N., Southern Finance Bldg., Augusta
Philpot, W. K., 1345 Greene St., Augusta
Phinizy, Irvine, Southern Finance Bldg., Augusta
Phinizy, Thomas, 501 Greene St., Augusta
Price, W. T., Montgomery Bldg., Augusta
Pund, Edgar R., Medical College, Augusta
Rhodes, R. L., Southern Finance Bldg., Augusta
Roberts, W. H., 828 Greene St., Augusta
Robertson, J. Righton, 1345 Greene St., Augusta
Ross, W. H., Wrightsville
Roule, J. Victor, Southern Finance Bldg., Augusta
Sanderson, E. S., Medical College, Augusta
Scharnitzky, E. O., Southern Finance Bldg., Augusta
Sherman, John H., 1122 Johns Road, Augusta
Sydenstricker, V. P., University Hospital, Augusta
Tessier, L. P., Masonic Temple, Augusta
Thurmond, J. W., 407 Seventh St., Augusta
Timmons, C. C., Marion Bldg., Augusta
Todd, L. N., Waverly Hills Sanatorium, Waverly Hills, Ky.
Traylor, Geo. A., Southern Finance Bldg., Augusta
Ward, S. D., 1345 Greene St., Augusta
Weeks, J. L., Harlem
Weeks, R. B., Southern Finance Bldg., Augusta
Wilcox, E. A., Southern Finance Bldg., Augusta
Williams, M. J., Southern Finance Bldg., Augusta
Wolfe, David M., Southern Finance Bldg., Augusta
Woodbury, Robert, Medical College, Augusta
Woods, E. D., Florida State Board of Health, Jacksonville, Fla.
Wright, Geo. W., Southern Finance Bldg., Augusta
Wright, R. B., 1345 Greene St., Augusta

ROCKDALE COUNTY
Officers
President . . . . Brown, P. J.
Vice-President . . . . Smith, P. S.
Secretary-Treasurer . . . . Griggs, H. E.
Delegate . . . . Ware, S. A.
Members
Brown, P. J., Conyers

Griggs. H. E., Conyers
Smith. P. S., Conyers
Ware. S. A., Conyers

SCREVEN COUNTY
Officer
Secretary-Treasurer..... Bennett, W. H.
Members
Bennett, W. H., Sylvania
Cail, Jno. C., Sylvania
Lanier, L. P., Sylvania
Rushing. W. E., Mlllhaven

SPALDING COUNTY
Officers
President.......... Hawkins, T. I.
Vice-President........ Walker, Geo. L.
Secretary-Treasurer...... Copeland, H. J.
Delegate................ Frye, A. H.
Alternate Delegate......... Miles, W. C.
Members
Anthony, J. R., Griffin
Carson, M. F., Griffin (Hon.)
Copeland, H. J., Griffin
Copeland, H. W., Griffin
Drewry, T. E., Griffin (Deceased)
English, R. E. L., Experiment
Forrer, D. A., Griffin
Frye, A. H., Griffin
Graves, J. R., Zebulon (Hon.)
Griffith, C. F., Griffin
Grubbs, J. H., Molena
Hawkins, T. I., Griffin
Head, D. L., Zebulon
Head, M. M., Zebulon
Howard, I. B., Williamson
Humphries, W. C., Griffin
Hunt, K. S., Griffin
Mallory, R. A., Concord (Hon.)
Miles, W. C., Griffin
Smaha, Tofey G., Griffin
Steele, W. H., Griffin (Hon.)
Walker, Geo. L., Griffin

STEPHENS COUNTY
Officers
President............. Terrell, J. H.
Vice-President.......... Chaffin, E. F.
Secretary-Treasurer..... Ayers, Clarence L.
Delegate.............. Schaefer, W. B.
Alternate Delegate..... Isbell, J. E. D.
Members
Ayers, Clarence L., Toccoa
Chaffin, E. F., Toccoa
Davis, Jeff, Toccoa (Hon.)
Edge, J. H., Toccoa (Hon.)
Heller, W. B., Toccoa
Isbell, J. E. D., Toccoa
Schaefer, W. B., Toccoa
Terrell, J. H., Toccoa

STEWART-WEBSTER COUNTIES
Officers
President................ Pickett, C. E.
Secretary-Treasurer....... Sims, A. R.
Delegate................ Lynch, C. S.
Alternate Delegate.......Kenyon, J. M.
Members
Kenyon, J. M., Richland
Lunsford, J. F., Preston (Hon.)
Lynch, C. S., Lumpkin
Miller, T. B., Richland (Hon.)
Pickett, C. E., Richland
Sims, A. R., Richland
Sims, W. C., Richland

SUMTER COUNTY
Officers
President............. Primrose, A. C.
Vice-President....... Pendergrass, R. C.
Secretary-Treasurer...... Avary, Arch, Jr.
Delegate................ Logan, J. C.
Members
Avary, Arch, Jr., Ellaville
Boyette, L. S., Ellaville
Cato, F. L., DeSoto (Hon.) (Deceased)
Chambliss, J. W., Americus
Jordan, A. P., Ellaville
Logan, J. C., Plains
McMath, J. F., Americus (Hon.)
Pendergrass, R. C., Americus
Prather, W. S., Americus
Primrose, A. C., Americus
Scruggs, S. A., Americus
Smith, Herschel A., Americus
Stukes, S. T., Americus
Wise, B. T., Americus
Wise, S. P., Americus
Wood, Kenneth, Leslie

TALBOT COUNTY
Member
Leonard, W. P., Talbotton

TALIAFERRO COUNTY
Officers
President.................. Nash, T. C.
Secretary-Treasurer..... Rhodes, Jno. A.
Delegate................. Nash, T. C.
Members
Nash, T. C., Philomath
Rhodes, John A., Crawfordville (Hon.)

TATTNALL COUNTY
Officers
President.............. Collins, J. C.
Vice-President......... Branch, A. C.
Secretary-Treasurer...... Hughes, J. M.
Delegate............ Strickland, L. V.
Alternate Delegate ...... Hughes, J. M.
Members
Bowen, J. H., Cobbtown (Hon.)
Branch, A. C., Glennville
Collins, J. C., Collins
Hughes, J. M., Glennville
Jelks, L. R., Reidsville
Jones, R. D., Eliza
Kennedy, J. J., Collins (Hon.)
Kicklighter, R. B., Glennville
Rountree, M. A., Reidsville (Deceased)
Smith, S. F., Glennville
Strickland, L. V., Cobbtown
Tootle, G. W., Denton
Walling, C. B., Collins

TAYLOR COUNTY
Officers
President.............. Besson, Lewis
Vice-President.......... Bryan, S. H.
Secretary-Treasurer..... Montgomery, R. C.
Delegate................ Bryan, S. H.
Members
Besson, Lewis, Butler
Bryan, S. H., Reynolds
Montgomery, R. C., Butler

TELFAIR COUNTY
Officers
President............. Parkerson, S. T.
Vice-President......... Born, W. H.
Secretary-Treasurer..... Harbin, F. P.
Delegate................ Mann, F. R.
Members
Born, W. H., McRae
Harbin, F. P., Lumber City
Kennon, B. M., McRae (Hon.)
Maloy, C. J., Helena
Maloy, D. W. F., Milan
Mann, Frank, McRae
Neal, J. W., Scotland (Hon.)
Parkerson, S. T., McRae
Powell, W. H., Hazlehurst
Youmans, C. R., Lumber City

TERRELL COUNTY
Officers
President.............. Chappell, Guy
Vice-President.......... Lewis, J. H.
Secretary-Treasurer...... Kenyon, Steve P.
Delegate............ Kenyon, Steve P.
Alternate Delegate ...... Arnold, J. T.
Members
Arnold, J. T., Parrott
Chappell, Guy, Dawson
Cranford, O. G., Sasser (Hon.)
Dean, J. C., Dawson (Hon.)
Kenyon, S. P., Dawson
Lamar, Lucius, Dawson
Lewis, J. H., Dawson (Hon.)

THOMAS COUNTY
Officers
President.............. Ainsworth, Harry
Vice-President.......... Isler, J. N.
Secretary-Treasurer...... Bell, Rudolph
Delegate................ Wall, C. K.
Alternate Delegate ...... Bell, Rudolph
Members
Ainsworth, Harry, Thomasville
Bell, Rudolph, Thomasville
Brinson, J. B., Monticello, Fla. (Hon.)
Brooks, Fletcher H., Thomasville (Hon.)
Cheshire, S. L., Thomasville
Dykes, J. R., Thomasville
Erickson, Mary J., Thomasville
Ferguson, C. H., Thomasville
Garrett, J. A., Meigs
Glover, G. B., Monticello, Fla. (Hon.)
Hill, Roy A., Thomasville
Isler, J. N., Meigs
Jarrell, W. W., Thomasville
Jones, Henry, Coolidge (Hon.)
King, J. T., Thomasville
Little, A. D., Thomasville
Lundy, L. L., Boston
Moore, H. M., Thomasville
Palmer, J. D., Thomasville
Reid, Jas. W., Thomasville

Reilly, C. J., Thomasville (Asso.)
Sanchez, S. E., Barwick
Wahl, Ernest F., Thomasville
Wall, C. K., Thomasville
Watt, C. H., Thomasville
Williams, J. F., Monticello. Fla. (Hon.)

TIFT COUNTY
Officers
President................ Shaw, M. F.
Vice-President......... Hendricks, W. H.
Secretary-Treasurer ...... Pittman, C. S.
Delegate................ Pittman, C. S.
Members
Dinsmore, V. F., Tifton
Evans, E. L., Tifton
Fleming, C. A., Tifton
Hendricks, W. H., Tifton
Little, Tom F., Tifton
Pittman, Carl S., Tifton
Shaw, M. F., Omega
Smith, W. T., Tifton
Webb, M. L., Tifton
Zimmerman, W. F., Tifton

TOOMBS COUNTY
Officers
President............... Mercer, J. E.
Vice-President........ Youmans, H. D.
Secretary-Treasurer....... Odom, W. W.
Delegate............. Youmans, H. D.
Members
Aiken, W. W., Lyons
Findley, C. W., Vidalia
Gross, O. S., Vidalia
Hall, J. K., Lyons
Meadows, Jno. M., Vidalia (Hon.)
Mercer, J. E., Vidalia
Odom, W. W., Lyons
Youmans, H. D., Lyons

TRI SOCIETY
(Calhoun, Early, Miller)
Officers
President............... Baughn, E. B.
Vice-President......... Barksdale, C. R.
Secretary-Treasurer...... Standifer, J. G.
Delegate.............. Shepard, W. O.
Alternate Delegate ...... Wall, W. H.
Members
Barksdale, C. R., Blakely
Baughn, E. B., Colquitt
Beard, J. S., Edison
Bridges, R. R., Leary
Cheshire, J. L., Damascus
Darden, Holt, Blakely
Ganter, G. O., Newton
Hattaway, J. C., Edison
Hays, W. C., Colquitt
Roberts, C. A., Leary
Sharp, C. K., Arlington
Shepard, W. O., Shelton
Simmons, B. K., Blakely
Standifer, J. G., Blakely
Standifer, W. B., Blakely (Hon.)
Wall, W. H., Blakely
Ward, L. C., Damascus

TRI SOCIETY
(Liberty, Long, McIntosh)
Officers
Secretary-Treasurer....... Gibson, B. H.
Delegate............. Armistead, I. G.
Alternate Delegate ...... Gibson, B. H.
Members
Armistead, I. G., Warsaw
Gibson, B. Harrison, Allenhurst
Long, Wm. J., Townsend
Ogden, I. K., Darien

TROUP COUNTY
Officers
President................ O'Neal, R. S.
Vice-President......... Morgan, J. C.
Secretary-Treasurer...... Holder, J. S.
Delegate............... Callaway, Enoch
Alternate Delegate ...... McCulloh, Hugh, Jr.
Members
Amis, Frank J., Jr., Hogansville
Avery, R. M., LaGrange
Byrd, M. M., West Point
Callaway, Enoch, LaGrange
Clark, W. H., LaGrange
Hadaway, W. H., LaGrange
Hammett, H. H., LaGrange
Harvey, C. W., Hogansville
Herman, E. C., LaGrange
Holder, J. S., LaGrange
Lee, R. O., LaGrange
McCall, W. R., LaGrange
McCulloh, Hugh, Jr., West Point
Morgan, D. E., LaGrange
Morgan, J. C., West Point
O'Neal, Rance, West Point

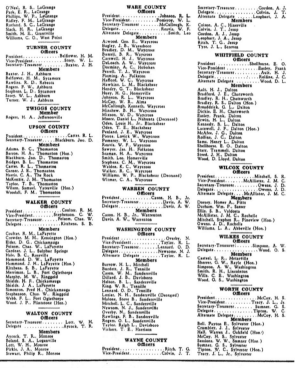

O'Neal, R. S., LaGrange
Park, E. R., LaGrange
Phillips, W. P., LaGrange
Ridley, F. M., LaGrange
Rutland, S. C., LaGrange
Slack, H. R., LaGrange
Smith, M. E., Grantville
Williams, C. O., West Point

TURNER COUNTY
Officers
President.............Belflower, H. M.
Vice-President.........Story, W. L.
Secretary-Treasurer.....Baxter, J. H.
Members
Baxter, J. H., Ashburn
Belflower, H. M., Sycamore
Rawlins, R. D., Rebecca
Rogers, F. W., Ashburn
Stephens, L. D., Sycamore
Story, W. L., Ashburn
Turner, W. J., Ashburn

TWIGGS COUNTY
Member
Rogers, H. A., Jeffersonville

UPSON COUNTY
Officers
President...............Carter, R. L.
Secretary-Treasurer....Blackburn, Jno. D.
Members
Adams, B. C., Thomaston
Barron, H. A., Thomaston (Hon.)
Blackburn, Jno. D., Thomaston
Bridges, B. L., Thomaston
Carter, R. L., Thomaston
Garner, J. E., Thomaston
Harris, C. A., The Rock
McKenzie, J. M., Thomaston
Taylor, T. B., Thomaston
Wilson, Samuel, Yatesville (Hon.)
Woodall, F. M., Thomaston

WALKER COUNTY
Officers
President............Coulter, R. M.
Vice-President........Stephenson, C. W.
Secretary-Treasurer....Folsom, Chas. W.
Delegate..............Kitchens, S. B.
Members
Coulter, R. M., LaFayette
Crowder, M. M., Kensington (Hon.)
Elder, D. G., Chickamauga
Folsom, Chas. W., Sulphur Springs
Gardner, J. L., Sulphur Springs
Hale, B. C., Rossville
Hammond, D. W., LaFayette
Hammond, J. H., LaFayette (Hon.)
Kitchens, S. B., LaFayette
Merriman, L. B., Fort Oglethorpe
Murphy, M. W., Ringgold
Shields, H. F., Chickamauga
Shields, J. A., LaFayette
Simonton, Fred H., Chickamauga
Stephenson, Chas. W., Ringgold
Webb, F. L., Fort Oglethorpe
Wood, J. P., Flintstone (Hon.)

WALTON COUNTY
Officers
Secretary-Treasurer..... Lott, W. H.
Delegate.............Aycock, T. R.
Members
Aycock, T. R., Monroe
Boland, S. A., Loganville
Lott, W. H., Monroe
Pirkle, J. A., Monroe
Stewart, Philip R., Monroe

WARE COUNTY
Officers
President.............Johnson, R. L.
Vice-President.........Pomeroy, W. L.
Secretary-Treasurer ......McCullough, K.
Delegate..............Reavis, W. F.
Alternate Delegate.........Smith, Leo
Members
Atwood, Geo. B., Waycross
Bagley, J. B., Waresboro
Bradley, D. M., Waycross
Bussell, B. R., Waycross
Caswell, H. J., Waycross
DeLoach, A. W., Waycross
Dormiay, A. C., Hoboken
Ferrell, T. J., Waycross
Fleming, A., Folkston
Hafford, W. C., Waycross
Hawkins, L. M., Blackshear
Hendry, G. T., Blackshear
Huey, H. G., Homerville
Johnson, R. L., Waycross
McCoy, W. R., Alma
McCullough, Kenneth, Waycross
Minchew, B. H., Waycross
Mixson, W. D., Waycross
Moore, Daniel L., Nahunta (Deceased)
Oden, Louis H., Jr., Blackshear
Oden, T. E., Blackshear
Penland, J. E., Waycross
Pierce, Lovick W., Waycross
Pomeroy, W. L., Waycross
Reavis, W. F., Waycross
Sawyer, Jas. H., Folkston
Seaman, H. A., Waycross
Smith, Leo, Homerville
Stephens, C. M., Waycross
Walden, R. C., Waycross
Walker, R. C., Waycross
Williams, W. P., Blackshear (Deceased)
Witmer, W. A., Waycross

WARREN COUNTY
Officers
President.........Cason, H. B., Jr.
Secretary-Treasurer ....Davis, A. W.
Delegate..............Davis, A. W.
Members
Cason, H. B., Jr., Warrenton
Davis, A. W., Warrenton

WASHINGTON COUNTY
Officers
President...............Overby, N.
Vice-President.........Taylor, R.
Secretary-Treasurer .....Lennard, O. D.
Delegate.............Newsome, N. J.
Alternate Delegate ....Taylor, R. L.
Members
Barrow, H. L., Mitchell
Burdett, J. R., Tennille
Casm, W. M., Sandersville
Dillard, J. B., Davisboro
Helton, B. L., Sandersville
King, W. R., Tennille
Lennard, O. D., Tennille
Lozier, H. M., Sandersville (Deceased)
Malone, Steve B., Sandersville
Mitchell, L. C., Sandersville
Newsom, N. J., Sandersville
Overby, N., Sandersville
Rawlings, F. B., Sandersville
Rogers, O. L., Sandersville
Taylor, Ralph L., Davisboro
Vickers, T. E., Harrison

WAYNE COUNTY
Officers
President.............Ritch, T. G.
Vice-President...........Colvin, J. T.

Secretary-Treasurer........Gordon, A. J.
Delegate.............Colvin, J. T.
Alternate Delegate ....Leophart, J. A.
Members
Colson, A. C., Hinesville
Colvin, J. T., Jesup
Gordon, A. J., Jesup
Leophart, J. A., Jesup
Ritch, T. G., Jesup
Tyre, J. L., Screven

WHITFIELD COUNTY
Officers
President...............Shellhorse, E. O.
Vice-President...........Easley, Frank
Secretary-Treasurer......Ault, H. J.
Delegate..............Rollins, J. C.
Alternate Delegate ....Wood, D. L.
Members
Ault, H. J., Dalton
Bradford, J. E., Chatsworth
Bradley, R. H., Chatsworth
Bradley, R. S., Dalton (Hon.)
Broaddrick, G. L., Dalton
Dickie, E. H., Chatsworth
Easley, Frank, Dalton
Erwin, H. L., Dalton
Kennedy, B. L., Dalton
Lacewell, J. P., Dalton (Hon.)
McAfee, J. G., Dalton
Rollins, J. C., Dalton
Sams, Henry L., Dalton
Shellhorse, E. O., Dalton
Starr, Trammell, Dalton
Steed, J. H., Dalton
Wood, D. Lloyd, Dalton

WILCOX COUNTY
Officers
President.............Mitchell, S. R.
Vice-President........McAllister, J. M. C.
Secretary-Treasurer.......Owens, J. D.
Delegate.............Owens, J. D.
Alternate Delegate ... McAllister, J. M. C.
Members
Dorsey, Homer A., Pitts
Durham, Wm. P., Sasser
Ellis, S. B., Valdosta
McAllister, J. M. C., Rochelle
Mitchell, Stephen R., Pineview (Hon.)
Owens, J. D., Rochelle
Williams, L. A., Abbeville (Hon.)

WILKES COUNTY
Officers
President.............Simpson, A. W.
Delegate..............Wood, O. S.
Members
Castell, L. R., Metasville
Sherrer, G. W., Rayle (Hon.)
Simpson, A. W., Washington
Smith, R. H., Lincolnton
Wills, C. E., Washington
Wood, O. S., Washington

WORTH COUNTY
Officers
President..............McCoy, H. S.
Vice-President.........Tracy, J. L., Jr.
Secretary-Treasurer........Sumner, G. S.
Delegate..............Tipton, W. C.
Alternate Delegate.......McCoy, H. S.
Members
Bell, Payton E., Sylvester (Hon.)
Crumbley, J. J., Sylvester
Hall, Warren J., Oakfield (Hon.)
McCoy, H. S., Sylvester
Sessions, W. W., Sumner (Hon.)
Sumner, G. S., Sylvester
Tipton, W. C., Sylvester (Hon.)
Tracy, J. L., Jr., Sylvester

GONOCOCCIC ENDOCARDITIS: REPORT OF CASE WITH POSITIVE BLOOD CULTURE

ISIDOR COHN's, Brooklyn (*Journal A. M. A.*, Nov. 14, 1936), case of gonorrheal endocarditis illustrates the difficulties often encountered in arriving at a diagnosis. In fact, were it not for the positive blood culture, in itself a rather rare observation, the diagnosis could not have been made, for there was no history nor anatomic evidence of gonorrhea except possibly the enlarged prostate and seminal vesicle. The positive complement fixation was contradicted by the equally positive Widal, so that the serologic reactions only confused the clinical picture, and the postmortem examination, while confirming the clinical diagnosis of ulcerative endocarditis, gave no hint of etiology. There was no evidence of previous cardiac damage or defect, so that this is one of those exceptional cases in which gonococci, invading the blood stream, have caused inflammation of a normal endocardium. Although the demonstration of gonococci in the valve would have been further evidence in this case, the failure to do so is explained by the fact that no active search was made for them until after the report of the last blood culture, by which time these fragile organisms could readily have been replaced by the secondary invaders found on culture—Bacillus coli and Staphylococcus aureus. The case illustrates the importance of repeated blood cultures, and·it·is interesting that growth was finally obtained on ordinary Savita agar and bouillon, after failure with special mediums.

MEDICAL ASSOCIATION OF GEORGIA
OFFICERS AND COMMITTEES
1936-1937

EIGHTY-EIGHTH ANNUAL SESSION, MACON
MAY 11, 12, 13, 14, 1937

OFFICERS

President..............B. H. Minchew, Waycross
President-Elect.........George A. Traylor, Augusta
First Vice-President........C. F. Holton, Savannah
Second Vice-President............J. B. Kay, Byron
Secretary-Treasurer.......Edgar D. Shanks, Atlanta
Parliamentarian...... John W. Simmons, Brunswick

DELEGATES TO THE A. M. A.

William H. Myers (1937-8)............Savannah
   Alternate, Wm. A. Mulherin..........Augusta
Chas. W. Roberts (1937-8)............Atlanta
   Alternate, Marion C. Pruitt............Atlanta
Olin H. Weaver (1936-7)................Macon
   Alternate, C. K. Sharp.............Arlington

COUNCIL

J. A. Redfearn, Chairman...............Albany
Grady N. Coker, Clerk..................Canton

Councilors

1. C. Thompson (1939)..............Millen
2. J. A. Redfearn (1939).............Albany
3. J. C. Patterson (1939)...........Cuthbert
4. Kenneth S. Hunt (1939)............Griffin
5. W. A. Selman (1937)..............Atlanta
6. H. G. Weaver (1937)..............Macon
7. M. M. McCord (1937)...............Rome
8. J. E. Penland (1937)............Waycross
9. Grady N. Coker (1938)............Canton
10. S. J. Lewis (1938)'...............Augusta

Vice-Councilors

1. R. V. Martin (1939)............Savannah
2. Chas. H. Watt (1939)..........Thomasville
3. J. Cox Wall (1939)............Eastman
4. Enoch Callaway (1939)..........LaGrange
5. Marion C. Pruitt (1937)..........Atlanta
6. H. D. Allen (1937)..........Milledgeville
7. H. J. Ault (1937)................Dalton
8. Wm. W. Turner (1937)...........Nashville
9. J. K. Burns (1938).............Gainesville
10. W. C. McGeary (1938)............Madison

Scientific Work

Geo. A. Traylor, Chairman (1937)......Augusta
H. C. Sauls (1938)...................Atlanta
Chas. H. Richardson (1939).............Macon
Edgar D. Shanks, Secretary-Treasurer.......Atlanta

Public Policy and Legislation

C. C. Aven, Chairman (1938)...........Atlanta
Dan Y. Sage (1937)..................Atlanta
J. O. Elrod (1939)..................Forsyth
C. L. Ayers...........................Toccoa
J. L. Campbell........................Atlanta
Edgar H. Greene.......................Atlanta
S. T. R. Revell.....................Louisville
Edgar D. Shanks, Secretary-Treasurer·······Atlanta
T. F. Abercrombie, Director, Department

of Public Health, State of Georgia......Atlanta

Medical Defense

Frank K. Boland, Chairman (1938)........Atlanta
Wm. A. Mulherin (1939)..............Augusta
A. R. Rozar (1941)....................Macon
J. A. Redfearn, Chairman of Council........Albany
Edgar D. Shanks, Secretary-Treasurer.......Atlanta

Hospitals

R. H. Oppenheimer, Chairman (1937)......Atlanta
Arthur D. Little (1941)............Thomasville
D. Henry Poer (1938)................Atlanta
C. D. Whelchel (1939)..............Gainesville
L. P. Holmes (1940)..................Augusta

Abner Wellborn Calhoun Lectureship

Jas. E. Paullin, Chairman (1938).........Atlanta
H. I. Reynolds (1939)................Athens
Eugene E. Murphey (1940)............Augusta
J. M. Smith (1941)..................Valdosta
Frank K. Boland (1937)................Atlanta

Economics

Lewis M. Gaines, Chairman (1940)........Atlanta
C. W. Roberts (1938)................Atlanta
C. L. Ridley (1941)....................Macon
Dan Y. Sage (1937)..................Atlanta
J. H. Downey (1939)................Gainesville

Sub-Committee on Compilation
Medical Economics

Jas. E. Paullin, Chairman...............Atlanta
C. W. Roberts........................Atlanta
L. M. Gaines.........................Atlanta
T. F. Abercrombie.'...................Atlanta
Edgar D. Shanks, Secretary-Treasurer.......Atlanta

Necrology

A. J. Mooney, Chairman..............Statesboro
Thos. J. McArthur....................Cordele
C. K. Sharp........................Arlington

Medical History of Georgia
Sub-Committee

Frank K. Boland, Chairman..............Atlanta
William R. Dancy......................Savannah
Arthur G. Fort........................Atlanta
V. H. Bassett........................Savannah
Allen H. Bunce........................Atlanta

Crawford W. Long Memorial Prize

William R. Dancy, Chairman............Savannah
Stewart R. Roberts....................Atlanta
V. P. Sydenstricker....................Augusta
George Bachmann......................Atlanta
Edgar R. Pund........................Augusta

Cancer Commission

Jas. L. Campbell, Chairman..............Atlanta
William H. Myers.....................Savannah
Charles H. Watt..................Thomasville
J. C. Patterson.....................Cuthbert
Kenneth S. Hunt.......................Griffin
Charles C. Harrold....................Macon
W. P. Harbin, Jr.......................Rome
Kenneth McCullough ....Waycross
Grady N. Coker......................Canton
Ralph H. Chaney......................Augusta

Advisory—State Board of Health
C. W. Roberts, Chairman................Atlanta
Craig Barrow ....Savannah
M. E. Winchester....................Brunswick
M. M. McCord.........................Rome
Marvin H. Head......................Zebulon
A. H. Hilsman.......................Albany
T. F. Abercrombie....................Atlanta

Sub-Committee
Advisory—State Board of Health
Social Security Act
J. R. McCord, Chairman...............Atlanta
O. R. Thompson......................Macon
Joseph Akerman ....Augusta

Advisory—Woman's Auxiliary
Jas. N. Brawner, Chairman............Atlanta
Wm. R. Dancy.......................Savannah
W. A. Selman........................Atlanta
W. R. Garner ....Gainesville
Benjamin Bashinski ....Macon

L. G. Hardman Loving Cup
W. A. Selman, Chairman..............Atlanta
Wm. A. Mulherin.....................Augusta
Chas. H. Watt.....................Thomasville
M. M. McCord........................Rome

Post-Graduate Study
G. Lombard Kelly, Chairman...........Augusta
Russell H. Oppenheimer.........Emory University
Chas. H. Watt.....................Thomasville
W. W. Chrisman......................Macon

Scientific Exhibit
Mark S. Dougherty, General Chairman......Atlanta
Thomas Harrold, Local Chairman...........Macon
Lee Howard ....Savannah
Everett L. Bishop ....Atlanta
J. L. Campbell......................Atlanta
W. L. Pomeroy......................Waycross
Wm. P. Harbin, Jr.....................Rome
Wm. F. Jenkins....................Columbus
Roy R. Kracke...............Emory University
Fred A. Mettler.....................Augusta
J. A. Redfearn......................Albany
T. F. Sellers.......................Atlanta
Ernest F. Wahl...................Thomasville

Prize for Hookworm Control*
W. F. Reavis, Chairman...............Waycross
E. F. Wahl.......................Thomasville
H. M. Tolleson.....................Eastman
*Award by the Ware County Medical Society.

Study of Maternal Mortality and Infant Deaths
H. F. Sharpley, Jr., Chairman...........Savannah

First District
A. J. Mooney......................Statesboro
A. J. Waring.......................Savannah

Second District
W. L. Wilkinson...................Bainbridge
W. W. Jarrell....................Thomasville

Third District
Herschel A. Smith...................Americus
J. C. Patterson.....................Cuthbert

Fourth District
H. J. Copeland.......................Griffin

Emory R. Park.......................LaGrange

Fifth District
E. D. Colvin........................Atlanta
J. R. McCord........................Atlanta

Sixth District
Otis R. Thompson....................Macon
T. C. Clodfelter....................Eatonton

Seventh District
P. O. Chaudron....................Cedartown
W. Mayes Gober.....................Marietta

Eighth District
M. E. Winchester...................Brunswick
C. M. Stephens.....................Waycross

Ninth District
Pratt Cheek ....Gainesville
Geo. C. Brooke.......................Canton

Tenth District
S. S. Smith.........................Athens
John W. Thurmond, Jr.................Augusta

ex officio
T. F. Abercrombie, Director, Department of
    Public Health for Georgia............Atlanta

Fraternal Delegate to the
Georgia Dental Association
R. Hugh Wood.......................Atlanta

Fraternal Delegate to the
Georgia Pharmaceutical Association
Glenville Giddings ....Atlanta

Fraternal Delegates to Other State Meetings
TO VISIT ALABAMA: Wallace H. Clark, LaGrange,
    and C. K. Sharp, Arlington.
TO VISIT FLORIDA: Wm. S. Goldsmith, Atlanta,
    and Arthur G. Fort, Atlanta.
TO VISIT NORTH CAROLINA: Clarence L. Ayers,
    Toccoa, and Grady N. Coker, Canton.
TO VISIT SOUTH CAROLINA: Wm. A. Mulherin,
    Augusta, and H. M. Michel, Augusta.

State Board of Health
First District—Cleveland Thompson, Millen, Sept. 1,
    1939.
Second District—C. K. Sharp, Arlington, Sept. 1,
    1939.
Third District—Mr. R. C. Ellis, Americus, Sept. 1,
    1942.
Fourth District—Marvin M. Head, Zebulon, Sept. 1,
    1937.
Fifth District—Mr. Robert F. Maddox, Atlanta, Sept.
    1, 1942.
Sixth District—A. R. Rozar, Macon, Sept. 1, 1938.
Seventh District—Mather M. McCord, Rome, Sept.
    1, 1938.
Eighth District—Henry W. Clements, Adel, Sept. 1,
    1938.
Ninth District—L. C. Allen, Hoschton, Sept. 1, 1939.
Tenth District—Wm. A. Mulherin, Augusta, Sept.
    1, 1937.

State of Georgia at Large
Pharmaceutical Association
T. C. Marshall, Atlanta, Sept. 1, 1941.
W. T. Edwards, Augusta, Sept. 1, 1941.

Georgia Dental Association
J. G. Williams, D.D.S., Atlanta, 1940.
Paul McGee, D.D.S., Waycross, Sept. 1, 1940

The Journal
Medical Association
of Georgia

INDEX

Volume XXV

January-December, 1936

PUBLICATION COMMITTEE

W. A. Selman, M.D., Chairman
Cleveland Thompson, M.D.
Edgar D. Shanks, M.D.

EDITOR

Edgar D. Shanks. M.D.

ASSOCIATE EDITORS

L. Minor Blackford, M.D.
T. C. Davison, M.D.
Daniel C. Elkin, M.D.
Jack C. Norris, M.D.
Carter Smith, M.D.
C. B. Upshaw, M.D.

BUSINESS MANAGER

H. L. Rowe

SUBJECT INDEX

A

ACNE VULGARIS
The Treatment of Acne Vulgaris. Cosby
Swanson, Atlanta, Sept., 1936 331
AMBLYOPIA
Toxic Amblyopia: Tobacco—Alcohol—Focal
Infection — Diabetes. Henry M. Moore,
Thomasville, Sept., 1936 333
ANASTOMOSIS
Uretero-Intestinal Anastomosis. George W.
Wright, Augusta, Aug., 1936 279
ANATOMY
Department of Gross Anatomy—Emory Uni-
versity School of Medicine. Homer Blincoe,
Emory University, Nov., 1936 ....: 401
ANEMIA
Fundamental Aspects of the Diagnosis and
Treatment of Anemia. Wm. Bosworth
Castle, Boston, Mass., Sept., 1936 307
ANESTHESIA
Sacral Anesthesia in Labor. Hugh J. Bicker-
staff, Columbus, May, 1936 148
ANEURYSM
Arteriovenous Aneurysm. Daniel C. Elkin,
Atlanta, Nov., 1936 417
APPENDICITIS
Charles Usher, Savannah, Sept., 1936 317
Acute Appendicitis — Factors Influencing the
Mortality. Daniel C. Elkin. Atlanta, Apr.,
1936 136
ANTENATAL
Antenatal Administration of Quinine. Linton
Smith, Atlanta, July, 1936 247
ARTHRITIS
Chronic Arthritis and Fibrositis. Hal M. Davi-
son, Mason I. Lowance and Crawford F.
Barnett, Atlanta, Dec., 1936 427

B

BADGE OF SERVICE
Presentation of the Badge of Service to the
President. F. Phinizy Calhoun, Atlanta,
Aug., 1936 292
Acceptance of the Badge of Service by the Presi-
dent. James E. Paullin. Atlanta, Aug.,
1936 294
BIOCHEMISTRY
Department of Biochemistry—Emory Univer-
sity School of Medicine. J. L. McGhee,
Ph.D., Emory University, Nov., 1936 409
BROMIDE
Bromide Intoxication—Report of Cases. W. G.
Elliott. Cuthbert, July, 1936 245

C

CANCER
Cancer of the Cervix. J. A. Fountain, Macon,
July, 1936 238
Cancer in Children. Everett L. Bishop. Atlanta,
May, 1936 164
Early Diagnosis of Cancer of the Mouth. J. L.
Campbell, Atlanta, July, 1936 252
Primary Bronchial Cancer and the Difficulty in
Early Diagnosis—Case Report. Stewart R.
Roberts. Atlanta, and J. Dewey Gray,
Augusta, Aug., 1936 275
Signs and Symptoms of Early Cancer. John F.
Denton, Atlanta, March, 1936 81
To What Extent May Hormones Be Blamed
for Cancer?—the Importance of Basal Gene-

tic Propensity. Charles Purcell Roberts,
Atlanta. July, 1936 242
CARCINOMA
Carcinoma of the Colon—Case Report. Frank
K. Boland. Atlanta, Feb., 1936 39
CARDIOVASCULAR
Cardiovascular Disease—Presentation of Case.
University of Georgia School of Medicine.
Augusta. Conducted by the Department of
Pathology and Clinical Departments. July,
1936 250
COMMITTEES
Maternal Mortality in Georgia During the
Year 1935—Report 205
Medical Economics—Report 207
Cancer Commission—Report 163
CHEST CONDITIONS
Chest Conditions in Infants and Children. Wm.
Willis Anderson. Atlanta, Jan., 1936 12
COLLEGES AND EDUCATION
Medical Colleges and Medical Education in
Georgia. J. L. Campbell, Atlanta, Nov.,
1936 385

CONSTITUTION AND BY-LAWS

Constitution

Article I.—Name of the Association 94
Article II.—Purposes of the Association 94
Article III.—Component Societies 94
Article IV.—Composition of the Association... 94
Article V.—House of Delegates 94
Article VI.—Council 94
Article VII.—Sessions and Meetings 94
Article VIII.—Sections and District Societies... 94
Article IX.—Officers 94
Article X.—Funds and Expenses 95
Article XI.—Ratification 95
Article XII.—The Seal 95
Article XIII.—Amendments 95

By-Laws

Chapter I.—Membership 95
Chapter II.—General Meetings 95
Chapter III.—House of Delegates 96
Chapter IV.—Duties of Officers 96
Chapter V.—Council 97
Chapter VI.—Committees 97
Chapter VII.—County Societies 98
Chapter VIII.—Rules and Ethics ....: 99
Chapter IX.—Amendments 100
Resolutions 100
Amendments 163

COUGH
The Chronic Cough. Robert C. Pendergrass,
Americus, Feb., 1936 60

D

DIAPHRAGM
The Problems of the Diaphragm. Arthur M.
Shipley, Baltimore, Md., Oct., 1936 345
DIRECTORY
Annual Directory, 1936 449

E

ECLAMPSIA
The Conservative Management of Eclampsia.
E. D. Colvin and R. A. Bartholomew, At-
lanta, Nov., 1936 423

EDITORIALS

American Medical Association
Official Call 134
The Kansas City Session. 210
ANEMIA
Anemia 64
ANNUAL SESSION
The Eighty-Seventh Annual Session. 170
APPENDICITIS
Appendicitis 133
CANCER
The Cancer Problem in Georgia. 65
Cancer of the Skin. 298
COMPENSATION ACT
The Georgia Workmen's Compensation Act . . 438
COOPERATION
Better Cooperation Among Physicians. 255
CREED
Osler's Creed 341
CORONARY
Coronary Insufficiency 336
DIARRHEA
Chronic Diarrhea 337
DISEASE
The Study of Disease. 337
ECLAMPSIA
Treatment of Eclampsia. 132
HEALTH
The State Department of Public Health. 298
HISTORY
History 174
HYGIENE
Mental Hygiene in Georgia. 298
INFECTION
Trichomonas Vaginalis Infection. 83
INSULINATE
Protamine Insulinate 296
INVITATION
Invitation to the Members of the Medical
Association of Georgia and Woman's Auxil-
iary 82
JOURNAL
The Journal 374
LETTERS
Don't Answer Threatening Letters. 170
MEDICAL DEFENSE
Medical Defense 254
MEDICAL ECONOMIC SURVEY
Questionnaire for Physicians. 29
MEDICAL SCHOOL
Admission to Medical School. 255
MALARIA
Malaria 372
OBLIGATIONS
Obligations to Our State Association. 373
OLEOTHORAX
Oleothorax 212
OPHTHALMOLOGY AND OTOLARYNGOLOGY
The General Practitioner in Relation to
Opthalmology and Otolaryngology. 297
OSTEOMYELITIS
Acute Osteomyelitis 254
PELLAGRA
Pellagra 376
PITYRIASIS CAPITIS
Pityriasis Capitis 375
PRESIDENT AND PRESIDENT-ELECT
Our President and President-Elect. 83
PROGRAM
Eighty-Seventh Annual Session, Savannah. . . 85
The Scientific Program for 1937. 213
PROBLEMS
Our Problems 166
PSYCHIATRY
Psychiatry 256
RENAL FUNCTION
Causative Factors of Inadequate Renal Function 339

RHINOLOGY
Changing Concepts in Rhinology. 376
SPINAL DRAINAGE
Forced Spinal Drainage. 29
STATUE
Statue of Crawford W. Long to Be Unveiled
at Danielsville 100
TRAYLOR
George Albert Traylor, Augusta, President-
Elect 168
TUBERCULOSIS
Tuberculosis in Adolescents 211
URINARY
Urinary Back Pressure as a Cause of Toxemia
in Pregnancy 338
VOMITING
Treatment of the Vomiting of Pregnancy. . . . 169
WELCOME
Welcome to Savannah. 132

**EMORY UNIVERSITY
SCHOOL OF MEDICINE**

Anatomy — Department of Gross Anatomy.
Homer Blincoe, Emory University, Nov.,
1936 401
Biochemistry — Department of Biochemistry.
J. L. McGhee, Ph.D., Emory University,
Nov., 1936 409
Education—Trend of Medical Education. Rus-
sell H. Oppenheimer, Emory University,
Nov., 1936 412
Emory University School of Medicine. Edgar
D. Shanks, Atlanta, Nov., 1936 389
Emory University School of Medicine. Glen-
ville Giddings, Atlanta, Nov., 1936. 390
Faculty—Emory University School of Medi-
cine, Nov., 1936 426
Histology—Department of Histology. P. E.
Lineback, Emory University, Nov., 1936. . 403
Medical Colleges and Medical Education in
Georgia. J. L. Campbell, Atlanta, Nov.,
1936 385
Pathology — Department of Pathology and
Bacteriology. Roy H. Kracke. Emory Uni-
versity, Nov., 1936. 406
Pharmacology—Department of Pharmacology.
Eugene L. Jackson, Ph.C., Emory Univer-
sity, Nov., 1936. 410
Physiology — Department of Physiology.
George Bachmann, Emory University, Nov.,
1936 405
Westmoreland, John G. 388

F

FEVER
The Use of Merthiolate Intravenously in Ty-
phoid Fever — Report of Nineteen Cases.
Lauren H. Goldsmith, Atlanta, in collabora-
tion with Inman Smith, Trion; Clarence D.
Fowler, Atlanta, and Harry Lange, Savan-
nah, June. 1936 197
FINANCIAL
Financial Statement 286
FISSURE
Scientific Management of Anal Fissure. Chas.
E. Hall, Atlanta, Feb., 1936. 57
FRACTURES
Five Unusual Fractures. J. H. Mull, Rome,
Oct., 1936 359
FUSOSPIROCHETAL
Fusospirochetal Diseases of the Lung. James P.
Tye, Albany, June, 1936. 192

G

GOITER
Goiter in Children. J. Gaston Gay, Atlanta,
July, 1936 228

GOITER AND IODINE
Ben Hill Clifton, Atlanta, July, 1936...... 230

H

HEALTH
Public Health Problems in Georgia. T. F.
Abercrombie, Atlanta, Aug., 1936....... 283
HISTOLOGY
Department of Histology—Emory University
School of Medicine. P. E. Lineback, Emory
University, Nov., 1936............... 403
HOUSE OF DELEGATES
Abstract of Proceedings, Eighty-Seventh An-
nual Session, April 21-24, 1936........ 162
HYPERPARATHYROIDISM
J. Reid Broderick, Savannah, July, 1936.... 232
HYPERTENSION
Stewart R. Roberts, Atlanta, Nov., 1936.... 413
HYPERTHYROIDISM
Chronic Hyperthyroidism with a Persistent
Low Basal Metabolic Rate. T. C. Davison,
Atlanta, July, 1936................. 225

I

INDEX
Authors' Index 465
Subject Index 462
INFANT FEEDINGS
A Yardstick to Measure Artificial Feedings for
Infants. Wm. A. Mulherin, Augusta, Aug.,
1936 265
INFECTION
Puerperal Infection — Report of Four Cases.
Grady N. Coker, Canton, May, 1936..... 158
INFECTIONS AND MENINGITIS
Antitoxin Treatment of Meningococcic Infec-
tions and Meningitis. Howard J. Morrison,
Savannah, Oct., 1936............... 365

L

LESIONS
Irradiation Versus Surgery in Breast Lesions.
William Perrin Nicolson, Jr., Atlanta, April,
1936 120
LEUKOPENIC STATE
Relation of Drugs to the Leukopenic State.
Roy R. Kracke, Emory University, Feb.,
1936 51
LIVE
Learning Better How to Live. James E.
Paullin, Atlanta, May, 1936.......... 145
LUMBAR PAIN
Left Lumbar Pain with Progressive Weakness
of Three Weeks Duration—Case Report No.
5. Medical Division University Hospital.
Augusta, Aug., 1936................ 294

M

MEDICINE
The Contributions of Crawford W. Long and
His Contemporaries to American Medicine.
Max Cutler, Chicago, Ill., March, 1936.. 75
MEMORIAM
In Memoriam. A. J. Mooney, Statesboro, Jan.,
1936 18
In Memoriam. A. J. Mooney, Statesboro, Oct.,
1936 368
MENINGITIS
Torula Meningitis—Report of Case. Edgar R.
Pund, Augusta, Feb., 1936........... 48
MENOPAUSE
Premenopause Ovarian Insufficiency. J. K.
Fancher, Atlanta, Sept., 1936.......... 328
MYOSARCOMA
Myosarcoma of Round Ligament—Report of
Case. J. D. Martin, Jr., and Fred F. Rudder,
Atlanta, June, 1936................. 202

N

NERVOUS SYSTEM
The Treatment by the General Practitioner of
the More Common Diseases of the Nervous
System. Lewellys F. Barker, Baltimore,
Md., Jan., 1936.................... 4

O

OFFICERS AND COMMITTEES, 1936-37.. 171
OFFICERS AND COMMITTEES, 1936-1937 459

P

PARALYTIC MUSCLES
The Treatment of Paralytic Muscles by Active
and Passive Exercise and the Importance of
Diet—Report of Case. M. F. Carson, Grif-
fin, Feb., 1936..................... 63
PATHOLOGY AND BACTERIOLOGY
Department of Pathology and Bacteriology—
Emory University School of Medicine. Roy
R. Kracke, Emory University, Nov., 1936 406
PERITONITIS
Septic Peritonitis Following Appendicitis.
Edgar Boling and Marvin Mitchell, Atlanta,
Apr., 1936 116
PHARMACOLOGY
Department of Pharmacology — Emory Uni-
versity School of Medicine. Eugene L. Jack-
son, Ph.C., Emory University, Nov., 1936 410
PHYSIOLOGY
Department of Physiology—Emory University
School of Medicine. George Bachmann,
Emory University, Nov., 1936......... 405
PNEUMONIA
Treatment of Acute Lobar Pneumonia—Re-
view of Five Year Records of Pneumonia in
Atlanta Hospitals. C. C. Aven and A. Worth
Hobby, Atlanta, Jan., 1936........... 15
POLIOMYELITIS
Anterior Poliomyelitis—A Review of Recent
Studies. William A. Smith, Atlanta, Sept.,
1936 324
PREGNANCY
Friedman's Modification of the Aschheim-
Zondek Test for Pregnancy. George F.
Klugh, Atlanta, Oct., 1936........... 362
PREJUDICE
The Psychology of Prejudice and Mob Action
in Tribes and Nations. Samuel Kahn, Apr.,
1936 130
PROSTATE
Examination of the Prostate. Rudolph Bell,
Thomasville, Sept., 1936............. 312

R

RHINOLARYNGOLOGY
The Present Day Practice of Rhinolaryngology
— Some Comments Based on Forty-two
Years Experience. Dunbar Roy, Atlanta,
Aug., 1936 271

S

SEPTICEMIA
A New Treatment for Septicemia. W. S. Dor-
ough, Atlanta, June, 1936........... 204
SLEEP
The Effect of Emotional Disturbances on Sleep.
Glenville Giddings, Atlanta, Oct., 1936.. 351
SYPHILIS
Complications of the Treatment of Syphilis in
Pregnancy — Report of Three Cases of
Arsenical Encephalitis Complicating Such
Treatment. E. Bryant Woods, Augusta
(Jacksonville, Fla.), Jan., 1936........ 23
Miliary Syphilis of the Intestine in the New-
Born — A Discussion of the Pathology of

Syphilis of the Gastro-Intestinal Tract in
Children. Joseph Yampolsky. May. 1936.. 154

TESTS OF KIDNEY FUNCTION
The Dilation and Concentration Tests of Kidney Function. W. Edward Storey, Columbus, June. 1936.................... 188
TUBERCULOSIS
Influence of Pregnancy on Tuberculosis. Walter W. Daniel, Atlanta, June. 1936...... 203
Pharyngeal Tuberculosis. Louis C. Rouglin, Atlanta, Feb., 1936................. 44
TUMORS
Early Diagnosis of Tumors of the Kidney, Earl Floyd and Jas. L. Pittman, Atlanta,

Oct., 1936 370
Intramedullary Tumors—Report of Case. J. Calvin Weaver, Atlanta, Feb., 1936 61
Malignant Tumors of Bone. Everett L. Bishop, Atlanta, April, 1936................ 124

U
ULCER
Perforated Peptic Ulcer—A Study of 32 Cases. J. C. Patterson, Cuthbert, Jan., 1936.... 20
VERTEBRA
The Fifth Lumbar Vertebra as a Cause of Low Back Pain. Thomas P. Goodwyn and H. Walker Jernigan, Atlanta, June, 1936 ... 185

W
WESTMORELAND, JOHN G., Atlanta...... 388

AUTHORS' INDEX

A

ABERCROMBIE, T. F., Atlanta
Public Health Problems in Georgia. Aug., 1936 283
ANDERSON, WM. WILLIS, Atlanta
Chest Conditions in Infants and Children. Jan., 1936 12
AVEN, C. C. Atlanta
HOBBY, A. WORTH, Atlanta
Treatment of Acute Lobar Pneumonia—Review of Five Year Records of Pneumonia in Atlanta Hospitals. Jan., 1936....... 15

B

BACHMANN, GEORGE, Emory University
Department of Physiology—Emory University School of Medicine. Nov., 1936 405
BARKER, LEWELLYS F., Baltimore, Md.
The Treatment by the General Practitioner of the More Common Diseases of the Nervous System. Jan., 1936................ 1
BARNETT, CRAWFORD F., Atlanta
DAVISON, HAL M., Atlanta
LOWANCE, MASON I., Atlanta
Chronic Arthritis and Fibrositis. Dec., 1936. 427
BARTHOLOMEW, R. A., Atlanta
COLVIN, E. D., Atlanta
The Conservative Treatment of Eclampsia. Nov., 1936 423
BELL, RUDOLPH, Thomasville
Examination of the Prostate. Sept., 1936 ... 312
BICKERSTAFF, HUGH J., Columbus
Sacral Anesthesia in Labor. May, 1936.... 148
BISHOP, EVERETT L., Atlanta
Cancer in Children. May, 1936........... 164
Malignant Tumors of Bone. April, 1936 ... 124
BLINCOE, HOMER, Emory University
Department of Gross Anatomy—Emory University School of Medicine. Nov., 1936.. 401
BOLAND, FRANK K., Atlanta
Carcinoma of the Colon — Case Report. Feb., 1936 39
BOLING, EDGAR, Atlanta
MITCHELL, MARVIN, Atlanta
Septic Peritonitis Following Appendicitis. Apr., 1936 116
BRODERICK, J. REID, Savannah
Hyperparathyroidism. July, 1936 232

C

CALHOUN, F. PHINIZY, Atlanta

Presentation of the "Badge of Service" to the President, James E. Paullin. Aug., 1936. 292
CAMPBELL, J. L., Atlanta
Early Diagnosis of Cancer of the Mouth. July, 1936 252
Medical Colleges and Medical Education in Georgia. Nov., 1936................. 385
CARSON, M. F., Griffin
The Treatment of Paralytic Muscles by Active and Passive Exercise. Feb., 1936 63
CASTLE, WM. BOSWORTH, Boston, Mass.
Fundamental Aspects of the Diagnosis and Treatment of Anemia. Sept., 1936...... 307
CLIFTON, BEN HILL, Atlanta
Goiter and Iodine. July, 1936............ 230
COKER, GRADY N., Canton
Puerperal Infection—Report of Four Cases. May, 1936 158
COLVIN, E. D., Atlanta
BARTHOLOMEW, R. A., Atlanta
The Conservative Management of Eclampsia. Nov., 1936 423
CUTLER, MAX, Chicago, Ill.
The Contributions of Crawford W. Long and His Contemporaries to American Medicine. March, 1936 75

D

DANIEL, WALTER W., Atlanta
Influence of Pregnancy on Tuberculosis. June, 1936 203
DAVISON, HAL M., Atlanta
LOWANCE, MASON I., Atlanta
BARNETT, CRAWFORD F., Atlanta
Chronic Arthritis and Fibrositis. Dec., 1936. 427
DAVISON, T. C., Atlanta
Chronic Hyperthyroidism with a Persistent Low Basal Metabolic Rate. July, 1936.. 225
DENTON, JOHN F., Atlanta
Signs and Symptoms of Early Cancer. March, 1936 81
DOROUGH, W. S., Atlanta
A New Treatment for Septicemia. June, 1936 204

E

ELKIN, DANIEL C., Atlanta
Arteriovenous Aneurysm. Nov., 1936...... 417
ELKIN, DANIEL C., Atlanta
GLENN, WADLEY, Atlanta
Acute Appendicitis—Factors Influencing the Mortality. April, 1936.............. 113
ELLIOTT, W. G., Cuthbert

Bromide Intoxication—Report of Cases. July,
1936 245

F

FANCHER, J. K., Atlanta
Premenopausal Ovarian Insufficiency. Sept.,
1936 328
FLOYD, EARL, Atlanta
PITTMAN, JAS. L., Atlanta
Early Diagnosis of Tumors of the Kidney.
Oct., 1936 370
FOWLER, CLARENCE D., Atlanta
SMITH, INMAN, Trion
LANGE, HARRY, Savannah
GOLDSMITH, LAUREN H., Atlanta
The Use of Merthiolate Intravenously in Ty-
phoid Fever — Report of Nineteen Cases.
June, 1936 197
FOWLER, CLARENCE D., Atlanta
YAMPOLSKY, JOSEPH, Atlanta
Miliary Syphilis of the Intestine in the New-
Born: A Discussion of the Pathology of
Syphilis of the Gastro-Intestinal Tract in
Children. May, 1936 154
FOUNTAIN, J. A., Macon
Cancer of the Cervix. July, 1936 238

G

GAY, J. GASTON, Atlanta
Goiter in Children. July, 1936 228
GIDDINGS, GLENVILLE, Atlanta
The Effect of Emotional Disturbances on Sleep.
Oct., 1936 351
Emory University School of Medicine. Nov.,
1936 390
GLENN, WADLEY, Atlanta
ELKIN, DANIEL C., Atlanta
Acute Appendicitis — Factors Influencing the
Mortality. April, 1936 113
GOLDSMITH, LAUREN H., Atlanta
SMITH, INMAN, Trion
FOWLER, CLARENCE D., Atlanta
LANGE, HARRY, Savannah
The Use of Merthiolate Intravenously in Ty-
phoid Fever — Report of Nineteen Cases.
June, 1936 197
GOODWYN, THOS. P., Atlanta
JERNIGAN, H. WALKER, Atlanta
The Fifth Lumbar Vertebra as a Cause of Low
Back Pain. June, 1936 185
GRAY, J. DEWEY, Augusta
ROBERTS, STEWART R., Atlanta
Primary Bronchial Cancer and the Difficulty
of Early Diagnosis — Case Report. Aug.,
1936 275

H

HALL, CHAS. E., Atlanta
Scientific Management of Anal Fissure. Feb.,
1936 57
HOBBY, A. WORTH, Atlanta
AVEN, C. C., Atlanta
Treatment of Acute Lobar Pneumonia—Re-
view of Five Year Records of Pneumonia in
Atlanta Hospitals. Jan., 1936 15

J

JACKSON, EUGENE L., Ph.C., Emory University
Department of Pharmacology—Emory Univer-
sity School of Medicine. Nov., 1936 410
JERNIGAN, H. WALKER, Atlanta
GOODWYN, THOS. P., Atlanta
The Fifth Lumbar Vertebra as a Cause of Low
Back Pain. June, 1936 185

K

KAHN, SAMUEL, Atlanta

The Psychology of Prejudice and Mob Action
in Tribes and Nations, April, 1936 130
KLUGH, GEORGE F., Atlanta
Friedman's Modification of the Aschheim-Zon-
dek Test for Pregnancy. Oct., 1936 362
KRACKE, ROY R., Emory University
Department of Pathology and Bacteriology—
Emory University School of Medicine.
Nov., 1936 408
KRACKE, ROY R., Emory University
PARKER, FRANCIS P., Emory University
Relation of Drugs to the Leukopenic State.
Feb., 1936 51

L

LANGE, HARRY, Savannah
FOWLER, CLARENCE D., Atlanta
SMITH, INMAN, Trion
GOLDSMITH, LAUREN H., Atlanta
The Use of Merthiolate Intravenously in Ty-
phoid Fever—Report of Nineteen Cases.
June, 1936 197
LINEBACK, P. E., Emory University
Department of Histology—Emory University
School of Medicine. Nov., 1936 403
LOWANCE, MASON I., Atlanta
BARNETT, CRAWFORD F., Atlanta
DAVISON, HAL M., Atlanta
Chronic Arthritis and Fibrositis. Dec., 1936. 427

M

MARTIN, J. D., JR., Atlanta
RUDDER, FRED F., Atlanta
Myosarcoma of Round Ligament—Report of
Case. June, 1936 202
McGHEE, J. L., Ph. D., Emory University
Department of Biochemistry—Emory Univer-
sity School of Medicine. Nov., 1936 409
MITCHELL, MARVIN, Atlanta
BOLING, EDGAR, Atlanta
Septic Peritonitis Following Appendicitis.
April, 1936 116
MOONEY, A. J., Statesboro
In Memoriam. Jan., 1936 18
In Memoriam. Oct., 1936 368
MOORE, HARRY M., Thomasville
Toxic Amblyopia: Tobacco—Alcohol—Fo-
cal Infection—Diabetes. Sept., 1936 333
MORRISON, HOWARD J., Savannah
Antitoxin Treatment of Meningococcic Infec-
tions and Meningitis. Oct., 1936 365
MULHERIN, WM. A., Atlanta
A Yardstick to Measure Artificial Feeding for
Infants. Aug., 1936 265
MULL, J. H., Rome
Five Unusual Fractures. Oct., 1936 359

N

NICOLSON, WILLIAM PERRIN, JR., Atlanta
Irradiation Versus Surgery in Breast Lesions.
April, 1936 120

O

OPPENHEIMER, RUSSELL H., Emory Univ.
Trend of Medical Education. Nov., 1936 ... 412

P

PARKER, FRANCIS P., Emory University
KRACKE, ROY R., Emory University
Relation of Drugs to the Leukopenic State.
Feb., 1936 51
PATTERSON, J. C., Cuthbert
Perforated Peptic Ulcer—A Study of 32
Cases. Jan., 1936 20
PAULLIN, JAMES E., Atlanta
Acceptance of the "Badge of Service" by the
President. Aug., 1936 294

Learning Better How to Live. May, 1936... 145
PENDERGRASS, ROBERT C., Americus
The Chronic Cough. Feb., 1936.......... 60
PITTMAN, JAMES L., Atlanta
FLOYD, EARL, Atlanta
Early Diagnosis of Tumors of the Kidney,
Oct., 1936 370
PUND, EDGAR R., Augusta
VAN WAGONER, FRANK H., Augusta
Torula Meningitis—Report of Case. Feb.,
1936 48

R

ROBERTS, CHARLES PURCELL, Atlanta
To What Extent May Hormones Be Blamed
for Cancer?—The Importance of Basal Gen-
etic Propensity. July, 1936.......... 242
ROBERTS, STEWART R., Atlanta
Hypertension. Nov., 1936............. 413
ROBERTS, STEWART ., Atlanta
GRAY, J. DEWEY, Augusta
Primary Bronchial Cancer and the Difficulty
of Early Diagnosis—Case Report. Aug.,
1936 275
ROUGLIN, LOUIS C., Atlanta
Laryngeal Tuberculosis. Feb., 1936....... 44
ROY, DUNBAR, Atlanta
The Present Day Practice of Rhinolaryngology
—Some Comments Based on Forty-two
Years Experience. Aug., 1936.......... 271
RUDDER, FRED F., Atlanta
MARTIN, J. D., JR., Atlanta
Myosarcoma of Round Ligament—Report of
Case. June, 1936 202

S

SHANKS, EDGAR D., Atlanta
Emory University School of Medicine. Nov.,
1936 389
SHIPLEY, ARTHUR M., Baltimore, Md.
The Problems of the Diaphragm. Oct., 1936. 345
SMITH, INMAN, Trion
GOLDSMITH, LAUREN H., Atlanta
FOWLER, CLARENCE D., Atlanta
LANGE, HARRY, Savannah
The Use of Merthiolate Intravenously in Ty-
phoid Fever—Report of Nineteen Cases.
June, 1936 197
SMITH, LINTON, Atlanta
Antenatal Administration of Quinine. July,
1936 247
SMITH, WILLIAM A., Atlanta
Anterior Poliomyelitis—A Review of Recent
Studies. Sept., 1936 324
STOREY, W. EDWARD, Columbus
The Dilution and Concentration Tests of
Kidney Function. June, 1936.......... 188
SWANSON, COSBY, Atlanta
The Treatment of Acne Vulgaris. Sept., 1936 331

T

TYE, JAMES P., Albany
Fusospirochetal Diseases of the Lung. June,
1936 192

U

UNIVERSITY OF GEORGIA
SCHOOL OF MEDICINE, Augusta
Cardiovascular Disease—Presentation of Case.
Conducted by the Department of Pathol-
ogy and Clinical Departments. July, 1936. 250
Left Lumbar Pain with Progressive Weakness
of Three Weeks Duration—Case Deport
No. 5. Aug., 1936. 294
USHER, CHARLES, Savannah
Appendicitis. Sept., 1936 317

V

VAN WAGONER, FRANK H., Augusta
PUND, EDGAR R., Augusta
Torula Meningitis—Report of Case. Feb.,
1936 48

W

WEAVER, J. CALVIN, Atlanta
Intramedullary Tumors—Report of Case.
Feb., 1936 61
WOODS, E. BRYANT, Augusta
(Jacksonville, Fla.)
Complications of the Treatment of Syphilis in
Pregnancy—Report of Three Cases of Ar-
senical Encephalitis Complicating Such
Treatment. Jan., 1936 23
WRIGHT, GEORGE W., Augusta
Uretero-Intestinal Anastomosis. Aug., 1936. 279

Y

YAMPOLSKY, JOSEPH, Atlanta
FOWLER, C. D., Atlanta
Miliary Syphilis of the Intestine in the New-
Born: A Discussion of the Pathology of
Syphilis of the Gastro-Intestinal Tract in
Children. May, 1936 154

NEW YORK POLYCLINIC
MEDICAL SCHOOL AND HOSPITAL

A special program was presented on October 2 at the Polyclinic Hospital for the American Academy of Ophthalmology and Otolaryngology and was well attended by doctors from many parts of the country. The program was as follows:

Radical Killian Operation with cadaver demonstration by Dr. Julius I. Klepper; Operative Nose and Throat Clinic by Dr. Nathan Settel; Nose and Throat (cadaver demonstration) by Dr. Max Halle; Cancer of the Larynx (lecture and demonstration of cases) by Dr. H. B. Orton; Operative Nose and Throat Clinic by Dr. William L. Gatewood; Diathermy in Throat Operations (lecture and demonstration) by Dr. Farel Jouard; Operative Nose and Throat Clinic by Dr. Lee M. Hurd; Demonstration of zin ionization in nasal allergy by Dr. W. W. Morrison; Radical Mastoid Surgery (cadaver demonstration) by Dr. Samuel J. Kopetzky and Dr. Ralph Almour.

The Polyclinic presented the following program for the Graduate Fortnight of the New York Academy of Medicine on October 19th and 26th. 1. Traumatic pudendal hernia (lantern slides) by Dr. Herbert C. Chase. 2. Tissue asphyxia and shock by Dr. Frederick M. Allen. 3. Traumas in the newborn as the pediatrician sees them, by Dr. W. Morgan Hartshorn. 4. Prevention of obstetric traumas (moving pictures) by Dr. Everett M. Hawks. 5. Physical therapy in traumatic conditions (demonstration and lantern slides) by Dr. Richard Kovacs. 6. Perforation of cervical esophagus (lantern slides) by Dr. H. B. Orton.

1. Traumas of the nose and face, by Dr. Lee M. Hurd. 2. Recurrent dislocation of shoulder by Dr. Toušick Nicola. 3. Traumatic lesions of short rotators of shoulder (lantern slides and presentation of cases) by Dr. D. M. Bosworth. 4. Trauma and optic atrophy by Dr. Ervin Torok. 5. Trauma of chest (lantern slides and moving pictures) by Dr. Pol N. Coryllos.

(Continued on page 470)

GEORGIA DEPARTMENT OF PUBLIC HEALTH
T. F. ABERCROMBIE, M.D., *Director*

COOPERATION

The splendid co-partnership that has existed for many years between the medical profession and the Georgia Department of Health is greatly appreciated by me and my fellow-laborers in the Department. Due to this support we have progressed, within a few years, under many handicaps, to a greatly enlarged department, one that compares favorably, in my opinion, with our sister states.

We are now in need of further expansion, and in consultation with the officers and committees of the MEDICAL ASSOCIATION OF GEORGIA we have outlined and adopted such a plan to present to our general assembly. We ask your support of this plan and your continued cooperation. It is vital that we procure a larger appropriation.

Illness and neglect of health services are factors in economic loss, sapping the vitality and productiveness of a community, a state and, in the last result, of a region—reducing earning power and hope of progress—increasing the cost of social security and all public operations—blighting the lot of all.

This is the message which has gone out over Georgia from a gathering held in Atlanta recently to recruit the State's business interests in a fight for adequate public health services. It bore a new appeal and significance.

The movement looks to building a health program through the Georgia State Board of Health which will result in organizing the State into 60 districts, with an expert personnel of health officers, sanitary engineers and nurses for each.

The first step will be an appeal to the Legislature at its next session for an increase of appropriations for health services in 1937. Pledge to work to this end was given recently by members of the state-wide group of business and professional men who gathered in Atlanta upon invitation of Robert F. Maddox, Chairman of the State Board of Health, to hear an outline of the program.

They heard of Georgia's needs, which were described as grave. Georgia, spending now from the State treasury for public health services *only three cents* for each inhabitant—Georgia, reaching at the first of this year only 28 per cent of its rural population through county or district health units operating on full time—lags far behind the other states.

Georgia, without means in many sections of the State to fight the encroachment of epidemics, preventable but devastating, has seen in the last year a steady increase of venereal diseases, of malaria which for the first time is invading North Georgia in virulent form; and the dreaded typhus fever, borne by infested rats.

The Director of the State Department of Public Health described the growth of these plagues and called attention to the alarming need of vigilance against typhoid fever, hookworm infection and its complications, against tuberculosis and other of the preventable diseases which crop out in deadly sporadic epidemics in places where there is no means of watchfulness or opposition against them—in localities now without organized services.

That only 33 counties among Georgia's 159 operate now under organized, full-time health departments was pointed out by Dr. B. H. Minchew of Waycross, President of the MEDICAL ASSOCIATION OF GEORGIA. In these counties, 43 per cent fewer deaths occur from preventable diseases than in the others. "Proper organization of our health services will prevent 2,600 deaths from illnesses easily avoidable in Georgia every ten years," he said.

The speakers, talking to business men with the message that good health is good business, drove home the facts that in 1935 the State government provided $9,481,106.78 for the common schools, $17,580,947.81 for the public roads, and only $104,375.00 for public health—in other words, $6.04 for each inhabitant for roads; $3.25 each for schools; three cents each for health services.

Other records which impressed the gathering included a chart showing that all the other Southern states appropriate for public health 2-2/3 to 7-2/3 times as much per capita as Georgia; that if the per capita expenditure of Georgia had equalled that of Maryland (the highest in the group), it would have amounted to $800,208; that Florida levies a half-mill tax for public health, on which basis in Georgia the amount available would have been $500,025.

Within the last year the State Board of Health has been enabled with aid of funds for federal projects to create in Georgia seven health districts, with health officers, engineers and nurses assigned to each. This marks an advance, but in the opinion of many it is spreading the health services "a little thin." *The necessity is for vigilance, constant contact with every center of existence — and above all, sanitation.*

Eventually, it is planned, the program which was sponsored at the Atlanta meeting and to which the gathering pledged support through adoption of formal resolutions, looks to the expenditure of $1,600,000 a year by the State government, which will make possible obtaining $400,000 from the Federal government.

It will provide in each of 60 districts a personnel consisting of a health officer (one to 50,000 population), two sanitary engineers (one to 25,000 population), five nurses (one to 10,000), and a clerk.

The prospect held out to the business leaders whose support for the plan was asked, was stated as follows: "It will create the means of better existence, higher standards of living and increased productivity, making a better State and a better people."

T. F. ABERCROMBIE, M.D.,
Director, Georgia Department of Public Health.

PHYSIOLOGIC EFFECTS OF BENZEDRINE

Myerson, Loman and Dameshek (Am. J. Med. Sci., Oct., 1936) report on the physiological effects of the sympathomimetic amine, benzyl methyl carbinamine ("Benzedrine") in adult humans. Administered parenterally in varying doses the average rise in systolic blood pressure was 29 mm. of mercury. The height of blood pressure was attained in an average time of 46 minutes and reached its normal level 2 to 8 hours after administration. Orally in rather large doses (40 mg.) the blood pressure increases were nearly identical with those after parenteral administration except that the action was delayed. Atropine when combined with Benzedrine markedly enhances its effects. A parasympathetic stimulant, mecholyl, when given with or during the period of Benzedrine action, exerted its depressor effect over a shorter period, temporarily nullifying the action of Benzedrine without being antagonistic to its continued prolonged action. Benzedrine has a definite stimulating action on the central nervous system as shown by the shortening of sodium amytal narcosis. A marked rise in both white and red blood cells, with a lowering of color index, was usually found. These increases were apparently mechanical and of no clinical significance. The authors state that they did not observe an increase in basal metabolic rate or blood sugar. Reference is made to the good effects of Benzedrine in lowered mood and in certain fatigue states; these are the subject of a separate study, as is the drug's action in relaxing gastro-intestinal spasm.

WHAT EVERY WOMAN DOESN'T KNOW— HOW TO GIVE COD LIVER OIL

Some authorities recommend that cod liver oil be given in the morning and at bedtime when the stomach is empty, while others prefer to give it after meals in order not to retard gastric secretion. If the mother will place the very young baby on her lap and hold the child's mouth open by gently pressing the cheeks together between her thumb and fingers while she administers the oil, all of it will be taken. The infant soon becomes accustomed to taking the oil without having its mouth held open. It is most important that the mother administer the oil in a matter-of-fact manner, without apology or expression of sympathy.

If given cold, cod liver oil has little taste, for the cold tends to paralyze momentarily the gustatory nerves. As any "taste" is largely a metallic one from the silver or silverplated spoon (particularly if the plating is worn), a glass spoon has an advantage.

On account of its higher potency in Vitamins A and D, Mead's Cod Liver Oil Fortified with Percomorph Liver Oil may be given in one-third the ordinary cod liver oil dosage, and is particularly desirable in cases of fat intolerance.

VITAMIN B₁ THERAPY IN NEUROLOGIC DISEASES

Both on the experimental side and the clinical side it has been repeatedly shown that vitamin B deficiency leads to severe derangements of the central and peripheral nervous systems, and evidence is rapidly accumulating that such deficiency may be of subclinical grade and cause considerable disability without being recognized. Just what the nature of the bio-chemical changes induced in nervous tissue by vitamin B is, is not clear, although a derangement of glucose metabolism appears to be involved.

"Betalin 1" (Vitamin B₁, Lilly) Pulvules have been found effective in the treatment of alcoholic polyneuritis and other forms of deficiency of this vitamin. They provide for an economical administration of vitamin B₁ to supplement dietary management and are frequently indicated where it is impossible for the patient to assimilate the necessary quantities of this accessory food substance.

KETOGENIC DIET

The ketogenic diet, introduced by Clark and Helmholz, of the Mayo Clinic, in 1931, has been highly successful in the treatment of certain types of infection of the urinary tract.

Variations in tolerance among different patients to this diet and the impossibility of sufficiently reducing the pH of the urine in some patients have led to the research for an adjunct to this treatment which would enhance the efficiency of the diet and reduce disturbing side-reactions.

Among the drugs now being studied for this purpose, mandelic acid has proved highly beneficial in a carefully controlled clinical series of cases. Originally introduced by Rosenheim, it has been used both as the sodium salt (sodium mandelate), combined with the administration of ammonium chloride, and as ammonium mandelate, obviating the simultaneous administration of ammonium chloride in many cases.

We are reliably informed that the Lilly Research Laboratories are co-operating with a limited number of clinical groups in the study of this new agent for increasing urinary acidity and the bacteriostatic and bactericidal power of the urine. In many cases it has been found unnecessary to continue the ketogenic diet in view of the beneficial results which can be obtained by the use of ammonium mandelate alone.

NEW YORK POLYCLINIC
MEDICAL SCHOOL AND HOSPITAL
(Continued from page 467)

6. Recent advances in tissue grafting (charts, photographs and moving pictures) by Dr. J. Eastman Sheehan. 7. Exhibition of pathological specimens by Dr. Aaron S. Price. Dr. E. L. Kellogg was chairman of the program committee.

At the October meeting of the Polyclinic Clinical Society there were notable contributions; namely: 1. The insulin treatment of non-diabetic tuberculosis, by Dr. James S. Edlin. The discussion was opened by Dr. George G. Ornstein and Dr. Frederick M. Allen. 2. B. Friedlander Infections, by Dr. George Baehr of Mount Sinai Hospital. The discussion was opened by Gregory Schwartman (by invitation) and Dr. Lee M. Hurd.

The following program was given at the Polyclinic Clinical Society on November 2nd: 1., Osteomyelitis of the skull by Dr. Joseph E. J. King. The discussion was opened by Dr. Foster Kennedy (by invitation) and Dr. S. Philip Goodhart. 2. Medical examiner's cases of surgical interest by Dr. Harrison S. Martland. Medical Examiner of Newark, N. J. The discussion was opened by Dr. Thomas A. Gonzales, Medical Examiner of New York City.

FOR SALE

X-Ray Machine in Good Condition. E. D. Highsmith, M.D., Trust Company of Georgia Bldg., Atlanta, Georgia.

PHYSICIAN WANTED

Want doctor to take over practice of deceased husband, live as one of family in the heart of the tobacco section in South Georgia and near turpentine industry. Mrs. E. A. Lambert, Denton, Ga.

FOR SALE

Florsheim Portable Diathermy Machine for $100.00, cost $600.00; Deep light therapy lamp at $55.00, cost $250.00; $40.00 table for $10.00; many medical and psychological books, intelligence tests and forms. S. Kahn, 80 Peachtree Place, Atlanta.

WANTS POSITION

Registered laboratory technician, experienced in x-ray, bookkeeping and stenographic work. Desires position in hospital or private laboratory. Good personality, energetic and thoroughly competent. Best references. Address "S", care of The Journal.

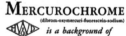